AF800434

Frontiers in Cardiovascular Drug Discovery

Editors

Prof. Dr. Atta-ur-Rahman, *FRS*

Prof. Dr. M. Iqbal Choudhary

Frontiers in Cardiovascular Drug Discovery

Bentham Science Publishers Ltd.
http://ebooks.benthamscience.com/book/9781608051601/

Volume 1

Contents

[†]"Cougulation Defects" AIEOP working group

PREFACE

Recent advances in drug discovery and development are based on post-genomic understanding of human diseases at the cellular as well as molecular levels. Cardiovascular disorders are among the most important group of diseases which have gone through major transformation, both in approach and techniques. The chapters contain in this volume are the updated version of articles published in ***Recent Patents on Cardiovascular Drug Discovery***. This volume comprises well-written reviews contributed by experts in the field of cardiovascular drug discovery and development. Each review summarizes cutting edge researches on a specific approach in CVD treatment. Many of these reviews are focused on the development of various classes of chemical compounds for cardiovascular disease management by interfering in the molecular mechanisms, which lead to atherosclerosis and hypertension.

Most reviews in this volume are written in a way to first introduce the topic and then gradually summarize the important developments in the field in a chronological manner. Thus each review should be of interest not only to professional scientists but also to research students. The references in each review are up-to-date, and represent state-of-the-art developments.

We are grateful to all contributors for their willingness to write short reviews on important aspects of cardiovascular drug discovery and development, as well as, submitting their articles in a timely manner. We are also grateful to the staff of Bentham Science Publishers, especially Mr. Mahmood Alam (Managing Director), Ms. Samina Khan (Senior Manager), Ms. Taqdees Malik (Assistant Manager) and Ms. Sadaf Idrees Khan (Composer), for their untiring efforts to make this assignment a success.

Prof. Dr. Atta-ur-Rahman, *FRS*
Prof. Dr. M. Iqbal Choudhary
Editors

Contributors

Carlos A. Feldstein	Hypertension Program, Hospital de Clínicas José de San Martín, Buenos Aires, Argentina, University of Buenos Aires, Av. Córdoba 2351, Buenos Aires, 1120, Argentina
Luca Puccetti	Department of Clinical Medicine and Immunology, Section of Internal Medicine, Centre for Atherosclerosis Research, University of Siena, Siena, Italy
Maurizio Acampa	Department of Clinical Medicine and Immunology, Section of Internal Medicine, Centre for Atherosclerosis Research, University of Siena, Siena, Italy
Marcello Pastorelli	Department of Clinical Medicine and Immunology, Section of Internal Medicine, Centre for Atherosclerosis Research, University of Siena, Siena, Italy
Vittoria Soldati	Department of Clinical Medicine and Immunology, Section of Internal Medicine, Centre for Atherosclerosis Research, University of Siena, Siena, Italy
Francesca Scarpini	Department of Clinical Medicine and Immunology, Section of Internal Medicine, Centre for Atherosclerosis Research, University of Siena, Siena, Italy
Alberto Auteri	Department of Clinical Medicine and Immunology, Section of Internal Medicine, Centre for Atherosclerosis Research, University of Siena, Siena, Italy
Mahesh T. Chhabria	Department of Pharmaceutical Chemistry and Quality Assurance, L M College of Pharmacy, Navrangpura, Ahmedabad – 380 009, Gujarat, India
Bhanubhai N. Suhagia	Department of Pharmaceutical Chemistry and Quality Assurance, L M College of Pharmacy, Navrangpura, Ahmedabad – 380 009, Gujarat, India
Pathik S. Brahmkshatriya	Department of Pharmaceutical Chemistry and Quality Assurance, L M College of Pharmacy, Navrangpura, Ahmedabad – 380 009, Gujarat, India
Jose Luis Pérez-Castrillon	Hospital Rio Hortega, University of Valladolid, Valladolid, Spain

Antonio Dueñas-Laita	Hospital Rio Hortega, University of Valladolid, Valladolid, Spain
Athanasios Tsatsaris	Laboratory for Experimental Surgery and Surgical Research, School of Medicine, University of Athens, Greece; Laboratory of Applied Mathematics, Department of Mathematics, University of Athens, Greece; Laboratory of Sanitary Police Department of Grevena, Greece
Efstathios Koukounaris	Mechanical Engineering Department of Hellenic Coast Guard, Hellenic Naval Academy, Greece
Theodoros Motsakos	Mechanical Engineering Department of Hellenic Coast Guard, Hellenic Naval Academy, Greece
Despina Perrea	Laboratory for Experimental Surgery and Surgical Research, School of Medicine, University of Athens, Greece
Harish Ramakrishna	Division of Cardiothoracic Anesthesiology, Department of Anesthesiology, Mayo Clinic, Phoenix, Arizona, USA
Manfredi Rizzo	Department of Clinical Medicine and Emerging Diseases, University of Palermo, Via Maqueda, 175, 90133 Palermo, Italy
Kaspar Berneis	Clinic for Endocrinology, Diabetes & Clinical Nutrition, University Hospital Zurich, Switzerland; and Zurich Center for Integrative Human Physiology, University of Zurich, Switzerland
Gian Luca Colussi	Division of Internal Medicine, Department of Experimental and Clinical Pathology and Medicine, University of Udine, Udine, Italy
Cristiana Catena	Division of Internal Medicine, Department of Experimental and Clinical Pathology and Medicine, University of Udine, Udine, Italy
Elisa Nadalini	Division of Internal Medicine, Department of Experimental and Clinical Pathology and Medicine, University of Udine, Udine, Italy
Alessandra Chiuch	Division of Internal Medicine, Department of Experimental and Clinical Pathology and Medicine, University of Udine, Udine, Italy

Alessandro Di Fabio	Division of Internal Medicine, Department of Experimental and Clinical Pathology and Medicine, University of Udine, Udine, Italy
Marica Valeri	Division of Internal Medicine, Department of Experimental and Clinical Pathology and Medicine, University of Udine, Udine, Italy
Leonardo A. Sechi	Division of Internal Medicine, Department of Experimental and Clinical Pathology and Medicine, University of Udine, Udine, Italy
Zia A. Khan	Department of Pathology, University of Western Ontario, London, Ontario N6G 2V4, Canada; Metabolism and Diabetes Research Program, Lawson Health Research Institute, London, Ontario N6G 2V4, Canada
Subrata Chakrabarti	Department of Pathology, University of Western Ontario, London, Ontario N6G 2V4, Canada; Metabolism and Diabetes Research Program, Lawson Health Research Institute, London, Ontario N6G 2V4, Canada; Department of Microbiology and Immunology, University of Western Ontario, London, Ontario N6G 2V4, Canada
Reiko Inagi	Division of Nephrology and Endocrinology, University of Tokyo, School of Medicine, Hongo, Bunkyo-ku, Tokyo 113-8655, Japan
Mario Cozzolino	Renal Division, San Paolo Hospital, University of Milan, Milan, Italy
Diego Brancaccio	Renal Division, San Paolo Hospital, University of Milan, Milan, Italy
Maqsood M. Elahi	Department of Cardiothoracic Surgery, Faculty of Medicine and Surgery, PIC, Lahore, Pakistan
Bashir M. Matata	Liverpool Heart and Chest Hospital NHS Trust, Thomas Drive, Liverpool, L14 3PE, United Kingdom
Dana Skultetyova	Dept. Cardiology, National Institute of Cardiovascular Diseases, Bratislava, Slovak Republic
Adriena Sakalova	Dept. Cardiology, Slovak Medical University, Bratislava, Slovak Republic

Pavol Chnupa	Dept. Cardiology, National Institute of Cardiovascular Diseases, Bratislava, Slovak Republic
Slavomira Filipova	Dept. Cardiology, Slovak Medical University, Bratislava, Slovak Republic
Marek Jankowski	Laboratory of Cardiovascular Biochemistry, Centre de Recherche, Centre Hospitalier de l'Université de Montréal (RCCHUM) and Department of Medicine, University of Montreal, 3850 Saint Urbain Street, Montréal, Québec, H2W 1T7, Canada
Adinarayana Kunamneni	Pharmaceutical Biotechnology Division, University College of Pharmaceutical Sciences, Andhra University, Visakhapatnam-530 003, India
Bhavani D. Ravuri	Pharmaceutical Biotechnology Division, University College of Pharmaceutical Sciences, Andhra University, Visakhapatnam-530 003, India
Vinjamuri Saisha	Pharmaceutical Biotechnology Division, University College of Pharmaceutical Sciences, Andhra University, Visakhapatnam-530 003, India
Poluri Ellaiah	Pharmaceutical Biotechnology Division, University College of Pharmaceutical Sciences, Andhra University, Visakhapatnam-530 003, India
Taadimalla Prabhakhar	Pharmaceutical Biotechnology Division, University College of Pharmaceutical Sciences, Andhra University, Visakhapatnam-530 003, India
Matthias Barton	University of Zurich, Molecular Internal Medicine, Institute of Laboratory Animal Science, Winterthurer Str. 190, 8057, Zurich, Switzerland
Philipp C. Nett	Department of Visceral and Transplantation Surgery, University Hospital Bern, Bern, Switzerland
Kerstin Amann	Abteilung für Nephropathologie, Klinikum der Friedrich-Alexander Universität Erlangen-Nürnberg, Glückstraße 11, 91054 Erlangen, Germany
Mauro M. Teixeira	Departamento de Bioquimica e Imunologia, Instituto Ciencias Biologicas, Universidade Federal de Minas Gerais, Belo Horizonte, Brazil

Charalambos Antoniades	1st Cardiology Department, Athens University Medical School, Athens, Greece
Michael Demosthenous	1st Cardiology Department, Athens University Medical School, Athens, Greece
Dimitris Tousoulis	1st Cardiology Department, Athens University Medical School, Athens, Greece
Costantinos Bakogiannis	1st Cardiology Department, Athens University Medical School, Athens, Greece
Nikolaos Koumallos	1st Cardiology Department, Athens University Medical School, Athens, Greece
Christodoulos Stefanadis	1st Cardiology Department, Athens University Medical School, Athens, Greece
Alessandro Pingitore	Institute of Clinical Physiology, C.N.R., Pisa, Italy
Giorgio Iervasi	Institute of Clinical Physiology, C.N.R., Pisa, Italy
Husnain K. Haider	Department of Pathology and Laboratory of Medicine, 231-Albert Sabin Way, University of Cincinnati, Ohio-45267-0529, USA
Lei Ye	National University Medical Institutes, National University of Singapore-117597, Singapore
Muhammad Ashraf	Department of Pathology and Laboratory of Medicine, 231-Albert Sabin Way, University of Cincinnati, Ohio-45267-0529, USA
Paola Giordano	Department of Biomedicine of Evolutive Age, University of Bari, Italy
Giovanni Carlo Del Vecchio	Department of Biomedicine of Evolutive Age, University of Bari, Italy
Paola Saracco	Hematology Unit, Department of Pediatrics, University of Torino, Italy
Marco Zecca	Department of Pediatric Sciences, University of Pavia, Italy

Angelo Claudio Molinari	Thrombosis and Haemostasis Unit, Department of Haematology and Oncology, Giannina Gaslini Children's Hospital, Genova, Italy
Domenico De Mattia[†]	Department of Biomedicine of Evolutive Age, University of Bari, Italy
Milagros Rocha	University Hospital Doctor Peset Foundation, Avda Gaspar Aguilar 90, 46017, Valencia, Spain; University Hospital Doctor Peset, Endocrinology Service, Avda Gaspar Aguilar 90, 46017, Valencia, Spain
Remedios García-Bou	University Hospital Doctor Peset, Endocrinology Service, Avda Gaspar Aguilar 90, 46017, Valencia, Spain
Raul Herance	High Technology Institute-PRBB, Barcelona, Spain
Antonio Hernandez-Mijares	University Hospital Doctor Peset, Endocrinology Service, Avda Gaspar Aguilar 90, 46017, Valencia, Spain; Department of Medicine, University of Valencia, and CIBER CB/06/02/0045 Research Group, CIBER Actions in Epidemiology and Public Health, Valencia, Spain
Victor M. Victor	University Hospital Doctor Peset Foundation, Avda Gaspar Aguilar 90, 46017, Valencia, Spain; University Hospital Doctor Peset, Endocrinology Service, Avda Gaspar Aguilar 90, 46017, Valencia, Spain; Department of Physiology and CIBERehd, University of Valencia, Valencia, Spain

[†]"Cougulation Defects" AIEOP working group

Statins in Hypertension

Carlos A. Feldstein*

Hypertension Program, Hospital de Clínicas José de San Martín, Buenos Aires, Argentina, University of Buenos Aires, Av. Córdoba 2351, Buenos Aires, 1120, Argentina

Abstract: Hypertension is highly prevalent in industrialized countries. Older age is associated with more uncontrolled hypertension New developments to reinforce antihypertensive drug effects include the use of statins. The beneficial effects of statins that are partly independent of their lipid-lowering actions are referred to as pleiotropic effects. These effects include the improvement of vascular endothelial function, inhibition of vascular smooth muscle cell prolife-ration and migration, anti-inflammatory actions, anti-oxidative effects or stabilization of vulnerable plaques, and enhancement of arterial compliance. So far, the available data support only a modest antihypertensive effect of statins that is most prominent in those patients with uncontrolled hypertension. Even though they only produce minor reduction in blood pressure, their effects may be relevant from the point of view of cardiovascular prevention. From trials results it appears consistent that statins may be useful in hypertensive subjects with high serum total cholesterol, in those whose hypertension is not well controlled with antihypertensive agents even without high serum total cholesterol, in hypertensive subjects well controlled with antihypertensives without high serum cholesterol when they have high PCR levels, in those with other concomitant cardiovascular risk factors, or when they require secondary prevention. Future research could further characterize the impact of statin use alone or in combination with antihypertensive agents to prevent the development of stage 1 hypertension in prehypertension.

Keywords: Statins, hypertension treatment.

INTRODUCTION

Hypertension is highly prevalent and a major risk factor for cardiovascular diseases in industrialized countries. In the United States the prevalence of uncontrolled hypertension has increased from 37 millions to 42 millions during the past two decades [1-3]. Older age is associated with more uncontrolled hypertension [4]. In the CardioMonitor 2004 survey, hypertension control was achieved by 53% of patients in the United States and 27% to 40% of patients across European countries [5]. There is considerable metabolic, epidemiological and clinical evidence that hypertension and dyslipidemia are inter-related [6,7]. A recent data analysis of the National Health and Nutrition Examination Survey 2003-2004 showed that the prevalence of hypertension ranged from 23.1% in subjects without cardiovascular comorbidities to 51.8% - 81.8% in those with cardiovascular comorbidities (chronic kidney disease: 81.8%; diabetics: 76.8%; peripheral artery disease: 73.7%; coronary artery disease: 73.0%; congestive heart disease: 71.4%; stroke: 69%; metabolic syndrome: 61.5%;

*Corresponding author: Tel: 54 114 982 9511; Fax: 54 114 982 9511; E-mail: carlfel@yahoo.com

Atta-ur-Rahman / M. Iqbal Choudhary (Eds.)

dyslipidemia: 51.8%). In spite of higher rates of hypertension treatment in patients with cardiovascular comorbidities (83.4%-89.3%) than in those without (66.5%), control rates for treatment remained low (23.2%-49.3%) [8]. The association between hypertension and dyslipidemia confers a greater increase in cardiovascular risk than would be expected with either risk factor alone [9]. The remarkable benefit achieved with statin treatment in patients with a wide range of cholesterol levels cannot be attributed only to their cholesterol lowering effect. The effectiveness and rapidity of statin-induced decreases in coronary events led to the assumption that these agents possess also cholesterol-independent effects. The beneficial effects of statins that are partly independent of their lipid-lowering actions are referred to as pleiotropic effects [10-18]. Table **1** summarizes the pleiotropic effects of statins. These effects are responsible for the improvement of vascular endothelial function, inhibition of vascular smooth muscle cell proliferation and migration, anti-inflammatory

Table 1. Pleiotropic Effects of Statins

Enhance of Endothelial Function and Increase Vascular Relaxation
Up regulate eNOS expression
Decrease release of reactive oxygen species (ROS)
Reduce levels of Endothelin-1
Decrease subunit P22 of NAD(P)H oxidase
Down-regulate Ang AT-1 receptor expression
Increase PI 3-kinase/Akt activity
Hyperpopolarize calcium-activated potassium channels
Inhibition of Inflammatory Responses
Decrease pro-inflammatory cytokines
Decrease MHC class II antigen expression
Inhibition of leukocyte function antigen-1
Decrease leukocyte-endothelial cell adhesion
Decrease nuclear factor- κB activation
Lower C-reactive protein levels
Lower Homocysteine levels
Antithrombotic Effects
Inhibition of platelet activation and adhesion
Increase t-PA
Decrease PAI-1
Decrease Tissue-Factor expression
Plaque Stabilization
Decreased macrophage cholesterol accumulation
Reduced production of matrix metalloproteinases
Decrease inflammatory cell infiltrate
Decrease collagen synthesis
Reduce angiogenesis
Improvement of coronary remodeling
Immunomodulation

actions, anti-oxidative effects or stabilization of vulnerable plaques, and improvement of arterial compliance. Nevertheless, it has been suggested that the mechanisms of pleiotropic effects could involve also the inhibition of 3-hydroxyl-3-methylglutaryl coenzyme A (HMG-CoA) reductase, a crucial enzyme for cholesterol synthesis. Statins reduce not only cholesterol but also non steroidal isoprenoid intermediates production. Since these isoprenoids, such as farnesyl pyrophosphate and geranylgeranyl pyrophosphate, regulate the small signaling proteins, Ras and Rho, inhibition of these prenylated proteins by statins might account for their non-lipid-related effects [10,11]. It has been suggested that other factors than those widely recognized, as chronic low-grade inflammation may also be implicated in the development of hypertension, either as a primary or secondary effect [12-14]. It has been reported increased levels of high-sensitivity C reactive protein (hsCRP), a sensitive marker of vascular inflammation is increased in patients with hypertension, even after adjustment for potential confounding factors [13,14]. Even more, elevated hsCRP levels were documented in subjects with prehypertension [19]. It has been demonstrated that statins reduce hsCRP levels independently of LDL-C levels [20]. Pleiotropic effects of statins raise the possibility that these agents may directly lower blood pressure in addition to reducing serum cholesterol levels. It would imply a further cardiovascular protective effect of these agents. Statins activate endothelial nitric oxid synthase [16, 20], downregulate angiotensin II type 1 receptors [17], reduce levels of endothelin-1 [18] and decrease the vascular production of reactive oxygen species [20]. There are controversies on the effect of statins on large artery stiffness in hypertension. While some studies reported an increase in systemic arterial compliance in subjects on statins [21-24], in the CAFE-LLA, a large substudy of the ASCOT there were not changes in central aortic pressures or hemodynamics in hypertensive subjects with coexisting three additional cardiovascular risk factors but no prior history of coronary heart disease, when treated with relatively low dose of atorvastatin [25].

The question about the possible antihypertensive effect of statins remains unanswered, and raises the possibility that statins may directly lower blood pressure in addition to reduce cholesterol levels. However, many gaps exist within our knowledge and there is limited guidance regarding the evaluation of statins as antihypertensive agents. Another aspect to analyze is the possible preventive action of statins alone or in combination with antihypertensive agents to avoid development of hypertension from prehypertension [26].

EXPERIMENTAL STUDIES

In normocholesterolemic, spontaneously hypertensive rats, 50 mg/kg per day of atorvastatin, a dose that produce plasma concentrations comparable to those achieved after administration of ordinary doses of atorvastatin in humans, caused a significant decrease in systolic blood pressure (SBP) [20]. This hemodynamic effect was accompanied by an improvement of endothelial dysfunction and a reduction of Ang II-induced vasoconstriction [27]. In atorvastatin-treated rats there was a decreased messenger RNA expression of aortic AT1 receptor and NAD(P)H oxidase subunit p22phox [27]. There is experimental evidence in angiotensin II hypertension model that statins may have a beneficial effect. In Sprague-Dawley rats, increases in heart weight index and carotid cross-sectional area induced by Ang II were inhibited by simvastatin [28].

EFFECTS OF STATINS ON BLOOD PRESSURE IN HYPERTENSIVE PATIENTS

Data on the blood pressure–lowering effects of statins in humans have been mixed and highly controversial. Whereas some studies have reported significant blood pressure reduction, others have not confirmed these results. Goode *et al.* [15] presented indirect evidence showing that cholesterol-lowering regimens may simultaneously reduce blood pressure by between 2 and 5 mm Hg. In a cross-sectional study of 2584 hypertensive patients with no known cardiovascular disease from the National Health and Nutrition Examination Survey 1999-2002 [29], significantly more statin users had blood pressure <140/90 mm Hg (52.2% *vs.* 38.0%), complied with low-salt diet, were using antihypertensive medication, and were non-smokers. A study in hypercholesterolemic subjects without hypertension showed no significant reduction in blood pressure [30]. Very few and relatively small, adequately designed studies have investigated the antihypertensive effect of statins in hypertensive patients with or without hypercholesterolemia [27-29, 31,32]. Only in few studies, hypertensive patients received only statins during the whole period of treatment [32-35] while the majority concomitantly received antihypertensive drugs. Furthermore these studies were not specifically designed to evaluate the antihypertensive effects of statins (Table **2**). Frequent methodological flaws in clinical trials were: inclusion

Table 2. Blood Pressure Effects of Statins in Studies that Included only Hypertensive Patients

Author (year)	Subjects	Duration	Statin (mg/d)	Change in BP (mm Hg)	Diagnosis
Straznicky, 1995	14	8 weeks	Pravastatin 40 *vs.* Placebo	No differences	HTN + HC
Ikeda, 2004	52	24 weeks	Pravastatin 10 *vs.* Probucol 500	-4.7/-0.7	Treated HTN + HC
Glorioso, 1999	25	32 weeks	Pravastatin 20-40	-8.0/-5.0	Untreated HTN + HC
Spósito, 1999	70	16 weeks	Lovastatin 20/Pravastatin 10+diet or only diet	-7.0/-4.0	Treated HTN +HC
Ferrier, 2002	22	12 weeks	Atorvastatin 80 *vs.* Placebo	-6.0/-2.0	Untreated Systolic HTN + NC
Fogari, 2004	45	12 weeks	Atorvastatin 20	-2.8/-3.8	Treated HTN + HC
Koh, 2004	47	8 weeks	Simvastatin 20	-3.0/-3.0	Treated HTN + HC
Zanchetti, 2001	508	2.6 years	Pravastatin 40	No Differences	Treated HTN +HC

HTN= hypertensive; HC= hypercholesterolemic.

of both normotensive and hypertensive subjects, absence of assessment of statistical significance, unblind nonrandomized design, the adjustment of antihypertensive medications during the treatment phase, and the short length of treatment. In hypercholesterolemic patients with controlled hypertension addition of statins to an ACE inhibitor, an ARB, a calcium channel blocker or a beta-blocker did not significantly decrease blood pressure levels [36]. On the other hand, in those patients with uncontrolled hypertension, addition of a statin to antihypertensive agents led to a further reduction in blood pressure [36]. In a double-blind, placebo-controlled crossover trial of untreated hypertensive patients with hypercholesterolemia, pravastatin significantly lowered blood pressure independently of age and gender. Importantly, this effect was unrelated to baseline plasma LDL-C and HDL-C levels [30]. Spósito *et al.* [34] compared blood pressure reduction between hypertensive subjects with hypercholesterolemia receiving ACE inhibitors (enalapril or lisinopril) alone or in combination with a statin (lovastatin or pravastatin). The statin–treated group showed a greater reduction in blood pressure. In another study that included patients with isolated systolic hypertension and normal levels of cholesterolemia that were treated with a high dose of atorvastatin (80 mg/d) or placebo without any antihypertensive, SBP was significantly lower after statin than on placebo (22). Ikeda *et al.* [38] reported an additional effect of pravastatin in decreasing SBP in patients undergoing long-term treatment with antihypertensive agents. However, this aspect remain controversial as several studies did not show any significant effect of statins on blood pressure. O´Gallaghan *et al.* did not find any significant short-term effect of low doses of pravastatin on blood pressure in hypertensive patients receiving ACE inhibitors or calcium channel blockers [35]. In the Plaque Hypertension Lipid Lowering Italian Study (PHYLLIS) [38], whose primary objective was to comparatively evaluate the effect of fosinopril and hydrochlorothiazide on carotid atherosclerosis progression in a large sample of hypertensive hypercholesterolemic patients followed up blindly for 2.6 years, there was no any additional effect of pravastatin (40 mg/d) on clinic or ambulatory blood pressure.

Studies Using Ambulatory Blood Pressure Monitoring (ABPM)

In the studies discussed above, blood pressure was measured employing the traditional clinic approach whose reproducibility and ability to consistently document small blood pressure differences may be limited. Results of studies using ABPM are displayed in Table **3** [31,39-42]. Terzoli *et al.* [39] compared the ABPM response to different statins versus soy lecithin in hypertensive subjects with hypercholesterolemia from both genders. They found that statins therapy resulted in a non statistically significant tendency to reduce casual SBP and DBP, a significant decrease in average daytime SBP and DBP without changes in nighttime blood pressure or in the circadian profile of blood pressure. In another study that compared the effects of adding a moderate dose of atorvastatin or diet to antihypertensive agents in hypertensive hypercholesterolemic patients, there was a striking reduction in SBP and DBP with the statin [40]. The addition of a moderate dose of atorvastatin to antihypertensive agents in hypercholesterolemic patients with resistant hypertension resulted in a significant decrease in 24- h SBP and DBP when compared to patients that were only added diet [41]. These findings are in contrast with the results from the largest double-blind trial in hypertensive patients with hyperlipidemia evaluated with ABPM comparing the ARB valsartan alone or in combination with low and high dose of simvastatin [42]. Valsartan /simvastatin combinations did not have an incremental effect on 24-hour ABPM compared with valsartan alone. Nevertheless, valsartan plus high–dose simvastatin lowered hs-CRP more effectively than valsartan alone or a combination of valsartan plus low dose of simvastatin [42].

Table 3. Statins Effects on Blood Pressure Measured by ABPM

Author (year)	Subjects	Duration	Statin (mg/d)	Change in BP (mm Hg)	Diagnosis
Abetel, 1998	23	12 weeks	Fluvastatin 40	-6.2/-5.3	Untreated HTN + HC
Magen, 2004	48	8 weeks	Atorvastatin 20 *vs.* Vitamin C 500 or Placebo	-13.7/-7.8	Resistant HTN + HC
Kanbay, 2005	49 placebo	12 weeks	Atorvastatin 20 *vs.* Diet	-5.1/-5.2	HTN + HC No
Terzoli, 2005	31	8 weeks	Simvastatin or Pravastatin 10-20, or Atorvastatin 5-10	in HTN: -6.5/-3.2	NT e HTN + HC
Rajagopalan, 2007	404	12 weeks	Valsartan 160 or Valsartan 160 plus Simvastatin 20 or 80	-0.36/-0.53	HTN+HC

HTN= hypertensive; NT= normotensive; HC= hypercholesterolemic.

Large Scale Clinical Studies

The majority of studies that included a large population were not specifically designed to determine the antihypertensive effects of statins. The studies that included a high proportion of normotensive subjects made the lowering blood pressure effects of statins difficult to detect. The possible heterogeneity of the blood pressure effects of statins in different groups of subjects according to their age, gender, cholesterolemia, well controlled or uncontrolled blood pressure with antihypertensives, etc, may also explain the discrepancies in the results of blood pressure lowering effects of statin. In the Brisighella Heart Study [43], hypertensive hypercholesterolemic patients in whom antihypertensive agents remained unchanged, treatment with low fat-diet, cholestyramine, gemfibrozil or simvastatin was added. Blood pressure decreased significantly only in those patients whose SBP at baseline were at the two highest quartiles. Subjects treated with statins had a greater reduction in blood pressure when compared to those receiving non-statin lipid-lowering agents[43]. In the UCSD statin study [44] normotensive and hypertensive subjects were included and not discriminatively analyzed. It was a randomized, double blind placebo controlled trial with equal allocation to simvastatin 20mg, pravastatin 40 mg, or placebo for 6 months. Statins significantly reduced blood pressure relative to placebo by 2.2 mm Hg for SBP and 2.4 mm Hg for DBP. The antihypertensive effect extended to subjects with prehypertension and subjects not receiving antihypertensive agents. Interestingly, at 2 months after statins were discontinued the difference in BP between the statin and placebo groups disappeared. In the Anglo-Scandinavian Cardiac Outcomes Trial-Lipid-Lowering-Arm (ASCOT-LLA) trial extra antihypertensive drug use in the placebo group obscured atorvastatin blood pressure effect [45]. Affected by the same limitations, the ALLHAT study [46] did not demonstrate any benefit on cardiovascular morbidity and mortality from addition of pravastatin 40 mg/d to antihypertensive agents.

Statins Treatment of Hypertensive Patients with Comorbidities

The importance of reducing the effects of hypertension in diabetic and in chronic kidney disease patients is widely recognized. The Seventh Report of the Joint National Committee on Prevention, Detection, Evaluation, and Treatment of High Blood Pressure (JNC 7) (1) and the 2007 European Society of Hypertension-European Society of Cardiology for the management of hypertension [47] have recommended a downward shift in target blood pressure to <130/80 mm Hg in both conditions. In a study performed in a group of type 2 diabetic patients with dyslipidemia and hypertension, receiving antihypertensive agents, the addition of low dose of atorvastatin (10 mg/d) lowered DBP levels [48]. In a long-term cross-over study in type 2 diabetic patients with hypertension and microalbuminuria, only simvastatin (20 mg/d) but not cholestyramine (6 g, three times a day) lowered DBP and microalbuminuria, though both hypolipidemic agents similarly decreased serum cholesterol levels [49]. Despite these favorable results, they are not in agreement with another study where statin did not result in significant additional blood pressure lowering when added to ramipril [50].

Meta-Analyses of the Antihypertensive Effects of Statins

A recent meta-analysis of 20 randomized, controlled trials including a total of 828 patients receiving concomitant antihypertensive treatment (if any), showed that SBP was only modestly but significantly lower in patients on statins when compared to patients who received placebo or control hypolipidemic agent. The antihypertensive effect of statins was greater when the analysis was restricted to studies with baseline SBP >130 mm Hg. There was also a non-significant trend for lower DBP in patients receiving statins compared with control [51]. These authors suggested that in general, the higher the baseline BP, the greater the effect of statins on BP. Even this well–performed meta-analysis study demonstrated significant heterogeneity between studies (e.g. diabetics, non diabetics, design protocols with different trial sizes and durations, crossover design, double blind or open-label trials). Furthermore the studies included a variety of settings, and employed different methodology of blood pressure determination, and different treatment regimens. These factors can greatly affect the interpretation of the results.

Another meta-analysis focused on the overall efficacy of statins in hypertensive and nonhypertensive patients. The results of fourteen major randomized clinical trials, at least following ≥1000 patients for ≥ 2 years were evaluated. This analysis showed that statin therapy effectively decreased cardiovascular morbidity and mortality to the same extent in hypertensive and nonhypertensive patients [52].

Benefits of Combination Therapy with Statins and Antihypertensive Agents

There are experimental evidences of the interaction between LDL-C and mediators of vasoconstriction. With regard to this, LDL-C up regulates the expression of both Ang AT-1 receptor [53] and the Endothelin-1 (ET B) receptor [54]. Statins increase the inhibitory effect of ACE inhibitors and ARBs on atherosclerosis through reduction of malondialdehide, monocyte chemoattractant protein-1 [55], and hsPCR. Besides, statins prevent heart alterations induced by Ang II [28]. In salt-loaded Dahl-sensitive hypertensive rats pravastatin and olmesartan improved endothelial function through different mechanisms. The statin increased eNOS activity through phosphatidylinositol-3-kinase (PI3K)-protein kinase B (Akt) phosphorylation, while the ARB produced downregulation on dihydrofolate reductase, regardless the serum cholesterol and blood pressure levels [56,57]. Experimental results suggested a potential benefit in combining statin with ARB for vascular diseases of salt-sensitive hypertension. Despite no synergistic impact of a combination of a statin with a renin-angiotensin system (RAS) inhibitor, it does seem to lower inflammatory mediator concentration like TNF-∝ and IL-6 as well as IL-6-induced CR54P and PAI-1 production in hepatocytes [58]. In spite of experimental evidences, the clinical benefit of the combination of a RAS blocker with a statin in hypertensive patients remains contradictory. Even though insulin resistance that is present in approximately 50% of patients with essential hypertension with or without obesity [58] decreases by the action of RAS inhibitors [59] the addition of simvastatin neither enhanced the blood pressure-lowering effect of losartan in hypertensive hypercholesterolemic patients nor ramipril lowering blood pressure effect in type 2 diabetics with hypertension [36].

In a double blind crossover study the combination of a calcium channel blocker and a statin in normocholesterolemic obese hypertensive patients resulted in greater reduction of BP, TNF- ∝, IL-6 and insulin resistance than that produced by the calcium channel blocker alone [60]. Those patients that received single-pill containing amlodipine/atorvastatin were 2 to 3 times more likely to be adherent than those receiving either co administered amlodipine and atorvastatin or other single-pill combination of a calcium channel blocker and a statin [61,62].

In the AVALON trial that included hypertensive subjects with hypercholesterolemia the combination of amlodipine with atorvastatin resulted in a greater improvement of small artery compliance than that obtained with either the calcium channel blocker or the statin alone [63].

CONCLUSIONS

So far it is unclear whether statins are effective in lowering blood pressure. The available data support only a modest blood pressure-lowering effect of statins that is most prominent in those patients with uncontrolled hypertension. Nevertheless they only produce minor reduction in blood pressure their effects may be relevant from the point of view of cardiovascular prevention. From the available results it appears consistent that statins may be useful in hypertensive subjects with high serum total cholesterol, in those whose hypertension is not well controlled with antihypertensive agents even without high serum total cholesterol, in hypertensive subjects well controlled with antihypertensives without high serum cholesterol when they have high PCR levels, in those who require preventive measures because other concomitant cardiovascular risk factors, or when they require secondary prevention.

Future research could further characterize the impact of statin use alone or in combination with antihypertensive agents to delay the development of stage 1 hypertension in prehypertension.

REFERENCES

[1] Chobanian AV, Bakris GL, Black HR, *et al.* The Seventh Report of the National Committee on Prevention, Detection, Evaluation, and Treatment of High Blood Pressure. The JNC 7 report. JAMA 2003; 289: 2560-2572.

[2] Cutler JA, Sorlie PD, Wolz M, Thom T, Fields LE, Roccella EJ. Trends in hypertension prevalence, awareness, treatment, and control rates in United States adults between 1988–1994 and 1999–2004. Hypertension 2008; 52: 818-827.

[3] Chobanian AV. The hypertension paradox — more uncontrolled disease despite improved therapy. N Engl J Med 2009; 361: 878-887.

[4] Plantinga LC, Miller, III ER, Stevens LA, *et al.* for the Centers for Disease Control and Prevention Chronic Kidney Disease Surveillance Team. Blood pressure control among persons without and with chronic kidney disease. US trends and risk factors 1999-2006. Hypertension 2009; 54: 47-56.

[5] Wang RY, Alexander GC, Stafford RS. Outpatient Hypertension Treatment, Treatment Intensification, and Control in Western Europe and the United States. Arch Intern Med 2007; 167: 141-147.

[6] Wilson PW, Kannel WB, Silbershatz H, D'Agostino RB Clustering of metabolic factors and coronary heart disease. Arch Intern Med 1999; 159: 1104-1109.

[7] Wilson PW, D'Agostino RB, Levy D, Belanger AM, Silbershatz H, Kannel WB. Prediction of coronary heart disease using risk factor categories. Circulation 1998; 97: 1837-1847.

[8] Wong ND, Lopez VA, L'Italien G, Chen R, Kline SE, Franklin SS. Inadequate control of hypertension in US adults with cardiovascular disease comorbidities in 2003-2004. Arch Intern Med 2007; 167: 2431-2436.

[9] Neaton JD, Blackburn H, Jacobs D, *et al.* Serum cholesterol level and mortality findings for men screened in the Multiple Risk Factor Intervention Trial. Multiple Risk Factor Intervention Trial Research Group. Arch Intern Med 1992; 152: 1490-1500.

[10] Faggiotto A, Paoletti R. State-of-the-Art lecture. Statins and blockers of the renin-angiotensin system: vascular protection beyond their primary mode of action. Hypertension 1999; 34: 987-996.

[11] Davignon J, Laaksonen R. Low-density lipoprotein-independent effects of statins. Curr Opin Lipidol 1999; 10: 543-559.

[12] Boos CJ, Lip GY. Is hypertension an inflammatory process? Curr Pharm Des 2006,12: 1623-1635.

[13] Sesso HD, Buring JE, Rifai N, Blake GJ, Gaziano JM, Ridker PM. C-reactive protein and the risk of developing hypertension. JAMA 2003; 290: 2945-2951.

[14] King DE, Egan BM, Mainous AG III; Geresey ME. Elevation of C-reactive protein in people with hypertension. J Clin Hypertens 2004; 6: 562-568

[15] Goode GK, Miller GP, Heagerty AM. Hyperlipidaemia, hypertension and coronary heart disease. Lancet 1995; 345: 362-364.

[16] Kaesemeyer WH, Caldwell RB, Huang J, Caldwell RW. Pravastatin sodium activates endothelial nitric oxide synthase independent of its cholesterol-lowering actions. J Am Coll Cardiol 1999; 33: 234-244.

[17] Nickenig G, Bäumer AT, Temur Y, Kebben D, Jockenhövel F, Böhm M. Statin-sensitive dysregulated AT1 receptor function and density in hypercholesterolemic men. Circulation 1999; 100: 2131-2134.

[18] Haug C, Schmid-Kotsas A, Zorn U, *et al.* Endothelin-1 synthesis and endothelin B receptor expression in human coronary artery smooth muscle cells and monocyte-derived macrophages is up-regulated by low density lipoproteins. J Mol Cell Cardiol 2001; 33: 1701-1712.

[19] King DE, Egan BM, Mainous AG 3rd, Geesey ME.Elevation of C-reactive protein in people with prehypertension. Clin Hypertens (Greenwich) 2004 ;6: 562-568.

[20] Wassmann S, Laufs U, Bäumer AT, *et al.* HMG-CoA reductase inhibitors improve endothelial dysfunction in normocholesterolemic hypertension via reduced production of reactive oxygen species. Hypertension 2001; 37: 1450-1457.

[21] Leibovitz E, Hazanov N, Zimlichman R, Shargorodsky M, Gavish D. Treatment with atorvastatin improves small artery compliance in patients with severe hypercholesterolemia. Am J Hypertens 2001; 14: 1096-1098.

[22] Ferrier KE, Muhlmann MH, Baguet JP, Cameron JD, Jennings GL, Dart AM, Kingwell BA. Intensive cholesterol reduction lowers blood pressure and large artery stiffness in isolated systolic hypertension. J Am Coll Cardiol 2002; 39: 1020-1025.

[23] Ichihara A, Hayashi M, Koura Y, Tada Y, Kaneshiro Y, Saruta T. Long-term effects of statins on arterial pressure and stiffness of hypertensives. J Hum Hypertens 2005;19: 103-109.

[24] Kool M, Lustermans F, Kragten H, *et al.* Does lowering of cholesterol levels influence functional properties of large arteries? Eur J Clin Pharmacol 1995; 48: 217-223.

[25] Williams B, Lacy PS, Cruickshank JK, *et al.* Impact of statin therapy on central aortic pressures and hemodynamics: principal results of the conduit artery function evaluation lipid-lowering arm (CAFE-LLA) study. Circulation 2009; 119: 53-61

[26] Julius S, Nesbitt S D, Egan BM, *et al.* for the Trial of Preventing Hypertension (TROPHY) Study Investigators. N Engl J Med 2006; 354: 1685-1697.

[27] Wassmann S, Laufs U, Müller K, Konkol C, Ahlbory K, Bäumer AT, Linz W, Böhm M, Nickenig G. Cellular antioxidant effects of atorvastatin *in vitro* and *in vivo*. Arterioscler Thromb Vasc Biol 2002 1; 22: 300-305.

[28] Delbosc S, Cristol JP, Descomps B, Mimran A, Jover B. Simvastatin prevents angiotensin II-induced cardiac alteration and oxidative stress. Hypertension 2002; 40: 142-147.

[29] King DE, Mainous III AG, Egab BM, Player M, Geesey ME. Use of statins and blood pressure Am J Hypertens 2007; 20: 937-941.

[30] Giannatasio C, Mangoni AA, Failla M, *et al.* Impaired radial artery compliance in normotensive subjects with familial hypercholesterolemia. Atherosclerosis 1996; 124: 249-260

[31] Abetel G, Poget PN, Bonnabry JP .Hypotensive effect of an inhibitor of cholesterol synthesis (fluvastatin). A pilot study] Schweiz Med Wochenschr 1998; 128: 272-277.

[32] Straznicky NE, Howes LG, Lam W, Louis WJ .Effects of pravastatin on cardiovascular reactivity to norepinephrine and angiotensin II in patients with hypercholesterolemia and systemic hypertension. Am J Cardiol 1995; 75: 582-586.

[33] Glorioso N, Troffa C, Filigheddu F, *et al.* Effect of the HMG-CoA reductase inhibitors on blood pressure in patients with essential hypertension and primary hypercholesterolemia. Hypertension 1999; 34: 1281-1286.

[34] Spósito AC, Mansur AP, Coelho OR, Nicolau JC, Ramires JA. Additional reduction in blood pressure after cholesterol-lowering treatment by statins (lovastatin or pravastatin) in hypercholesterolemic patients using angiotensin-converting enzyme inhibitors (enalapril or lisinopril). Am J Cardiol 1999; 83: 1497-1499, A8.

[35] O'Callaghan CJ, Krum H, Conway EL, *et al.* Short term effects of pravastatin on blood pressure in hypercholesterolaemic hypertensive patients. Blood Press1994; 3: 404-406.

[36] Koh KK, Quon MJ, Han SH, *et al.* Additive beneficial effects of losartan combined with simvastatin in the treatment of hypercholesterolemic, hypertensive patients. Circulation 2004; 110: 3687-3692.

[37] Ikeda T, Sakurai J, Nakayama D, *et al.* Pravastatin has an additional depressor effect in patients undergoing long-term treatment with antihypertensive drugs. Am J Hypertens 2004; 17: 502-506.

[38] Zanchetti A, Crepaldi G, Bond MG, *et al.* Different effects of antihypertensive regimens based on fosinopril or hydrochlorothiazide with or without lipid lowering by pravastatin on progression of asymptomatic carotid atherosclerosis: principal results of PHYLLIS—a randomized double-blind trial. Stroke 2004; 35: 2807-2812

[39] Terzoli L, Mircoli L, Raco R, Ferrari AU Lowering of elevated ambulatory blood pressure by HMG-CoA reductase inhibitors. J Cardiovasc Pharmacol 2005; 46: 310-315.

[40] Kanbay M, Yildirir A, Bozbas H, *et al.* Statin therapy helps to control blood pressure levels in hypertensive dyslipidemic patients. Ren Fail 2005; 27: 297-303.

[41] Magen E, Viskoper R, Mishal J, *et al.* Resistant arterial hypertension and hyperlipidemia: atorvastatin, not vitamin C, for blood pressure control. Isr Med Assoc J 2004; 6: 742-746.

[42] Rajagopalan S, Zannad F, Radauceanu A, *et al.* Effects of valsartan alone versus valsartan/simvastatin combination on ambulatory blood pressure, C-reactive protein, lipoproteins, and monocyte chemoattractant protein-1 in patients with hyperlipidemia and hypertension. Am J Cardiol 2007; 100: 222-226.

[43] Borghi C, Dormi A, Veronesi M, Sangiorgi Z, Gaddi A. Brisighella Heart Study Working Party. Association between different lipid-lowering treatment strategies and blood pressure control in the Brisighella Heart Study. Am Heart J 2004; 148: 285-292

[44] Golomb BA, Dimsdale J, White HL, Ritchie JB, Criqui MH. Reduction in blood pressure with statins. Results from the UCSD statin study. A randomized trial. Arch Intern Med 2008; 168: 721-727.

[45] Sever PS, Dahlöf B, Poulter NR, *et al.* ASCOT investigators. Prevention of coronary and stroke events with atorvastatin in hypertensive patients who have average or lower-than-average cholesterol concentrations, in the Anglo-Scandinavian Cardiac Outcomes Trial--Lipid Lowering Arm (ASCOT-LLA): a multicentre randomised controlled trial. Lancet 2003; 361: 1149-1158.

[46] ALLHAT Officers and Coordinators for the ALLHAT Collaborative Research Group. The Antihypertensive and Lipid-Lowering Treatment to Prevent Heart Attack Trial. ALLHAT-LLT Major outcomes in high-risk hypertensive patients randomized to angiotensin-converting enzyme inhibitor or calcium channel blocker vs. diuretic: The Antihypertensive and Lipid-Lowering Treatment to Prevent Heart Attack Trial (ALLHAT). JAMA 2002; 288: 2981-2997.

[47] Mancia G, De Backer G, Dominiczak A, *et al.* 2007 Guidelines for the management of arterial hypertension.The Task Force for the Management of Arterial Hypertension of the European Society of Hypertension (ESH) and of the EuropeanSociety of Cardiology (ESC).Eur Heart J 2007; 28: 1462-1536.

[48] Velussi M, Cernigoi AM, Tortul C, Merni M. Atorvastatin for the management of Type 2 diabetic patients with dyslipidaemia. A mid-term (9 months) treatment experience. Diabetes Nutr Metab 1999; 12: 407-1412.

[49] Tonolo G, Melis MG, Formato M, *et al.* Additive effects of Simvastatin beyond its effects on LDL cholesterol in hypertensive type 2 diabetic patients. Eur J Clin Invest 2000; 30: 980-987.

[50] Koh KK, Quon MJ, Han SH, *et al.* Vascular and metabolic effects of combined therapy with ramipril and simvastatin in patients with type 2 diabetes. Hypertension 2005; 45: 1088-1093.

[51] Strazzullo P, Kerry SM, Barbato A, Versiero M, D'Elia L, Cappuccio FP. Do statins reduce blood pressure?: a meta-analysis of randomized, controlled trials. Hypertension 2007; 49: 792-798.

[52] Messerli FH, Pinto L, Tang SS, Thakker KM, Cappelleri JC, Sichrovsky T, Dubois RW. Impact of systemic hypertension on the cardiovascular benefits of statin therapy--a meta-analysis. Am J Cardiol 2008; 101: 319-325.

[53] Strehlow K, Wassmann S, Böhm M, Nickenig G. Angiotensin AT1 receptor over-expression in hypercholesterolaemia. Ann Med 2000; 32: 386-389.

[54] Best PJ, Lerman LO, Romero JC, Richardson D, Holmes DR Jr, Lerman A. Coronary endothelial function is preserved with chronic endothelin receptor antagonism in experimental hypercholesterolemia *in vitro*. Arterioscler Thromb Vasc Biol 1999; 19: 2769-2775.

[55] Yamamoto E, Yamashita T, Tanaka T,*et al*. Pravastatin enhances beneficial effects of olmesartan on vascular injury of salt-sensitive hypertensive rats, via pleiotropic effects. Arterioscler Thromb Vasc Biol 2007; 27: 556-563.

[56] Zhou MS, Jaimes EA, Raij L. Atorvastatin prevents end-organ injury in salt-sensitive hypertension: role of eNOS and oxidant stress. Hypertension 2004; 44: 186-190.

[57] Arnaud C, Burger F, Steffens S, *et al*. Statins reduce interleukin-6-induced C-reactive protein in human hepatocytes: new evidence for direct antiinflammatory effects of statins. Arterioscler Thromb Vasc Biol 2005; 25: 1231-1236.

[58] Reaven GM, Lithell H, Landsberg L. Hypertension and associated metabolic abnormalities--the role of insulin resistance and the sympathoadrenal system. N Engl J Med 1996; 334: 374-381.

[59] Perkins JM, Davis SN. The renin-angiotensin-aldosterone system: a pivotal role in insulin sensitivity and glycemic control. Curr Opin Endocrinol Diabetes Obes 2008; 15: 147-152.

[60] Fogari R, Preti P, Zoppi A, *et al*. Effects of amlodipine-atorvastatin combination on inflammation markers and insulin sensitivity in normocholesterolemic obese hypertensive patients. Eur J Clin Pharmacol 2006; 62: 817-822.

[61] Chapman RH, Benner JS, Petrella AA, *et al*. Predictors of adherence with antihypertensive and lipid-lowering therapy. Arch Intern Med 2005; 165: 1147-1152.

[62] Flack JM, Victor R, Watson K, *et al*. Improved attainment of blood pressure and cholesterol goals using single-pill amlodipine/atorvastatin in African Americans: the CAPABLE trial. Mayo Clin Proc 2008; 83: 35-45.

[63] Cohn JN, Wilson DJ, Neutel J, *et al*. Coadministered amlodipine and atorvastatin produces early improvements in arterial wall compliance in hypertensive patients with dyslipidemia. Am J Hypertens 2009; 22: 137-144.

New Insights into Pharmacogenetics of Statins Therapy

Luca Puccetti*, Maurizio Acampa, Marcello Pastorelli, Vittoria Soldati, Francesca Scarpini and Alberto Auteri

Department of Clinical Medicine and Immunology, Section of Internal Medicine, Centre for Atherosclerosis Research, University of Siena, Siena, Italy

Abstract: Cardiovascular disease has become the global leading cause of death worldwide, representing the most frequent cause of morbidity and mortality in the developed world.

Statins, the most widely prescribed cholesterol-lowering drugs, are considered to be first-line therapeutics for the prevention of coronary heart disease and atherosclerosis. Meta-analyses from several primary and secondary intervention studies have clearly shown that cholesterol-lowering medication, significantly reduces cardiovascular events, mortality, and morbidity, but considerable interindividual variation exists in response to statin therapy.

Pharmacogenomics can provide important insights into statins therapy through elucidation of the genetic (or genomic) contribution to variable response for these drugs. The search for genetic polymorphisms may enable us to identify novel determinants of drug responsiveness by means of the study of three candidate genes groups: (1) genes encoding proteins involved in metabolism or drug transport, or both, that influence drug pharmacokinetics; (2) genes encoding proteins involved in mechanism of action and/or metabolic pathways on which drugs operate (that influence pharmacodynamics); (3) genes encoding proteins involved in the underlying disease condition or intermediate phenotype.

This review briefly summarizes the recent pharmacogenomic and pharmacogenetic patents and the potential contributions of genetic variations in candidate genes related to lipid and lipoprotein metabolism and statins efficacy.

Keywords: Statins, pharmacogenomic, genetic polymorphisms, apolipoprotein E, hydroxy-methylglutaryl-coenzyme A reductase, cholesteryl ester transfer protein, sterol regulatory element-binding factors, Lipoprotein lipase, P450 cytochrome.

INTRODUCTION

Cardiovascular disease (CVD) has become the global leading cause of death worldwide. Despite major progress in diagnosis and treatment over the past 25 years, CVD represents the most frequent cause of morbidity and mortality (37% of all deaths annually) in the developed world, according to a report of American Heart Association statistics Committee [1].

*Corresponding author: Tel: +39(0)577585741; Fax: +39(0)57744114; E-mail: puccetti@unisi.it

Since the 2001 update of the American Heart Association (AHA)/American College of Cardiology (ACC) consensus statement on secondary prevention, important evidence from clinical trials has emerged that further supports and broadens the merits of aggressive risk-reduction therapies for patients with established coronary and other atherosclerotic vascular disease, including peripheral arterial disease, atherosclerotic aortic disease, and carotid artery disease. This growing body of evidence confirms that aggressive comprehensive risk factor management improves survival, reduces recurrent events and the need for interventional procedures, and improves quality of life for these patients [2].

Current treatment guidelines stress the importance of compre-hensive risk factor management in such patients. Furthermore, arterial hypertension, hypercholesterolemia, and smoking lead the list of risk factors associated with mortality.

Statins, the most widely prescribed cholesterol-lowering drugs, are considered to be first-line therapeutics for the prevention of coronary heart disease and atherosclerosis. As inhibitors of hepatic hydroxy-methylglutaryl-coenzyme A reductase (HMG-CoA reductase), the enzyme catalyzing the rate-limiting step in hepatic cholesterol synthesis, statins decrease synthesis of cholesterol by the liver, which results in two important effects: the up-regulation of LDL receptors by hepatocytes and the consequent increased removal of apolipoprotein (apo) E- and B-containing lipoproteins from the circulation, and a reduction in the synthesis and secretion of lipoproteins from the liver. The net effect of statin therapy is to lower plasma concentrations of cholesterol-carrying lipoproteins, the most prominent of which is low density lipoprotein (LDL). Importantly, however, statins also increase the removal and reduce the secretion of remnant particles, i.e., very low density lipoprotein (VLDL) and intermediate-density lipoprotein (IDL). Although all statins share a common mechanism of action, they differ in terms of their chemical structures, pharmacokinetic profiles, and lipid-modifying efficacy [3]. The chemical structures of statins govern their water solubility, which in turn influences their absorption, distribution, metabolism and excretion. Lovastatin, pravastatin and simvastatin are derived from fungal metabolites and have elimination half-lives of 1–3 h. Atorvastatin, cerivastatin (with-drawn from clinical use in 2001), fluvastatin, pitavastatin and rosuvastatin are fully synthetic compounds, with elimination half-lives ranging from 1 h for fluvastatin to 19 h for rosuvastatin. At maximum approved doses, the LDL-cholesterol-lowering effects have been reported to range from 30% to 55% and the incidence of CVD can be reduced by 25–60%. All statins lower triglyceride levels up to 20–30%, and therefore, they are also useful in the treatment of moderate hypertriglyceridemia [4].

Pharmacological management of CVD is largely based on evidence from clinical trials and guidelines from expert consensus panels. Meta-analyses from several primary and secondary intervention studies have clearly shown that cholesterol-lowering medication, significantly reduces cardiovascular events, mortality, and morbidity [5-7], but considerable inter-individual variation exists in response to statin therapy.

Important factors in inter-individual variation assessment can be the patient's disease severity, low compliance to treatment, physiological and biological conditions and genetic profile.

This results in treatment recommendations for the population, with recognition that not all individuals will derive the benefit seen in large samples. Pharmacogenomics can provide important insights into statins therapy through elucidation of the genetic (or genomic) contribution to variable response for these drugs. Pharmacogenomics holds the promise of allowing further refinement in the management of patients, by enabling clinicians to individualize cardiovascular drug therapy based on a person's genetic make up. Such an approach has the potential to lead to greater efficacy in treated patients, fewer adverse effects and better disease management, which might in turn lead to a reduction in cardiovascular events (i.e. better outcomes) and reduced health care costs [8].

The search for genetic polymorphisms or DNA sequence variations may enable us to identify novel determinants of drug responsiveness by means of the study of three candidate genes groups: (a) genes encoding proteins involved in metabolism or drug transport, or both, that influence drug pharmacokinetics; (b) genes encoding proteins involved in mechanism of action and/or metabolic pathways on which drugs operate (that influence pharmacodynamics); (c) genes encoding proteins involved in the underlying disease condition or intermediate phenotype [9].

This review briefly summarizes the recent pharmacogenomic and pharmacogenetic studies and the potential contributions of genetic variations in candidate genes related to lipid and lipoprotein metabolism and statins efficacy.

PHARMACOGENETICS OF STATINS EFFICACY

Genes Encoding Proteins Involved in Lipid Cholesterol Metabolism, Lipoprotein Secretion and Clearance

Multiple genetic polymorphisms have been investigated in relation to their potential effect on plasma lipid-lowering response to statins treatment; among them, *apoE polymorphisms* have been studied extensively.

Apolipoprotein E plays a key role in the metabolisms of cholesterol and triglyceride by serving as a receptor-binding ligand mediating the clearance of chylomicron and remnants of VLDL cholesterol from plasma. The ApoE gene is located at the long arm of chromosome 19; the polymorphic locus shows three common alleles (ε2, ε3 and ε4) that codes for the 3 common isoforms E2, E3, and E4 that has been studied extensively. Compared with ε3 homozygotes, carriers of the ε2 allele, which has defective receptor-binding ability, have lower circulating cholesterol levels and higher triglyceride levels, whereas carriers of the ε4 allele appear to have higher plasma levels of total and low-density lipoprotein cholesterol [10].

A meta-analysis of 15 492 CVD case-patients and 32965 controls pooled from 48 studies supports the notion that the ε 4 allele is significantly related to an increased risk for CVD while the ε2 allele has no effect [11].

In a substudy of the Scandinavian Simvastatin Survival Study (4S) [12], Gerdes *et al.* shows that patients survivors of myocardial infarction, carrying the ε4 allele, have about twice the risk of dying during a follow-up period of 5.5 years, compared with patients who are not ε4 carriers and that these ε4 carriers seem to benefit particularly well from treatment with simvastatin.

Judging from the available data, it can be concluded that carriers of the E4 (ε4) allele tend to have a greater percent reduction in LDL cholesterol in response to statin therapy than subjects carrying the wild-type apoE allele (E3 or ε3). Conversely, carriers of the E2 (ε2) allele show a smaller reduction. These differences remain significant, even after adjustment for age and baseline LDL cholesterol, both of which are well-known nongenetic determinants of the LDL-lowering response to statin therapy.

It has been suggested that lipoproteins containing the apoE4 isoform are cleared more efficiently from the circulation, leading to a more pronounced down-regulation of hepatic cholesterol synthesis [13], which could take part in the patented functional relationship between plasma levels of ApoE and cardiovascular disease as suggested by Mooijaart *et al.* [14]. ApoE2 containing lipoproteins display attenuated plasma clearance resulting in up-regulation of HMG-CoA synthesis. Such a condition could influence statins effectiveness as ApoE4 carriers have low HMG-CoA reductase levels resulting in costitutively decreased biological target for their mechanism of action.

However, other studies show contrasting data as Peña *et al.* [15] suggest that ApoE genotype appears not to influence the hypolipidaemic effect of pravastatin in patients monitored in a general outpatient setting. This discrepancy could be related to the complexity of lipid metabolic pathway in which ApoE exerts a relevant role also independently of HMG-CoA reductase. In this setting the observation that other lipidic fractions such as HDL changes during statin treatment are influenced by ApoE polymorphisms in relation with the cholesteryl ester transfer protein polymorphism (B2 allele) [16,17].

Apolipoproteins genes coding for major structural proteins in LDL, as *ApoB gene*, may also alter lipid response to statins treatment: polymorphisms of ApoB at XbaI locus show a relative high frequency in patients with hyperlipidemia, in whom the total cholesterol-lowering efficacy is decreased following treatment of simvastatin [18] or fluvastatin [19]. However, Ojala *et al.* [20] observed that the apoB XbaI genotype did not affect the hypocholesterolaemic efficacy of lovastatin in any patient.

It is of interest that the patients with the APOB R3500Q muta-tion tend to respond extremely well to statins therapy, probably because the up-regulation of their two normal LDL receptor genes allows clearance of their LDL (whether or not it has the APOB 3500 R or 3500 Q), but also clears IDL and other remnant particles before they can be metabolized into LDL [21].

Apolipoprotein A-I gene (APOA1) polymorphisms have been also associated with variations in serum LDL- and HDL-cholesterol: Sorkin *et al.* [22] suggested that APOA1 polymorphisms are associated with variations of baseline serum concentrations of triglyceride and VLDL-cholesterol and in response to atorvastatin in a gender-specific manner; in particular APOA1+83 variant allele was associated with higher basal LDL cholesterol levels in men as well, but not in women, with significant interactions between the polymorphisms in the estrogen receptor alpha and the APOA1+83 variant allele regarding both HDL and LDL cholesterol responses to atorvastatin therapy [23].

Because they encode for proteins with key roles in cholesterol metabolism, the *HMG CoA reductase (HMGCR)* gene is an obvious candidate to explore in pharmacogenetic (pharmacogenomic) studies of statins response. In a large pharmacogenomic study, Chasman *et al.* [24] analyzed 148 single nucleotide polymorphisms (SNPs) in 10 candidate genes, including genes relevant for cholesterol biosynthesis such as HMG-CoA reductase and squalene synthase (farnesyldiphosphate farnesyltransferase 1, FDFT1) in 1536 participants of the Pravastatin Inflammation/CRP Evaluation (PRINCE) study.

Chasman observed that two common and tightly linked intronic SNPs (SNP 12 and 29) in the gene coding for HMG-CoA reductase were significantly associated with reduced efficacy of pravastatin therapy: in fact, individuals with a single copy of the minor allele had a 22% smaller reduction in total cholesterol and a 19% smaller reduction in LDL cholesterol suggesting that individuals heterozygous for a genetic variant in the HMG-CoA reductase gene may experience significantly smaller reductions in cholesterol when treated with pravastatin.

Presumably, the intron variants are marking a functional SNP that could be altering transcription of the gene, or messenger RNA stability or enzyme activity or drug binding.

In the remaining genes, the polymorphism SNP4 in the *squalene synthase gene* had differential effects of pravastatin on lipid reduction. However, most of these variations were also significantly associated with baseline lipid levels. Furthermore pharmacogenetic influence for pravastatin clearly has been established only in specific populations [25, 26]. Medina et al. also demonstrated that alternative splicing in HMG.CoA reductase modifies the lipid-lowering efficacy of simvastatin; particularly influenced by the rs3846662 snp located within intron 13 [27]. Moreover single nucleotide polymorphism of HMGCoA-reductase gene (RS 17238540) influences simvastatin action also in patients with other relevant metabolic disease such us diabetes mellitus [28]. However contrasting data have been described for other statins in association with several clinical pictures and/or associated treatments [29].

Another well-characterized association between statins response and genetic variations has been described for the *cholesteryl ester transfer protein (*CETP) gene. CETP is a plasma glycoprotein that mediates the transfer of neutral lipids between lipoproteins, in particular cholesteryl ester (CE) from HDL is transferred to VLDL and LDL (which then transport cholesteryl ester back to the liver) with the reciprocal transfer of triacylglycerol (TG); CETP also mediates the transfer of phospholipids (PLs) from TG-rich lipoproteins to HDL, principally during lipolysis of the former when excess surface is generated (Table **1**). Growing evidence indicates that CETP significantly modulates lipoprotein metabolism, including the multi-step process known as reverse cholesterol transport. Genetic alterations in CETP levels in humans are associated with impairment of important steps involved in reverse cholesterol transport [30].

Several DNA polymorphisms of the *CETP* gene have been described [31] (alterations that cause multiple or single aminoacid changes or significant truncations, alterations that do not affect the coding sequence of CETP but could potentially affect expression levels of the protein). Two single-nucleotide polymorphisms, TaqIB, which do not alter the sequence of CETP, and I405V, which results in a single aminoacid change, have been studied sufficiently.

Of these, the restriction polymorphism TaqIB located in intron 1 of the *CETP* gene is one of the most intensively studied: the term B1 was used to denote the presence of TaqI while B2 was used to denote absence of TaqI. The TaqIB polymorphism is very frequent, with the heterozygous B1B2 state being the most common in most populations.

B1 allele carriers (presence of the restriction site) have higher CETP concentrations, lower HDL cholesterol levels and homozy-gote individuals with the B1B1 genotype have been reported to show a fast progression of coronary arteriosclerosis [32].

The less-common B2 allele generally is associated with a reduction in CETP activity and increased HDL level in the homozygous B2B2 state relative to the homozygous B1B1 state.

In the Regression Growth Evaluation Statin Study (REGRESS) Kuivenhoven *et al.* [33] examined the relation between the TaqlB polymorphism of the CETP gene and the

Table 1. Genetic Polymorphisms Influencing Pharmacodynamic and Pharmacokinetic of Statin Therapy

Gene	SNP	Drugs	Effect on Drug Therapy
Lipid metabolism			
Apolipoprotein E (ApoE)	E2, E3, E4 A 491-T	All statins	E2 allele more frequent in responders, greater reduction of LDL-C in male E2 carriers; reduced mortality risk but less compliance in E4 carriers [10]. Greater reduction in LDL-C in A-491T carriers.
Apolipoprotein B (ApoB)	XbaIins/del	Lovastatin, Fluvastatin	Greater reduction in LDL-C (34% vs. 27%) in ins-homozygotes [15-18].
Apolipoprotein A1 (ApoA1)	G-75A (MspI) +83 (MspI)	Pravastatin, Atorvastatin	Higher increase in HDL-C in GG carriers [20]. Gender-difference in HDL-C increase in +83 variant carriers [21].
HMG-CoA reductase (HMGCR)	SNP12, SNP29 Rs384662	Pravastatin Simvastatin	22% smaller reduction in total cholesterol and 19% smaller reduction in LDL-C in heterozygotes [22]. 6-15% difference in reduction of total cholesterol and Apo-B [27]
Squalene synthase (FDFT1)	SNP4	Pravastatin	Variable reduction in total cholesterol in men [22].
Cholesteryl ester transfer protein (CETP)	TaqI B (B1,B2), I405V Haplotypes, SNP15	Atorvastatin Pravastatin	Greatest HDL response and TG reduction in B2 carriers [24], Reduced HDL and TG response [35] More angiographic disease progression in B2B2 [31]. SNPs1-6 associated with variable increase in HDL-C and SNPs4-9 with decrease in TG [33]. Hap SNPs 1-6 are associated with variable HDL-C increase and SNPs 4-9 with TG decrease [33]. SNP15 reduces HDL-C baseline and response in men [33].
ATP-binding cassette transporter A1 (ABCA1)	C-477T G-320C	Fluvastatin	-477C/T variant associated with less apoA-I increase, more coronary events in -477TT or CT carriers [46].

(Table 1) Contd.....

Gene	SNP	Drugs	Effect on Drug Therapy
ATP-binding cassette transporter G8 (ABCG8)	D19H	Atorvastatin	D19H variant determines 36% vs. 40% reduction in LDL-C and interacts with CYP7A1 A-204C [44].
Sterol regulatory element binding protein 1 (SREBF1)	-36del/G	Fluvastatin	Largest response in apoA-I and apoC-III levels in GG carriers [36-39].
SCAP	A2386G	Simvastatin	Increased TC, TG and LDLC response by carriers [36, 38].
Peroxisome proliferator activated receptor δ/γ (PPAR δ/γ)	Haplotypes	Fluvastatin	PPARδ haplotype 2 determines TG and apo CIII response and coronary lesions PPARγ haplotype 7 associated with reduced mean lumen diameter [40].
Lipoprotein lipase (LPL)	D9N	Pravastatin	Attenuated response in mutation carriers [41].
Hepatic lipase (LIPC)	C-514T	Lovastatin	96% of patients in the CC group, 60% in the CT group and 0% in the TT group displayed CAD regression [42,43].
CYP7A1	A-204C	Atorvastatin	Marginally smaller reduction in LDLC by carriers, greater response in interaction with ABCG8 D19H [44].
MTP	G-493T	Pravastatin	Increased CHD risk in placebo group by mutation carriers, which is eliminated by pravastatin treatment [45].
PON-1	C-107T	Simvastatin	Reduced PON activity [51]
Drug metabolism and transporters			
Cytochrome P450 3A4 (CYP3A4)	A-290G	Atorvastatin	Increased LDL-C in variant carriers [52].
Cytochrome P450 3A5 (CYP3A5)	CYP3A5 *1, *3	Atorvastatin Lovastatin Simvastatin	Greater reduction in TC(34% vs. 17%) in CYP3A5 expressors (CYP3A5 *1) than non-expressors (CYP3A5 *3) [55].
Cytochrome P450 2D6 (CYP2D6)	CYP2D6 *3, *4, *5, *2xN	Simvastatin Atorvastatin	Carriers of CYP2D6 homozygous mutant alleles had stronger decrease in total cholesterol and higher incidence of intolerability [57]. Carriers of CYP2D6*4 had increased rate of myopathy [72]

(Table 1) Contd.....

Gene	SNP	Drugs	Effect on Drug Therapy
ATP-binding cassette transporter B1 (ABCB1, MDR1)	C3435T	Atorvastatin	Female CC homozygotes had smaller reduction in LDL-C, but larger increase in HDL-C [58].
Organic anion transporter-C (OATP-C)	A388G (*1b), T521C (*5), V174A, G-11187A (*17 with *1b and*5)	Pravastatin	Increased statin plasma level in V174A homozygotes [59]. *15B and *17 heterozygote carriers have higher statin plasma levels [60].

progression of coronary atherosclerosis, as well as its influence on cholesterol-lowering therapy: in REGRESS patients treated with pravastatin or placebo individuals with the B2B2 genotype did not adequately respond with a decrease in disease progression to pravastatin treatment as assessed by angiographic determination of coronary luminal diameters. According to these findings, Mohrschladt *et al.* [34] found that the Taq1B polymorphism is a significant predictor of future CVD events in statin-treated (simvastatin, pravastatin, atorvastatin) patients with familial hypercholesterolemia; in fact the relative risk for CVD events was 1.8 for B2B2 carriers compared to B1 allele carriers, despite the fact that B2B2 patients had higher baseline HDL cholesterol levels; these results suggested that in spite of similar improvement of the lipoprotein profile during statin therapy, these patients with the B2B2 genotype have a higher CVD risk in comparison with the B1 allele carriers. Furthermore the CETP I405V polymorphism was associated with a reduced effect of simvastatin on TG and HDL-c [35].

Single SNPs and haplotypes in the CETP gene were analyzed by Winkelmann *et al.* [36] in 98 patients with untreated dyslipidemias receiving three different statins: pravastatin, atorvastatin, and cerivastatin. Analysis of several SNPs as haplotypes, SNPs1-6 and SNPs4-9 significantly predict HDL-cholesterol increase and triglyceride decrease, respectively; This results indicates that haplotypes of informative SNPs rather than single genetic variations may be much more effective in predicting the effects of lipid-modifying therapy with statins. Moreover CETP genotype (TaqIB2 allele) associated with lower CETP level and higer HDL-c adversely affects clinically outcome in the course of statin treatment. These data provide a furthen basis for the hypothesis that reducing CETP activity by statins with genetically determined low CETP levels may have adverse effects in term of vascular protection [37].

Another promising pathway for pharmacogenetics studies is related to the cholesterol synthesis pathway and its control through transcription factors such as the sterol regulatory element-binding factors (SREBFs) and SCAP protein (SREBF cleavage-activating protein), responsible for SREBF activation and peroxisome proliferator-activated receptors (PPARs).

The sterol regulatory element-binding protein (SREBP) family of transcription factors control cholesterol and lipid metabolism and play critical roles during adipocyte differentiation and insulin-dependent gene expression [38]. Use of compounds that activate the pathway of SREBP has been patented by Berger *et al.* [39]. The family consists of three different SREBP proteins, SREBP1a, SREBP1c/ADD1 and SREBP2. The SREBPs are synthesized as large precursor proteins that are inserted into the endoplasmic reticulum (ER) membrane through two membrane-spanning domains. The membrane-associated proteins are transcriptionally inactive. In the ER, the C terminus of the SREBP interacts with a protein called Scap (SREBP-cleavage-activating protein), which functions as a sterol sensor. In sterol-depleted cells, Scap escorts the SREBPs from the ER to the Golgi, where they are processed by two membrane-associated proteases, the site 1 (S1P) and site 2 (S2P) proteases, which release the mature forms of the proteins. These transcriptionally active fragments of the SREBPs are translocated to the nucleus, where they bind to the promoters of SREBP target genes, including genes involved in the synthesis and metabolism of cholesterol. Once in the nucleus, the active fragments of SREBPs bind to the promoters of target genes as dimers and affect their expression (the list of genes regulated includes many genes involved in synthesis and uptake of cholesterol, triglycerides, fatty acids, including the *HMG-CoA reductase* gene itself). SREBPs belong to the basic helix-loop-helix leucine zipper family of transcription factors and their unique DNA binding domains allow them to recognize both classical E-boxes and distinct promoter motifs known as sterol regulatory elements (SREs).

In the Lipoprotein and Coronary Atherosclerosis Study (LCAS), individuals homozygous for the G allele of SREBP1a-G-36del variation had the greatest apoA-I increase (16.5%), whereas homozygous deletion allele carriers showed no response to fluvastatin [40]. In the same study in subjects treated with simvastatin 20 mg/day, polymorphisms in the related SCAP gene (2386A/ G) were significantly associated with total cholesterol LDL-cholesterol and triglyceride levels reduction; but these results were not observed in two other studies including patients treated with fluvastatin [41] and pravastatin [42].

In the same patient collection, Chen *et al.* demonstrate that the PPAR δ haplotype 2 showed strong interactions with response of plasma triglycerides and to a lesser extent with HDL cholesterol levels after fluvastatin therapy, whereas the PPAR γ haplotype 7 was associated with reduced changes in mean lumen diameter [43].

Other studies reported associations of lipid modulating proteins and response to statin treatment. These include: lipoprotein lipase (LPL), hepatic lipase (HL), cholesterol-hydroxylase (CYP7A1), ATP binding cassette transporters G5 and G8 (ABCG5/G8), microsomal triglyceride transfer protein (MTP) and ATP-binding cassette transporter A1.

LPL is a multifunctional protein that is involved in the breakdown of triglycerides in lipoproteins such as chylomicrons and (VLDL). Common mutations in the LPL gene leading to deficient LPL activity have been associated with hypertriglyceridemia and low levels of HDL, the presence of the Asp9Asn LPL mutation in a given patient would confer increased susceptibility to atherosclerosis and therefore be associated with more progression of CVD. In patients who received pravastatin, carriers of the Asp9Asn LPL mutation were associated with a 41% attenuation in reduction of both total cholesterol and LDL-C when compared to noncarriers associated with an increased adjusted relative risk for a clinical event [44].

Hepatic lipase (HL) is a plasma lipolytic enzyme that plays an important role in the metabolism of triglycerides, LDL, and HDL. However, controversial evidence exists concerning whether hepatic lipase is pro or anti-atherogenic. Twenty to 30% of individual variation of hepatic lipase activity is accounted for by the presence of a common polymorphism in the promoter region (-514 C to T) of the HL gene. This polymorphism, *via* its impact on hepatic lipase synthesis and activity, appears to contribute to individual susceptibility to CVD (the presence of the T allele with low hepatic lipase activity, may carry a marginally increased risk of atherosclerosis) and to response of CVD patients to lipid-lowering therapy (patients with the CC genotype have the greatest clinical benefit from intensive lipid-lowering therapy) [45].

Lipid-lowering therapy was associated with a 18% decrease in HL activity and a 12% increase in LDL buoyancy in patients with the CC genotype while HL activity and LDL buoyancy did not significantly change in patients with the TT genotype [46].

Cholesterol excretion by ATP binding cassette transporters G5 and G8 (ABCG5/G8) and bile acid biosynthesis by cholesterol 7 alpha-hydroxylase (CYP7A1) are major pathways for the removal of cholesterol into bile. Kajinami *et al.* [47] investigating the interactions between common polymorphisms in ABCG5/G8 and CYP7A1 and statin response concluded that the ABCG8 H19 and CYP7A1 C-204 alleles appear to interact in a dose-dependent manner on atorvastatin response.

The microsomal triglyceride transfer protein (MTP) transfers lipids into apolipoprotein B-containing lipoproteins for secretion from liver, intestine, and heart. The T-variant of a functional polymorphism in the MTP promoter, MTP-493G/T, has been associated with reduced low-density lipoprotein cholesterol concentrations; in particular, the MTP-493T variant confers an increased risk of CVD that is unrelated to plasma lipids and lipoproteins, but eliminated by pravastatin treatment [48].

Luctuta *et al.* [49] studied polymorphisms in the ABCA1 gene in subjects participants in the prospective Lipoprotein Coronary Atherosclerosis Study (LCAS) treated with fluvastatin: this study showed that heterozygous subjects for -477C/T polymorphisms had a modest reduction in HDL-C and apoA1 levels and a lesser response of apoA1 to treatment with fluvastatin; furthermore the mean number of coronary lesions was greater in subjects with the TT or CT genotype than in subjects with the CC genotype.

Among HDL protective effects, the activity of HDL-associated paraoxonase enzyme (PON) could be extremely relevant for vascular protection although the specific effect of statins on PON activity is still under investigastion [50]. Deakin *et al.* have shown that the effect of simvastatin on PON-1 activity is influenced by C(-107T) polymorphism of PON-1 gene so further studies should elucidate how this putative specific ant-atherogenic mechanism is really induced by different statins [51].

Genes Encoding Proteins Involved in Drug Metabolism and/or Drug Transport

In addition to genes directly connected to lipid metabolism, candidate genes influencing pharmacokinetics of HMG-CoA reductase inhibitors are of potential relevance for therapy response and adverse effects of statins. Many statins are metabolized in the intestine and in the liver by the cytochrome P450-system (CYP450) and are substrates for organic anion-transporting polypeptide C (OATP-C) [52]. Polymorphism of human OATP-C affects statin pharmacokinetics in humans, especially rosuvastatin as described by Lee [53]. A significant number of the CYP450 isoenzymes has yet to be identified. CYP3A4 is the most abundant CYP450 isoenzyme in humans and is the primary metabolic pathway for lovastatin, simvastatin and atorvastatin, whereas CYP2C9 metabolizes fluvastatin. In contrast, pravastatin, rosuvastatin, and pitavastatin do not appear to be metabolized through the CYP450 system.

Lovastatin, simvastatin, and pravastatin, which are produced from fungi like Aspergillus terreus by fermentation, are present as lacton prodrugs and must be converted into the active acid form by hydrolysis [54]. The resulting mevalonic acid side chain anologon is the common structural characteristic by which HMG-CoA reductase is inhibited. CYP450 isoenzymes selectively transform statins into hydroxylated products (phase 1 metabolism) [55]. In phase 2 metabolism, the hydroxylated statins are conjugated with glucuronic acid to form hydrophilic, negatively charged glucuronides which are bound to the canalicular multispecific organic anion transporter cMOAT (ABCC2, MRP2). The statin-glucuronide complexes are then excreted via ABCC2 into the bile (phase 3 metabolism).

CYP3A4, CYP3A5, and CYP2C9 are the most important phase 1 enzymes for statin metabolism and CYP2D6 and CYP2C8 seem to be of minor importance.

Kajinami *et al.* [56] tested whether genetic variation in the CYP system may influence the statin response, analyzing a promoter (A-290G) and 2 nonsynonymous polymorphisms (F189S and M445T) in the CYP3A4 gene locus of 340 hypercholesterolemic patients treated with atorvastatin 10 mg: the A-290G variant allele was significantly associated with higher levels of post-treatment LDL cholesterol, whereas the M445T variant was associated with lower levels of LDL cholesterol before and after treatment. Recently, Wang *et al.* observed the impact of CYP3A4 (I118V) genetic polymorphism on the lipid-lowering effects of simvastatin [57].

CYP3A5 is a recently identified protein that can contribute to the biotransformation of certain statins. Hustert investigated the expression of CYP3A5 and its genetic determinants in a panel of 183 Caucasian liver samples, reporting that a SNP within intron 3 (g.6986G>A) is the primary cause of the CYP3A5 protein polymorphism [58].

CYP3A5 results a genetic determinant of interindividual differences in response to certain statins: lovastatin, simvastatin and atorvastatin were significantly less effective in CYP3A5 polymorphism expressors (CYP3A5*1 carriers) than in non-expressors (CYP3A5*3 homozygotes) [59]; Of interest, no relation between CYP3A5 polymorphisms and LDL-cholesterol response or total cholesterol levels was observed among 23 subjects receiving pravastatin or fluvastatin, which do not undergo CYP3A mediated biotransformation to a significant extent.

The polymorphic CYP3A5 gene affects also the disposition of simvastatin and provides a plausible explanation for interindividual variability of simvastatin disposition.

Moreover, CYP2D6 has also been demonstrated to metabolize simvastatin, and there is evidence that the cholesterol-lowering effect of simvastatin is influenced by CYP2D6 [60]: in fact, subjects carrying 1 or 2 CYP2D6 mutant alleles, which results in decreased metabolism, had greater reductions in LDL cholesterol than those having 2 wild-type alleles. However, another group reported no significant difference in LDL cholesterol reduction in response to simvastatin among different CYP2D6 allele groups known to be less effective, intermediate, highly efficient, or ultrarapid metabolizers [61].

Statin pharmacokinetics is also influenced by transporter proteins, such as the adenosine triphosphate- binding cassette transporter (ABC transporters) ABCB1 (MDR1), ABCC2 (MRP2), and the organic anion transporting peptide- C (OATP-C). ABC, also known as multidrug resistance–1 (MDR1) or P-glycoprotein is a transmembrane protein. Hepatic cholesterol synthesis is associated with ATP binding cassette transporter G5 and G8 (ABCG5/8) activities. ATP binding cassette transporters G5 and G8 (ABCG5/8) are unique proteins located in the plasma membrane, as well as in the intracellular membranes of enterocytes and hepa-tocyte. In the same patient cohort as for the CYP3A4 study, Kajjinami *et al.* investigated in 338 hypercholesterolemic patients the effects of two prevalent polymorphisms in the ABCB1 gene (G2677T/A, C3435T) on lipid response to atorvastatin treatment [62]. The C allele of the C3435T SNP was significantly and independently associated with less reduction in LDL-cholesterol and with a larger increase in HDL relative to variant carriers in women, but not in men.

The OATPs can mediate the cellular uptake of a large number of structurally divergent compounds including drugs. Pravastatin, rosuvastatin, and cerivastatin have been shown to be transported by one of these OATPs, OATP-C (OATP1B1, *SLCO1B1*), and pitavastatin by another, OATP2. It is now becoming apparent that SNPs in the genes encoding these transporters have functional conequences: Nishizato *et al.* [63] observed that certain commonly occurring single-nucleotide polymorphisms in OATP-C, such as T521C (Val174Ala), are likely to be associated with altered pharmacokinetics of pravastatin. Mwinyi and Niemi *et al.* [64] observed also that there is a significant effect of OATP-C variant haplotypes on pravastatin disposition: whereas *5 (T521C) haplotypes expression delayed the hepatocellular uptake of pravastatin, *1b (A388G) expression seemed to accelerate OATP-C-dependent uptake of the drug [65].

Pasanen [66] observed also that SLCO1B1 polymorphism markedly affects the pharmacokinetics of active simvastatin acid, but has no significant effect on parent simvastatin. Raised plasma concentrations of simvastatin acid in patients carrying the SLCO1B1 c.521C variant allele may enhance the risk of systemic adverse effects during simvastatin treatment. In addition, reduced uptake of simvastatin acid by OATP1B1 into the liver in patients with the c.521C allele could reduce its cholesterol-lowering efficacy.

PHARMACOGENETICS AND ADVERSE DRUG REACTIONS

Although safe and well tolerated by most patients statins have also been rarely associated with severe adverse reactions. Common adverse reactions include gastrointestinal disturbances, dyspepsia, headaches, myalgia, central nervous system disturbances and sleep disorders. There are only two uncommon but potentially serious adverse effects related to HMG-CoA reductase inhibitor therapy: hepatotoxicity and myopathy [67].

Statins are associated with skeletal muscle complaints [68], including clinically important myositis and rhabdomyolysis, mild serum creatine kinase (CK) elevations, myalgia with and without elevated CK levels, muscle weakness, muscle cramps, and persistent myalgia and CK elevations after statin withdrawal. Few data are available regarding the frequency of less-serious events such as muscle pain and weakness, which may affect 1% to 5% of patients. Sewright has recently patented predictive biomarkers of statin-induced muscle toxicity [69]. The risk of rhabdomyolysis and other adverse effects with statin use can be exacerbated by several factors, including compromised hepatic and renal function, hypothyroidism, diabetes, and concomitant medications. Medications such as the fibrate gemfibrozil alter statin metabolism and increase statin plasma concentration. How statins injure skeletal muscle is not clear, although recent evidence suggests that statins reduce the production of small regulatory proteins that are important for muscle cells maintenance [70].

The fundamental mechanism of statin muscle toxicity remains elusive but is believed to be a class effect. The most common explanation for the cause of toxic muscle injury invokes the deficiency of one of three main synthetic products in the 3-hydroxy-3-methyl-glutaryl-coenzyme A reductase pathway. Recent studies have revealed several patients with statin-induced rhabdomyolysis who also have metabolic muscle defects, indicating that statin use may unmask presymptomatic metabolic myopathies. Although statin-related muscle toxicity is believed to be a non-inflammatory, toxic myopathy, experimental evidence suggests that it may be triggered by an autoimmune reaction or, conversely, initiate an autoimmune process.

Wilke *et al.* [71] studied the possible relationship between CYP3A gene polymorphisms and atorvastatin-induced muscle damage demonstrating that patients who develop myalgia while taking atorvastatin are more likely to experience a greater degree of muscle damage if they express two copies of CYP3A5*3. Furthermore Frudakis *et al.* showed that CYP2D6*4 allele was associated with myopathy in patients treated with atorvastatin [72].

Ruano *et al.* [73] observed that SNPs in the angiotensin II Type 1 receptor (AGTR1) and nitric oxide synthase 3 (NOS3) genes were significantly associated with CK activity. These results demonstrate a strong association between CK activity during statin treatment and variability in genes related to vascular function, and suggest that vascular smooth muscle function may contribute to the muscle side effects of statins.

Fiegenbaum [74] observed that ABCB1 (1236C>T, 2677G> A/T, and 3435C>T) allelic variants correlate with adverse drug reactions: haplotype analyses demonstrated a reduction of the T-non-G-T haplotype frequency (20%) in patients in whom myalgia developed during simvastatin treatment, as compared with the non- adverse drug reactions.

Another mechanism which could be involved in statin- induced myopathy has been described in rats by Dorajo *et al.* [75]. The involvement of multi-drug resistence associated protein-1 transporter suggest a relevant role for transport mechanism that could be susceptible of genetic modulation [76].

Recently a large study by the SEARCH Collaborative Group confirmed the strong association between myopathy and the SLCO1B1 rs4149056 Genotype in subjects treated with high dose of simvastatin (80 mg/day) [77].

PHARMACOGENETICS OF STATINS PLEIOTROPIC EFFECTS

The positive effect of statin therapy in cardiovascular acute events could be related with the possible involvement of mechanisms at least partially independent from LDL-lowering. Animal, and clinical studies have all shown that statins may also have important pleiotropic properties, such as the reduction of endothelial dysfunction, inhibition of inflammatory responses, stabilization of atherosclerotic plaques, and modulation of procoagulant activity and platelet function, all of which can be useful in treating both cardiovascular and non-cardiovascular diseases [78].

Interestingly, restoration of endothelial function preceded substantial reductions in serum cholesterol levels, suggesting that there are additional effects on endothelial function beyond that of cholesterol reduction. Statins exert many favorable effects on the endothelium and attenuate endothelial dysfunction by means of endothelial NO synthase (eNOS) stimulation and increased expression of this enzymatic activity. However, a functional polymorphism in the promoter of the eNOS gene (T-786C) reduces its activity and could modulate the response to statins. Nagassaki *et al.* [78] genotyped 200 healthy subjects for this polymorphism, and 15 subjects with the TT genotype and 15 with the CC genotype were selected to receive placebo or atorvastatin 10 mg/day p.o. for 14 days and suggested that the T-786C polymorphism modulates the effects of atorvastatin on NO bioavailability and oxidative stress [79] (Table **2**).

Table 2. Genetic Polymorphisms Influencing Pleiotropic Effects of Statin Therapy

Pleiotropic Effects			
Endothelial nitric oxide synthase (eNOS)	T-786C	Atorvastatin Fluvastatin	Increased transcriptional activity of the eNOS stronger in the 786C/C than in the 786T/T genotype [79-80]. Anti-inflammatory effect [89].
Lectin-like oxidized receptor 1 (LOX-1)	3'UTR (188C>T)	Atorvastatin	In 3'UTR/T carriers, atorvastatin reduced platelet activity by LDL and ox-LDL lowering and not by rapid CD36 and LOX-1 downregulation as in C carriers [83].
Angiotensin-I converting enzyme (ACE)	Intron 16 ins/del	Fluvastatin	Greater reduction in TC, LDL-C and apoB and lesion regression in DD genotypes [87].
Glycoprotein III A (GPIIIA)	PI (A1/A2)	Pravastatin	Decreased risk of recurrent event in A2 carriers, linked to ACE D genotype [85].

Furthermore Abe *et al.* [80] examined eNOS mRNA levels, mRNA stability and the transcriptional activities of the eNOS gene in human umbilical vein endothelial cells treated with fluvastatin and simvastatin: fluvastatin significantly increased the transcriptional activity of the eNOS gene and this effect was stronger in the -786C/C genotype than in the -786T/T genotype. suggesting that fluvastatin increases endothelial NO activity and thus may be more beneficial to patients with the -786C allele.

Recently, we studied the influence of lectin-like oxidized LDL receptor-1 (LOX-1) polymorphisms on statins activity [81]. In fact, it seems that atorvastatin and simvastatin, beyond lipid-lowering action, decreased platelet activity as detected by P-selectin levels (sensitive marker of platelet activation) and one of the putative factors involved in this pleiotropic action could be the rapid modulation of specific receptors for ox-LDL (CD36 and LOX-1) that are potent platelet activators [82].

In particular, evaluating a SNP in 3′ untranslated region (3′UTR) (188C>T) of LOX-1 gene of hypercholesterolemic patients treated with atorvastatin, Puccetti observed that in 3'UTR/T carriers atorvastatin reduced platelet activity by LDL and ox-LDL lowering and not by rapid CD36 and LOX-1 downregulation as in C carriers. These results suggest that in T carriers LDL lowering is needed to achieve anti-platelet action [83]. Furthermore LOX-1 polymorphisms induce increased risk of cardiovascular events independently of NOS polymorphisms when evaluated in a specific population of hypercholesterolemic subjects treated with atorvastatin [84]. Mainly, the LOX-1 3'UTR/T polymorphisms select a specific population whom cardiovascular protection is achieved only by LDL-lowering whereas in C carriers the statin is able to offer a protective effect by antithrombotic mechanisms regardless of magnitude in lipid profile changes [84].

Bray *et al.* [85] studied platelet glycoprotein IIIa and polymorphic alleles Pl(A2) in 767 patients (treated with pravastatin) of Cholesterol And Recurrent Events (CARE) trial followed prospectively for 5 years suggesting a potential role of these genotypes in therapeutic decision making.

Previous studies showed also a reduction in blood pressure associated with the use of statins, reported in patients with untreated hypertension and in patients treated with antihypertensive drugs, particularly angiotensin-converting enzyme inhibitors and calcium channel blockers. The mechanism responsible for the hypotensive effect seems to be largely independent of the effect of statins on plasma cholesterol, and probably is related to the interaction of the medications with endothelial function or angiotensin II receptors [86].

Marian *et al.* [87] showed that angiotensin-1 converting enzyme I/D polymorphism is associated with the response of plasma lipids and coronary atherosclerosis to treatment with fluvastatin: subjects with DD genotype had a greater reduction in LDL-C, a higher rate of regression and a lower rate of progression of coronary artery disease; however a recent study [88] found no evidence that the ACE ID genotype was a major modifier of the efficacy of pravastatin in reducing the risk of cardiovascular events.

Inflammatory mediators share a relevant role in the pathogenesis of atherotrombosis ant anti-inflammatory action of statins has been described as a relevant anti-atherothrombotic mechanism. Souza-Costa DC *et al.* have shown a modulation of anti-inflammatory effect of atorvastatin induced by the T-876C polymorphism in the endothelial NOS gene [89]. Such an evidence confirm that diferrent SNPs could influence several anti-atherothrombotic mechanisms induced by statins, thus confirming a multi-gene influence [90].

CURRENT AND FUTURE DEVELOPMENTS

Aggressive reduction of LDL-C is a cornerstone of preventive cardiovascular care, but additional therapeutic approaches to reduce atherosclerosis progression (or induce its regression) and prevent cardiovascular events are still needed. Pharmacological management of cardiovascular diseases is largely based on evidence from clinical trials and guidelines from expert consensus panels. This results in treatment recommendations for the population, with recognition that not all individuals will derive the benefit seen in large samples. Pharmacogenomics holds the promise of allowing further refinement in the management of patients, by enabling clinicians to individualize cardiovascular drug therapy based on a person's genetic make up, reducing also adverse drug reactions.

However, while much has been learned through candidate gene-driven studies, there are certain limitations to this approach, the greatest of which is that gene selection is based on our present understanding of the mechanism of action of the drug, its pharmacokinetics and the disease state. Thus, the candidate gene approach precludes identification of novel genes that might contribute to variable drug response. One advantage of a genomic approach is that it requires no previous knowledge of gene function, proteins involved in disease biology or drug effects. Since a genome-wide approach has the potential to identify unsuspected genetic associations with drug response, it may provide insight into previously unknown disease mechanisms, drug effects and/or targets for disease intervention.

Since different ethnic groups display distinct allele distributions for several drug metabolizing enzymes, the influence of ethnicity on pharmacogenetic responses must be taken into account by performing and comparing clinical trials in various ethnic groups. In the near future, pharmacogenomics may allow the identification of patient subgroups which most likely profit from lipid-lowering therapy. A multigene haplotype approach rather than a single gene analysis could likely to adequately characterize the effects of common polymorphisms on the response to therapy. Furthermore, genotyping of highrisk patients may prevent adverse effects in individuals with genetic predisposition.

Finally, a relevant issue that future studies should improve is how much of a statin failure is pharmacogenomics related. At present time, available data can only suggest a putative influence of pharmacogenetics in statins effectiveness. However, especially multigene studies could provide reliable data concerning individual safety and efficacy of each single statin [91,92].

REFERENCES

[1] Goff DC Jr, Brass L, Braun LT, *et al.* Essential features of a surveillance system to support the prevention and management of heart disease and stroke: a scientific statement from the american heart association councils on epidemiology and prevention, stroke, and cardiovascular nursing and the interdisciplinary working groups on quality of care and outcomes research and atherosclerotic peripheral vascular disease. Circulation 2007; 115: 127-155.

[2] Smith SC Jr, Allen J, Blair SN, *et al.* AHA/ACC guidelines for secondary prevention for patients with coronary and other atherosclerotic vascular disease: 2006 update: endorsed by the National Heart, Lung, and Blood Institute. Circulation 2006; 113: 2363-2372.

[3] Michael S. Chemical, pharmacokinetic and pharmacodynamic properties of statins: an update. Fund Clin Pharmacol 2005; 19: 117-125.

[4] Davidson MH, Toth PP. Comparative effects of lipid-lowering therapies. Prog Cardiovasc Dis 2004; 47: 73-104.

[5] Kreisberg RA, Oberman A. Clinical review 141: lipids and atherosclerosis: lessons learned from randomized controlled trials of lipid lowering and other relevant studies. J Clin Endocrinol Metab 2002; 87: 423-437.

[6] Baigent C, Keech A, Kearney PM, *et al.* Cholesterol Treatment Trialists' (CTT) Collaborators. Efficacy and safety of cholesterol-lowering treatment: prospective meta-analysis of data from 90,056 participants in 14 randomised trials of statins. Lancet 2005; 366: 1267-1278.

[7] Thavendiranathan P, Bagai A, Brookhart MA, Choudhry NK. Primary prevention of cardiovascular diseases with statin therapy: a meta-analysis of randomized controlled trials. Arch Intern Med 2006; 166: 2307-313.

[8] Johnson JA, Cavallari LH. Cardiovascular pharmacogenomics. Exp Physiol 2005; 90: 283-289.

[9] Kajinami K, Akao H, Polisecki E, *et al.* Pharmacogenomics of statin responsiveness. Am J Cardiol 2005; 96 (Suppl 1): 65K-70K.

[10] Chasman DI, Paré G, Zee RY, *et al.* Genetic loci associated with plasma concentration of LDL-C, HDL-C, triglycerides, ApoA1, and ApoB among 6382 Caucasian women in genome-wide analysis with replication. Circ Cardiovasc Genet 2008; 1: 21-30.

[11] Song Y, Stampfer MJ, Liu S. Meta-analysis: apolipoprotein E genotypes and risk for coronary heart disease. Ann Int Med 2004; 141: 137-147.

[12] Gerdes LU, Gerdes C, Kervinen K, *et al.* The apolipoprotein epsilon 4 allele determines prognosis and the effect on prognosis of simvastatin in survivors of myocardial infarction: a substudy of the Scandinavian simvastatin survival study. Circulation 2000; 101: 1366-1371.

[13] Kypreos KE, van Dijk KW, van Der Zee A, Havekes LM, Zannis VI. Domains of apolipoprotein E contributing to triglyceride and cholesterol homeostasis *in vivo*. Carboxyl-terminal region 203-299 promotes hepatic very low density lipoprotein-triglyceride secretion. J Biol Chem 2001; 276: 19778-19786.

[14] Mooijaart SP, Berbee JF, Van HEW, *et al.* ApoE plasma levels and risk of cardiovascular mortality in older age. Plos Med 2006; 3: e176.

[15] Peña R, Lahoz C, Mostaza JM, *et al.* Effect of apoE genotype on the hypolipidaemic response to pravastatin in an outpatient setting. J Intern Med 2002; 251: 518-525.

[16] Sorlí JV, Corella D, Francés F, *et al.* The effect of the APOE polymorphism on HDL-C concentrations depends on the cholesterol ester transfer protein gene variation in a Southern European population. Clin Chim Acta 2006; 366: 196-203.

[17] Nieminen T, Kähönen M, Viiri LE, Grönroos P, Lehtimäki T. Pharmacogenetics of apolipoproyein E gene during lipid-lowering therapy: lipid levels and prevention of coronary heart disease. Pharmacogenomics 2008; 9: 1475-1486.

[18] Ye P, Shang Y, Ding X. The influence of apolipoprotein B and E gene polymorphisms on the response to simvastatin therapy in patients with hyperlipidemia. Chin Med Sci J 2003; 18: 9-13.

[19] Guzman EC, Hirata MH, Quintao EC, Hirata RD. Association of the apolipoprotein B gene polymorphisms with cholesterol levels and response to fluvastatin in Brazilian individuals with high risk for coronary heart disease. Clin Chem Lab Med 2000; 38: 731-736.

[20] Ojala JP, Helve E, Ehnholm C, *et al.* Effect of apolipoprotein E polymorphism and XbaI polymorphism of apolipoprotein B on response to lovastatin treatment in familial and non-familial hypercholesterolaemia. J Intern Med 1991; 230: 397-405.

[21] Heath KE, Gudnason V, Humphries SE, Seed M. The type of mutation in the low density lipoprotein receptor gene influences the cholesterol-lowering response of the HMG-CoA reductase inhibitor simvastatin in patients with heterozygous familial hypercholesterolaemia. Atherosclerosis 1999; 143: 41-54.

[22] Sorkin SC, Forestiero FJ, Hirata MH, *et al.* APOA1 polymorphisms are associated with variations in serum triglyceride concentrations in hypercholesterolemic individuals. Clin Chem Lab Med 2005; 43: 1339-1345.

[23] Kajinami K, Brousseau ME, Lamon-Fava S, Ordovas JM, Schaefer EJ. Gender-specific effects of estrogen receptor α gene haplotype on high-density lipoprotein cholesterol response to atorvastatin: interaction with apolipoprotein AI gene polymorphism. Atherosclerosis 2005; 178: 331-338.

[24] Chasman DI, Posada D, Subrahmanyan L, *et al.* Pharmacogenetic study of statin therapy and cholesterol reduction. JAMA 2004; 291: 2821-2827.

[25] Peters B, Maitland-van der Zee AH. Pharmacogenomic importance of pravastatin. Pharmacogenomics 2008; 9: 1207-1210.

[26] Zhang W, Chen BL, Ozdemir V, He YJ, Zhou G, Peng DD, Deng S, Xie QY, Xie W, Xu LY, Wang LC, Fan L, Wang A, Zhou HH. SLCO1B1 521T-->C functional genetic polymorphism and lipid-lowering efficacy of multiple-dose pravastatin in Chinese coronary heart disease patients. Br J Clin Pharmacol 2007; 64: 346-352.

[27] Medina MW, Gao F, Ruan W, Rotter JI, Krauss RM. Alternative splicing of 3-hydroxy-3-methylglutaryl coenzyme A reductase is associated with plasma low-density lipoprotein cholesterol response to simvastatin. Circulation 2008; 118: 355-362.

[28] Donnelly LA, Doney AS, Dannfald J, Whitley AL, Lang CC, Morris AD, Donnan PT, Palmer CN. A paucimorphic variant in the HMG-CoA reductase gene is associated with lipid-lowering response to statin treatment in diabetes: a GoARTS study. Pharmacogenet Genomics 2008; 18; 1021-1026.

[29] Singer JB, Holdaas H, Jardine AG, fellstrom B, Os I, Bermann G, Meyer JM. Assessment of Lescol in renal Transplantation (ALERT) Study Investigators. Genetic Analysis of fluvastatin response and dyslipidemia in renal transplant recipients. J Lipid Res 2007; 48: 2072-2078.

[30] Izem L, Morton RE. Cholesteryl ester transfer protein biosynthesis and cellular cholesterol homeostasis are tightly interconnected. J Biol Chem 2001; 276: 26534-26541.

[31] Kuivenhoven JA, de Knijff P, Boer JM, *et al.* Heterogeneity at the *CETP* gene locus: influence on plasma CETP concentrations and HDL cholesterol levels. Arterioscler Thromb Vasc Biol 1997; 17: 560-568.

[32] Ordovas JM, Cupples LA, Corella D, *et al.* Association of cholesteryl ester transfer protein-TaqIB polymorphism with variations in lipoprotein subclasses and coronary heart disease risk: the Framingham study. Arterioscler Thromb Vasc Biol 2000; 20: 1323-1329.

[33] Kuivenhoven JA, Jukema JW, Zwinderman AH, *et al.* The role of a common variant of the cholesteryl ester transfer protein gene in the progression of coronary atherosclerosis. N Engl J Med 1998; 338: 86-93.

[34] Mohrschladt MF, van der Sman-de Beer F, Hofman MK, van der Krabben M, Westendorp RG, Smelt AH. TaqIB polymorphism in CETP gene: the influence on incidence of cardiovascular disease in statin-treated patients with familial hypercholesterolemia. Eur J Hum Genet 2005; 13: 877-882.

[35] Anagnastopoulou K, Kolovou G, Kostakou P, Mihas C, Mikhailidis D, Cokkinos DV. Pharmacogenetic study of cholesteryl ester transfer protein gene and simvastatin treatment in hypercholesterolaemic subjects. Expert Opin Pharmacother 2007; 8: 2459-863.

[36] Winkelmann BR, Hoffmann MM, Nauck M, *et al.* Haplotypes of the cholesteryl ester transfer protein gene predict lipidmodifying response to statin therapy. Pharmacogenomics J 2003; 3: 284-296.

[37] Regieli JJ, Jukema JW, Grobbee DE, *et al.* CETP genotype predicts increased mortality in statin-treated men with proven cardiovascular disease: an adverse pharmacogenetic interaction. Eur Heart J 2008; 29: 2792-2799.

[38] Bengoechea-Alonso MT, Ericsson J. SREBP in signal transduction: cholesterol metabolism and beyond. Curr Opin Cell Biol 2007; 19: 215-222.

[39] Weinhofer I, Forss-Petter S, Zigman M, Berger J. Cholesterol regulates ABCD2 expression. Hum Mol Genet 2002; 11: 2701-2708.

[40] Fiegenbaum M, Silveira FR, Van der Sand CR, *et al.* Determinants of variable response to simvastatin treatment: the role of common variants of SCAP, SREBF-1a and SREBF-2 genes. Pharmacogenomics J 2005; 5: 359-364.

[41] Salek L, Lutucuta S, Ballantyne CM, *et al.* Effects of SREBF-1a and SCAP polymorphisms on plasma levels of lipids, severity, progression and regression of coronary atherosclerosis and response to therapy with fluvastatin. J Mol Med 2002; 80: 737-744.

[42] Fan YM, Laaksonen R, Janatuinen T, *et al.* Effects of pravastatin therapy on serum lipids and coronary reactivity are not associated with SREBP cleavage activating protein polymorphism in healthy young men. Clin Genet 2001; 60: 319-321.

[43] Chen S, Tsybouleva N, Ballantyne CM, *et al.* Effects of PPARα, γ and Δ haplotypes on plasma levels of lipids, severity and progression of coronary atherosclerosis and response to statin therapy in the lipoprotein coronary atherosclerosis study. Pharmacogenetics 2004; 14: 61-71.

[44] Jukema JW, van Boven AJ, Groenmeijer B, *et al.* The Asp9 Asn mutation in the lipoprotein lipase gene is associated with increased progression of coronary atherosclerosis. Circulation 1996; 94: 1913-1918.

[45] Zambon A, Deeb SS, Pauletto P, Crepaldi G, Brunzell JD. Hepatic lipase: a marker for cardiovascular disease risk and response to therapy. Curr Opin Lipidol 2003; 14: 179-189.

[46] Zambon A, Deeb SS, Hokanson JE, *et al.* Common variants in the promoter of the hepatic lipase gene are associated with lower levels of hepatic lipase activity, buoyant LDL, and higher HDL2 cholesterol. Arterioscler Thromb Vasc Biol 1998; 18: 1723-1729.

[47] Kajinami K, Brousseau ME, Ordovas JM, Schaefer, EJ. Interactions between common genetic polymorphisms in ABCG5/G8 and CYP7A1 on LDL-cholesterol-lowering response to atorvastatin. Atherosclerosis 2004; 175: 287-293.

[48] Ledmyr H, McMahon AD, Ehrenborg E, *et al.* The microsomal triglyceride transfer protein gene-493T variant lowers cholesterol but increases the risk of coronary heart disease. Circulation 2004; 109: 2279-2284.

[49] Lutucuta S, Ballantyne CM, Elghannam H, Gotto Jr AM, Marian AJ. Novel polymorphisms in promoter region of atp binding cassette transporter gene and plasma lipids, severity, progression, and regression of coronary atherosclerosis and response to therapy. Circ Res 2001; 88: 969-873.

[50] Bergheanu SC, Van Tol A, dallinga-Thie GM, Dunselman PH, Van der Bom Jg, Jukema JW. Effect of rosuvastatin versus atorvastatin treatment on paraoxonase-1 activity in men with established cardiovascular disease and a low HDL-cholestarol. Curr Med Res Opin 2007; 23: 2235-2240.

[51] Deakin S, Guernier S, James RW. Pharmacogenetic interaction between paraoxonase-1 gene promoter polymorphism C-107T and statin. Pharmacogenetic interaction between paraoxonase -1 gene promoter polymorphism C-107T and statin. Pharmacogenet Genomics 2007; 17: 451-457.

[52] Worz CR, Bottorff M. The role of cytochrome P450-mediated drug-drug interactions in determining the safety of statins. Expert Opin Pharmacother 2001; 2: 1119-1127.

[53] Lee E, Ryan S, Birmingham B, Zalikowski J, March R, Ambrose H, Moore R, Lee C, Chen Y, Schneck D. Rosuvastatin pharmacokinetics and pharmacogenetics in white and Asian subjects residing in the same environment. Clin Pharmacol Ther 2005; 78: 330-341.

[54] Ucar M, Mjornda T, Dahlqvist R. HMG-CoA reductase inhibitors and myotoxicity. Drug Saf 2000; 22: 441-457.

[55] Corsini A, Bellosta S, Baetta R, Fumagalli R, Paoletti R, Bernini F. New insights into the pharmacodynamic and pharmacokinetic properties of statins. Pharmacol Ther 1999; 84: 413-428.

[56] Kajinami K, Brousseau ME, Ordovas JM, Schaefer EJ. CYP3A4 genotypes and plasma lipoprotein levels before and after treatment with atorvastatin in primary hypercholesterolemia. Am J Cardiol 2004; 93: 104-107.

[57] Wang A, Yu BN, Luo CH, *et al.* Ile118Val genetic polymorphism of CYP3A4 and its effects on lipid-lowering efficacy of simvastatin in Chinese hyperlipidemic patients. Eur J Clin Phamacol 2005; 60: 843-848.

[58] Hustert E, Haberl M, Burk O, *et al.* The genetic determinants of the CYP3A5 polymorphism. Pharmacogenetics 2001; 11: 773-779.

[59] Kivistö KT, Niemi M, Schaeffeler E, *et al.* Lipid-lowering response to statins is affected by CYP3A5 polymorphism. Pharmacogenetics 2004; 14: 523-525.

[60] Mulder AB, van Lijf HJ, Bon MA, *et al.* Association of polymorphism in the cytochrome CYP2D6 and the efficacy and tolerability of simvastatin. Clin Pharmacol Ther 2001; 70: 546-551.

[61] Geisel J, Kivisto KT, Griese EU, Eichelbaum M. The efficacy of simvastatin is not influenced by CYP2D6. Clin Pharmacol Ther 2002; 72: 595-596.

[62] Kajinami K, Brousseau ME, Nartsupha C, Ordovas JM, Schaefer EJ ATP binding cassette transporter G5 and G8 genotypes and plasma lipoprotein levels before and after treatment with atorvastatin. J Lipid Res 2004; 45: 653-656.

[63] Nishizato Y, Ieiri I, Suzuki H, *et al.* Polymorphisms of OATP-C (SLC21A6) and OAT3 (SLC22A8) genes: consequences for pravastatin pharmaco-kinetics. Clin Pharmacol Ther 2003; 73: 554-565.

[64] Mwinyi J, Johne A, Bauer S, Roots I, Gerloff T. Evidence for inverse effects of OATP-C (SLC21A6) 5 and 1b haplotypes on pravastatin kinetics. Clin Pharmacol Ther 2004; 75: 415-421.

[65] Niemi M, Schaeffeler E, Lang T, Fromm MF, Neuvonen M, Kyrklund C, Backman JT, Kerb R, Schwab M, Neuvonen PJ, Eichelbaum M, Kivistö KT.High plasma pravastatin concentrations are associated with

single nucleotide polymorphisms and haplotypes of organic anion transporting polypeptide-C (OATP-C, SLCO1B1). Pharmacogenetics. 2004; 14: 429-440.
[66] Pasanen MK, Neuvonen M, Neuvonen P, *et al.* SLCO1B1 polymorphism markedly affects the pharmacokinetics of simvastatin acid. Pharmacogenet Genomics 2006; 16: 873-879.
[67] Vasudevan AR, Hamirani YS, Jones PH. Safety of statins: effects on muscle and the liver. Cleve Clin J Med 2005; 72: 990-993.
[68] Thompson PD, Clarkson P, Karas RH. Statin-associated myopathy. JAMA 2003; 289: 1681-1690.
[69] Sewright Ka, Clarkson PM, Thompson PD. Statin myopathy: incidence, risk factors and pathophysiology.Curr Atherosclr rep 2007; 9: 389-396
[70] Baer AN, Wortmann RL. Myotoxicity associated with lipid-lowering drugs. Curr Opin Rheumatol 2007; 19: 67-73.
[71] Wilke RA, Moore JH, Burmester JK. Relative impact of CYP3A genotype and concomitant medication on the severity of atorvastatin-induced muscle damage. Pharmacogenet Genomics 2005; 15: 415-421.
[72] Frudakis TN, Thomas MJ, Ginjupalli SN, Handelin B, Gomez HJ. CYP2D6*4 polymorphism is associated with statin-induced muscle effects. Pharmacogenetic Genomics 2007; 17: 695-707.
[73] Ruano G, Thompson PD, Windemuth A, *et al.* Physiogenomic analysis links serum creatine kinase activities during statin therapy to vascular smooth muscle homeostasis. Pharmacogenomics 2005; 6: 865-872.
[74] Fiegenbaum M, da Silveira FR, Van der Sand CR, *et al.* The role of common variants of ABCB1, CYP3A4, and CYP3A5 genes in lipid-lowering efficacy and safety of simvastatin treatment. Clin Pharmacol Ther 2005; 78: 551-558.
[75] Dorajo R, Pereira BP, Yu Z, Gopalakrishnakone P, Leong CC, Wee A. Lee E. Role of multi-drug resistance-associated protein -1 transporter in statin-induced myopathy. Life Sci 2008; 82: 823-830.
[76] Vladutiu GD. Genetic predisposition to statin myopathy. Curr Opin Rheumatol 2008; 20: 648-655.
[77] The SEARCH Collaborative Group. SLCO1B1 Variants and Statin-Induced Myopathy - A Genomewide Study. N Engl J Med 2008;359:789-799
[78] Calabrò P, Yeh ETH. The pleiotropic effects of statins. Curr Opin Cardiol 2005; 20: 541-546.
[79] Nagassaki S, Sertorio JT, Metzger IF, Bem AF, Rocha JB, Tanus-Santos JE. eNOS gene T-786C polymorphism modulates atorvastatin-induced increase in blood nitrite. Free Radic Biol Med 2006; 41: 1044-1049.
[80] Abe K, Nakayama M, Yoshimura M, *et al.* Increase in the transcriptional activity of the endothelial nitric oxide synthase gene with fluvastatin: a relation with the -786T>C polymorphism. Pharmacogenet Genomics 2005; 15: 329-336.
[81] Puccetti L, Pasqui AL, Bruni F, *et al.* Lectin-like oxidized-LDL receptor-1 (LOX-1) polymorphisms influence cardiovascular events rate during statin treatment. Int J Cardiol 2007; 119: 41-47.
[82] Damas JK, Puccetti L, Aukrust P. Early anti-thrombotic and anti-inflammatory actions of statins and fibrates-time for adjuvant therapy in acute coronary syndromes? Thromb Haemost 2005; 94: 1-3.
[83] Puccetti L, Pasqui AL, Pastorelli M, *et al.* 3'UTR/T polymorphism of lectin-like oxidized low-density lipoprotein receptor-1 (LOX-1) is associated with modified anti-platelet activity of atorvastatin in hypercholesterolemic subjects. Atherosclerosis 2005; 183: 322-328.
[84] Puccetti L, Bruni F, Pasqui AL, Pastorelli M, Ciani F, Palazzuoli A, Acampa M, Auteri A. Genetic influence in antithrombotic actions of atorvastatin in hypercholesterolaemia. Eur J Clin Invest 2008; 38: 11-16.
[85] Bray PF, Cannon CP, Goldschmidt-Clermont P, *et al.* The platelet Pl(A2) and angiotensin-converting enzyme (ACE) D allele polymorphisms and the risk of recurrent events after acute myocardial infarction. Am J Cardiol 2001; 88: 347-352.
[86] Borghi C, Dormi A, Veronesi M, Immordino V, Ambrosioni E. Use of lipid-lowering drugs and blood pressure control in patients with arterial hypertension. J Clin Hypertens (Greenwich) 2002; 4: 277-285.
[87] Marian AJ, Safavi F, Ferlic L, *et al.* Interactions between angiotensin-I converting enzyme insertion/deletion polymorphism and response of plasma lipids and coronary atherosclerosis to treatment with fluvastatin: the lipoprotein and coronary atherosclerosis study. J Am Coll Cardiol 2000; 35: 89-95.
[88] Maintland-van der Zee AH, Boerwinkle E, Arnett DK, *et al.* Absence of an interaction between the angiotensin-converting enzyme insertion-deletion polymorphism and pravastatin on cardiovascular disease in high-risk hypertensive patients: The Genetics of Hypertension-Associated Treatment (GenHAT) study. Am Heart J 2007; 153: 54-58.
[89] Souza-Costa eDC, Sandrim VC, Lopes LF et al. Anti-inflammatory effects of atorvastatin: modulation by the T-876C polymorphism in the endothelial nitric oxide synthase gene. Atherosclerosis 2007; 193: 438-444.
[90] Puccetti L, Capati E, Auteri A. Genetic modulation of anti-inflammatory effects of atorvastatin; probably a multi-gene condition. Atherosclerosis 2008; 197: 469-470.
[91] Mangravite LM, Krauss RM. Pharmacogenomics of statin response. Curr Opin Lipidol 2007; 18: 409-414.

[92] Knouff CW, Lim N, Song K, *et al*. Pharmacological effects of lipid-lowering drugs recapitulate with a larger amplitude the phenotype effects of common variants within their target genes. Pharmacogenet Genomics 2008; 18: 1051-1057.

HDL Elevation and Lipid Lowering Therapy: Current Scenario and Future Perspectives

Mahesh T. Chhabria*, Bhanubhai N. Suhagia and Pathik S. Brahmkshatriya

Department of Pharmaceutical Chemistry and Quality Assurance, L M College of Pharmacy, Navrangpura, Ahmedabad – 380 009, Gujarat, India

Abstract: High density lipoprotein (HDL) has proven its role in reverse cholesterol transport and cellular cholesterol efflux thus acting as a protective factor against atherogenic cardiovascular diseases. The article focuses primarily on structure and function of genes influencing HDL metabolism. Various novel targets involve liver X receptor, retinoid X receptor and peroxisome proliferators activated receptor agonists and apoA-I mimetics. New molecules targeting these receptors are described. Phospholipid transfer protein and scavenger receptor B1 are also attractive targets in HDL metabolism. ATP-Binding Cassette transporter A1 and several lipases also play a crucial role in HDL metabolism and are very useful target for atherogenic dyslipidemia. Several cholesterol ester transfer protein inhibitors have shown great promise as possible drug candidates of future. Notably, JTT-705 (Japan Tobacco, Roche) is of great interest in spite of withdrawal of torcetrapib. Considering modest effect of currently available therapeutic options on HDL, these novel HDL elevating targets are doubtlessly the target for future atherosclerotic intervention.

Keywords: HDL elevation, coronary artery disease, ATP-binding cassette transporter A1, liver X receptor, retinoid X receptor, peroxisome proliferators activated receptor, phospholipids transfer protein, scavenger receptor B1, lipoprotein lipase, hepatic lipase, endothelial lipase, cholesteryl ester transfer protein, apolipoprotein A-I.

INTRODUCTION

It is well established that a mere control of cholesterol levels in the blood is inadequate for even an approximate assessment of lipid alterations, 60–70% of the cardiovascular events continue to manifest despite the lipid-lowering therapy and surprisingly it is observed that atherosclerosis can affect even individuals whose cholesterol values are within the normal range [1]. Moreover, studies suggest that the most frequent lipid alteration in patients with coronary artery disease (CAD) is not hypercholesterolemia but low HDL values. It has been observed that more than 40% of patients that survived after a myocardial infarction have low HDL plasma concentrations as their most relevant cardiovascular risk factor [2]. Four different mechanisms suggesting importance of HDL are: (i) HDL removes cholesterol from the artery wall *via* a process called reverse cholesterol transport (RCT) [3];

*Corresponding author: Tel: 91-79-26302746; Fax: 91-79-26304865; E-mail: mahesh.chhabria@rediffmail.com

(ii) HDL is an inverse marker for the atherogenic triglyceride rich lipoproteins [4]; (iii) HDL acts as a sink for oxidized lipid [5] (iv) HDL interacts with atherogenic triglyceride-rich lipoprotein remnants to decrease their atherogenicity and/or to enhance their rate of clearance [6].

The association between low levels of HDL-cholesterol (HDL-C) and an increased risk for cardiovascular disease has been well established through epidemiological and clinical studies [7]. Although low HDL levels may result from factors such as diabetes, obesity, cigarette smoking, physical inactivity, carbohydrate-rich diets or certain drugs (β-blockers, corticosteroids, anabolic steroids, androgenic progestins) [8], the phenotype of low HDL concentrations can be produced by the mutation of genes involved in lipid metabolism (ABCA1, CETP, ApoA-I, etc.) [9]. The term *hypoalphalipoproteinemia* is still employed to identify the condition characterized by extremely low HDL concentrations, associated with reduced or normal low density lipoprotein (LDL) levels [10,11].

It is well established that dietary management of hyperlipidemia is a safer and effective alternative to blockbuster drugs. Omega-3 fatty acids (4 g per day) reduced triglyceride levels by 30% [12,13]. However, at this dosage, omega-3 elevated LDL-C by 5% to 10% and had no effect on the HDL-C [13]. Traditional HDL elevating agents, niacin and fibric acid derivatives like fenofibrate significantly increased plasma HDL-C and decreased plasma triglyceride concentrations [14,15]. Also, studies have demonstrated significant role of physical exercise in management of hyperlipidemia and CAD. However, all the above mentioned means to manage hyperlipidemia are not therapeutically significant. The present review focuses on the current scenario of HDL elevation and lipid lowering therapy. Major targets for HDL elevation and medicinal agents in preclinical and clinical trials acting on the said targets are also reviewed.

ABCA1

ATP-Binding Cassette transporters are the largest membrane transporter superfamily, with members in all phyla [16]. Seven subclasses labeled ABCA through ABCG belong to this family. ABCA1 mediates the transport of cholesterol, phospholipids, and other lipophilic molecules across cellular membranes, where they are removed from cells by lipid-poor HDL apolipoproteins [17]. ABCA1 has been shown to regulate cholesterol movement from the periphery to the liver, which is responsible for facilitating HDL formation by adding phospholipids and cholesterol to free apoA-I [18,19]. ABCA1 appears to target specific membrane domains for lipid secretion. These are regions that are sensitive to accumulation of cholesterol and other lipophilic compounds. This same source of cholesterol feeds into intracellular compartments that are the preferred substrate for enzyme responsible for esterification, i.e. acyl CoA: cholesterol acyltransferase (ACAT) [20,21]. Thus, ABCA1 helps remove cholesterol that would otherwise accumulate as cytosolic cholesteryl ester lipid droplets. ABCA1 has been shown to promote phospholipids efflux from cells even when membranes are depleted of cholesterol [22,23], consistent with phospholipids being the primary substrate for ABCA1. Studies have demonstrated function of ABCA1 as cholesterol efflux regulatory protein [23]. One study revealed that ABCA1 is the major protein mediating the efflux of cellular cholesterol to lipid-free apoproteins from murine macrophages, and that it is up-regulated by increasing cellular cAMP levels [24]. A recent review focusing on the role of ABC transporter in cholesterol efflux and the complications associated with the altered levels has recently been published [25].

Mutations in ABCA1 can cause an autosomal recessive genetic transfer disorder, characterized by very low levels of plasma HDL and deposition of sterols in tissue macrophages, called as Tangier disease [26]. It has proved that the defective Tangier disease gene is ABCA1 [27-30]. Moreover, over 70 mutations in ABCA1 have been identified in subjects with very low plasma HDL levels [31-33].

Animal studies have provided additional evidence that ABCA1 is a major determinant of plasma HDL levels. The only naturally occurring animal model of Tangier disease is the Wisconsin Hypoalpha Mutant (WHAM) chicken. Reports show that ABCA1 in these chickens has a missense mutation near the NH_2 terminus that produces a defective protein [34]. Targeted disruption of the ABCA1 gene in mice has been shown to produce a phenotype similar to that of human Tangier disease [35-37], along with an HDL deficiency and accumulation of sterols in some tissues. Conversely, overexperessing ABCA1 in mice have shown to raise HDL levels significantly [38-40]. Reports imply that the liver ABCA1 pathway in mice is responsible for generating most of the plasma HDL and selective overexpression of ABCA1 in the liver using adenovirus transgenes markedly raises plasma HDL levels [39]. Also, targeted disruption of liver ABCA1 in chow-fed mice dropped plasma HDL levels upto 80% [41]. These observations suggest that the major cause of the HDL deficiency in Tangier patients and ABCA1 knockout mice is an impaired liver ABCA1 pathway.

Tangier disease homozygotes over the age of 30 have a sixfold higher than normal incidence of CAD in both the sexes [42]. Evidences suggest strong link between dysfunctional ABCA1 mutations and greater intima-media thickness of the carotid arteries [43]. Moreover, polymorphisms in ABCA1 are strongly linked with either increased or decreased CVD [33]. Differential expression of ABCA1 also has been reported in mice liver and in nonhepatic tissues through alternate promoters, resulting in increased cholesterol efflux from macrophages [44]. Overexpression of human ABCA1 in transgenic C57B1/6 mice significantly reduced diet-induced atherosclerosis, suggesting possible atherorotective effects of ABCA1 [45]. A number of data have suggested that an increased expression of ABCA1 in macrophages or other tissues can activate movement of cholesterol to HDL and thus retard development of atherosclerosis [46,47]. Moreover, selective adenovirus-mediated overexpression of ABCA1 gene in the liver resulted in a remarkable increase in plasma HDL-C level in conjunction with an up-regulation of LDL receptor, HMG Co-A reductase, and LDL receptor-related protein (LRP) genes involved in cellular cholesterol homeostasis [48].

Well proven atheroprotective activity of ABCA1 signifies this transporter as an attractive new therapeutic target for treating CVDs [49]. Such a target would prevent foam-cell atherosclerotic lesion formation along with raised plasma HDL levels. Most of the attention has been drawn towards the following three targets:

LXR Agonists

The liver X receptor (LXR) α and β isoforms [50] are members of type II nuclear receptor family that includes peroxisome proliferators activated receptor (PPAR), farnesoid X receptor (FXR) and pregnane X receptor (PXR) [51-55]. LXRα is expressed primarily in liver, adipose tissue, intestine, and macrophages, whereas LXRβ is expressed in many cell types. A physiological requirement for LXRs in the maintenance of cholesterol homeostasis is exemplified by the finding that LXRα-null mice fed with a high-cholesterol diet developed massive hepatic accumulation of cholesterol, whereas wild-type mice are highly resistant to cholesterol feeding [56]. Consistent with this, induction of other proteins involved in several steps along with reverse cholesterol transport pathway, viz. *ABCG1* [57], which mediates cholesterol efflux to HDL particles [58]; *apoE* [59], which promotes cholesterol efflux from macrophages by both ABCA1-dependent and -independent mechanisms [60]; and liver and intestinal *ABCG5* and *ABCG8* [61], which promote excretion of liver and dietary cholesterol into the bile, is also an added advantage.

Studies of *Lxra*$^{-/-}$ and *Lxrb*$^{-/-}$ mice have shown that the hepatic lipogenic activity of LXRs is predominantly under the control of LXR-α, which suggests that selective LXR-β agonists could have substantial therapeutic benefit without the undesirable side effects associated with LXR-α activation [62,63]. A recent series of studies has begun to address the issue of selective LXR-β activation to ameliorate atherosclerosis and the closely related question of whether selective inactivation of LXR-α exacerbates atherosclerosis in susceptible mice [64]. Interestingly, ageing *Apoe*$^{-/-}$*Lxra*$^{-/-}$ mice accumulated significantly more lipids in peripheral tissues and developed atherosclerosis faster than *Apoe*$^{-/-}$ mice. These data suggest that LXR-α is essential for optimal reverse cholesterol transport.

Oxidized derivatives of cholesterol such as 24(S),25-epoxycholesterol, 22(*S*)-hydroxycholesterol and 24(*S*)-hydroxycholesterol have been shown to act as activators of LXRs at physiologically relevant concentrations [65-70]. Thus LXR agonists have the potential for activating multiple processes that coordinate excretion of excess cholesterol from the body. Most of therapeutic approaches of ABCA1 induction have focused on LXR agonists that induce ABCA1 transcription due to the robust induction of ABCA1 by sterols.

In addition, LXRs directly and indirectly regulate genes involved in fatty acid metabolism, including sterol response element binding protein-1c (SREBP-1c), fatty acid synthase, acyl-CoA carboxylase and stearoyl-CoA desaturase [71] and regulate genes that control the secretion and metabolism of triglyceriderich lipoproteins, including LPL [72], CETP, PLTP [73], and the apolipoprotsein E/C-I/C-IV/C-II gene cluster [74]. The overall impact of administration of LXR agonists to mice is to stimulate fatty acid biosynthesis in liver and cause an increase in circulating triglyceride levels, at least in part as a consequence of inducing the expression and activity of SREBP-1c [71,75]. Also, stearoyl-CoA desaturase has been shown to convert saturated fatty acids to unsaturated fatty acids that destabilize ABCA1 protein [76]. In consistent with the proven antiatherogenic role of LXRs, LXR agonists may be of therapeutic utility in humans if undesirable effects on circulating triglyceride levels can be reduced or eliminated through the development of selective modulators [75].

Two distinct non-steroidal LXR ligands GW3965 (**1**) [77] and TO901317 (**2**) [75] have been developed which are shown to increase plasma HDL levels and reduce or even reverse atherosclerotic processes in mouse models.

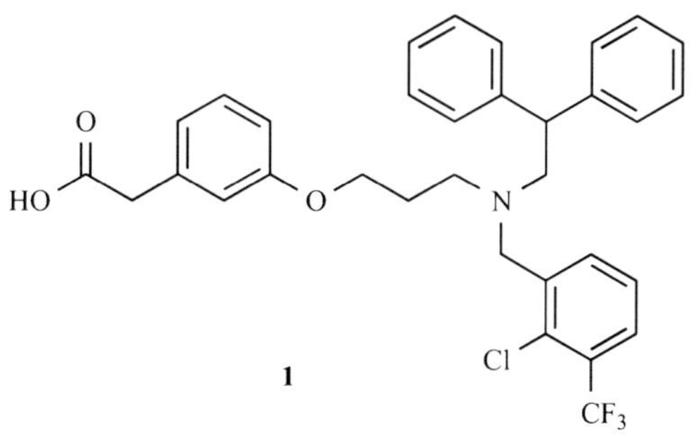

1

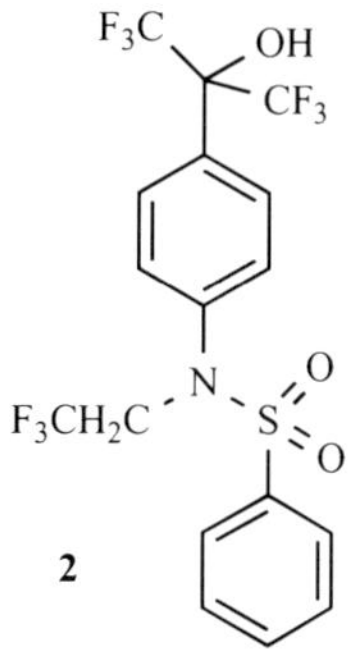

2

Recently, identification and optimization of some novel phenyl acetic acid substituted quinolines as potent LXR agonists were reported [78]. The series was further explored and optimized to get some more derivatives by the same group, from which two compounds **3** and **4** displayed good binding affinity for LXRβ and LXRα with IC_{50} values of 5.0 and 21.0 nM for **3** and 1.4 and 5.0 nM for **4**, for LXRβ and LXRα, respectively. The compounds also had desirable pharmacokinetic properties in mice and displayed *in vivo* efficacy in a 12-week Apo E knockout mouse lesion model [79].

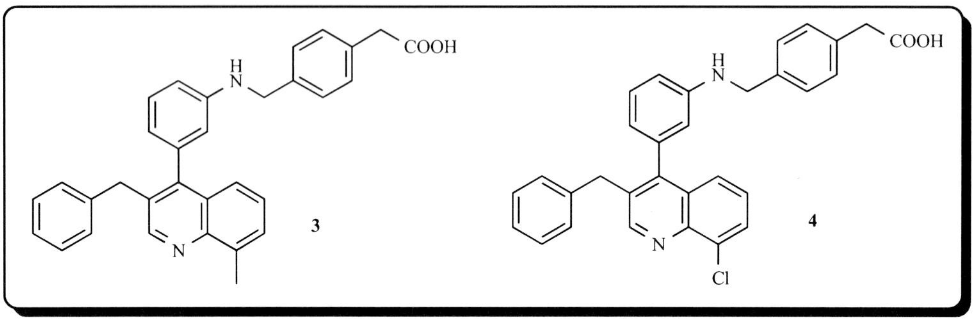

AstraZeneca reported a series of pyrrole-2,5-dithione derivatives as LXR modulators [80], where compounds **5** and **6** displayed EC_{50} of 0.09 and 0.14 μmol/l in coactivator recruitment assays, respectively.

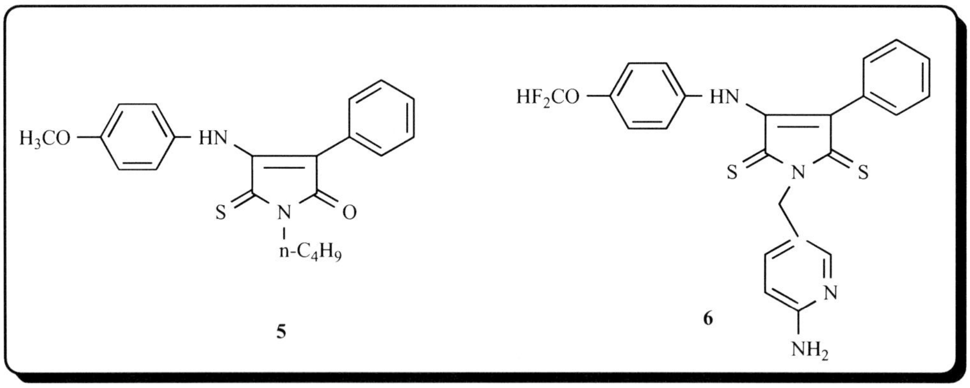

Merck invented novel LXR ligands where compounds **7** and **8** were found to be potent than the others [81]. Very good binding with EC_{50} between 0.001 μM to 1.5 μM along with % efficacy between 20% and 150% in transcriptional assay for LXRβ was found in a new series of LXR modulators [82].

Recently, novel indolyl derivatives were invented as LXR modulators with compounds showing EC_{50} values in range of 0.1 nM to 1 μM in either radioligand binding assay or luciferase transcriptional reporter gene assay [83].

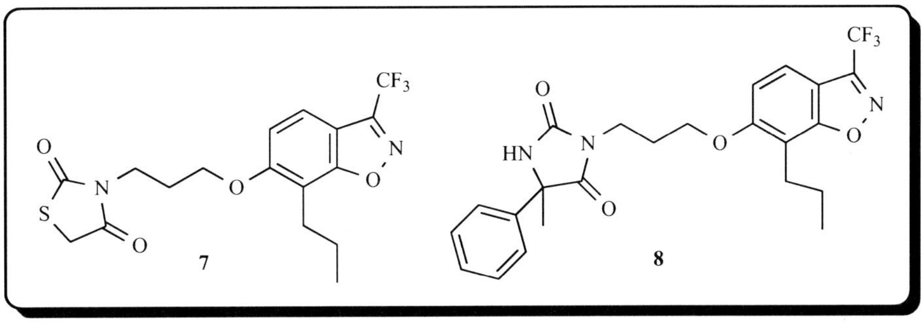

RXR Agonists

Retinoid X receptor (RXR) is considered "promiscuous" as it forms heterodimers with several other family members of nuclear receptors that can be further classified as permissive or nonpermissive binding partners. Heterodimers formed by RXR and permissive binding partners (PPARs, LXR, and FXR) can be activated by RXR specific ligands or by ligands specific for the binding partner. It has been shown that heterodimers formed by RXR and nonpermissive partners (vitamin D and thyroid hormone receptors) can only be activated by ligands specific for the partner, but not by ligands specific for RXR [84].

Briefly, there are 3 RXR isotypes: RXRα, RXRβ, and RXRγ. Each isotype is encoded by a distinct gene, and each gene is capable of generating at least 2 distinct transcripts due to alternative promoter utilization and alternative splicing. The isotypes also exhibit different patterns of tissue specific expression. RXRα is expressed in liver, kidney, spleen, placenta, and the epidermis; RXRβ is expressed ubiquitously; and RXRγ is expressed in cardiac muscles and skeletal muscles, the anterior pituitary, and to a lesser extent in brain. Importantly, the pattern of tissue-specific expression varies widely during development. The homology of the isotypes suggests that these receptors regulate common target sequences and respond to common ligands [85-87].

RXR has been shown to have diverse physiological functions using RXR knockout (KO) mouse models [85,86]. Loss of RXRα results in much more severe phenotype than the loss of either RXRβ or RXRγ. Loss of RXRα function in adipose tissue has been shown to result in altered preadipocyte differentiation and resistance to obesity, though this is thought to be attributable to the absence of functional RXRα/PPARγ heterodimers in adipose tissue. Loss of RXR*α* in the liver perturbs multiple metabolic pathways mediated by LXR*α*, PPAR*α*, CAR*β*, PXR, and FXR. Interestingly, many, but not all, of the defects in lipid metabolism in liver-specific $RXR\alpha^{-/-}$ mice are similar to those in $LXR^{-/-}$ mice, suggesting that RXR*α*:LXR plays an important role in hepatic lipid metabolism [85,86].

Agonists for RXR also have shown to stimulate ABCA1 transcription in cultured cells [88,89]. Significant decrease in atherosclerotic lesions was seen by administration of an LXR agonist to atherosclerotic mice [90].

Because RXR has been shown to play a role in diverse physiological processes including cell proliferation, differentiation, apoptosis and metabolism, RXR isotypes have been referred to as "master regulators" [85,86]. Therefore, compounds that alter the activity of RXR also have the potential to alter multiple physiological and metabolic pathways, with the potential of both beneficial as well as harmful effects. Indeed, in animal models of insulin resistance and diabetes, these modulators have been shown to have beneficial glucose lowering, insulin-sensitizing, and antiobesity effects, while at the same time raising TG levels and suppressing the thyroid hormone axis. These side effects have greatly limited the development of these compounds as therapeutic agents mainly for the treatment of diabetes and metabolic syndrome. It was reported, however, that RXR activators can induce ABCA1 without affecting other LXR-targeted genes [91], raising the possibility of selective drug therapy through the RXR system.

Smithkline Beecham Co. recently filed patent claiming novel fused heterocycles as selective RXRα, RXRβ or RXRγ modulators [92]. Johnson & Johnson filed a patent application featuring novel class of dihydro-[1H]-quinolin-2-one as potential dyslipidemic and hypocholesterolemic agent acting through RXR modulation where compound **9** was shown to be most potent with EC_{50} 1 nM for RXR co-transfection [93].

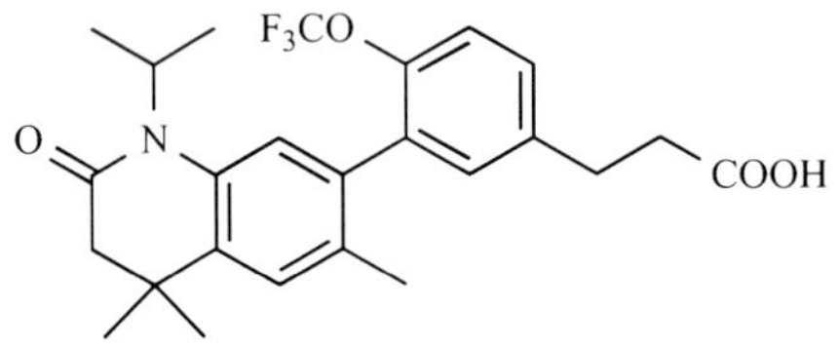

9

Takeda also filed a patent claiming novel 5-membered N-heterocyclic hypoglycemic and hypolipidemic compounds with EC_{50} in the range of 0.22 to 320 nM for PPARγ-RXRα heterodimer ligand activity with compounds **10** and **11** being the preferred compounds [94].

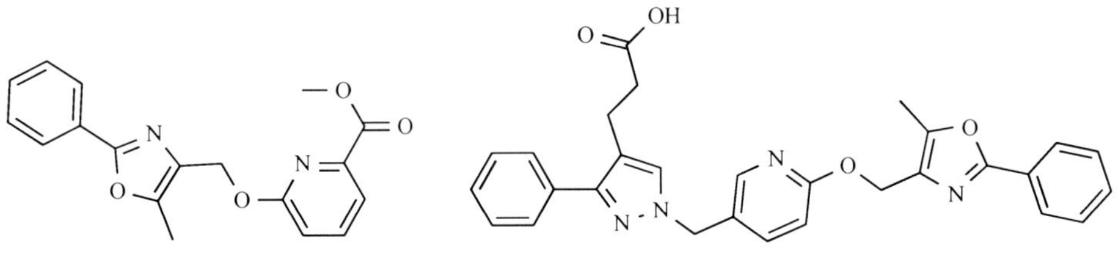

10 **11**

PPAR Agonists

PPARα (NR1C1), PPAR β/δ (NR1C2), and PPARγ (NR1C3) belong to the PPAR subfamily of nuclear receptors. The cloning of PPARα cDNAs proved PPARα as the molecular target of fibrates, such as gemfibrozil, drugs widely used in the treatment of hypertriglyceridemia [95,96].

Several studies have shown that activation of PPARα increase apoA-I and apoA-II and decrease apoC-III, an inhibitor of LPL [97,98]. These effects would tend to increase HDL levels and decrease triglyceride levels and are thought to contribute to the beneficial effects of fibrates on lipoprotein levels in hypertriglyceridemic patients. PPARα agonists have also been shown to regulate cholesterol homeostasis in cultured macrophages. Activation of PPARα can lead to the induction of expression of LXRα, which can then stimulate ABCA1 expression and promote efflux of cholesterol to apoA-I [99]. PPARα can inhibit esterification of free cholesterol by ACAT-1 and increase the efflux of free cholesterol by increasing the expression of scavenger receptor class B type 1 [100,101].

Also, the effects of PPARα agonists on carbohydrate and lipid metabolism would be expected to result in protection against the development of atherosclerosis. Consistent with this, a clinical trial studying effects of the PPARα agonist gemfibrozil in men with a history of CHD and low HDL levels demonstrated a significant decrease in the incidence of fatal and nonfatal myocardial infarction [102].

Surprisingly, PPARα$^{-/-}$/apoE$^{-/-}$ mice exhibited less atherosclerosis than control apoE$^{-/-}$ mice, suggesting a possible atherogenic role of PPARα [103]. In another study of apoE$^{-/-}$ mice, treatment with ciprofibrate worsened diet-induced hyperlipidemia and increased atherosclerosis [104]. In these studies, ciprofibrate treatment was associated with an increase in apoB-48-containing lipoproteins, demonstrating an effect of PPARα on editing of the apoB mRNA. Other studies have found that PPARα agonists are antiatherogenic. In one study, fenofibrate had minimal antiatherogenic effects in apoE$^{-/-}$ mice [90,105] but exerted a more pronounced effect in apoE$^{-/-}$ mice carrying a fenofibrate-inducible human apoA-I transgene. Other studies also demonstrated that activation of PPARα by a highly specific and potent agonist (GW7647, **12**) inhibited atherosclerosis by nearly 50% throughout the aortas of hyperlipidemic LDLR$^{-/-}$ mice [106].

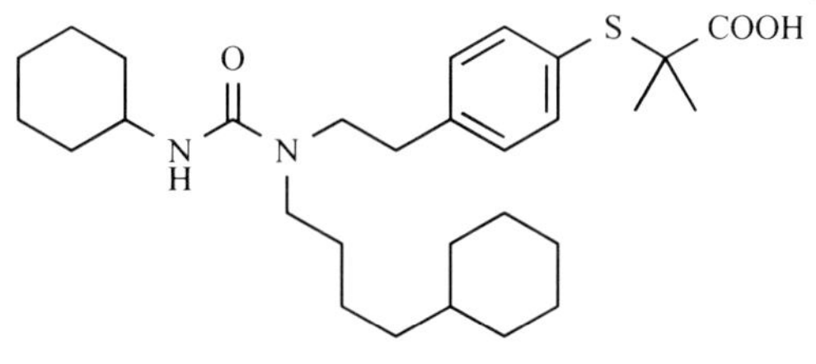

12

The nuclear receptor PPARγ regulates transcription of multiple genes involved in cell differentiation and lipid metabolism. Two isoforms of PPARγ have been identified and are derived from the same gene by alternative promoter usage [107,108]. PPARγ promotes adipocyte differentiation *in vitro* and has been shown to be crucial for the development of adipose tissue *in vivo* [109-112]. PPARγ plays a critical role in glucose homeostasis and is the molecular target of thiazolidinediones, a class of drugs developed for treating insulin resistance and type 2 diabetes [113]. A patent has been filed claiming isolation, cloning and identification of the promoters and other regulatory elements of the PPARγ gene [114].

Cholesterol loading of macrophages induces PPARγ [115], which has several effects on cholesterol trafficking. PPARγ directly stimulates transcription of a scavenger receptor (CD36) that promotes uptake of oxidized lipoproteins [116]. PPARγ also stimulates cholesterol efflux from cells by increasing ABCA1 expression, an effect that is secondary to inducing LXRα [99,117]. A comprehensive review that highlights role of PPARδ in metabolic disease has been recently published [118]. In mice, PPARγ activators retard atherosclerosis [117,119], suggesting that they have a favorable effect on macrophage cholesterol balance. Large-scale clinical trials examining the effects of PPARγ agonists on cardiovascular complications are yet to be explored. Two small clinical studies observed a decrease in carotid intimal thickening by the treatment of diabetic patients with thiazolidinediones

[120,121]. Studies of the effects of PPARγ agonists in hypercholesterolemic male mice have consistently demonstrated anti-atherogenic effects despite an increased expression of CD36 in atherosclerotic lesions [119,122,123]. Thus, PPARγ activators have the potential of both improving insulin sensitivity and reducing the atherosclerosis that is often associated with diabetes.

Eli Lilly recently filed a patent claiming novel heterocycles as potential PPAR modulators. IC_{50} of compounds were typically in range of 1 nM to 1000 nM for either PPAR alpha, gamma or delta, preferably below about 50 nM for PPARδ and below 500 nM for PPARγ [124]. Also, phenoxyether derivatives were also patented as PPAR modulators by Eli Lilly [125] where upto 50% mean reduction in TG was observed.

PHOSPHOLIPIDS TRANSFER PROTEIN (PLTP)

Phospholipids are a major and essential lipid component of HDL. HDL phospholipid composition is an important factor determining cholesterol efflux capacity from cells to human serum. The regulatory role of PLTP is achieved via its two main functions, phospholipid transfer activity [126,127] and the capability to modulate HDL size and composition in a process called HDL conversion [128-130]. In the process of reverse cholesterol transport (RCT), a subpopulation of HDL, called preβ-HDL, has been shown to act as efficient acceptors in the cholesterol efflux process at the plasma membrane of peripheral cells [131]. PLTP is capable of generating preβ-HDL through HDL conversion, and on the other hand, it has a major role in maintaining the HDL levels in the circulation due to its ability to transport surface remnants after lipolysis of triglyceride-rich lipoproteins. Thus, PLTP is likely to play an important role in atherosclerotic prevention [132-134].

PLTP displays sequence homology to three other proteins: CETP, lipopolysaccharide binding protein (LBP) and bactericidal permeability increasing protein (BPI); these proteins together comprise the LPS-binding: lipid transfer protein family [135]. The crystal structure of PLTP is still unsolved. However, based on the known structure of one of the members of the LPS-binding:lipid transfer protein family BPI [136], a molecular model of PLTP was constructed [137]. Cloning of the PLTP cDNA revealed that the sequence contains four cysteine residues and six potential N-glycosylation sites [135]. Using cell-culture studies and site-directed mutagenesis, the authors and others demonstrated that the cysteine residues 146 and 185 form a disulphide bridge in PLTP which is essential for the correct folding and secretion of the protein [137-139].

PLTP is a non-specific lipid transfer protein. Several studies have indicated that PLTP is capable of transferring all common phospholipid species [127,140,141]. Besides phospholipids, diacylglycerol, a significant lipid constituent of HDL particles, is also transferred efficiently [127]. The PLTP KO mouse model best illustrates the importance of PLTP-mediated phospholipid transfer *in vivo*. The plasma of homozygous PLTP KO-mice showed total absence of ability to transfer various phospholipid species in an *in vitro* assay [134]. In order to investigate if CETP can compensate for PLTP deficiency *in vivo*, the PLTP KO-mice were bred with human CETP transgenic mice [142]. Interestingly, PL transfer activity (measured both *in vitro* and *in vivo*) in PLTP KO-mice carrying a human CETP gene was similar to that of PLTP KO-mice alone, which strongly suggests that the plasma PL transfer activity *in vivo* is mainly due to PLTP. Consistent with the information obtained from the mouse model, PLTP appears to account for most of the phospholipid transfer in human plasma. When the majority (85–96%) of PLTP in plasma was removed by immunoprecipitation with anti-PLTP antibodies, 50–70% of PL transfer between

VLDL:LDL and HDL was abolished [143]. The remaining phospholipid transfer activity in plasma is suggested to be due to CETP [144], and possibly to other factors, such as LBP and CD14 [145]. In contrast to the above mentioned studies, results from several other studies are interesting [146,147]. One study has actually shown that macrophage PLTP is a significant contributor to plasma PLTP activity and deficiency of PLTP in macrophages leads to lowered atherosclerotic lesion development in low-density lipoprotein receptor KO mice on Western-type diet [148].

HDL Conversion by PLTP

Human plasma PLTP is able to convert *in vitro* HDL3 particles into larger particles with a concomitant release of lipid-poor apoA-I [129,130]. The physiological significance of this process was suggested by a study wherein plasma incubated with purified PLTP showed enhanced production of preβ-HDL and an increased capacity to accept cellular cholesterol [132]. Pig and mouse PLTP proteins also show HDL conversion activity [149,150]. Furthermore, PLTP was demonstrated to mediate conversion of HDL2 particles with a concomitant release of lipid-poor apoA-I [151] and to transform reconstituted discoidal HDL particles into vesicular structures [152]. The *in vivo* relevance of PLTP-mediated HDL conversion is evident in both recombinant adenovirus-infected and transgenic mouse models of PLTP [133,153-157]. High overexpression of PLTP either with adenovirus (4–40-fold PL transfer activity compared to controls) or by a transgene (2.5–4.5-fold activity) resulted in a significant decrease in HDL levels [133,153,154]. Increased capacity of the plasma of mice overexpressing PLTP to produce preβ-HDL is demonstrated in several studies [133,153]. Furthermore, in mice expressing both human PLTP and apoA-I, generation of large buoyant HDL particles was observed [154].

In contrast to findings made in high-expressing animals, a more modest increase in PLTP activity in the human apoA-I transgenic background (47% increase in PLTP activity compared to controls) resulted in a parallel increase in HDL lipid and apoA-I levels [156]. Importantly, a major increase of apoA-I in preβ-HDL (56% increase compared to controls) was also observed [156]. Even though no increase in PLTP activity was observed in one of the transgenic PLTP strains, the lipoprotein pattern of the mice showed an increased HDL:non- HDL cholesterol ratio [155]. Thus, it is likely that a mild increase in PLTP levels leads to elevation of HDL, whereas marked overexpression of PLTP decreases plasma HDL level.

SCAVENGER RECEPTOR B1

Scavenger receptors (SRs) are defined as cell surface membrane proteins that bind chemically modified lipoproteins, such as acetylated LDL and oxidized LDL, and often many other types of ligands [158-160]. In 1996, SR-BI, a member of the CD36 protein superfamily [161], was reported as the first molecularly well-defined and functionally active cell-surface HDL receptor [162]. SR-BI plays an important role in mediating selective uptake of HDL cholesterol by hepatocytes and steroidogenic cells [163]. Hepatic overexpression of SR-BI in mice results in markedly reduced HDL cholesterol levels [164]. The absence of SR-BI in KO mice dramatically accelerates the onset of atherosclerosis [165,166], whereas atherosclerosis is suppressed by hepatic overexpression of SR-BI [167-169]. Also, mice with homozygous null mutations in the SR-BI gene [170] or those bearing an insertion in the promoter region of the SR-BI gene, which results in about 50% of normal hepatic SR-BI expression [171], exhibit increased plasma HDL cholesterol levels.

In addition to HDL binding, SR-BI has also been shown to interact with LDL [161, 172], VLDL [172] and modified LDL [152], suggesting a multilipoprotein-binding activity. The cloning [173] and further characterization [172,174] of the human homologue of SR-BI has proved that human SR-BI is also an active HDL receptor in cultured cells.

Additional studies correlating importance of SR-BI in HDL metabolism have been reported [175, 176]. SR-BI is most abundant in the liver and steroidogenic tissues – the main sites of selective lipid uptake from HDL *in vivo*. SR-BI is also found in the brush border membrane of the small intestine, where it might mediate absorption of dietary cholesterol [177]. Also, SR-BI expression is coordinately regulated in steroidogenic cells in response to trophic hormones, which modulate HDL-C uptake and steroid hormone synthesis. Moreover, SR-BI not only mediates HDL-CE uptake, but also stimulates free cholesterol efflux from cells into HDL, suggesting that SR-BI expression in the vessel wall might play a role in removal of excess cholesterol [178]. Thus, SR-BI might ultimately facilitate both the initial step (HDL-mediated cholesterol efflux from the arterial wall) as well as the final step (hepatic uptake of HDL-C) of the reverse cholesterol transport pathway. Thus, upregulation of hepatic SR-BI expression might be expected to enhance the rate of reverse cholesterol transport and hence reduce atherosclerosis despite reducing the steady state plasma level of HDL cholesterol.

LIPASES

Several members of the family of triglyceride lipase genes influence the metabolism of HDL. Following are the principle lipases which play a key role in HDL catabolism.

Lipoprotein Lipase

Lipoprotein lipase (LPL) is a key enzyme in hydrolysis of chylomicron and VLDL triglyceride [179-181]. Due to the large size of its substrates, the physiological site of LPL action is at the luminal surface of blood vessels, to which the enzyme is attached via highly charged heparin sulphate proteoglycans (HSPG) [179, 180]. Through its lipolytic action, LPL generates free fatty acids for conversion to triglyceride for the storage in adipocytes, and for energy use by skeletal and cardiac myocytes, thus playing an important role in energy homeostasis [180]. Zilversmit was the first to propose the importance of LPL in the atherosclerotic process [182]. Subsequent research was directed towards role of macrophage LPL in the development of atherosclerosis. Studies have demonstrated lesser atherosclerosis in mice lacking macrophage LPL [183]. High LPL activity was found by Zilversmit in aortae of cholesterol fed rabbits [184], and this observation found support by the marked increase in LPL mass and immunoreactivity in the neointima after deendothelization of aorta and in rabbit carotid arteries after silastic collar injury [185]. Mice that only express LPL in skeletal muscle have normal triglycerides but reduced HDL cholesterol [186], whereas mice expressing LPL only in cardiac muscle have normal TG and HDL cholesterol levels [187].

Antiatherogenic Role of LPL

Before around a decade, the first studies on the atheroprotective effect of plasma LPL were studied on mice overexpressing hepatic LPL (hLPL) [188,189]. In one study, in the LDL-$R^{-/-}$ mice overexpressing hLPL, plasma cholesterol and TG levels were lowered by 40 and 90%, respectively, than in LDL-$R^{-/-}$ controls along with around 18-fold decrease in atherosclerosis in the LPL overexpressing mice [188]. Also, several homozygous LPL-deficient patients have been found to develop relatively advanced atherosclerosis [190].

Moreover, overexpression of LPL is highly effective in normalizing the atherosclerotic lipoprotein profiles of both apoE-deficient and LDL receptor-deficient mice and protects wild-type mice against diet-induced hyperlipidaemia [191,192]. Post-heparin plasma LPL activity has also been linked directly to HDL levels in humans [193] with a heterozygous LPL genotype associated with decreased HDL-cholesterol levels [194]. Equally, administration of the compound NO-1886 (**13**), which increases tissue LPL activity, protects against atherosclerosis via elevation of HDL levels [195].

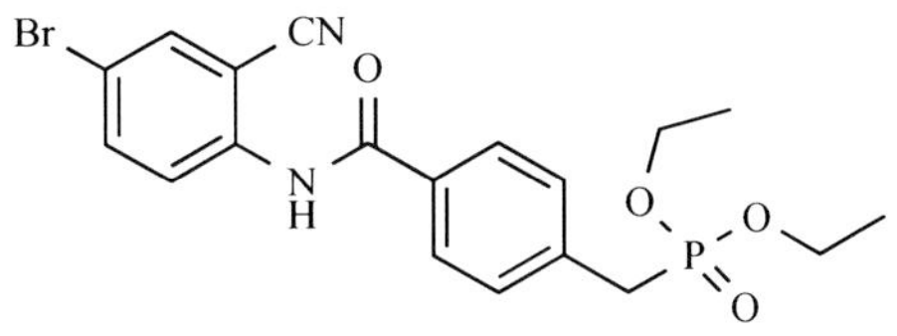

13

Moreover, statins and fibrates have been shown to enhance LPL activity in adipose tissue and heart as well as decreasing plasma levels of apolipoprotein C-III, an LPL inhibitor [196,197]. Pharmacologic upregulation of LPL in rats was found to raise HDL cholesterol levels and reduce atherosclerosis [195] and therapies designed to increase LPL expression could potentially be of therapeutic value in humans [see ref 198-202 for more detailed reviews].

Hepatic Lipase

Hepatic lipase (HL) is a member of the same triglyceride lipase gene family as LPL [181]. HL is synthesized primarily in hepatocytes and is found to bind mostly to endothelial HSPGs in the hepatic sinusoids [203]. Like LPL, HL has substantial triglyceride lipase activity, but, unlike LPL, HL also has substantial phospholipase activity [203]. In cultured hepatoma cells, an inverse relation has been described between the cell cholesterol content and the levels of HL mRNA and activity [204].

Transgenic mice [205-207] and rabbits [208,209] that overexpress the gene encoding HL (*Lipc*) have reduced levels of HDL-C and smaller HDL particles. Overexpression of *Lipc* in the liver using adenoviral-mediated gene transfer decreased HDL-C levels by ~65% in *Lipc*-deficient mice [210], 63% in *Lcat*-transgenic mice [211] and 41% in *Apoe*-deficient mice [212].

In humans, high plasma HL activity is associated with reduced HDL-C levels and smaller HDL particles [193]. Conversely, genetic HL deficiency is associated with modestly elevated HDL-C levels and larger HDL particles [213,214]. The relationship between HL and atherosclerosis is quite complex. Overexpression of *Lipc* in mice has been reported to reduce atherosclerosis as assessed by aortic cholesterol content [205]. Conversely, KO of *Lipc* expression in mice is associated with decreased atherosclerosis in *ApoE*-deficient mice [215]. HL-deficient humans have been reported to be at an elevated risk for atherosclerotic vascular disease [214], but also have augmented levels of atherogenic lipoproteins. Humans with CHD have been reported to have increased [216] or decreased [217] post-heparin plasma HL activity levels compared with control subjects in cross sectional studies. The regression of coronary atherosclerosis resulting from intensive lipid lowering therapy is associated with a decrease in HL activity and favorable changes in LDL buoyancy [218].

The involvement of HL in a novel proatherogenic pathway was first inferred from the unexpected finding that despite increased levels of the proatherogenic apoB containing lipoproteins, HL deficiency reduces aortic lesion formation in apoE-KO mice [219] and LCAT triglyceride mice [220]. These findings suggested the possibility that this lipase might have a localized effect on the arterial wall that could overwhelm the HL-mediated effects on the plasma lipoproteins. Aviram *et al.* [221] reported that HL enhances the uptake and accumulation of LDL-C by macrophages, and Nong *et al.* [220] have shown that the uptake of oxidized LDL-C differed significantly in peritoneal macrophages isolated from HL KO mice compared with control mice.

Endothelial Lipase

In 1999, Jaye *et al.* reported the isolation and functional characterization of a new member of the LPL gene family [222]. The sequence of this gene revealed substantial homology with LPL and HL, indicating that it was a new member of the triacylglycerol lipase family. Unlike LPL and HL, this new member of the gene family is synthesized by endothelial cells and hence was termed endothelial lipase (EL).

EL has the ability to hydrolyze triglycerides, yet this activity is substantially lower relative to its phospholipase activity compared with HL and especially LPL [223]. Therefore, these three lipases should be considered as defining a spectrum of lipase activities, with LPL acting primarily as a triglyceride hydrolase, EL acting primarily as a phospholipase, and HL acting in between.

In addition to the differences in lipid substrate specificity, EL has distinct lipoprotein preferences *in vitro* compared with LPL and HL. LPL and HL preferentially hydrolyze triglyceride-rich lipoproteins such as chylomicrons, VLDL and IDL, whereas EL is more active against HDL [223] but is not HDL specific; EL is also capable of hydrolyzing apoB-containing lipoproteins *in vitro* [223]. Independent of their lipolytic activities, LPL and HL mediate bridging between lipoproteins and HSPGs on the cell surface [199,224]. Like LPL and HL, EL significantly enhances the binding of VLDL and LDL to cell-surface HSPGs *in vitro* [225]. LPL and HL have relatively little ability to bridge HDL to cellular HSPGs, whereas EL effectively mediates binding of HDL to cell-surface HSPGs *in vitro* [225].

When EL was overexpressed by intravenous injection of adenovirus containing human EL cDNA, there was a marked decrease in plasma HDL levels [222].

Transgenic overexpression of EL under the control of the endogenous promoter resulted in moderately (~15%) reduced HDL-C levels [226]. Conversely, antibody inhibition of mouse EL activity in wild-type, apoA-I-transgenic and HL deficient mice resulted in significantly increased (>40%) HDL cholesterol and phospholipid levels associated with increased HDL particle size and reduced HDL phospholipid turnover [226]. Moreover, HDL-C levels were significantly increased (>42%) in the EL KO mouse [227]. The catalytic activity of EL is by far the most important mechanism by which EL modulates metabolism of HDL [228]. Therefore, inhibition of EL activity could be a novel strategy for raising HDL cholesterol levels.

CHOLESTERYL ESTER TRANSFER PROTEIN (CETP)

Plasma CETP has 476 amino acid residues and a 74-kDa molecular mass, of which 28% is attributed to N-glycosylation at residues 88, 240, 341 and 396 [229]. Plasma cholesteryl ester transfer protein (CETP) is a hydrophobic glycoprotein that is secreted mainly from the liver and that circulates in plasma, bound mainly to HDL. It promotes the redistribution of cholesteryl esters, triglycerides, and, to a lesser extent, phospholipids between plasma lipoproteins. CETP transfers lipids from one lipoprotein particle to another in a process that results in equilibration of lipids between lipoprotein fractions [230]. Although various dyslipidemias have been linked with increased CETP concentrations [231-233], it is possible that elevated CETP is the result of dyslipidemia rather than its cause [234]. By transferring CEs from HDLs to VLDLs and LDLs, CETP reduces the concentration of antiatherogenic HDLs while increasing the concentration of LDL-C [235].

Mice transduced with the human CETP gene displayed a dose-related decrease in HDL, accompanied by an increase in LDL and VLDL [236]. Plump *et al.* [237] transduced atherosclerosis prone, apoE-KO mice with human CETP and apoA-I transgenes, thereby inducing plasma CETP levels to rise to 5 to 10 times that of healthy normal humans. This increase in CETP was linked with a 76% reduction in HDL cholesterol. Inhibition of CETP expression has been studied in high- CETP animals, such as the hypercholesterolemic rabbit, a model that more closely models the human condition. Homozygous deficiency of CETP owing to at least two common mutations has been reported in the Japanese population, and leads to a marked increase in HDL cholesterol and apoA-I levels [238] and a marked delay in the catabolism of apoA-I [239].

Sugano *et al.* [240, 241] used antisense oligodeoxynucleotides against CETP. Total cholesterol and CETP were significantly reduced at 12 and 16 weeks compared with controls. HDL cholesterol, measured by ultracentrifugation and column chromatography, increased significantly. Aortic cholesterol content and the percentage of surface area with atherosclerosis were markedly decreased. Similar effects on CETP and HDL levels have been observed with anti-CETP antibodies [242].

Several thiol-modifying inhibitors of CETP have been identified, and their sites of action have been mapped to specific CETP Cys residues [243,244]. Several hydrophobic disulfides, including the dithiobis(nicotinic ester) [245] derivative (SC-19752, Monsanto/Searle, **14**) and the bis(o-amidophenyl)disulfides [246] (Japan Tobacco), have been identified as low-micromolar CETP inhibitors *in vitro*.

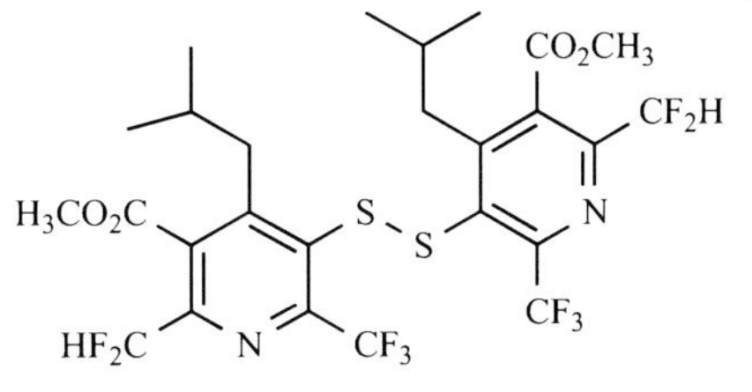

14

The most extensively studied and advanced of these sulfur based inhibitors is the thiol ester (JTT-705, Japan Tobacco, **15**) [246]. Additional SAR studies of **15** have been reported that explored modifications to the central benzene ring and identified the related 4,5-dichloropivaloyl thioester analogue **16** (IC_{50} = 2M, human plasma) having the extended α-

(3-methylbutyl)cyclohexyl side chain as a slightly more potent inhibitor than **15**, although only *in vitro* data were disclosed [247].

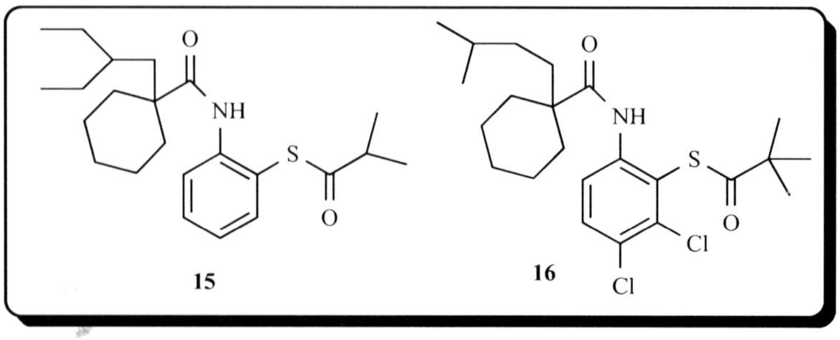

Bayer has described the discovery, key SAR findings, and lead optimization efforts for both their first- and second-generation 5,6,7,8-tetrahydroquinolines and related CETP inhibitors [248]. Starting from an initial series of highly functionalized 5-hydroxymethyl-pyridine based [249] and benzyl alcohol based [250] leads, the pentasubstituted pyridine **17** was identified as a lead candidate with nanomolar potency (IC_{50} = 0.013 μM, buffer).

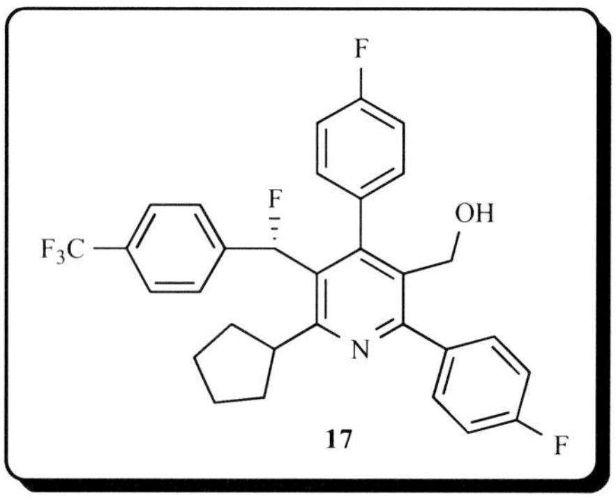

Multiple series of related fused bicyclic heterocycles were investigated, and early patented examples include both the 5-hydroxyquinoline **18** (IC_{50} =0.18 μM) [251] and the naphthyridine derivative **19** [252], having submicromolar activity against CETP under buffered conditions and oral activity in animals.

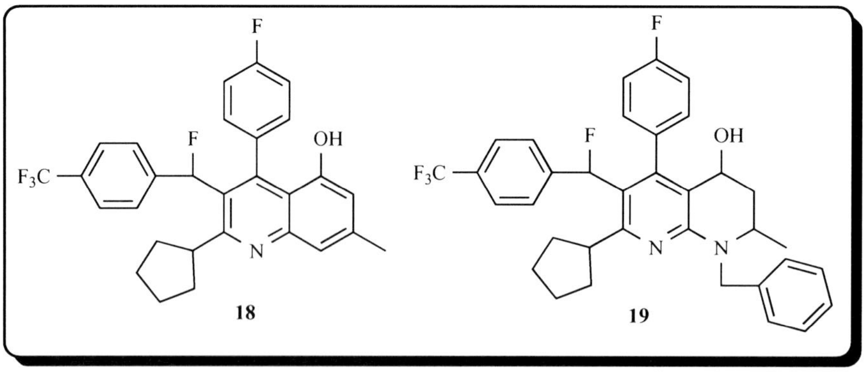

These have been further optimized to provide unresolved racemic examples of the related highly substituted secondary and tertiary tetrahydroquinolinols **20** and **21** (IC_{50} = 0.006 μM) with cyclic aliphatic groups at the 2-position and containing geminal small aliphatic groups at the 7-position of the saturated ring that exhibit significantly greater potency than either **18** or **19** [253].

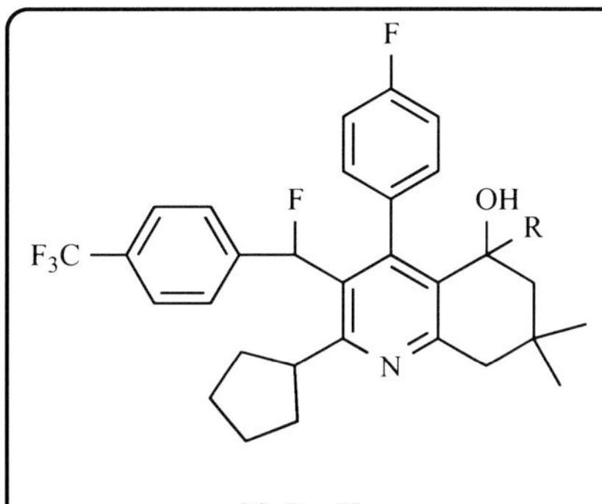

20: R = H,
21: R = CH_3

Researchers at Pfizer have identified a completely distinct but related series of 4-amino-substituted-1,2,3,4-tetrahydroquinoline carbamates where the partial saturation occurs in the heterocyclic ring rather than the carbocyclic ring found in the Bayer leads. Optimization of this series led to an exciting new potent (IC_{50} = 0.05 μM, human plasma) chiral CETP inhibitor torcetrapib (CP-529,414, **22**), for clinical development. Recently, torcetrapib has been withdrawn from further clinical trials due to 82 deaths in the group taking torcetrapib along with lipitor (Atorvastatin) in the ILLUMINATE study. Since torcetrapib was known to elevate blood pressure, the deaths are possibly linked with severe hypertension.

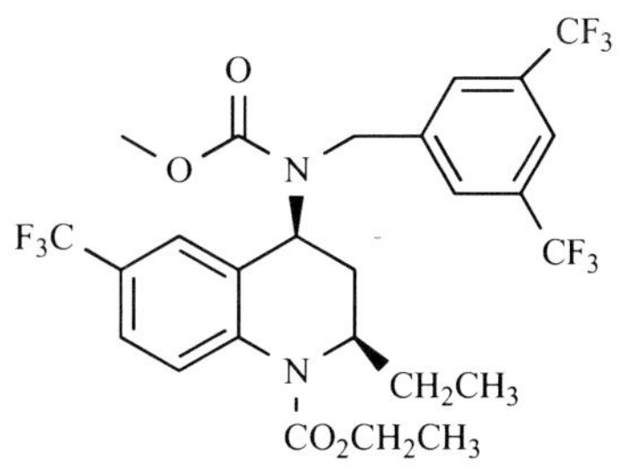

22

The discovery and early optimization of torcetrapib have been reported [254] starting from the initial lead 6,7-dimethoxy-4-aminotetrahedroquinoline **(23)** that had micromolar potency (IC_{50} = 10 μM) under buffered conditions and retained its activity in the presence of human plasma (IC_{50} = 25 μM) [255].

Torcetrapib became the first CETP inhibitor to enter a large-scale, prospective, placebo-controlled interventional trial—the Investigation of Lipid Level Management to Understand its Impact in Atherosclerotic Events (ILLUMINATE). This trial was prematurely terminated

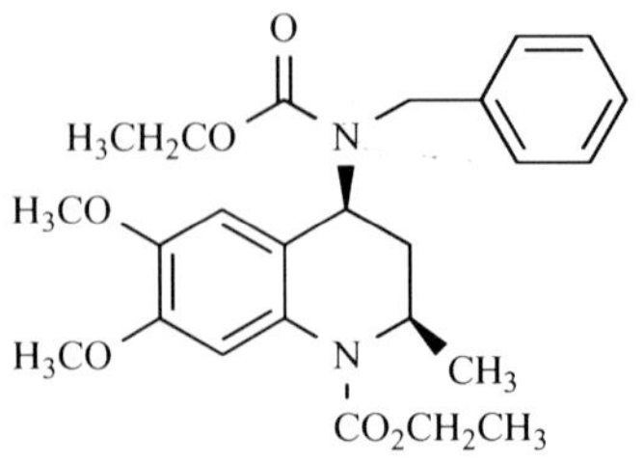

23

in December 2006 as a consequence of excess mortality in the active treatment group relative to the placebo group [256]. Since termination of ILLUMINATE, however, new data have clearly demonstrated that torcetrapib treatment was associated with a substantial increase in aldosterone levels, changes in serum electrolytes indicative of mineralocorticoid excess, and elevated blood pressure [256]. These findings strongly suggest that torcetrapib has off-target toxic effects unrelated to its HDL-raising actions that involve the activation of mineralocorticoid receptors by aldosterone and the subsequent induction of hypertension. Importantly and in contrast with torcetrapib, other CETP inhibitors such as JTT-705 and MK-0859 (anacetrapib) do not increase blood pressure in humans [257]. These findings indicate that the adverse effects observed with torcetrapib cannot be attributed to a class effect of CETP inhibitors resulting from alterations in steroid metabolism through elevated delivery of HDL cholesterol to the adrenals.

APOLIPOPROTEIN A-I (APOA-I)

Apo A-I is a 243-residue protein that contains a globular (possibly lipid-binding) N-terminal domain (residues 1–43) and a lipid-binding C-terminal domain (residues 44–243) [258]. ApoA-1 is synthesized by the liver and intestine and plays a key role in the formation, metabolism, and catabolism of HDL cholesterol esters. Human apoA-I is markedly associated to HDL particles and it seems to regulate HDL particle size distribution [259]. This protein also promotes cellular cholesterol efflux [260] and interacts with several proteins such as SR-B1 [261] and ABCA1 [262]. Decades of epidemiological studies have repeatedly demonstrated that low plasma HDL apoA-I levels are a major risk factor for the development of CAD [263]. A recent study suggested that very high plasma HDL-C and very large HDL particles may represent increased CAD risk when levels of apoA-I and apoB remain unaffected. In contrast, apoA-I appears not to turn into a significant risk factor at high plasma concentrations [264].

ApoA-I Milano is a naturally occurring variant of apoA-I wherein arg173 is replaced by a cysteine residue. Individuals expressing this protein have significantly lower than average HDL-C. However, the subpopulation expressing apoA-I Milano shows a much reduced frequency of atherosclerosis than would be anticipated based on their HDL levels [265]. In a small, placebo controlled clinical trial, recombinant apoA-I Milano/phospholipids complex was intravenously administered once per week for 5 weeks to individuals with CAD. Intravascular ultrasound imaging studies were used to assess the development of the atherosclerosis. At the end of the trial, the treated group had a small but marked decrease in atheroma volume while the untreated group had a small increase in plaque size [266].

One of the more intriguing approaches under investigation is the use of synthetic peptides, the so-called apoA-I mimetic peptides, that mimic the function of apoA-I without bearing any sequence homology to apoA-I [267]. Synthesis and characterization of a number of amphipathic peptides as potential apoA-I mimetics has been reported. The first *in vivo* efficacy was demonstrated when intraperitoneal administration of 5F peptide at 20 μg/day for 16 weeks reduced diet-induced aortic sinus atherosclerosis in C57B6J mice [268]. Interestingly, 2.5 times the amounts of mouse apoA-I had no effect on lesions in this study.

The next major development in this field was the demonstration that 4F peptide could be made orally bioavailable if synthesized from d-amino acids (D-4F) rather than l-amino acids (L-4F) [269]. D-4F is an 18 residue peptide comprised of D-amino acids. Oral administration of D-4F to apoE KO mice resulted in low (picomolar) plasma concentrations of the peptide. These animals displayed an increase in preβ-HDL enriched in antioxidant activity. As a control, scrambled D-4F was administered and resulted in no detectable plasma levels nor any effects on blood lipids [270]. Studies on the effect of D-4F on atherosclerosis in apoE KO mice resulted in reduction of atherosclerotic plaque size in evolving lesions while no significant effect was observed on established atherosclerosis [271].

FUTURE HDL BASED THERAPIES

Phospholipids

Phospholipid liposomes mediate RCT and promote cholesterol efflux [272]. Liposomes are too large to cross the endothelium and instead accept cholesterol that has been shuttled across the endothelium by HDL. The interaction of the liposome with HDL creates a cholesterol-poor, phospholipid-rich particle that is thought to have enhanced cholesterol efflux capability [273]. Anionically charged phosphatidylinositol (PI), which is a small component of the phospholipid layer, inhibited LCAT activity, reduced synthesis and storage of cholesteryl esters, increased cholesterol efflux and decreased cholesterol synthesis and esterification [274,275]. In patients, PI administration increased HDL-C and ApoA-1 levels by up to 18% and 6%, respectively (without apparent side effects) after two weeks [276].

Reconstituted HDL

Reconstituted HDL not only induces effective cholesterol efflux but also inhibits proinflammatory changes and platelet aggregation [277, 278]. Infusion of reconstituted HDL in cholesterol-fed rabbits significantly reduced atheroma size compared with oral atorvastatin. Mean HDL-C levels were increased by 69% and 225% among patients with hypercholesterolaemia and Tangier disease, respectively, and intravenous infusion of reconstituted HDL normalized endothelium-mediated vasodilation through increased nitric oxide bioavailability [279,280]. Reconstituted HDL *in vitro* directly induced endothelial progenitor-cell differentiation and increased angiogenesis within ischaemic muscle [281]. Theoretically, these activities make reconstituted HDL an ideal agent for patients with acute coronary syndromes. Indeed, reconstituted HDL infusion in patients with acute coronary syndrome was associated with reduced atheroma volume when compared with baseline (pre-infusion) values, and with an improvement of plaque quality compared with placebo [282].

CONCLUSION

Well established experimental and clinical studies clearly demonstrated HDL as an attractive target for lipid lowering therapy. Complex HDL metabolism represents various attractive targets to combat hyperlipidemia in a rationalized manner. Among several targets reviewed, CETP has received most of the attention. Roche laboratory is currently pursuing further development of CETP inhibitor JTT 705. Also, failure of torcetrapib has raised an alarming concern for biologists and medicinal chemists. On the other hand, discovery of crystal structure of CETP would definitely facilitate design of new CETP inhibitors. Notably, the focus on HDL is beginning to shift towards improving HDL function rather than simply increasing HDL-C levels, although the two are certainly not mutually exclusive. HDL and ApoA-I also have anti-inflammatory, antioxidant and nitric-oxide promoting properties, which could contribute to their atheroprotective effects. Thus, development of therapies that directly enhance these properties of HDL might be expected to have a beneficial effect in reducing progression of atherosclerosis. Out of the other targets described, ABCA1 targeting agents, specifically PPAR agonists and apoA-I mimetic peptides are of considerable potential. There has not been sufficient work on LPL activators except NO-1886. Medicinal chemistry efforts are not upto the mark in many targets possibly because of poor understanding of biochemical role of the target or lack of crystal structure of the target. Significant research is required in the design of various HDL elevating entities as marked output from biochemistry and molecular biologists would greatly aid the design process. Notably, crystal structure of CETP has opened doors of all explorations including molecular simulations, docking and ligand binding assays. Computational chemistry along with medicinal chemistry research is required to synthesize novel potent and safe lipid lowering entities.

REFERENCES

[1] Shah PK, Kaul S, Nilsson J, *et al.* Exploiting the vascular protective effects of high-density lipoprotein and its apolipoproteins: an idea whose time for testing is coming, part I. Circulation 2001; 104(19): 2376-2383.

[2] Genest J, McNamara J, Salem D, *et al.* Prevalence of risk factors in men with premature coronary artery disease. Am J Cardiol 1991; 67: 1185-1189.

[3] Fluiter K, van Berkel TJ. Scavenger receptor B1 (SR-B1) substrates inhibit the selective uptake of high-density-lipoprotein cholesteryl esters by rat parenchymal liver cells. Biochem J 1997; 326: 515-519.

[4] Gianturco SH, Ramprasad MP, Song R, *et al.* Apolipoprotein B-48 or its apolipoprotein B-100 equivalent mediates the binding of triglyceride-rich lipoproteins to their unique human monocyte-macrophage receptor. Arterioscler Thromb Vasc Biol 1998; 18: 968-976.

[5] Watson AD, Berliner JA, Hama SY, *et al.* Protective effect of high density lipoprotein associated paraoxonase. Inhibition of the biological activity of minimally oxidized low density lipoprotein. J Clin Invest 1995; 96: 2882-2891.

[6] Chung BH, Tallis G, Yalamoori V, *et al.* Liposome-like particles isolated from human atherosclerotic plaques are structurally and compositionally similar to surface remnants of triglyceride-rich lipoproteins. Arterioscler Thromb 1994; 14: 622-635.

[7] Gordon DH, Rifkind BM. High-density lipoprotein: the clinical implications of recent studies. N Engl J Med 1989; 321: 1311-1316.

[8] Moti L, Kashyap MD. Mechanistic studies of high density lipoprotein. Am J Cardiol 1998; 82: 42U-48U.

[9] Calabresi L, Franceschini G. High density lipoprotein and coronary heart disease: insights from mutations leading to low high density lipoprotein. Curr Opin Lipidol 1997; 8(4): 219-224.

[10] Vergani C, Bettale G. Familial hypoalphalipoproteinemia. Clin Chim Acta 1981; 114: 42–52.

[11] Third JL, Montag J, Flynn M, *et al.* Primary and familial hypoalphalipoproteinemia. Metabolism 1984; 33: 136-146.

[12] Harris WS. N-3 fatty acids and serum lipoproteins: human studies. Am J Clin Nutr 1997; 65: 1645S-54S.

[13] Covington MB. Omega 3 fatty acids. Am Fam Physician 2004; 70: 133-40.

[14] Capuzzi DM, Guyton JR, Morgan JM, *et al.* Efficacy and safety of an extended-release niacin (Niaspan): a long-term study. Am J Cardiol 1998; 82: 74U-81U.

[15] Forcheron F, Cachefo A, Thevenon S, Pinteur C, Beylot M. Mechanisms of the triglyceride- and cholesterol-lowering effect of fenofibrate in hyperlipidemic type 2 diabetic patients. Diabetes 2002; 51: 3486-3491.

[16] Dean M, Hamon Y, Chimini G. The human ATP-binding cassette (ABC) transporter superfamily. J Lipid Res 2001; 42: 1007-1017.

[17] Oram JF. HDL apolipoproteins and ABCA1: partners in the removal of excess cellular cholesterol. Arterioscler Thromb Vasc Biol 2003; 23: 720-727.

[18] Schmitz G, Langmann T. Structure, function and regulation of the ABC1 gene product. Curr Opin Lipidol 2001; 12: 129-140.

[19] Brewer Jr. HB, Remaley AT, Neufeld EB, *et al.* Regulation of plasma high-density lipoprotein levels by the ABCA1 transporter and the emerging role of high-density lipoprotein in the treatment of cardiovascular disease. Arterioscler Thromb Vasc Biol 2003; 24: 1755-1760.

[20] Mendez AJ, Anantharamaiah GM, Segrest JP, *et al.* Synthetic amphipathic helical peptides that mimic apolipoprotein A-I in clearing cellular cholesterol. J Clin Invest 1994; 94: 1698-1705.

[21] Yamauchi Y, Chang CC, Hayashi M, *et al.* Intracellular cholesterol mobilization involved in the ABCA1/apolipoprotein-mediated assembly of high density lipoprotein in fibroblasts. J Lipid Res 2004; 45: 1943-1951.

[22] Vaughan AM, Oram JF. ABCA1 redistributes membrane cholesterol independent of apolipoprotein interactions. J Lipid Res 2003; 44:1373-1380.

[23] Wang N, Silver DL, Thiele C, *et al.* ATP-binding cassette transporter A1 (ABCA1) functions as a cholesterol efflux regulatory protein. J Biol Chem 2001; 276: 23742-23747.

[24] Bortnick AE, Rothblat GH, Stoudt G, *et al.* The correlation of ATP-binding cassette 1 mRNA levels with cholesterol efflux from various cell lines. J Biol Chem 2000; 275: 28634-28640.

[25] Tall AR, Yvan-Charvet L, Terasaka N, Pagler T, Wang N. HDL, ABC transporters, and cholesteol efflux: implications for the treatment of atherosclerosis. Cell Metbol 2008; 7: 365-375.

[26] Assman G, von Eckardstein A, Brewer HB. Familial high density lipoprotein deficiency: Tangier disease. In: Scriver CR, Beaud AL, Sly WS, Valle D, Eds. The metabolic and molecular bases of inherited disease. New York: McGraw-Hill 1995; 2053-2072.

[27] Bodzioch M, Orso E, Klucken J, *et al.* The gene encoding ATP-binding cassette transporter 1 is mutated in Tangier disease. Nat Genet 1999; 22: 347-351.

[28] Brooks-Wilson A, Marcil M, Clee SM, *et al.* Mutations in ABC1 in Tangier disease and familial high-density lipoprotein deficiency. Nat Genet 1999; 22: 336-345.

[29] Lawn RM, Wade DP, Garvin MR, *et al.* The Tangier disease gene product ABC1 controls the cellular apolipoproteinmediated lipid removal pathway. J Clin Invest 1999; 104: R25-R31.

[30] Rust S, Rosier M, Funke H, *et al.* Tangier disease is caused by mutations in the gene encoding ATP-binding cassette transporter 1. Nat Genet 1999; 22: 352-355.

[31] Cohen JC, Kiss RS, Pertsemlidis A, *et al.* Multiple rare alleles contribute to low plasma levels of HDL cholesterol. Science 2004; 305: 869-872.

[32] Frikke-Schmidt R, Nordestgaard BG, Jensen GB, *et al.* Genetic variation in ABC transporter A1 contributes to HDL cholesterol in the general population. J Clin Invest 2004; 114: 1343-1353.

[33] Singaraja RR, Brunham LR, Visscher H, *et al.* Efflux and atherosclerosis: the clinical and biochemical impact of variations in the ABCA1 gene. Arterioscler Thromb Vasc Biol 2003; 23: 1322-1332.

[34] Attie AD, Brooks-Wilson A, Gray-Keller ME, *et al.* Massive cholesterol ester accumulation in hepatocytes and intestinal epithelial cells caused by ABC1 mutation in WHAM chickens. Circulation 2000; 102: II-312.

[35] Orso E, Broccardo C, Kaminski WE, *et al.* Transport of lipids from Golgi to plasma membrane is defective in tangier disease patients and Abc1-deficient mice. Nat Genet 2000; 24: 192-196.

[36] McNeish J, Aiello RJ, Guyot D, *et al.* High density lipoprotein deficiency and foam cell accumulation in mice with targeted disruption of ATP-binding cassette transporter-1. Proc Natl Acad Sci USA 2000; 97: 4245-4250.

[37] Aiello RJ, Brees D, Francone OL. ABCA1-deficient mice: insights into the role of monocyte lipid efflux in HDL formation and inflammation. Arterioscler Thromb Vasc Biol 2003; 23: 972-980.

[38] Singaraja RR, Fievet C, Castro G, *et al.* Increased ABCA1 activity protects against atherosclerosis. J Clin Invest 2002; 110: 35-42.

[39] Wellington CL, Brunham LR, Zhou S, *et al.* Alterations of plasma lipids in mice *via* adenoviral-mediated hepatic overexpression of human ABCA1. J Lipid Res 2003; 44: 1470-1480.

[40] Joyce C, Freeman L, Brewer HB Jr, *et al.* Study of ABCA1 function in transgenic mice. Arterioscler Thromb Vasc Biol 2003; 23: 965-971.

[41] Lee JY, Parks JS. ATP-binding cassette transporter AI and its role in HDL formation. Curr Opin Lipidol 2005; 16: 19-25.

[42] Serfaty-Lacrosniere C, Civeira F, Lanzberg A, *et al.* Homozygous Tangier disease and cardiovascular disease. Atherosclerosis 1994; 107: 85-98.

[43] Van Dam MJ, de Groot E, Clee SM, *et al.* Association between increased arterial-wall thickness and impairment in ABCA1-driven cholesterol efflux: an observational study. Lancet 2002; 359: 37-42.

[44] Cavelier LB, Qiu Y, Bielicki JK, *et al.* Regulation and activity of the human ABCA1 gene in transgenic mice. J Biol Chem 2001; 276: 18046-18051.

[45] Joyce CW, Amar MJ, Lambert G, *et al.* The ATP binding cassette transporter A1 (ABCA1) modulates the development of aortic atherosclerosis in C57BL/6 and apoE-knockout mice. Proc Natl Acad Sci USA 2002; 99: 407-412.

[46] Wang N, Tall AR. Regulation and mechanisms of ATP-binding cassette transporter A1-mediated cellular cholesterol efflux. Arterioscler Thromb Vasc Biol 2003; 23: 1178-1184.

[47] Vaisman BL, Lambert G, Amar M, *et al.* ABCA1 overexpression leads to hyperalphalipoproteinemia and increased biliary cholesterol excretion in transgenic mice. J Clin Invest 2001; 108: 303-309.

[48] Basso FP, Freeman L, Knapper CL, *et al.* Role of the hepatic ABCA1 transporter in modulating intrahepatic cholesterol and plasma HDL cholesterol concentrations. J Lipid Res 2003; 44: 296-302.

[49] Oram JF. The cholesterol mobilizing transporter ABCA1 as a new therapeutic target for cardiovascular disease. Trends Cardiovasc Med 2002; 12(4): 170-175.

[50] Peet DJ, Janowski BA, Mangelsdorf DJ. The LXRs: a new class of oxysterol receptors. Curr Opin Genet Dev 1998; 8(5): 571-575.

[51] Jaye M. LXR Agonists for the treatment of atherosclerosis. Curr Opin Invest Drugs 2003; 4(9): 1053-1058.

[52] Repa JJ, Mangelsdorf DJ. The liver X receptor gene team: Potential new players in atherosclerosis. Nat Med 2002; 8(11): 1243-1248.

[53] Karpen SJ. Nuclear receptor regulation of hepatic function. J Hepatol 2002; 36: 832-850.

[54] Torchia J, Glass C, Rosenfeld MG. Co-activators and co-repressors in the integration of transcriptional responses. Curr Opin Cell Biol 1998; 10(3): 373-378.

[55] Moras D, Gronemeyer H. The nuclear receptor ligand-binding domain: structure and function. Curr Opin Cell Biol 1998; 10(3): 384-391.

[56] Peet DJ, Turley SD, Ma W, *et al.* Cholesterol and bile acid metabolism are impaired in mice lacking the nuclear oxysterol receptor LXRα. Cell 1998; 93: 693-704.

[57] Schmitz G, Langmann T, Heimerl S. Role of ABCG1 and other ABCG family members in lipid metabolism. J Lipid Res 2001; 42: 1513-1520.

[58] Wang N, Lan D, Chen W, *et al.* ATP-binding cassette transporters G1 and G4 mediate cellular cholesterol efflux to high-density lipoproteins. Proc Natl Acad Sci USA 2004; 101: 9774-9779.

[59] Laffitte BA, Repa JJ, Joseph SB, *et al.* LXRs control lipid-inducible expression of the apolipoprotein E gene in macrophages and adipocytes. Proc Natl Acad Sci USA 2001; 98: 507-512.

[60] Huang ZH, Lin CY, Oram JF, *et al.* Sterol efflux mediated by endogenous macrophage ApoE expression is independent of ABCA1. Arterioscler Thromb Vasc Biol 2001; 21: 2019-2025.

[61] Repa JJ, Berge KE, Pomajzl C, *et al.* Regulation of ATP-binding cassette sterol transporters ABCG5 and ABCG8 by the liver X receptors alpha and beta. J Biol Chem 2002; 277: 18793-18800.

[62] Bensinger SJ, Tontonoz P. Integration of metabolism and inflammation by lipid-activated nuclear receptors. Nature 2008; 454: 470-477.

[63] Alberti S, Schuster G, Parini P, *et al.* Hepatic cholesterol metabolism and resistance to dietary cholesterol in LXRβ-deficient mice. J Clin Invest 2001; 107: 565-573.

[64] Bradley MN, Hong C, Chen M, *et al.* Ligand activation of LXRβ reverses atherosclerosis and cellular cholesterol overload in mice lacking LXRα and apoE. J Clin Invest 2007; 117: 2337-2346.

[65] Fu X, Menke JG, Chen Y, *et al.* 27-Hydroxycholesterol is an endogenous ligand for liver X receptor in cholesterol-loaded cells. J Biol Chem 2001; 276: 38378-38387.

[66] Spencer TA, Li D, Russell JS, *et al.* Pharmacophore analysis of the nuclear oxysterol receptor LXRα. J Med Chem 2001; 44(6): 886-897.

[67] Song C, Liao S. Cholestenoic acid is a naturally occuring ligand for liver X receptor α. Endocrinology 2000; 141(11): 4180-4184.

[68] Janowski BA, Grogan MJ, Jones SA, *et al.* Structural requirements of ligands for the oxysterol liver X receptors LXRalpha and LXRbeta. Proc Natl Acad Sci USA 1999; 96: 266-271.

[69] Lehmann JM, Kliewer SA, Moore LB, *et al.* Activation of the nuclear receptor LXR by oxysterols defines a new hormone response pathway. J Biol Chem 1997; 272: 3137-3140.

[70] Janowski BA, Willy PJ, Devi TR, *et al.* An oxysterol signalling pathway mediated by the nuclear receptor LXRa. Nature 1996; 383: 728-731.

[71] Repa JJ, Liang G, Ou J, *et al.* Regulation of mouse sterol regulatory elementbinding protein-1c (SREBP-1c) by oxysterol receptors LXRα and LXRβ. Genes Dev 2000; 14: 2819-2830.

[72] Zhang Y, Repa JJ, Gauthier K, *et al.* Regulation of lipoprotein lipase by the oxysterol receptors, LXRalpha and LXRbeta. J Biol Chem 2001; 276: 43018-43024.

[73] Mak PA, Kast-Woelbern HR, Anisfeld AM, *et al.* Identification of PLTP as an LXR target gene and apoE as an FXR target gene reveals overlapping targets for the two nuclear receptors. J Lipid Res 2002; 43: 2037-2041.

[74] Mak PA, Laffitte BA, Desrumaux C, *et al.* Regulated expression of the apolipoprotein E/C-I/C-IV/C-II gene cluster in murine and human macrophages. A critical role for nuclear liver X receptors alpha and beta. J Biol Chem 2002; 277: 31900-31908.

[75] Schultz, JR, Tu H, Luk A, *et al.* Role of LXRs in control of lipogenesis. Genes Dev 2000; 14: 2831-2838.

[76] Ntambi JM, Miyazaki M. Recent insights into stearoyl-CoA desaturase-1. Curr Opin Lipidol 2003; 14: 255-261.

[77] Collins JL, Fivush AM, Watson MA, *et al.* Identification of a nonsteroidal liver X receptor agonist through parallel array synthesis of tertiary amines. J Med Chem 2002; 45: 1963-1966.

[78] Hu B, Collini M, Unwalla R, *et al.* Discovery of phenyl acetic acid substituted quinolines as novel liver x receptor agonists for the treatment of atherosclerosis. J Med Chem 2006; 49: 6151-6154.

[79] Hu B, Jetter J, Kaufman D, *et al.* Further modification on phenyl acetic acid based quinolines as liver X receptor modulators. Bioorg Med Chem 2007; 15: 3321-3333.

[80] Holm, P.: US20060189663A1 **(2006)**.

[81] Jones, A.B,, Adams, A.D., Green, A.I., Huang, S.Y, Tse, B., Gutteridge, C.E., Cheng, Y.: US7125865B2 **(2006)**.

[82] Molteni, V., Li, X., Liang, F., Nabakka, J., Saez, E., Wityak, J.: WO2005077122A2 **(2005)**.

[83] Dehmlow, H., Kuhn, B., Panday, N., Ratni, H., Schulz-Gasch, T., Wright, M.B.: US7173048B2 (**2007**).

[84] Desvergne B, Michalik L, Wahli W. Transcriptional regulation of metabolism. Physiol Rev 2006; 86(2): 465-514.

[85] Ahuja HS, Szanto A, Nagy L, *et al.* The retinoid X receptor and its ligands: versatile regulators of metabolic function, cell di.erentiation and cell death. J Biol Regul Homeost Agents 2003; 17(1): 29-45.

[86] Szanto A, Narkar V, Shen Q, *et al.* Retinoid X receptors: X-ploring their (patho)physiological functions. Cell Death Differ 2004; 11(2): S126-S143.

[87] Bastien J, Rochette-Egly C. Nuclear retinoid receptors and the transcription of retinoid-target genes. Gene 2004; 328(1-2): 1-16.

[88] Costet P, Luo Y, Wang N, *et al.* Sterol-dependent transactivation of the ABC1 promoter by the liver X receptor/retinoid X receptor. J Biol Chem 2000; 275: 28240-28245.

[89] Schwartz K, Lawn RM, Wade DP. ABC1 gene expression and ApoA-I-mediated cholesterol efflux are regulated by LXR. Biochem Biophys Res Commun 2000; 274: 794-802.

[90] Claudel T, Leibowitz MD, Fievet C. Reduction of atherosclerosis in apolipoprotein E knockout mice by activation of the retinoid X receptor. Proc Natl Acad Sci USA 2001; 98: 2610-2615.

[91] Costet P, Lalanne F, Gerbod-Giannone MC, *et al.* Retinoic acid receptor-mediated induction of ABCA1 in macrophages. Mol Cell Biol 2003; 23: 7756-7766.

[92] Haffner, C.D., Istvan, K., McDougald, D.L., Miller, A.B.: US7173134B2 **(2007)**.

[93] Lagu, B., Lebedev, R., Pio, B.: US20070078160A1 **(2007)**.

[94] Momose, Y., Maekawa, T., Odaka, H., Kimura, H.: US7179823B1 **(2007)**.

[95] Schoonjans K, Watanabe M, Suzuki H, *et al.* Induction of the acyl-coenzyme A synthetase gene by fibrates and fatty acids is mediated by a peroxisome proliferator response element in the C promoter. J Biol Chem 1995; 270: 19269-19276.

[96] Motojima K, Passilly P, Peters JM, *et al.* Expression of putative fatty acid transporter genes are regulated by peroxisome proliferator-activated receptor alpha and gamma activators in a tissue- and inducer-specific manner. J Biol Chem 1998; 273: 16710-16714.

[97] Berthou L, Duverger N, Emmanuel F, *et al.* Opposite regulation of human versus mouse apolipoprotein A-I by fibrates in human apolipoprotein A-I transgenic mice. J Clin Invest 1996; 97: 2408-2416.

[98] Vu-Dac N, Chopin-Delannoy S, Gervois P, *et al.* The nuclear receptors peroxisome proliferator-activated receptor alpha and Rev-erbalpha mediate the species-specific regulation of apolipoprotein A-I expression by fibrates. J Biol Chem 1998; 273: 25713-25720.

[99] Chinetti G, Lestavel S, Bocher V, *et al.* PPAR-alpha and PPARgamma activators induce cholesterol removal from human macrophage foam cells through stimulation of the ABCA1 pathway. Nat Med 2001; 7: 53-58.

[100] Chinetti G, Gbaguidi FG, Griglio S, *et al.* CLA-1/SR-BI is expressed in atherosclerotic lesion macrophages and regulated by activators of peroxisome proliferator-activated receptors. Circulation 2000; 101: 2411-2417.

[101] Chinetti G, Lestavel S, Fruchart JC, *et al.* Peroxisome proliferator-activated receptor alpha reduces cholesterol esterification in macrophages. Circ Res 2003; 92: 212-217.

[102] Robins SJ, Collins D, Wittes JT, *et al.* Relation of gemfibrozil treatment and lipid levels with major coronary events. VA-HIT: a randomized controlled trial. J Am Med Assoc 2001; 285: 1585-1591.

[103] Tordjman K, Bernal-Mizrachi C, Zemany L, *et al.* PPARalpha deficiency reduces insulin resistance and atherosclerosis in apoE-null mice. J Clin Invest 2001; 107: 1025-1034.
[104] Fu T, Kashireddy P, Borensztajn J. The peroxisomeproliferator- activated receptor alpha agonist ciprofibrate severely aggravates hypercholesterolaemia and accelerates the development of atherosclerosis in mice lacking apolipoprotein E. Biochem J 2003; 373: 941-947.
[105] Duez H, Chao YS, Hernandez M, *et al.* Reduction of atherosclerosis by the peroxisome proliferator-activated receptor alpha agonist fenofibrate in mice. J Biol Chem 2002; 277: 48051-48057.
[106] Li AC, Binder CJ, Gutierrez A, *et al.* Differential inhibition of macrophage foam-cell formation and atherosclerosis in mice by PPARα, β/δ, and γ. J Clin Invest 2004; 114: 1564-1576.
[107] Tontonoz P, Hu E, Graves RA, *et al.* mPPAR gamma 2: tissue-specific regulator of an adipocyte enhancer. Genes Dev 1994; 8: 1224-1234.
[108] Zhu Y, Qi C, Korenberg JR, *et al.* Structural organization of mouse peroxisome proliferator-activated receptor gamma (mPPAR gamma) gene: alternative promoter use and different splicing yield two mPPAR gamma isoforms. Proc Natl Acad Sci USA 1995; 92: 7921-7925.
[109] Tontonoz P, Hu E, Spiegelman BM. Stimulation of adipogenesis in fibroblasts by PPARγ2, a lipid-activated transcription factor. Cell 1994; 79: 1147-1156.
[110] Barak Y, Nelson MC, Ong ES, *et al.* PPARγ is required for placental, cardiac, and adipose tissue development. Mol Cell 1999; 4: 585-595.
[111] Kubota N, Terauchi Y, Miki H, *et al.* PPARγ mediates high-fat diet-induced adipocyte hypertrophy and insulin resistance. Mol Cell 1999; 4: 597-609.
[112] Rosen ED, Sarraf P, Troy AE, *et al.* PPARγ is required for the differentiation of adipose tissue *in vivo* and *in vitro*. Mol Cell 1999; 4: 611-617.
[113] Lehmann JM, Moore LB, Smith-Oliver TA, *et al.* An antidiabetic thiazolidinedione is a high affinity ligand for peroxisome proliferatoractivated receptor gamma (PPARgamma). J Biol Chem 1995; 270: 12953-12956.
[114] Auwerx, J., Fajas, L., Briggs, M.R., Saladin, R.: US20060276426A1 **(2006)**.
[115] Nagy L, Tontonoz P, Alvarez JG, *et al.* Oxidized LDL regulates macrophage gene expression through ligand activation of PPARgamma. Cell 1998; 93: 229-240.
[116] Tontonoz P, Nagy L, Alvarez JG, *et al.* PPARgamma promotes monocyte/macrophage differentiation and uptake of oxidized LDL. Cell 1998; 93: 241-252.
[117] Chawla A, Boisvert WA, Lee CH, *et al.* A PPAR gamma-LXR-ABCA1 pathway in macrophages is involved in cholesterol efflux and atherogenesis. Mol Cell 2001; 7: 161-171.
[118] Reilly SM, Chih-Hao L. PPARδ as a therapeutic target in metabolic disease. FEBS Lett 2008; 582: 26-31.
[119] Li AC, Brown KK, Silvestre MJ, *et al.* Peroxisome proliferator-activated receptor gamma ligands inhibit development of atherosclerosis in LDL receptor-deficient mice. J Clin Invest 2000; 106: 523-531.
[120] Koshiyama H, Shimono D, Kuwamura N, *et al.* Inhibitory effect of pioglitazone on carotid arterial wall thickness in type 2 diabetes. J Clin Endocrinol Metab 2001; 86: 3452-3456.
[121] Minamikawa J, Tanaka S, Yamauchi M, *et al.* Potent inhibitory effect of troglitazone on carotid arterial wall thickness in type 2 diabetes. J Clin Endocrinol Metab 1998; 83: 1818-1820.
[122] Chen Z, Ishibashi S, Perrey S, *et al.* Troglitazone inhibits atherosclerosis in apolipoprotein E-knockout mice: pleiotropic effects on CD36 expression and HDL. Arterioscler Thromb Vasc Biol 2001; 21: 372-377.
[123] Collins AR, Meehan WP, Kintscher U, *et al.* Troglitazone inhibits formation of early atherosclerotic lesions in diabetic and nondiabetic low density lipoprotein receptor-deficient mice. Arterioscler Thromb Vasc Biol 2001; 21: 365-371.
[124] Canada, E.J., Gossett, L.S., Mantlo, N.B., Shi, Q., Wang, M., Warshawsky, A.M., Xu, Y.: US20070082907A1 **(2007)**.
[125] Winneroski, L.L. Jr., Xu, Y., York, J.S.: US20070037812A1 **(2007)**.
[126] Tall AR, Abreu E, Shuman J. Separation of a plasma phospholipid transfer protein from cholesterol ester:phospholipid exchange protein. J Biol Chem 1983; 258: 2174-2180.
[127] Rao R, Albers JJ, Wolfbauer G, *et al.* Molecular and macromolecular specificity of human plasma phospholipid transfer protein. Biochemistry 1997; 36: 3645-3653.
[128] Rye KA, Barter PJ. Changes in the size and density of human high-density lipoproteins promoted by a plasma-conversion factor. Biochim Biophys Acta 1986; 875: 429-438.
[129] Tu AY, Nishida HI, Nishida T. High density lipoprotein conversion mediated by human plasma phospholipid transfer protein. J Biol Chem 1993; 268: 23098-23105.
[130] Jauhiainen M, Metso J, Pahlman R, *et al.* Human plasma phospholipid transfer protein causes high density lipoprotein conversion. J Biol Chem 1993; 268: 4032-4036.
[131] Castro GR, Fielding CJ. Early incorporation of cell-derived cholesterol into pre-beta-migrating high-density lipoprotein. Biochemistry 1988; 27: 25-29.
[132] von Eckardstein A, Jauhiainen M, Huang Y, *et al.* Phospholipid transfer protein mediated conversion of high density lipoproteins generates prebeta 1-HDL. Biochim Biophys Acta 1996; 1301: 255-262.

[133] van Haperen R, van Tol A, Vermeulen P, *et al.* Human plasma phospholipid transfer protein increases the antiatherogenic potential of high density lipoproteins in transgenic mice. Arterioscler Thromb Vasc Biol 2000; 20: 1082-1088.

[134] Jiang XC, Bruce C, Mar J, *et al.* Targeted mutation of plasma phospholipid transfer protein gene markedly reduces high-density lipoprotein levels. J Clin Invest 1999; 103: 907-914.

[135] Day JR, Albers JJ, Lofton-Day CE, *et al.* Complete cDNA encoding human phospholipid transfer protein from human endothelial cells. J Biol Chem 1994; 269: 9388-9391.

[136] Beamer LJ, Carroll SF, Eisenberg D. Crystal structure of human BPI and two bound phospholipids at 2.4 angstrom resolution. Science 1997; 276: 1861-1864.

[137] Huuskonen J, Wohlfahrt G, Jauhiainen M, *et al.* Structure and phospholipid transfer activity of human PLTP: analysis by molecular modeling and site-directed mutagenesis. J Lipid Res 1999; 40: 1123-1130.

[138] Huuskonen J, Jauhiainen M, Ehnholm C, *et al.* Biosynthesis and secretion of human plasma phospholipid transfer protein. J Lipid Res 1998; 39: 2021-2030.

[139] Qu SJ, Fan HZ, Kilinc C, *et al.* Role of cysteine residues in human plasma phospholipid transfer protein. J Prot Chem 1999; 18: 193-198.

[140] Massey JB, Hickson D, She HS, *et al.* Measurement and prediction of the rates of spontaneous transfer of phospholipids between plasma lipoproteins. Biochim Biophys Acta 1984; 794: 274-280.

[141] Huuskonen J, Olkkonen VM, Jauhiainen M, *et al.* Acyl chain and headgroup specificity of human plasma phospholipid transfer protein. Biochim Biophys Acta 1996; 1303: 207-214.

[142] Kawano K, Qin S-C, Lin M, *et al.* CETP and PLTP have non-overlapping functions *in vivo*. J Biol Chem 2000; 275: 29477-29841.

[143] Cheung MC, Wolfbauer G, Albers JJ. Plasma phospholipid mass transfer rate: relationship to plasma phospholipid and cholesteryl ester transfer activities and lipid parameters. Biochim Biophys Acta 1996; 1303: 103-10.

[144] Brown ML, Hesler C, Tall AR. Plasma enzymes and transfer proteins in cholesterol metabolism. Curr Opin Lipidol 1990; 1: 122-7.

[145] Yu B, Hailman E, Wright SD. Lipopolysaccharide binding protein and soluble CD14 catalyze exchange of phospholipids. J Clin Invest 1997; 99: 315-24.

[146] Ehnholm S, Willems K, Belinda H, *et al.* Adenovirus mediated overexpression of human phospholipid transfer protein alters plasma HDL levels in mice. J Lipid Res 1998; 39: 1248-53.

[147] Yang XP, Yan D, Qiao C, *et al.* Increased atherosclerotic lesions in apoE mice with plasma phospholipid transfer protein overexpression. Arterioscler Thromb Vasc Biol 2003; 23:1601-7.

[148] Vikstedt R, Ye D, Metso J, *et al.* Macrophage phospholipid transfer protein contributes significantly to total plasma phospholipid transfer activity and its deficiency leads to diminished atherosclerotic lesion development. Arterioscler Thromb Vasc Biol 2007; 27: 578-86.

[149] Albers JJ, Wolfbauer G, Cheung MC, *et al.* Functional expression of human and mouse plasma phospholipid transfer protein: effect of recombinant and plasma PLTP on HDL subspecies. Biochim Biophys Acta 1995; 1258: 27-34.

[150] Pussinen P, Jauhiainen M, Metso J, *et al.* Pig plasma phospholipid transfer protein facilitates HDL interconversion. J Lipid Res 1995; 36: 975-985.

[151] Marques-Vidal P, Jauhiainen M, Metso J, *et al.* Transformation of high density lipoprotein 2 particles by hepatic lipase and phospholipid transfer protein. Atherosclerosis 1997; 133: 87-95.

[152] Nishida HI, Klock DG, Guo Z, *et al.* Phospholipid transfer protein can transform reconstituted discoidal HDL into vesicular structures. Biochim Biophys Acta 1997; 1349: 222-232.

[153] Föger B, Santamarina-Fojo S, Shamburek RD, *et al.* Plasma phospholipid transfer protein. Adenovirus-mediated overexpression in mice leads to decreased plasma high density lipoprotein (HDL) and enhanced hepatic uptake of phospholipids and cholesteryl esters from HDL. J Biol Chem 1997; 272: 27393-27400.

[154] Ehnholm S, van Dijk KW, van't Hof B, *et al.* Adenovirus mediated overexpression of human phospholipid transfer protein alters plasma HDL levels in mice. J Lipid Res 1998; 39: 1248-1253.

[155] Albers JJ, Tu AY, Paigen B, *et al.* Transgenic mice expressing human phospholipid transfer protein have increased HDL:non-HDL cholesterol ratio. Int J Clin Lab Res 1996; 26: 262-267.

[156] Jiang X, Francone OL, Bruce C, *et al.* Increased prebeta-high density lipoprotein, apolipoprotein AI, and phospholipid in mice expressing the human phospholipid transfer protein and human apolipoprotein AI transgenes. J Clin Invest 1996; 98: 2373-80.

[157] van Tol A, Jauhiainen M, de Crom R, *et al.* Role of phospholipid transfer protein in high-density lipoprotein metabolism: insights from studies in transgenic mice. Int J Tissue React 2000; XXII: 79-84.

[158] Krieger M. The other side of scavenger receptors: pattern recognition for host defense. Curr Opin Lipidol 1997; 8: 275-280.

[159] Brown MS, Goldstein JL. Lipoprotein metabolism in the macrophage: implications for cholesterol deposition in atherosclerosis. Annu Rev Biochem 1983; 52: 223-261.

[160] Krieger M, Herz J. Structures and functions of multiligand lipoprotein receptors: macrophage scavenger receptors and LDL receptor- related protein (LRP). Annu Rev Biochem 1994; 63: 601-637.

[161] Acton SL, Scherer PE, Lodish HF, *et al.* Expression cloning of SR-BI, a CD36-related class B scavenger receptor. J Biol Chem 1994; 269: 21003-21009.

[162] Acton S, Rigotti A, Landschulz KT, *et al.* Identification of scavenger receptor SR-BI as a high density lipoprotein receptor. Science 1996; 271: 518-520.

[163] Williams DL, Connelly MA, Temel RE, *et al.* Scavenger receptor BI and cholesterol trafficking. Curr Opin Lipidol 1999; 10: 329-339.

[164] Kozarsky KF, Donahee MH, Rigotti A, *et al.* Overexpression of the HDL receptor SR-BI alters plasma HDL and bile cholesterol levels. Nature 1997; 387: 414-417.

[165] Trigatti B, Rayburn H, Viñals M, *et al.* Influence of the high density lipoprotein receptor SR-BI on reproductive and cardiovascular pathophysiology. Proc Natl Acad Sci USA 1999; 96: 9322-9327.

[166] Huszar D, Varban ML, Rinninger F, *et al.* Increased LDL cholesterol and atherosclerosis in LDL receptor-deficient mice with attenuated expression of scavenger receptor B1. Arterioscler Thromb Vasc Biol 2000; 20: 1068-1073.

[167] Arai T, Wang N, Bezouevski M, *et al.* Decreased atherosclerosis in heterozygous low density lipoprotein receptor- deficient mice expressing the scavenger receptor BI transgene. J Biol Chem 1999; 274: 2366-2371.

[168] Ueda Y, Gong E, Royer L, *et al.* Relationship between expression levels and atherogenesis in scavenger receptor class B, type I transgenics. J Biol Chem 2000; 275: 20368-20373.

[169] Kozarsky KF, Donahee MH, Glick JM, *et al.* Gene transfer and hepatic overexpression of the HDL receptor SRBI reduces atherosclerosis in the cholesterol-fed LDL receptor-deficient mouse. Arterioscler Thromb Vasc Biol 2000; 20: 721-727.

[170] Rigotti A, Trigatti BL, Penman M, *et al.* A targeted mutation in the murine gene encoding the high density lipoprotein (HDL) receptor scavenger receptor class B type I reveals its key in HDL metabolism. Proc Natl Acad Sci USA 1997; 94: 12610-12615.

[171] Varban ML, Rinninger F, Wang N, *et al.* Targeted mutation reveals a central role for SR-BI in hepatic selective uptake of high density lipoprotein cholesterol. Proc Natl Acad Sci USA 1998; 95: 4619-4624.

[172] Calvo D, Gomez-Coronado D, Lasuncion MA, *et al.* CLA-1 is an 85-kD plasma membrane glycoprotein that acts as a high-affinity receptor for both native (HDL, LDL, and VLDL) and modified (OxLDL and AcLDL) lipoproteins. Arterioscler Thromb Vasc Biol 1997; 17: 2341-2349.

[173] Calvo D, Vega MA. Identification, primary structure, and distribution of CLA-1, a novel member of the CD36/LIMPII gene family. J Biol Chem 1993; 268: 18929-18935.

[174] Murao K, Terpstra V, Green SR, *et al.* Characterization of CLA-1, a human homologue of rodent scavenger receptor BI, as a receptor for high density lipoprotein and apoptotic thymocytes. J Biol Chem 1997; 272: 17551-17557.

[175] Rigotti A, Trigatti B, Babitt J, *et al.* Scavenger receptor BI. A cell surface receptor for high density lipoprotein. Curr Opin Lipidol 1997; 8: 181-188.

[176] Krieger M. The 'best' of cholesterols, the 'worst' of cholesterols: a tale of two receptors. Proc Natl Acad Sci USA 1998; 95: 4077-4080.

[177] Compassi S, Gemperli A, Boffelli D, *et al.* Identification of a receptor mediating absorption of dietary cholesterol in the intestine. Biochemistry 1998; 37: 17843-17850.

[178] Rothblatt GH, Llera-Moya M, Atger V, *et al.* Cell cholesterol efflux: integration of old and new observations provides new insights. J Lipid Res 1999; 40: 781-796.

[179] Braun JEA, Severson DL. Regulation of the synthesis, processing and translocation of lipoprotein lipase. Biochem J 1992; 287: 337-347.

[180] Enerback S, Gimble JM. Lipoprotein lipase gene expression: physiological regulators at the transcriptional and post-transcriptional level. Biochim Biophys Acta 1993; 1168: 107-125.

[181] Zechner R. The tissue-specific expression of lipoprotein lipase: implications for energy and lipoprotein metabolism. Curr Opin Lipidol 1997: 8: 77-88.

[182] Zilversmit DB. A proposal linking atherogenesis to the interaction of endothelial lipoprotein lipase with triglyceride-rich lipoproteins. Circ Res 1973; 33(6): 633-8.

[183] Van Eck M, Zimmermann R, Groot PH, *et al.* Role of macrophage-derived lipoprotein lipase in lipoprotein metabolism and atherosclerosis. Arterioscler Thromb Vasc Biol 2000; 20(9): E53-E62.

[184] Corey JE, Zilversmit DB. Effect of cholesterol feeding on arterial lipolytic activity in the rabbit. Atherosclerosis 1977; 27(2): 201-12.

[185] Werba JP, Martinet V, Abulafia DP, *et al.* Marked neointimal lipoprotein lipase increase in distinct models of proclivity to atherosclerosis: a feature independent of endothelial layer integrity. Atherosclerosis 2001; 156(1): 91-101.

[186] Levak-Frank S, Weinstock PH, Hayek T, *et al.* Induced mutant mice expressing lipoprotein lipase exclusively in muscle have subnormal triglycerides yet reduced high density lipoprotein cholesterol levels in plasma. J Biol Chem 1997; 272: 17182-17190.

[187] Levak-Frank S, Hofmann W, Weinstock PH, *et al.* Induced mutant mouse lines that express lipoprotein lipase in cardiac muscle, but not in skeletal muscle and adipose tissue, have normal plasma triglyceride and high-density lipoprotein-cholesterol levels. Proc Natl Acad Sci USA 1999; 96: 3165-3170.

[188] Shimada M, Ishibashi S, Inaba T, *et al.* Suppression of diet-induced atherosclerosis in low density lipoprotein receptor knockout mice overexpressing lipoprotein lipase. Proc Natl Acad Sci USA 1996; 93(14): 7242-7246.

[189] Yagyu H, Ishibashi S, Chen Z, *et al.* Overexpressed lipoprotein lipase protects against atherosclerosis in apolipoprotein E knockout mice. J Lipid Res 1999; 40(9): 1677-1685.

[190] Benlian P, De Gennes JL, Foubert L, *et al.* Premature atherosclerosis in patients with familial chylomicronemia caused by mutations in the lipoprotein lipase gene. N Engl J Med 1996; 335: 848-854.

[191] Clee SM, Bissada N, Miao F, *et al.* Plasma and vessel wall lipoprotein lipase have different roles in atherosclerosis. J Lipid Res 2000; 41: 521-531.

[192] Zsigmond E, Kobayashi K, Tzung KW, *et al.* Adenovirus-mediated gene transfer of human lipoprotein lipase ameliorates the hyperlipidemias associated with apolipoprotein E and LDL receptor deficiencies in mice. Hum Gene Ther 1997; 8: 1921-1933.

[193] Blades B, Vega GL, Grundy SM. Activities of lipoprotein lipase and hepatic triglyceride lipase in postheparin plasma of patients with low concentrations of HDL cholesterol. Arterioscler Thromb Vasc Biol 1993; 13: 1227-1235.

[194] Hokanson JE. Lipoprotein lipase gene variants and risk of coronary disease: a quantitative analysis of population-based studies. Int J Clin Lab Res 1997; 27: 24-34.

[195] Tsutsumi K, Inoue Y, Shima A, *et al.* The novel compound NO-1886 and on lipase increases lipoprotein lipase activity with resulting elevation of high density lipoprotein cholesterol, and long-term administration inhibits atherogenesis in the coronary arteries of rats with experimental atherosclerosis. J Clin Invest 1993; 92: 411-417.

[196] Schoonjans K, Peinado-Onsurbe J, Fruchart JC, *et al.* 3-Hydroxy-3- methylglutaryl CoA reductase inhibitors reduce serum triglyceride levels through modulation of apolipoprotein C-III and lipoprotein. FEBS Lett 1999; 452: 160-164.

[197] Fruchart JC, Staels B, Duriez P. The role of fibric acids in atherosclerosis. Curr Atheroscler Rep 2001; 3: 83-92.

[198] Mead JR, Cryer A, Ramji DP. Lipoprotein lipase, a key role in atherosclerosis. FEBS Lett 1999; 462(1-2): 1-6.

[199] Olivecrona G, Olivecrona T. Triglyceride lipases and atherosclerosis. Curr Opin Lipidol 1995; 6(5): 291-305.

[200] Goldberg IJ. Lipoprotein lipase and lipolysis: central roles in lipoprotein metabolism and atherogenesis. J Lipid Res 1996; 37(4): 693-707.

[201] Beisiegel U. New aspects on the role of plasma lipases in lipoprotein catabolism and atherosclerosis. Atherosclerosis 1996; 124(1): 1-8.

[202] Markku O, Pentikainen MO, Oksjoki R, *et al.* Lipoprotein lipase in the arterial wall: linking LDL to the arterial extracellular matrix and much more. Arterioscler Thromb Vasc Biol 2002; 22(2): 211-217.

[203] Santamarina-Fojo S, Haudenschild C, Amar M. The role of hepatic lipase in lipoprotein metabolism and atherosclerosis. Curr Opin Lipidol 1998: 9: 211-219.

[204] Ragab A, Rittner U, Danet C, *et al.* Competitive PCR as a tool to study hepatic lipase regulation in Hep G2 cells. Bull Mol Biol Med 1995; 20: 19-21.

[205] Busch SJ, Barnhart RL, Martin GA, *et al.* Human hepatic triglyceride lipase expression reduces high density lipoprotein and aortic cholesterol in cholesterol-fed transgenic mice. J Biol Chem 1994; 269: 16376-16382.

[206] Dichek HL, Brecht W, Fan J, *et al.* Overexpression of hepatic lipase in transgenic mice decreases apolipoprotein B-containing and high density lipoproteins. Evidence that hepatic lipase acts as a ligand for lipoprotein uptake. J Biol Chem 1998; 273: 1896-1903.

[207] Braschi S, Couture N, Gambarotta A, *et al.* Hepatic lipase affects both HDL and ApoB-containing lipoprotein levels in the mouse. Biochim Biophys Acta 1998; 1392: 276-290.

[208] Fan J, Wang J, Bensadoun A, *et al.* Overexpression of hepatic lipase in transgenic rabbits leads to a marked reduction of plasma high density lipoproteins and intermediate density lipoproteins. Proc Natl Acad Sci USA 1994; 91: 8724-8728.

[209] Barbagallo CM, Fan J, Blanche PJ, *et al.* Overexpression of human hepatic lipase and ApoE in transgenic rabbits attenuates response to dietary cholesterol and alters lipoprotein subclass distributions. Arterioscler Thromb Vasc Biol 1999; 19: 625-632.

[210] Applebaum-Bowden D, Kobayashi J, Kashyap VS, *et al.* Hepatic lipase gene therapy in hepatic-lipase deficient mice. Adenovirus-mediated replacement of a lipolytic enzyme to the vascular endothelium. J Clin Invest 1996; 97: 799-805.

[211] Dugi KA, Vaisman BL, Sakai N, *et al.* Adenovirus-mediated expression of hepatic lipase in LCAT transgenic mice. J Lipid Res 1997; 38: 1822-1832.

[212] Amar MJ, Dugi KA, Haudenschild CC, *et al.* Hepatic lipase facilitates the selective uptake of cholesteryl esters from remnant lipoproteins in apoE-deficient mice. J Lipid Res 1998; 39: 2436-2442.

[213] Connelly PW, Maguire GF, Lee M, *et al.* Plasma lipoproteins in familial hepatic lipase deficiency. Arteriosclerosis 1990; 10: 40-48.

[214] Hegele R, Little JA, Vezina C, *et al.* Hepatic lipase deficiency: clinical, biochemical, and molecular genetic characteristics. Arterioscler Thromb 1993; 13: 720-728.

[215] Descamps V, Blumenfeld N, Villeval J-L, *et al.* Erythropoientin gene transfer and expression in adult normal mice: use of an adenovirus vector. Hum Gene Ther 1994; 5: 979-985.

[216] Katzel LI, Coon PJ, Busby MJ, *et al.* Reduced HDL2 cholesterol subspecies and elevated postheparin hepatic lipase activity in older men with abdominal obesity and asymptomatic myocardial ischemia. Arterioscler Thromb 1992; 12: 814-823.

[217] Dugi KA, Brandauer K, Schmidt N, *et al.* Low hepatic lipase activity is a novel risk factor for coronary artery disease. Circulation 2001; 104: 3057-3062.

[218] Zambon A, Brown BG, Deeb SS, *et al.* Hepatic lipase as a focal point for the development and treatment of coronary artery disease. J Invest Med 2001; 49: 112-118.

[219] Mezdour H, Jones R, Dengremont C, *et al.* Hepatic lipase deficiency increases plasma cholesterol but reduces susceptibility to atherosclerosis in apolipoprotein E-deficient mice. J Biol Chem 1997; 272: 13570-13575.

[220] Nong Z, Gonzalez-Navarro H, Amar M, *et al.* Hepatic lipase expression in macrophages contributes to atherosclerosis in apoEdeficient and LCAT-transgenic mice. J Clin Invest 2003; 112: 367-378.

[221] Aviram M, Bierman EL, Chait A. Modification of low-density lipoprotein by lipoprotein lipase or hepatic lipase induces enhanced uptake and cholesterol accumulation in cells. J Biol Chem 1988; 263: 15416-15422.

[222] Jaye M, Lynch KJ, Krawiec J, *et al.* A novel endothelial-derived lipase that modulates HDL metabolism. Nat Genet 1999; 21: 424-428.

[223] McCoy MG, Sun GS, Marchadier D, *et al.* 2002. Characterization of the lipolytic activity of endothelial lipase. J Lipid Res 43: 921-929.

[224] Ji ZS, Lauer SJ, Fazio S, *et al.* Enhanced binding and uptake of remnant lipoproteins by hepatic lipase-secreting hepatoma cells in culture. J Biol Chem 1994; 269: 13429-13436.

[225] Fuki IV, Blanchard N, Jin W, *et al.* Endogenously produced endothelial lipase enhances binding and cellular processing of plasma lipoproteins via HSPG-mediated pathway. J Biol Chem 2003; 278: 34331-34338.

[226] Jin W, Millar JS, Broedl U, *et al.* Inhibition of endothelial lipase causes increased HDL cholesterol levels *in vivo*. J Clin Invest 2003; 111: 357-362.

[227] Ma K, Cilingiroglu M, Otvos JD, *et al.* Endothelial lipase is a major genetic determinant for high-density lipoprotein concentration, structure, and metabolism. Proc Natl Acad Sci USA 2003; 100: 2748-2753.

[228] Broedl UC, Maugeais C, Marchadier D, *et al.* Effects of nonlipolytic ligand function of endothelial lipase on HDL metabolism *in vivo*. J Biol Chem 2003; 278: 40688-40693.

[229] Qiu X, Mistry A, Ammirati MJ, *et al.* Crystal structure of cholesteryl ester transfer protein reveals a long tunnel and four bound lipid molecules. Nat Struct Mol Biol 2007; 14: 106-113.

[230] Barter PJ, Hopkins CJ, Calvert GD. Transfers and exchanges of esterified cholesterol between plasma lipoproteins. Biochem J 1982; 208: 1-7.

[231] de Grooth GJ, Smilde TJ, Van Wissen S, *et al.* The relationship between cholesteryl ester transfer protein levels and risk factor profile in patients with familial hypercholesterolemia. Atherosclerosis 2004; 173: 261-267.

[232] McPherson R, Mann CJ, Tall AR, *et al.* Plasma concentrations of cholesteryl ester transfer protein in hyperlipoproteinemia. Relation to cholesteryl ester transfer protein activity and other lipoprotein variables. Arterioscler Thromb 1991; 11: 797-804.

[233] Moulin P, Appel GB, Ginsberg HN, *et al.* Increased concentration of plasma cholesteryl ester transfer protein in nephrotic syndrome: role in dyslipidemia. J Lipid Res 1992; 33: 1817-22.

[234] Van Tol A. CETP-catalysed transfer of cholesterylesters from HDL to apo B-containing lipoproteins in plasma from diabetic patients. Eur J Clin Invest 1993; 23: 856.

[235] de Grooth GJ, Klerkx AH, Stroes ES, *et al.* A review of CETP and its relation to atherosclerosis. J Lipid Res 2004; 45: 1967-74.

[236] Agellon LB, Walsh A, Hayek T, *et al.* Reduced high density lipoprotein cholesterol in human cholesteryl ester transfer protein transgenic mice. J Biol Chem 1991; 266: 10796-10801.

[237] Plump AS, Masucci-Magoulas L, Bruce C, *et al.* Increased atherosclerosis in apoE and LDL receptor gene knock-out mice as a result of human cholesteryl ester transfer protein transgene expression. Arterioscler Thromb Vasc Biol 1999; 19: 1105-1110.

[238] Inazu A, Brown ML, Hesler CB, *et al.* Increased high-density lipoprotein levels caused by a common cholesteryl-ester transfer protein gene mutation. N Engl J Med 1990; 323: 1234-1238.

[239] Ikewaki K, Rader DJ, Sakamoto T, *et al.* Delayed catabolism of high density lipoprotein apolipoprotein A-I and A-II in human cholesteryl ester transfer protein deficiency. J Clin Invest 1993; 92: 1650-1658.

[240] Sugano M, Makino N, Sawada S, *et al.* Effect of antisense oligonucleotides against cholesteryl ester transfer protein on the development of atherosclerosis in cholesterol-fed rabbits. J Biol Chem 1998; 273: 5033-5036.

[241] Sugano M, Sawada S, Tsuchida K, *et al.* Low density lipoproteins develop resistance to oxidative modification due to inhibition of cholesteryl ester transfer protein by a monoclonal antibody. J Lipid Res 2000; 41: 126-133.

[242] Whitlock ME, Swenson TL, Ramakrishnan R, *et al.* Monoclonal antibody inhibition of cholesteryl ester transfer protein activity in the rabbit. J Clin Invest 1989; 84: 129-137.

[243] Connolly DT, Heuvelman D, Glenn KC. Inactivation of cholesteryl ester transfer protein by cysteine modification. Biochem Biophys Res Commun 1996; 223: 42-47.

[244] Epps DE, Vosters AF. The essential role of a free sulfhydryl group in blocking the cholesteryl site of cholesteryl ester transfer protein (CETP). Chem Phys Lipids 2002; 114: 113-122.

[245] Hope HR, Heuvelman D, Duffin K, *et al.* Inhibition of cholesteryl ester transfer protein by substituted dithiobis-nicotinic acid dimethyl ester: involvement of a critical cysteine. J Lipid Res 2000; 41: 1604-1610.

[246] Shinkai H, Maeda K, Yamasaki T, *et al.* Bis-[2-(acylamino)-phenyl] disulfides, 2-(acylamino)benzenethiols, and S-[2-(acylamino)phenyl] alkane-thioates as novel inhibitors of cholesteryl ester transfer protein. J Med Chem 2000; 43: 3566-3572.

[247] Maeda K, Okamoto H, Shinkai H. S-[2-(Acylamino)phenyl] 2,2-dimethylpropane-thioates as CETP Inhibitors. Bioorg Med Chem Lett 2004; 14: 2589-2591.

[248] Paulsen H, Schmeck C, Brandes A, *et al.* Fluorine-substitution in cholesteryl ester transfer protein inhibitors (CETP-inhibitors): biology, chemistry, SAR, and properties. Chimia 2004; 58: 123-127.

[249] Schmidt, G., Angerbauer, R., Brandes, A., Logers, M., Muller-Gliemann, M., Bischoff, H., Schmidt, D., Wohlfeil, S.: US6127383 **(2000)**.

[250] Mueller-Gliemann, M., Angerbauer, R., Brandes, A., Loegers, M., Schmeck, C., Schmidt, G., Bremm, K.D., Bischoff, H., Schmidt, D.: US6121330 **(2000)**.

[251] Mueller-Gliemann, M., Angerbauer, R., Brandes, A., Loegers, M., Schmeck, C., Schmidt, G., Bremm, K.D., Bischoff, H., Schmidt, D.: WO9839299 **(1998)**.

[252] Schmeck, C., Mueller-Gliemann, M., Schmidt, G., Brandes, A., Angerbauer, R., Loegers, M., Bremm, K.D., Bischoff, H., Schmidt, D., Schuhmacher, J.: US5932587 **(1999)**.

[253] Schmidt, G., Stoltefuss, J., Loegers, M., Brandes, A., Schmeck, C., Bremm, K.-D., Bischoff, H., Schmidt, D.: US6562976 **(2003)**.

[254] Ruggeri RB, Wester RT, Magnus-Aryitey G. Discovery of CP- 529,414: A potent synthetic inhibitor of human plasma cholesteryl ester transfer protein (CETP). *225th ACS Meeting*, Washington, DC, USA (2003).

[255] Goldstein, S.W., Makowski, M.R., Ruggeri, R.B., Wester, R.T.: US6362198 **(2002)**.

[256] Barter PJ, Caulfield M, Eriksson M, *et al.* Effects of torcetrapib in patients at high risk for coronary events. N Engl J Med 2007; 357: 2109-2122.

[257] Chapman MJ. Therapeutic elevation of HDLcholesterol to prevent atherosclerosis and coronary heart disease. Pharmacol Ther 2006; 111: 893-908.

[258] Segrest JP, Garber DW, Brouillette CG, *et al.* The amphipathic alpha helix: a multifunctional structural motif in plasma apolipoproteins. Adv Protein Chem 1994; 45: 303-369.

[259] Reschly EJ, Sorci-Thomas MG, Davidson WS, *et al.* Apolipoprotein A-I a-helices 7 and 8 modulate high density lipoprotein subclass distribution. J Biol Chem 2002; 277: 9645-9654.

[260] Fielding CJ, Fielding PE. Molecular physiology of reverse cholesterol transport. J Lipid Res 1995; 36: 211-228.

[261] Liu T, Krieger M, Kan HY, *et al.* The effects of mutations in helices 4 and 6 of ApoA-I on scavenger receptor class B type I (SR-BI)-mediated cholesterol efflux suggest that formation of a productive complex between reconstituted high density lipoprotein and SR-BI is required for efficient lipid transport. J Biol Chem 2002; 277: 21576-21584.

[262] Arakawa R, Yokoyama S. Helical apolipoproteins stabilize ATP-binding cassette transporter A1 by protecting it from thiol protease-mediated degradation. J Biol Chem 2002; 277: 22426-22429.

[263] Kwiterovich PO. The antiatherogenic role of high-density lipoprotein cholesterol. Am J Cardiol 1998; 82: 13Q-21Q.

[264] Van der Steeg WA, Holme I, Boekholdt SM, *et al.* High-density lipoprotein cholesterol, high-density lipoprotein particle size, and apolipoprotein-A-I: Significance for cardiovascular risk. J Am Coll Cardiol 2008; 51(6): 634-42.

[265] Sirtori CR, Calabresi L, Franceschini G, *et al.* Cardiovascular status of carriers of the apolipoprotein A-I_{Milano} mutant: the limone sul Garda study. Circulation 2001; 103: 1949-1954.

[266] Nissen SE, Tsunoda T, Tuzcu EM, *et al.* Effect of recombinant ApoA-I milano on coronary atherosclerosis in patients with acute coronary syndromes. JAMA 2003; 290: 2292-2300.

[267] Navab M, Anantharamaiah GM, Reddy ST, *et al.* Apolipoprotein A-I mimetic peptides. Arterioscler Thromb Vasc Biol 2005; 25:1325-1331.

[268] Garber DW, Datta G, Chaddha M, *et al.* A new synthetic class a amphipathic peptide analogue protects mice from diet-induced atherosclerosis. J Lipid Res 2001; 42: 545-552.

[269] Navab M, Anantharamaiah GM, Hama S, *et al.* Oral administration of an Apo A-I mimetic Peptide synthesized from d-amino acids dramatically reduces atherosclerosis in mice independent of plasma cholesterol. Circulation 2002; 105: 290-292.

[270] Navab M, Anantharamaiah GM, Reddy ST, *et al.* Oral D-4F causes formation of Pre-ß high-density lipoprotein and improves high-density lipoprotein–mediated cholesterol efflux and reverse cholesterol transport from macrophages in apolipoprotein E–Null mice. Circulation 2004; 109: 3215-3220.

[271] Li X, Chyu K-Y, Neto JRF, *et al.* Differential effects of apolipoprotein A-I–mimetic peptide on evolving and established atherosclerosis in apolipoprotein E-Null mice. Circulation 2004; 110: 1701-1705.

[272] Rodrigueza WV, Mazany KD, Essenburg AD, *et al.* Large *versus* small unilamellar vesicles mediate reverse cholesterol transport *in vivo* into two distinct hepatic metabolic pools. Implications for the treatment of atherosclerosis. Arterioscler Thromb Vasc Biol 1997; 17: 2132-2139.

[273] Newton RS, Krause BR. HDL therapy for the acute treatment of atherosclerosis. Atheroscler Suppl 2002; 3: 31-38.

[274] Stamler CJ, Breznan D, Neville T, Viau FJ, Camlioglu E, Sparks DL. Phosphatidylinositol promotes cholesterol transport *in vivo*. J Lipid Res 2000; 41: 1214-1221.

[275] Burgess JW, Boucher J, Neville T, *et al.* Phosphatidylinositol promotes cholesterol transport and excretion. J Lipid Res 2003; 44: 1355-1363.

[276] Burgess JW, Neville T, Rouillard P, Harder Z, Beanlands DS, Sparks DL. Phosphatidylinositol increases HDL-C levels in humans. J Lipid Res 2005; 46: 350-355.

[277] Nicholls SJ, Dusting GJ, Cutri B, *et al.* Reconstituted high-density lipoproteins inhibit the acute pro-oxidant and proinflammatory vascular changes induced by aperiarterial collar in normocholesterolemic rabbits. Circulation 2005; 111: 1543-1550.

[278] Lerch PG, Spycher MO, Doran JE. Reconstituted high density lipoprotein (rHDL) modulates platelet activity *in vitro* and *ex vivo*. Thromb Haemost 1998; 80: 316-320.

[279] Bisoendial RJ, Hovingh GK, Levels JHM, *et al.* Restoration of endothelial function by increasing high-density lipoprotein in subjects with isolated low high-density lipoprotein. Circulation 2003; 107: 2944-2948.

[280] Spieker LE, Sudano I, Hurlimann D, *et al.* High-density lipoprotein restores endothelial function in hypercholesterolemic men. Circulation 2002; 105: 1399-1402.

[281] Sumi M, Sata M, Miura S, *et al.* Reconstituted high-density lipoprotein stimulates differentiation of endothelial progenitor cells and enhances ischemia-induced angiogenesis. Arterioscler Thromb Vasc Biol 2007; 27: 813-818.

[282] Tardif JC, Gregoire J, Lallier PL, *et al.* Effects of reconstituted high-density lipoprotein infusions on coronary atherosclerosis: a randomized controlled trial. JAMA 2007; 297: 1675-1682.

Frontiers in Cardiovascular Drug Discovery, **2010**, *1*, 61-72

New Approaches to Atherosclerotic Cardiovascular Disease: The Potential of Torcetrapib

Jose Luis Pérez-Castrillon* and Antonio Dueñas-Laita

Hospital Rio Hortega, University of Valladolid, Valladolid, Spain

Abstract: Atherosclerosis is the leading cause of death and disability in the developed world. Although low-density lipoprotein (LDL) cholesterol lowering drugs reduce the mortality and morbidity associated with coronary artery disease, mortality and morbidity remain high. Reverse cholesterol transport mediated by high-density lipoproteins (HDL) may provide an independent pathway for lipid removal from atheroma. The current NCEP ATPIII include HDL-cholesterol ≥1.6 mmol/l as a negative risk factor. Torcetrapib is an inhibitor of cholesteryl ester-transfer protein (CETP) that increases HDL-cholesterol levels. Published studies show a favourable lipid profile of torcetrapib but no clinical efficacy, with greater mortality, lack of antiatherosclerotic action and increased blood pressure and aldosterone, leading to its use being abandoned. However, these detrimental effects are related to the molecule itself and not to CETP inhibition.Raising HDL-cholesterol by CETP inhibition could be a new approach to atherosclerotic cardiovascular disease, although trials based on hard clinical end points are necessary.

Keywords: Atherosclerosis, HDL-cholesterol, LDL-cholesterol, Statins, Torcetrapib, CETP.

INTRODUCTION

Atherosclerosis is an important cause of death in developed countries and is associated with high morbidity and health costs. Cardiovascular diseases cause 38 % of deaths in North America and are the main cause of death in European men under 65 years and the second cause in women [1]. Studies have demonstrated the beneficial effect of statins through their action of lowering total cholesterol and LDL-cholesterol levels, together with other pleiotropic mechanisms unrelated to dyslipemia. However, despite this and the use of aggressive therapies, high levels of morbidity and mortality of vascular origin persist. Therefore, the search for new, complementary therapeutic objectives to solve this health problem is ongoing.

The aim of this review is to describe reported data on the utility of increasing HDL-cholesterol in order to reduce cardiovascular morbidity and mortality, the antiatherogenic mechanisms of HDL-cholesterol and the characteristics of the drug torcetrapib, especially its mechanism of action through CETP (cholesterol ester transfer protein) inhibition and the results of the use of torcetrapib in humans.

*Corresponding author: Tel: +34 983420400; E-mail: castrv@terra.es

HDL-CHOLESTEROL. PROTECTIVE EFFECT

The HDL-cholesterol particle is a protein complex constituted of different apolipoproteins, of which the most abundant, apoA-I and apoA-II, are present in 2/3 of HDL particles, plus associated enzymes such as paraxonase, platelet-activated factor acetylhydrolase (PAF-AH), lecithin- cholesterolacyltransferase (LCAT) and plasma glutathione seleneperoxidase (GPX3) [2-6]. The outer layer is amphipathic and contains free cholesterol, apolipoproteins and phospholipids. The inner layer is hydrophobic and contains cholesteryl esters. ApoA-I plays an important protective role against atheroesclerosis as, a cholesterol acceptor whereas the role of apoA-II has not been clearly established.

The protective role of HDL-cholesterol has been demonstrated in various demographic studies and clinical trials. In one case-control study [7] of 6859 men and women from different ethnic groups, mean HDL-cholesterol levels were lower in subjects with coronary disease than in healthy controls: the differences remained significant after adjusting for levels of LDL-cholesterol and triglycerides. In the Framingham Study [8], lower levels of HDL-cholesterol were the main risk factor of lipidic origin [9] and remained so when the analysis was repeated after 12 years of monitoring. In four prospective American studies (Framingham Heart Study -FHS-, Lipid Research Clinics Prevalence Mortality Follow-up Study - LRCF-, Coronary Primary Prevention Trial -CPPT-, and Multiple Risk Factor Intervention Trial - MRFIT) an increase of 1 mg/dl in HDL-cholesterol led to a significant reduction in coronary disease of between 2 % and 4.7 % [10]. The Tromso Heart Study [11] prospectively assessed the relationship between HDL-cholesterol and coronary risk, and found an inverse relationship between the two parameters in men aged 20-49 years. In older men, low levels of HDL-cholesterol increased coronary mortality after 21-years of follow up [12]. The effect persisted after adjusting for other risk factors and was particularly intense in diabetics.

In the German PROCAM study, the relative risk of coronary disease was six-fold higher in patients with HDL-cholesterol < 35 mg/dl [13]. In two prospective studies using gemfibrozil, the Helsinki Heart study [14] in primary prevention and the Va-Hit study [15] in secondary prevention, a reduction in cardiovascular events was associated with an increase in HDL-cholesterol in the treated group. The Bezafibrate Coronary Atherosclerosis Intervention Trial (BECAIT) assessed the protective effect of bezafibrate on the progression of focused atherosclerosis measured by coronary angiography in patients with recent heart attack [16]. The treated group showed an increase in HDL-cholesterol of 90 % with a reduction in disease progression. The HDL Intervention Trial (HIT) evaluated the benefits obtained by increased HDL-cholesterol in patients with normal values of triglycerides and LDL-cholesterol [17]. A reduction in the incidence of heart attack, death of cardiovascular origin and ictus in the group treated with gemfibrozil was observed.

Studies evaluating the effect of statins on the reduction of coronary events show similar results. Five of six published studies showed an inverse relationship between HDL-cholesterol levels and coronary risk [18]. In some of those studies, specifically the LIPID and 4S studies [19, 20], part of the beneficial effect of statins was attributed to the increase in HDL or apoA-I, the main apolipoprotein of HDL. Recently, the EPIC study showed that lower levels of HDL-cholesterol were a risk factor for the recurrence of cardiovascular events [21].

These data, corroborated by the presence of lowered HDL-cholesterol in patients with metabolic syndrome [22], suggest a possible protective effect of HDL-cholesterol with increased levels being necessary in order to reduce coronary disease. Statins have successfully reduced coronary events in both primary and secondary prevention, even though marked morbidity and mortality persists, even when very-low levels of LDL-cholesterol are achieved [23]. The above evidence suggests that increasing HDL-cholesterol levels is an effective therapeutic option.

ANTIATHEROGENIC MECHANISMS OF HDL-CHOLESTEROL

Various epidemiological studies have shown a protective role of HDL-cholesterol in cardiovascular diseases. The mechanisms involved, although not clearly established, include [24]:

- Efflux of cholesterol from macrophages located in the vascular walls
- Inhibition of LDL-cholesterol oxidation
- Inhibition of inflammation
- Stabilization of endothelial tissue by nitric oxide (NO)

Efflux of Cholesterol from Cholesterol Loaded Macrophages

Atherosclerosis is a chronic inflammatory disease characterized by the accumulation of macrophages and T lymphocytes in arteries accompanied by an increase in plasma concentrations of inflammatory markers [25, 26]. Monocytes reach the arterial wall where they become macrophages expressing scavenger receptors with the ability to uptake LDL-cholesterol originating foam cells. These activated macrophages initiate the inflammatory mechanisms that perpetuate the inflammatory process, comprising the fatty grooves [27].

HDL-cholesterol participates by easing the outflow of cholesterol excess from peripheral tissues (macrophages in this case), which are transported to the liver and removed by bile excretion. This process is named reverse cholesterol transport [28]. The efflux of cholesterol from macrophages occurs through three different mechanisms. The ATP-binding cassette (ABC) transporter superfamily are membrane proteins which employ ATP as an energy source and are used to pass various elements through them. Macrophages are rich in ABCA1, whose expression is controlled by intracellular cholesterol levels [29]. It is sterified to oxysterol, which is attached to a transcription factor of LXR, which forms a dimeric structure with the X-retinoid receptor. The formed complex stimulates the expression of the carrier gene. Lack of function of this carrier, due to diverse mutations, causes Tangier disease, characterized by an absence of HDL-cholesterol and reduction in LDL-cholesterol with no marked increase in the risk of atherosclerosis [30]. This system contributes to the efflux of cholesterol from the macrophages located in the vascular wall but has little influence on plasmatic levels of HDL [31]. However, it plays an important role as an antiatherogenic agent. Independent mechanisms other than the ABCA1 system also contribute to plasmatic levels of HDL (ABCG1 and ABCG4) and help its incorporation to major HDL-2 and HDL-3 particles, which determine plasmatic levels [32].

Other mechanisms also play a role, including aqueous diffusion to phospholipid-containing acceptors [33] and the SR-B1 system, which promotes a bidirectional flow of cholesterol between cells and HDL, assisting efflux when the HDL are rich in phospholipids and poor in cholesterol [34].

Cholesterol from peripheral tissues is captured by nascent-HDL particles (rich in triglycerides and poor in cholesterol) synthesized in the liver and small bowel or by hydrolysis of rich particles in triglycerides with later shape modifications into spherical particles named HDL-2 and HDL-3. These particles are sterified by lecithin-cholesterol acyltransferase (LCAT), creating cholesterol esters which are transferred to the liver by three routes: CETP, which transfers cholesterol from HDL to triglycerides rich in lipoproteins, which are subsequently catabolized by the LDL receptor route; scavenger receptor B1 (SR-B1), which mediates the selective uptake of cholesterol esters by the liver; and, endocytosis of HDL holoparticles by a catabolic hepatic receptor [35].

Inhibition of LDL Oxidation

LDL-cholesterol particles penetrate the macrophages located in the vascular walls, where they are oxidized, producing their proatherogenic effect. This oxidation occurs when the lipidic hydroperoxides produced by the metabolic route of lipooxygenase and mieloperoxidase achieve a specific threshold [27]. The oxidized LDL penetrates the vessel walls and binds to it by means of VCAM-1 and E-selectin. They are captured by two scavenger receptors (CD-36 and SR-B1) located in the macrophage, leading to their activation. This activation determines the synthesis of adhesion and chemotactic molecules. The oxidation performed by HDL-cholesterol is inhibited by apoA-I, which removes hydroperoxides, and by various enzymes (paraoxonases, platelet-activated factor acetyl-hydrolase -PAF-AH-, LCAT, plasma glutathione selenoperoxidase) which destroy the lipidic hydroperoxides and hydrolyze the oxidized phospholipids [36].

Inhibition of Inflammation

An early event in atherogenesis is the adhesion of monocytes to the endothelium through adhesion molecules (VCAM-1, ICAM-1, E-selectin), which are rapidly synthesized in response to cytokines and C-reactive protein [37,38]. Native and reconstituted HDL-cholesterol can inhibit the expression of both these adhesion molecules and MCP-1 through blockade of an endothelial enzyme, sphingosine kinase, acting in the NF-kB pathway, used by TNF-α to stimulate the expression of adhesion molecules [27,39].

Stabilization of Endothelial Tissue through Nitric Oxide (NO)

Vascular endothelial injuries perform a key role in the pathogenesis of atherosclerosis. The integrity of endothelia maintains a series of activities that generate an atheroprotective effect, with NO playing a key role in maintaining this function. HDL-cholesterol particles take part by inhibiting the effects of oxidized LDL-cholesterol and lead to vasodilatation through the release of NO after attaching to SR-B1. NO activation is mediated by NOS (endothelial nitric oxide synthetase) [40].

TORCETRAPIB

Low HDL-cholesterol levels are a lipid abnormality frequently observed in patients with known coronary disease and therapies that increase the level of HDL-cholesterol and decrease vascular risk have been searched for. Cholestyramine increases HDL-cholesterol levels by 3 to 5%, statins by 5 to 15% and fibrates by 10 to 15%. The magnitude these effects is not considerable, especially when compared with LDL-cholesterol reduction, which ranges from 15 to 30% for cholestyramine, 30 to 50% for statins and 10 to 15% for fibrates [41]. Apart from these therapies, clinical information on three types of drugs is also available: agonists of nuclear receptors (PPARα, PPARδ, PPARγ), CETP inhibitors and infusion of apolipoproteins or synthetic HDL particles, which could act as cholesterol acceptors [42]. Many therapeutic alternatives have been designed to inhibit CETP: immunological modulators of protein activity [43,44], JTT705, a drug which binds to protein through disulfide bridges [45] and torcetrapib [46-51], which is objective of this review.

Torcetrapib is a molecule with the chemical formula 4-[3,5-Bis-trifluoromethybenzyl-methoxycarbonyl-amino]-2-ethyl-6-trifluoromehtyl-3,4-dihydro-2H-quinoline-1-carbo-xylic acid ethyl ester. It acts by inhibiting CETP. This mechanism increases HDL-cholesterol and reduces LDL-cholesterol and apolipoprotein B. Low HDL-cholesterol levels are the most-frequently seen lipid abnormality in patients with known coronary disease, and currently available drugs have only a moderate effect. Statins increase HDL levels by only 5-10%, while fibrates and niacines rarely achieve more than 25%. This justifies the need for new drugs such as torcetrapib. Therefore, we will analyse the effect of CETP, the target protein of torcetrapib, on vascular risk, and review studies carried out using torcetrapib.

Cholesteryl Ester Transfer Protein

CETP is a glycoprotein physically associated with HDL particles. It helps transport cholesterol ester from HDL to lipoproteins that contain apolipoprotein B (very low density lipoprotein - VLDL -, VLDL remnants, intermediate density lipoprotein - IDL - and low density lipoprotein - LDL -). This process is followed by the transfer of triglycerides in the opposite direction [52].

Plasma CETP levels range between 1 and 3 μg/ml in healthy individuals and may be twice or three times as high in patients with hypercholesterolemia, especially if triglyceride levels are high. As mentioned, it has been shown that a human CETP genetic deficit is associated with high levels of HDL, which have a possible protective effect on atherosclerosis. Therefore, the possibility of using CETP inhibitors as a therapeutic option has been suggested. Theoretically, CETP inhibition could have a proatherogenic effect by reducing the metabolic pathway of reverse cholesterol. However, small population-based studies have not shown this effect, and no relationship between mass and CETP activity and cardiovascular diseases [53,54] has been observed. Chinese subjects with myocardial infarction or ictus had CETP levels and activities higher than those of controls [55].

Recently, Boekholdt *et al.* [56] analysed the relationship between CETP plasmatic levels and posterior risk for coronary disease in a prospective case-control study including 735 cases and 1400 controls. A positive lineal correlation with cholesterol-LDL and a negative lineal correlation with cholesterol-HLD were observed. After adjusting for non lipidic risk factors, the study found that the risk of coronary artery disease was increased in subjects with triglyceride levels above the median, especially those in the highest quintile. The benefit of low levels of CETP and its relationship to increases was also confirmed by a meta-analysis carried out by the same authors. These results justify research into its therapeutic use.

Effect of Torcetrapib on Cholesterol Metabolism: Human Studies

Currently, there are few reported studies on torcetrapib. A summary of published studies is shown in Table **1**. The first study was a clinical trial carried out in forty healthy volunteers [57]. Five groups of 8 subjects were created and each was randomised to placebo (n=2) or torcetrapib (n=6) at 10, 30, 60, and 120 mg daily and 120 mg twice-daily for 14 days. Plasma CETP activity, plasma CEPT concentrations, plasma lipids and apolipoproteins were determined. Torcetrapib at the different study doses was accepted by all patients. Mean inhibition of CEPT activity was 12±17, 35+17, 53+8 and 80+6 for the 30, 60, 120 mg daily and 120 mg twice-daily groups respectively.

Table 1. Summary of Results in Clinical Trials with Torcetrapib

Study type	Number of subjects	Dose/day	Weeks of treatment	HDL-C increase	LDL-C decrease
Healthy volunteers, different doses [57]	6 per dose (total=40)	10 to 120 mg and 120 mg b.i.d	2	16 to 91%	21 to 42%
Single-blind, placebo-controlled [58]	19 (part associated with atorvastatin* n=9)	120 mg and 120 mg b.i.d (n=6)	4 - 8	46 to 106% (61% in association with atorvastatin)	NS (17% in association with atorvastatin)
Multi-centre, double-blind, placebo-controlled, different doses [62]	~30 per dose, total=236 (part associated with atorvastatin*)	10 to 90 mg	8	9 to 54.5% (up to 40.2% in association with atorvastatin)	16.5% (up to 18.9 % in association with atorvastatin)

Reference between brackets.
NS= No significant difference with respect to placebo.
*Dose of atorvastatin was 20 mg/day in all the studies where it was employed.

A dose- and time-dependent increase in CEPT plasma concentrations was observed. HDL-C increased significantly (between 16 and 91%) at all doses with respect to placebo, with no substantial changes in TPC (Total Plasma Cholesterol) .The lack of effect on TPC is due to a decrease in non HDL-C, with LDL-C decreasing 21% with 120 mg daily and 42% with 120 mg twice-daily. At the highest dose, apoA-I and apoE increased by 27% and 66%, respectively whereas apoB decreased by 26%. Cholesteryl ester content decreased and triglycerides increased in the non HDL plasma fraction, with the opposite occurring in HDL.

A single blind, placebo-controlled study included subjects with HDL-C below 40 mg per decilitre [58]. Nineteen patients (17 men and 2 women) were enrolled: 9 were also treated with 20 mg of atorvastatin [59,60]. All participants received placebo for 4 weeks, followed by torcetrapib 120 mg per day for 4 weeks. A subgroup (n=6) that did not take atorvastatin received 120 mg of torcetrapib twice daily for the next 4 weeks. TPC, triglycerides, LDL-C, HDL-C and subclasses, nonsterified and sterified cholesterol, phospholipids, apolipoproteins and CEPT activity were determined. Only minor and moderate side effects were observed during the trial and therefore treatment was not interrupted. The side effects perceived were headache, asthenia, dyspepsia, sweating, aching, herpes simplex, herpes zoster, amnesia and cognitive alterations. With respect to placebo, CETP activity was less than 28±16 and 65±16 percent in patients receiving 120 mg daily and 120 mg twice daily, respectively. Treatment with torcetrapib 120 mg daily increased plasma HDL-C concentrations by 46% and 120 mg twice daily by 106%, without substantial changes in TPC. Torcetrapib alone did not significantly modify LDL-C, with a 17% decrease only observed in association with atorvastatin. Apolipoproteins A-I and A-II increased by between 12% and 36% and apolipoprotein B was reduced by between 10% and 17% in patients taking the minimum and maximum torcetrapib doses, respectively. Triglycerides decreased 26% only in patients receiving 120 mg twice daily.

Another study carried out in the same patients analyzed the effect of torcetrapib on apolipoprotein A-I (apoA-I) containing HDL subspecies, apoA-I turnover and markers of reverse cholesterol transport. Torcetrapib 120 mg daily increased the amount of apoA-I in α1-migrating HDL in the atorvastatin (136 %, $p < 0.001$) and nonatorvastatin (153 %, $p < 0.01$) cohorts with respect to placebo, but an increase of 382 % ($p< 0.01$) was observed in the 120 mg twice daily group. HDL apoA-I pool increased in the nonatorvastatin cohort (16 + 7 %, $p < 0.0001$ y 34 + 8 %, $p > 0.0001$). These changes were attributable to reductions in HDL apoA-I fractional catabolic rates. In addition, torcetrapib did not significantly change serum markers of cholesterol or bile acid synthesis or fecal sterol excretion [61].

Multicentre, double-blind clinical studies (n=162 y n=174, respectively) have been carried out in patients with HDL-C < 44 mg/dl in men and <54 mg/dl in women [62]. One study used various doses of torcetrapib alone (10, 30, 60 and 90 mg) or placebo and the other used atorvastatin 20 mg per day. The study using torcetrapib found a reduction in HDL-C of between 9 and 54.5% in the 30 mg and 90mg dose groups, respectively. LDL-C decreased 16.5% only at the 90 mg dose. In the study using atorvastatin, HDL-C was reduced by 8.3 to 40.2% in the torcetrapib 30 mg and maximum dose groups, respectively. LDL-C decreased 18.9% in the torcetrapib 90 mg group. Neither study found dose-dependent increases in side effects, although small increases in systolic and diastolic blood pressure were observed.

Effect of Torcetrapib in Patients at High Risk of Cardiovascular Events

After the previously-mentioned initial studies, which evaluated the beneficial effect of torcetrapib, studies were initiated to determine its efficacy in reducing clinical events.

The pivotal study on the effectiveness of torcetrapib, the ILLUMINATE (Investigation of Lipid Level Management to Understand its Impact in Atherosclerotic Events, ClinicalTrials.gov number, NCT00134264) study [63], was suspended prematurely by the independent safety committee due to higher mortality in the torcetrapib arm. This was a randomized, controlled trial in parallel groups that included patients aged 45-75 years, with a history of cardiovascular disease or diabetes type 2. Initially, patients received progressive doses of atorvastatin until cholesterol-LDL levels <100 mg/dl were achieved. Patients were then randomized to atorvastatin alone or in association with torcetrapib 60 mg/day. A total of 15067 patients, 7534 in the atorvastatin arm and 7533 in the combination arm, were included, with a mean follow-up of 552 days. The primary endpoint was the reduction in major cardiovascular events, including death of coronary origin, nonfatal myocardial infarction, stroke and hospitalization for unstable angina. The results showed a very favourable response of lipids, with an increase in HDL-cholesterol of 72.1%, and a reduction of 24.9% in LDL-cholesterol and 9% in triglycerides. However, the risk of major cardiovascular events was 1.25 for torcetrapib, with 93 deaths compared with 59 in the atorvastatin arm (hazard ratio 1.58, 95% CI 1.14-2.19, $p=0.006$). The increased mortality was of cardiovascular and noncardiovascular origin. In the torcetrapib arm, a reduction of 0.08 nmol in potassium was observed, with 2.3% of patients having hypokalemia, compared with 0.6% in the atorvastatin arm. In addition, there was an increase in sodium and bicarbonate. The most striking adverse effects included a higher risk of hypertension (18.7% versus 7.5%, $p= 0.001$), peripheral edema (12% *versus* 4.7%, $p= 0.001$), angina (6% *versus* 4.8%, $p= 0.001$) and dyspnea (4.2% *versus* 3.2%, $p= 0.003$). Increased mortality in the torcetrapib arm, together with the higher number of secondary effects, lead to the suspension of the trial.

Simultaneously, three studies tried to evaluate the antiatherosclerotic effect of torcetrapib evaluated by coronary and carotid echography using similar methods to the ILLUMINATE trial. Patients began treatment with progressive doses of atorvastatin until previously-established levels of LDL cholesterol were achieved and were then divided into parallel, randomized groups receiving atorvastatin alone and atorvastatin plus torcetrapib. The studies lasted 24 months. Nissen *et al.* [64] evaluated the efficacy of torcetrapib in reducing the progression of coronary atherosclerosis (Investigation of Lipid Level management USing coronary ultrasound To assess Reduction in ATherosclerosis by CETP inhibition and HDL elevation (ILLUSTRATE). ClinicalTrials.gov number, NCT00134173). A total of 1188 patients with previous coronary disease demonstrated by cardiac catheterization were included. The primary efficacy measure was the change in percent atheroma volume. The lipid response was very favourable but no changes in the primary outcome were observed (0.12% *versus* 0.19%, p= 0.72). A favourable effect was observed for normalized total atheroma volume, a secondary efficacy measure. The combination caused a reduction of 9.5 mm^3 compared with 6.3 mm^3 in the atorvastatin arm, p= 0.02. The torcetrapib arm also showed an increased risk of hypertension (21.3% *versus* 8.2%).

Two studies, RADIANCE 1 (ClinicalTrials. Gov number, NCT00136981) [65] and RADIANCE 2 (ClinicalTrials.gov number 66 2 NCT00134238) [66] evaluated the efficacy of the combination of atorvastatin and torcetrapib in reducing atheroma plaque at the carotid level. RADIANCE 1 included 850 patients with familial hypercholesterolemia and RADIANCE 2 included 752 patients with mixed dyslipemia. The primary objective was to evaluate changes in carotid intima thickness. Neither study found a beneficial effect and both found an increase in blood pressure in the torcetrapib arm.

These studies uniformly showed an improvement in the lipid profile when torcetrapib was added to atorvastatin but a lack of efficacy associated with increased blood pressure. The ionic profile shown (reduction in potassium and increase in sodium and bicarbonate) was suggestive of hyperaldosteronism.

Mechanisms Explaining the Prejudicial Effect of Torcetrapib

Two possible hypotheses could explain the lack of clinical efficacy of torcetrapib: A possible vasculotoxic effect of torcetrapib and secondly an adverse effect of CETP inhibition, with the possible generation of dysfunctional or even proatherogenic HDL-cholesterol.

All studies have shown an increase in blood pressure with the use of torcetrapib. This increase could be responsible for the lack of efficacy and higher mortality observed with torcetrapib. Studies have shown a relationship between changes in blood pressure and the progression of atherosclerosis [67]. The ILLUMINATE study found an increase in blood pressure was associated with changes in ions suggestive of hyperaldosteronism. Post-hoc studies showed a trend to raised aldosterone levels with the use of torcetrapib. To confirm this evidence, Hu *et al.* [68] made cultures with cell lines derived from human adrenal carcinoma. They found that torcetrapib increased the synthesis of aldosterone and cortisol dose-dependently, with a behaviour similar to that of angiotensin II. In addition, they found that the effect was independent of CETP inhibition and was mediated by the induction of two enzymes, CYP11B2 and CYP11B1. Enzyme induction was regulated by a series of genes that are induced by angiotensin II and torcetrapib. The biochemical mediators intervening in the liberation of cortisol and aldosterone were analyzed and showed that the effect was mediated by intracellular calcium and that calcium antagonists were able to block the effect.

Forrest *et al.* [69] carried out a series of experiments in rats to clarify the hypertensor mechanism of torcetrapib using two CETP inhibitors (torcetrapib and anacetrapib). They found that increased blood pressure was not associated with CETP inhibition using two models, rats not expressing CETP and transgenic rats with CETP. Blood pressure rose in both models but HDL-cholesterol increased only in the second model. On the other hand, anacetrapib raised HDL-cholesterol in a similar way to torcetrapib without increasing blood pressure. Acute administration of anacetrapib raised blood pressure and aldosterone levels but the use of epleronone, an aldosterone receptor antagonist, did not correct the hypertensive effect torcetrapib and neither did trilostane, a 3 β-hydroxysteroid dehydrogenase inhibiter, which blocks aldosterone synthesis completely. These data indicate that acute blood pressure elevation is not mediated by aldosterone which, however, probably plays an important role in chronic BP elevation. The mechanism of this acute elevation is not clear, since the authors ruled out the intervention of a central mechanism, direct action on vascular tone, and the activation of angiotensin-1 receptors, endothelin receptors and α-adrenoreceptors.

Haan *et al.* [70] compared the efficacy of atorvastatin, torcetrapib and atorvastatin plus torcetrapib in reducing atheroma plaque using APOE3-Leiden.CETP mice. Unusually, one arm was assigned to torcetrapib alone without atorvastatin. Torcetrapib and atorvastatin reduced the size of the atherosclerotic lesion. However, the combination of torcetrapib and atorvastatin did not reduce the lesion compared with atorvastatin alone and lacked potentiating effect. In addition, torcetrapib increased the recruitment of monocytes and the expression of monocyte chemoattractant protein-1, giving rise to a more-inflammatory, less stable injury, an effect contrary to that caused by HDL-cholesterol.

The previously-mentioned studies indicate two possible mechanisms of injury induced by torcetrapib, the elevation of blood pressure and aldosterone and an inflammatory action on atheroma plaque which would block the possible beneficial effect of HDL-cholesterol.

The possible detrimental effect of CETP inhibition *per se* does not seem likely. The detrimental effects derived from torcetrapib are not mediated by CETP inhibition. In addition, inhibitors do not elevate blood pressure. A revision of the ILLUSTRATE data [71] found that the percent volume atheroma was reduced in patients with the highest HDL-cholesterol levels. It is possible that very-high HDL-cholesterol levels may overcome the detrimental effects derived from raised blood pressure and aldosterone.

CURRENT AND FUTURE DEVELOPMENT

The epidemiological studies mentioned and the therapeutic studies carried out with gemfibrozil have shown the relationship between low levels of HDL-cholesterol and cardiovascular morbidity and mortality, and also the benefit obtained from increases in HDL-cholesterol. The use of an CETP inhibitor, torcetrapib, to increase HDL-cholesterol might therefore be thought to be a good therapeutic alternative. Published studies show a favourable lipid profile of torcetrapib but no clinical efficacy, with greater mortality, lack of antiatherosclerotic action and increased blood pressure and aldosterone, and has led to its use being abandoned. However, the detrimental effects are related to the molecule itself and not to CETP inhibition. The search for therapeutic alternatives that raise HDL-cholesterol levels seem reasonable and CETP inhibition may be a useful alternative.

REFERENCES

[1] Hansson GR. Inflammation, atherosclerosis and coronary artery disease. N Engl J Med 2005; 352: 1685-1695.

[2] Schultz JR, Verstuyft JG, Gong EL, Nichols AV, Rubim EM. Protein composition determines the anti-atherogenic properties of HDL in transgenic mice. Nature 1993; 365: 762-764.

[3] Watson AD, Berliner JA, Hama SY, *et al.* Protective effect of high density lipoprotein associated paraoxonase. Inhibition of the biological activity of minimally oxidized low density lipoprotein. J Clin Invest 1995; 96: 2882-2891.

[4] Watson AD, Navab M, Hama SY, *et al.* Effect of platelet activating factor-acetylhydrolase on the formation and action of minimally oxidized low density lipoprotein. J Clin Invest 1995; 95: 774-782.

[5] Vohl MC, Neville TA, Kumarathasen R, Braschi S, Sparks DL. A novel lecithin-cholesterol acyltransferase antioxidant activity prevents the formation of oxidized lipids during lipoprotein oxidation. Biochemistry 1999; 38: 5976-5981.

[6] Meddipati KR, Marnett LJ. Characterization of the major hydroperoxide-reducing activity of human plasma. Purification and properties of a selenium-dependent glutathione peroxidase. J Biol Chem 1987; 262: 17398-17403.

[7] Castelli WP, Doyle JT, Gordon T, *et al.* HDL cholesterol and other lipids in coronary heart disease. The cooperative lipoprotein phenotyping study. Circulation 1977; 55: 767-772.

[8] Gordon T, Castelli WP, Hjortland MC, Kannel WD, Dawber TR. High density lipoprotein as a protective factor against heart disease. The Framingham Study. Am J Med 1977; 62: 707-714.

[9] Castelli WP, Garrison RJ, Wilson WP, Abbot RD, Kalousdian S, Kannel WB. Incidence of coronary heart disease and lipoprotein cholesterol levels. The Framingham Study. JAMA 1986; 256: 2835-2838.

[10] Gordon DJ, Probstfield JL, Garrison RJ, *et al.* High-density lipoprotein cholesterol and cardiovascular disease. Four prospective American studies. Circulation 1989; 79: 8-15.

[11] Miller NE, Thelle DS, Forde OH, Mjos OD. The Tromso heart-study. High-density lipoprotein and coronary heart-disease: a prospective case-control study. Lancet 1977; 1: 965-968.

[12] Goldbourt U, Yaari S, Medalie JH. Isolated low HDL cholesterol as a risk factor for coronary heart disease mortality. A 21-year follow-up of 8000 men. Arterioscler Thromb Vasc Biol 1997; 17: 107-113.

[13] Assmann G, Schulte H. Relation of high density lipoprotein cholesterol and triglycerides to incidence of atherosclerotic coronary artery disease (The PROCAM experience). Am J Cardiol 1992; 70: 732-737.

[14] Manninem V, Tenkanen L, Koskinien P, *et al.* Joint effects of serum triglycerides and LDL cholesterol and HDL cholesterol concentration on coronary heart disease risk in the Helsinki Heart Study: implications for treatment. Circulation 1992; 85: 37-45.

[15] Rubins HB, Robins SJ, Collins D, *et al.* Gemfibrozil for the secondary prevention of coronary heart disease in men with low levels of high-density lipoprotein cholesterol. N Engl J Med 1999; 341: 410-418.

[16] Ericsson CG, Hamsten A, Nilsson J, *et al.* Angiographic assessment of effects of bezafibrate on progression of coronary artery disease in young male postinfarction patients. Lancet 1996; 347: 849-853.

[17] Bloomfield H, Davenport J, Babikian V, *et al.* Reduction in stroke with gemfibrozil in men with coronary heart disease and low HDL cholesterol: The Veterans Affairs HDL Intervention Trial (VA-HIT). Circulation 2001; 103: 2828-2833.

[18] Sacks FM. The role of high-density lipoprotein (HDL) cholesterol in the prevention and treatment of coronary heart disease: Expert Group recommendations. Am J Cardiol 2002; 90: 139-143.

[19] Simes RJ, Marschner IC, Hunt D, *et al.* Relationship between lipid levels and clinical outcomes in the Long-Term Intervention with Pravastatin in ischemic disease (LIPID). Circulation 2003; 105: 1162-1169.

[20] Pedersen TR, Olsson AG, Faergemen O, *et al.* Lipoprotein changes and the reduction in the incidence of major coronary events. Circulation 1998; 97: 1453-1460.

[21] Wattanakit K, Folson AR, Chambless LE, Nieto J. Risk factors for cardiovascular event recurrence in the Atherosclerosis Risk in communities (ARIC). Am Heart J 2005; 149: 606-612.

[22] Grundy SM, Brewer B, Cleemen JI, Smith SC, Lenfant C. Definition of metabolic syndrome. Circulation 2004; 109: 433-438.

[23] Larosa JC, Grundy SM, Waters DD, *et al.* Intensive lipid lowering with atorvastatin in patients with stable coronary disease. N Engl J Med 2005.

[24] Brewer HB. High-density lipoproteins: a new potential therapeutic target for the prevention of cardiovascular disease. Arterioscler Thromb Vasc Biol 2004; 24: 387-391.

[25] Osterud B, Bjorklid E. Role of monocytes in atherogenesis. Physiol Rev 2003; 83: 1069-1112.

[26] Libby P, Ridker PM, Maseri A. Inflammation and atherosclerosis. Circulation 2002; 105: 1135-1143.

[27] Barter PJ, Nicholls S, Rye KA, Anantharamaiah GM, Navab M, Fogelman AM. Anti-inflammatory properties of HDL. Circ Res 95: 764-772.

[28] Rader DJ. Regulation of reverse cholesterol transport and clinical implications. Am J Cardiol 2003; 92: 42S-49S.

[29] Aiello RJ, Brees D, Bourassa PA, *et al.* Increased atherosclerosis in hyperlipidemic mice with inactivation of ABCA1 in macrophages. Arterioscler Thromb Vas Biol 2002; 22: 630-637.
[30] Schoefer EJ, Blum CB, Levy RI, *et al.* Metabolism of High-density lipoprotein apolipoproteins in Tangier Disease. New Engl J Med 1978; 299: 905-910.
[31] Haghpassand M, Bourassa PA, Fancone OL, Aiello RJ. Monocyte/macrophage expression of ABCA1 has minimal contribution to plasma HDL levels. J Clin Invest 2001; 108: 1315-1320.
[32] Wang N, Lan D, Chen W, Matssura F, Tall AR. ATP-binding cassette transporters G1 and G4 mediated cellular cholesterol efflux to high-density lipoproteins. Proc Natl Acad Sci USA 2004; 101: 9774-9779.
[33] Rothblat GH, De la LLera M, Atger V, *et al.* Cell cholesterol efflux integration of old and new observations provides new insights. J Lipid Res 1999; 40: 781-796.
[34] Ji Y, Jian B, Wang N, *et al.* Scavenger receptor BI promotes high density lipoprotein-mediated cellular cholesterol efflux. J Biol Chem 1997; 272: 20892-20895.
[35] Mayers CD, Kashyap ML. Pharmacological elevation of high-density lipoproteins, recent insights on mechanism of action and atherosclerosis protectors. Curr Opin Cardiol 2004; 19: 366-373.
[36] Ribas V, Sanchez-Quesada JC, Anton R, *et al.* Human apolipoprotein AII enrichment displaces paraoxonase from HDL and impairs its antioxidant properties. Circ Res 2004; 95: 789-797.
[37] Cockerill GW, Rye KA, Gamble JR, Vadas MA, Barter PJ. High-density lipoprotein inhibit cytokine-induced expression of endothelial cell adhesion molecules. Arterioscler Thromb Vasc Biol 1995; 15: 1987-1994.
[38] Wadham C, Albanese N, Roberts J, *et al.* High-Density lipoproteins neutralize C-reactive protein proinflammatory activity. Circulation 2004; 109: 2116-2122.
[39] Xia P, Vadas MA, Rye KA, Barter PJ, Gamble JR. High density lipoprotein (HDL) interrupt the sphingosine kinase signaling pathway. A possible mechanism for protection against atherosclerosis by HDL. J Biol Chem 1999; 274: 33143-33147.
[40] Nofer JR, Van der Giet M, Tolle M, *et al.* HDL induces NO-dependent vasorelaxation *via* the lysophospholipid receptor S1P3. J Clin Invest 2004; 113: 569-581.
[41] Fredenrich A, Bayer P. Reverse cholesterol transport, high density lipoprotein and HDL cholesterol: recent data. Diabetes Metab 2003; 29: 201-205.
[42] Linsel-Nitschke P, Tall A. HDL as a target in the treatment of atherosclerotic cardiovascular disease. Nat Rev Drug Discov 2005; 4:193-205.
[43] Thomas, L.J.: US6846808 **(2005).**
[44] Rittershaus, C.W., Thomas, L.J.: USA6555113 **(2003).**
[45] Glombik, H., Falk, E., Frick, W., *et al.*: US6884812 **(2005).**
[46] Robl, J.A., Chen, B.-C., Sun C.-Q.: US6812345 **(2004).**
[47] Sato, N., Ando, M., Ishikawa, S., Nagai, K., Kanatani, A.: US6869966 **(2005).**
[48] Sikorski, J.A., Durley, R.C., Massa, M.A., Wang, J.L., Mischke, D.A., Parnas, B.L., Rueppel, M.L.: US6861561 **(2005).**
[49] Cheng, P.T.W., Chen, S., Ding, C.Z., Herpin, T.F.: US6875782 **(2005).**
[50] Sulsky, R., Robl, J.A.: US6919323 **(2005).**
[51] Sirkorski, J.A., Durley, R.C., Rueppel, M.L., Mischke, D.A., Parnas, B.L.: US6924313 **(2005).**
[52] Le Goff W, Guerin M, Chapman MJ. Pharmacological modulation of cholesteryl ester transfer protein, a new therapeutic target in atherogenic dyslipemia. Pharmacol Ther 2004; 101: 17-38.
[53] Blakenberg S, Rupprecht HJ, Bickel C, *et al.* Common genetic variation of the cholesteryl ester transfer protein gene strongly predicts future cardiovascular death in patients with coronary artery disease. J Am Coll Cardiol 2003; 41: 1983-1989.
[54] Goto A, Sasai K, Suzuki S, *et al.* Cholesteryl ester transfer protein and atherosclerosis in Japanese subjects: a study basal on coronary angiography. Atherosclerosis 2001; 159: 153-163.
[55] Zhuang Y, Wang J, Quiang H, *et al.* Cholesteryl ester transfer protein levels and gene deficiency in Chinese patients with cardio-cerebrovascular disease. Chin Med J 2002; 115: 371-374.
[56] Boekholdt SM, Kuivenhoven JA, Wareham NJ, *et al.* Plasma levels of cholesteryl ester transfer protein and the risk of future coronary artery disease in apparently healthy men and women. Circulation 2004; 110: 1418-1423.
[57] Clark RW, Suftin TA, Ruggeri RB, *et al.* Raising high-density lipoprotein in human through inhibition of cholesteryl ester transfer protein: an initial multidose study of torcetrapib. Arterioscler Thromb Vasc Biol 2004; 24: 490-497.
[58] Brousseau ME, Schaefer EJ, Wolfe ML, *et al.* Effects of an inhibitor of cholesteryl ester transfer protein on HDL Cholesterol. N Engl J Med 2004; 350: 1505-1515.
[59] Brousseau ME, Diffenderfer MR, Miller JS, *et al.* Effects of cholesteryl ester transfer protein inhibition on high-density lipoprotein subspecies, apolipoprotein A-I metabolism and fecal sterol excretion. Arterioscler Thromb Vasc Biol 2005; 25: 1-8.
[60] Sikorski, J.A., Glenn, K.C.: US6890958 **(2005).**

[61] Mylari, B.L.: US6894047 **(2005).**

[62] Davidson M, Mckenney J, Revkin J, Shear Ch. Efficacy and safety of a novel cholesteryl ester transfer protein inhibitor Torcetrapib when administered with and without atorvastatin to subjects with a low level of high-density lipoprotein cholesterol. JACC 2005; 394A.

[63] Barter PJ, Caulfield M, Eriksson M, *et al.* Effects of torcetrapib in patients at high risk for coronary events. N Engl J Med 2007; 357: 2109-2122.

[64] Nissen S, Tardiff JC, Nicholls SJ, *et al.* Effect of torcetrapib on the progression of coronary atherosclerosis. N Engl J Med 2007; 356: 13: 1304-1316.

[65] Kastelein JP, Van Leuven SI, Burgess L, *et al.* Effect of torcetrapib on carotid atherosclerosis in familial hypercholesterolemia. N Engl J Med 2007; 356: 1620-1630.

[66] Bots ML, Visseren FL, Evans GW, *et al.* Torcetrapib and carotid intima-media thickness in mixed dyslipidaemia (RADIANCE 2 study): a randomised, double-blind trial. Lancet 2007; 370: 153-160.

[67] Sipahi I, Tuzcu EM, Schoenhagen P, *et al.* Effects of normal, pre-hypertensive, and hypertensive blood pressure levels on progression of coronary atherosclerosis. J Am Coll Cardiol 2006; 48: 833-888.

[68] Hu X, Dietz JD, Xia C, *et al.* Torcetrapib induces aldosterone and cortisol production by an intracellular calcium-mediated mechanism independently of cholesteryl ester transfer protein inhibition. Endocrinology 2009; 150: 2211-2219.

[69] Forrest MJ, Bloomfield D, Briscoe RJ, *et al.* Torcetrapib-induced blood pressure elevation is independent of CETP inhibition and is accompanied by increased circulating levels of aldosterone. Br J Pharmacol 2008; 154: 1465-1473.

[70] de Haan W, de Vries-van der Weij J, van der Hoorn JW, *et al.* Torcetrapib does not reduce atherosclerosis beyond atorvastatin and induces more proinflammatory lesions than atorvastatin. Circulation 2008; 117: 2515-2522.

[71] Nicholls SJ, Tuzcu EM, Brennan DM, Tardif JC, Nissen SE. Cholesteryl esters transfer protein inhibition, high-density lipoprotein raising, and progression of coronary atherosclerosis. Circulation 2008; 118: 2506-2514.

Role of Infrasound Pressure Waves in Atherosclerotic Plaque Rupture: A Theoretical Approach

Athanasios Tsatsaris[*,1,2,3], Efstathios Koukounaris[4], Theodoros Motsakos[4] and Despina Perrea[1]

[1]*Laboratory for Experimental Surgery and Surgical Research, School of Medicine, University of Athens, Greece;* [2]*Laboratory of Applied Mathematics, Department of Mathematics, University of Athens, Greece;* [3]*Laboratory of Sanitary Police Department of Grevena, Greece;* [4]*Mechanical Engineering Department of Hellenic Coast Guard, Hellenic Naval Academy, Greece*

Abstract: *Objective*: To investigate the role of infrasound aortic pressure waves (IPW) in atherosclerotic plaque rupture. *Methods*: Atherosclerotic plaques have been simulated partly, in two dimensions, as being short or long Conical Intersections(CIS) , that is to say elliptic, parabolic or hyperbolic surfaces. Consequently, the course and reflection of the generated aortic pressure wave (infrasound domain-less than 20Hz) has been examined around the simulated plaques. *Results*: The incidence of IPW on plaque surface results in reflection and "refraction" of the wave. The IPW course within tissue, seems to be enhanced by high Cu-level presence at these areas according to recent evidence (US2003000388213). The "refracted", derived wave travels through plaque tissue and is eventually accumulated to the foci of the respective CIS-plaque geometry. *Conclusions*: The foci location within or underneath atheroma declares zones where infrasound energy is mostly absorbed. This process, among other mechanisms may contribute to plaque rupture through the development of local hemorrhage and inflammation in foci areas. In future, detection of foci areas and repair (i.e. *via* Laser Healing Microtechnique) may attenuate atherosclerotic plaque rupture behavior.

Keywords: Atherosclerosis, plaque rupture, conical intersections.

INTRODUCTION

During the last decades, aorta has emerged as an independent, and unique organ of cardiovascular system [1]. Left ventricular systole generates an Infrasound Pressure Wave (IPW-frequency less than 20Hz) which runs along the circulatory frame. The IPW interacts in its course with the surrounding environment, that is to say, with branch points, curved regions and atherosclerotic stenoses, resulting in reflection and "refraction" of the wave [2-3]. The "refracted" wave is nothing more than the derived infrasound wave which travels within arterial wall. In case of atherosclerotic tissue, a variety of plaque formation could be approximated by Conical Intersections (CIS), that take partly, the form of Elliptic, Parabolic or Hyperbolic areas. CIS occupy certain properties-such as the Reflecting Property which

*Corresponding author: E-mail: tsapol@otenet.gr

have found application in different scientific domains, such as Mathematics, Quantum Chemistry, Telecommunication systems etc. The Reflecting Property (RP) determines that, if a light beam or waves such as electromagnetic waves, infrasound waves etc, fell onto a CIS-surface then they would be reflected or refracted towards the respective foci or focus.

The present study explores the involvement of Reflecting Property (RP) in plaque rupture mechanism, suggesting that RP property may contribute to plaque rupture initiation due to the development of local hemorrhage and inflammation at foci areas.

METHODS

CIS can be obtained by crossing a cone with a plane at different angles, producing the curves of Ellipse, Parabola or Hyperbola. Ellipse is a plane algebraic curve, where the sum of the distances from any point on the curve to two fixed points is constant. The two fixed points are called the **foci**. An Ellipse curve in the Cartesian plane can be defined by an equation of the form:

$$A \cdot x^2 + B \cdot x \cdot y + C \cdot y^2 + D \cdot x + E \cdot y + F = 0 ..... (A, B, C, D, E, F) \in \Re$$

such that $B^2<4AC$, where all the coefficients are real and where more than one solution, defining a pair of points (x,y) on the Ellipse, exists. The line segment that passes through the foci and terminates on the Ellipse is called the major axis. Virtually, the major axis passes along the longest segment of the Ellipse (Fig. **1**). If the foci coincide then the Ellipse becomes a circle. Hyperbola is a plane curve consisting of points so that the difference between the distances from any point on the curve to two fixed points (foci) is the same for all points. A Hyperbola can be obtained by a plane cutting both napes of a cone; thus, it has two parts. The center of Hyperbola is the point halfway between its foci, while the principal axis is the straight line through the foci. Algebraically, a Hyperbola is a curve in the Cartesian plane defined by an equation of the form:

$$A \cdot x^2 + B \cdot x \cdot y + C \cdot y^2 + D \cdot x + E \cdot y + F = 0 ..... (A, B, C, D, E, F) \in \Re$$

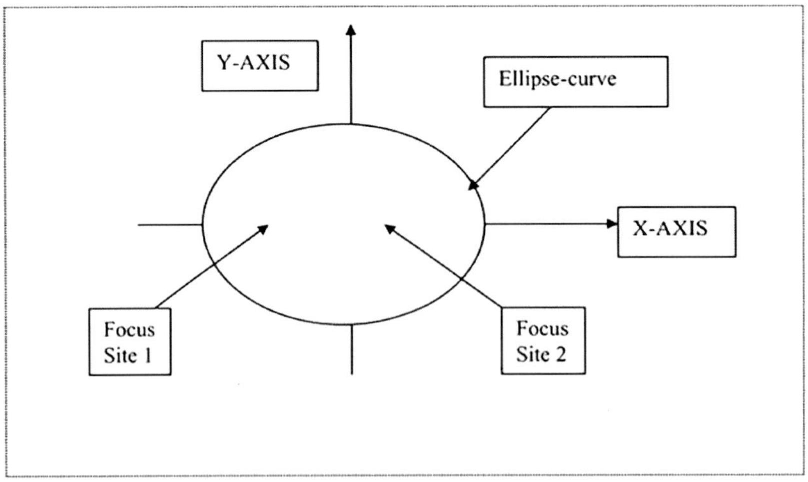

Fig. (1). An Ellipse is presented in Cartesian X-Yplane.

such that $B^2>4AC$, where all of the coefficients are real, and where more than one solution, defining a pair of points (x,y) on the Hyperbola, exists. Parabola is a plane curve formed by the intersection of a right circular cone and a plane parallel to an element of the cone, or by the locus of points equidistant from a fixed line (named directrix) and a fixed point (focus) not on the line (Fig. **2**). Algebraically, a Parabola is a curve in Cartesian plane defined by an irreducible equation of the form:

$$A \cdot x^2 + B \cdot x \cdot y + C \cdot y^2 + D \cdot x + E \cdot y + F = 0.....(A, B, C, D, E, F) \in \Re$$

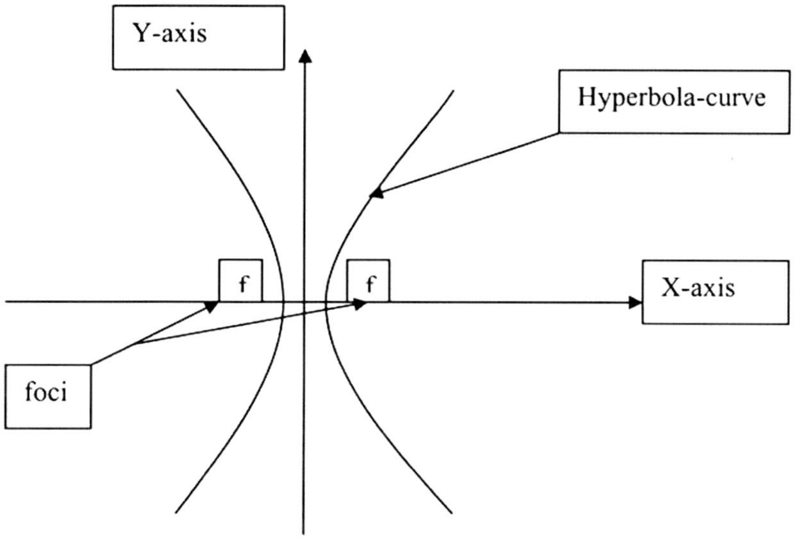

Fig. (2). A Hyperbola is presented in Cartesian X-Y plane.

such that $B^2=4AC$, where all the coefficients are real, where A or/and C is non-zero, where more than one solution, giving a pair of points (x,y)on the Parabola, exists (Fig. **3**).

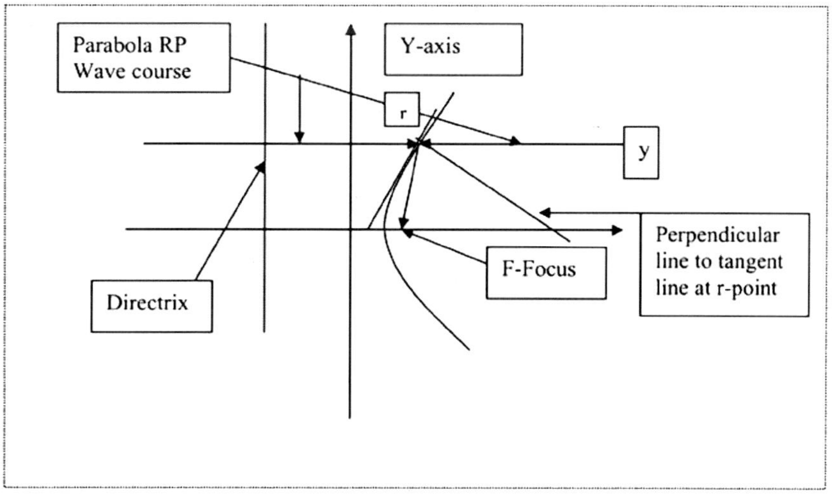

Fig. (3). A Parabola is presented in Cartesian X-Y plane

Arteries represent cylindrical vessels around branch points are degenerated to the curved CIS-regions on the account of being intersected by other cylindrical vessels. Accordingly, atheroma is an abnormal curved formation which emerges in artery tube, taking the form of short or long surfaces that are very similar to CIS-formations (i.e. based on histological findings in most of the cases, stable atheromatic plaques can be simulated by Elliptic, Hyperbolic or Parabolic surfaces [4,5] (Fig. **4**). Furthermore, extensive mathematical elaboration of CIS-equations gave the following results.

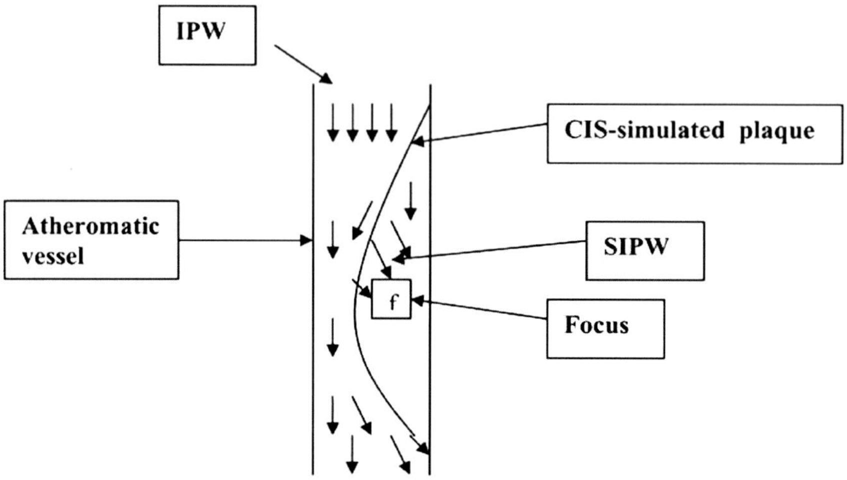

Fig. (4). A CIS-simulation of an atheromatic stenose is illustrated. IPW, SIPW and Focus represent Infrasound Pressure Waves, Secondary Infrasound Pressure Waves, and wave concentration centre respectively.

RESULTS

Analytic Geometry proved that CIS curves exhibit one very important attribute, the so-called Reflecting Property (RP). Generally speaking, RP determines that if a light beam or waves, such as electromagnetic waves, infrasound waves etc, fell onto a CIS-surface then they would be reflected or refracted towards the respective foci or focus (Figs. **3** and **4**). Mathematically this property could also be stated as: the perpendicular line to the tangent line at a certain point r(x,y) of parabola, bisects the angle **Fry** (Fig. **3**). For the first time, this property was proved in 5th century B.C by the Greek mathematician Euklidis. Similarly, and other conical intersections occupy the reflecting property adapted each time to the specified curve.

DISCUSSION

The most life-threatening event an atherosclerotic patient may face, is the plaque rupture. So far, many scientific attempts have been made in order to elucidate and modify the underlying mechanisms which could lead to this dangerous situation [6-10]. The prevalent rupture mechanisms [11-13] are outlined below: i) hemodynamic factors such as, turbulence, increased shear stress and pressure gradient ii) rupture of vasa vasorum, subintimal hemorrhage and inflammation iii) fibrous cap mechanical stress behavior and iv) biochemical degradation of matrix. It is worth mentioning that the plaque tissue also exhibits complex mechanical behavior due to its anisotropy, heterogeneity, nonlinearity and the activity of smooth muscle cells [13]. Moreover, recent patents in area of atherosclerosis

(ATH) research, such as: 1) Trientine-therapy against high copper (Cu) level in atheromatic tissues [14, 2] the inhibiting action of N-terminal dipeptide nitriles to Cathepsins B, K, L, S [15, 3] the use of proteinaceous or non proteinaceous agents to block M-CSF activation [16], have brought new treatment methods against ATH and its complications. In connection with the present study, it is worth mentioning that elevated Cu-concentration also facilitates IPW traveling via aortic tissue.

In the present research, stable atherosclerotic plaques have been approximated by CIS-surfaces because stenoses are very similar to the average CIS-surfaces according to macro and microscopic evidence. Moreover, CIS-surfaces are degenerated to CIS-curves in two dimensions and so it is deduced that properties of CIS-curves will be possessed by plaques as well. But how this hypothesis is connected to plaque rupture which can be easily decipherable is explained below:

IPW is produced during cardiac circle and travels along circulatory system. Furthermore, infrasound is characterized by an ability to cover long distances and get around obstacles with little dissipation. Aortic infrasound frequency is usually lower than 17Hz and once IPW starts traveling, many secondary waves (SIPW) are born due to reflection of mother-IPW on branch points or curved regions. These SIPW have lower velocity than their mother-IPW but the same frequency. SIPW may also be reflected and/or "refracted" within aortic tissue and travel as long as their mechanical energy permits. Additionally, taking into account the RP of atheromatic plaques it is easily deduced that SIPW may concentrate on respective plaque focus or foci, which always dwell within pathological aortic tissue. Moreover, IPW have been proved to transfer energy at areas which are concentrated and cause inflammation and hemorrhage [17-19]. In our case, this energy concentration on plaque foci may raise topically tissue temperature and cause hemorrhage (i.e rupture of vasa vasorum) and inflammation, and since hemorrhage and inflammation are the cornerstone of an aortic lesion [20,21] from the mechanical point of view SIPW might significantly contribute to the initiation of plaque rupture.

CURRENT AND FUTURE DEVELOPMENTS

In this research, plaques have been considered to be stable, covered by a fibrous cap overlying a central core of lipid and cellular debris. The central core contains foamy macrophages, cholesterol clefts and mononuclear inflammatory cells. An intact endothelial layer covers the intimal surface of the fibrous cap while neovascularization occurs at the base of atheroma due to the proliferation of thin-walled small blood vessels. We hypothesize that, complications, such as intraplaque hemorrhage among other reasons may also take place under the influence of IPW during ATH-progression creating an unstable plaque. However, it should be addressed that RP-property has been proved for the theoretical CIS-curves and not directly for atherosclerotic tissues.

Furthermore, intravascular ultrasound could give information about the geometric characteristics of the examined atheroma and declaring, which CIS simulation is more suitable for that. Thus, the focus or foci location could be estimated.

Additionally, current research considering snoring [22], have revealed the significant impact of vibration parameters on carotid atherosclerosis, an outcome which is consistent with our hypothesis.

In conclusion, although the study needs further experimental verification since no human data are available theoretically, it is certain that the foci location within or underneath atheroma declares zones of highly absorbed infrasound energy which might lead to hemorrhage and inflammation. Among other mechanisms, CIS-mechanism seems to elucidate the important role of foci areas, and early detection (i.e. *via* a suitable Ultra Sound method) and repair of these areas (i.e. possibly *via* Intravascular Laser Healing Microtechiques) may attenuate plaque rupture behavior.

REFERENCES

[1] Boudoulas H, Wooley CF. Aortic Function. In: Boudoulas H, Toutouzas PK, Wooley CF, Eds. Functional abnormalities of the aorta. New York: Futura 1996; pp. 3-36.

[2] Marchais SJ, Guerin AP, Pannier BM, Levy BI, Safar ME, London GM. Wave reflections and cardiac hypertrophy in chronic uremia: influence of body size. Hypertension 1993; 22: 876-883.

[3] Pannier BM, Guerin AP, Marchais SJ, London GM. Different aortic reflection wave responses following long-term angiotensin-converting enzyme inhibition and beta-blocker in essential hypertension. Clin Exp Pharmacol Physiol 2001; 28(12): 1074-1077.

[4] Aidinian G, Weiswasser JM, Arora S, Abularrage CJ, Singh N, Sidawv AN. Carotid plaque morphologic characteristics. Perspect Vasc Surg Endovasc Ther 2006; 18(1): 63-70.

[5] Amel E, Prathiba D, Kumar S. Morphological and morphometric analysis of coronary atherosclerosis—an autopsy study. Indian J Pathol Microbiol 2006; 49(2): 239-242.

[6] Ratcliffe NR, Kennedy SM, Morganelli PM. Immunocytochemical detection of Fcgamma receptors in human atherosclerotic lesions. Immunol Lett 2001; 77(3): 169-174.

[7] Johnstone MT, Perez AS, Nasser I, *et al.* Angiotensin receptor blockade with candesartan attenuates atherosclerosis, plaque disruption, and macrophage accumulation within the plaque in a rabbit model. Circulation 2004; 110(14): 2060-2065.

[8] Oh GT, Choi JH, Hong JJ, *et al.* Dietary hematein ameliorates fatty streak lesions in the rabbit by the possible mechanism of reducing VCAM-1 and MCP-1 expression. Atherosclerosis 2001; 159(1): 17-26.

[9] Lemay J, Hamet P, deBlois D. Losartan-induced apoptosis as a novel mechanism for the prevention of vascular lesion formation after injury. J Renin Angiotensin Aldosterone Syst 2000; 1(1): 46-50.

[10] Ikeda N, Torii R. When does atherosclerosis become irreversible? Chronological change from an early to an advanced atherosclerotic lesion observed by angioscopy. Angiology 2005; 56(4): 361-370.

[11] Binns RL, Ku KN. Effect of stenosis on wall motion: A possible mechanism of stroke and transient ischemic attack. Arteriosclerosis 1989; 9: 842-847.

[12] Loree HM, Kamm RD, Stringfellow RG, *et al.* Effects of fibrous cap thickness on peak circumferential stress in model atherosclerotic vessels. Circ Res 1992; 71: 850-858.

[13] Barger AC, Beeuwkes R, Lainey LL, *et al.* Hypothesis: Vasa vasorum and neovascularization of human coronary arteries. A possible role in the pathophysiology of atherosclerosis. N Engl J Med 1991; 88: 8154-8158.

[14] Cooper, GJS, Baker, JR.: US2003000388213(**2005**).

[15] Missbach, M.: US2006000374995(**2006**).

[16] Goldsschimidt-Clermont, PJ, Kereiakes, DJ, Sheshlah P.: US2003000342330(**2003**).

[17] Gavreau V. Infra sons: generateurs, detecteurs, proprietes physiques, effets biologiques. Acustica 1966;17(1): 1-10.

[18] Gavreau V. Infrasound Sci J 1968; 4(1): S.33.

[19] Gavreau V. "Sons graves intenses et infrasons". Scientific Progres – la Nature 1968; 336-344.

[20] Lee RT, Grodznisky AJ, Frank EH, *et al.* Structure-dependent dynamic mechanical behavior of fibrous cap from human atherosclerotic plaques. Circulation 1991; 83: 1764-1770.

[21] Rao DS, Goldin JG, Fishbein MC. Determinants of plaque instability in atherosclerotic vascular disease. Cardiovasc Pathol 2005; 14(6): 285-293.

[22] Sharon A Lee, Terence C, Amis Karen Byth, *et al.* Heavy Snoring as a Cause of Carotid Artery Atherosclerosis. Wheatley Sleep 2008; 31(9): 1207-1213.

Advances in the Perioperative Management of Pulmonary Hypertension

Harish Ramakrishna*

Division of Cardiothoracic Anesthesiology, Department of Anesthesiology, Mayo Clinic, Phoenix, Arizona, USA

Abstract: Cardiovascular anesthesiologists have traditionally resorted to using intravenous therapy in the operating room to manipulate hemodynamics and the determinants of cardiac output and systemic vascular resistance during cardiac surgery. General anesthesia involves the administration of both intravenous and inhaled drug therapy to achieve the desired goals, i.e. analgesia, amnesia, muscle relaxation and blockade of autonomic activity. Anesthesiologists are the experts in the use and titration of drugs that are administered through the inhaled route. However, this method of drug delivery presents many challenges, notably timing, dosage accuracy, rapid titratability and consistency of drug delivery. Arguably the most rapid method of treating acute reactive pulmonary vasculature would be by drugs that directly act upon the pulmonary endothelium. In the operating room, pulmonary hypertension and right ventricular failure are high predictors of morbidity and mortality and present significant challenges to the anesthesiologist. In this article, we will focus on advances in inhaled therapy of these conditions, including concerned recent patents. This review will focus on some of the advances in the pharmacology of inhaled drugs that are being used to treat pulmonary hypertension, right and left ventricular failure in the perioperative setting.

Keywords: Pulmonary hypertension, right ventricular failure, inotropes, pulmonary vasodilators, nitric oxide.

PULMONARY HYPERTENSION IN THE PERIOPERATIVE PERIOD

Pulmonary hypertension (PH) was initially described by Romberg in 1881 as pulmonary arterial sclerosis. There have been many classifications and modifications since then, but the World Health Organization in 1998 put forth the definitive nomenclature which is still the gold standard in the classification and has gained widespread acceptance. This was revised in 2003 and is outlined in (Table **1**). The three fundamental pathologic processes determined to be responsible for increasing pulmonary vascular resistance in PH are vasoconstriction, remodeling of the pulmonary arteries and in –situ thrombus formation. The pulmonary vasculature is typically a low pressure environment since the pulmonary endothelium tightly regulates the production of vasodilators (prostacyclin, nitric oxide) and vasoconstrictors (endothelin-1, thromboxane and serotonin). PH results when there is an imbalance of

*Corresponding author: Tel: 480-342-1800; Fax: 480-342-2319; E-mail: ramakrishna.harish@mayo.edu

Atta-ur-Rahman / M. Iqbal Choudhary (Eds.)

mediators with an overproduction of vasoconstricting agents and decreased level of vasodilators.

Table 1. Pulmonary Hypertension Classification

Group I.	Pulmonary arterial hypertension (PAH)
	Idiopathic (IPAH)
	Familial (FPAH)
	Associated with (APAH):
	Connective tissue disease
	Congenital systemic-to-pulmonary shunts
	Portal hypertension
	HIV infection
	Drugs and toxins
	Other (thyroid disorders, glycogen storage disease, Gaucher's disease, hereditary haemorragic telangiectasia, haemoglobinopathies, myeloproliferative disorders, splenectomy)
	Associated with significant venous or capillary involvement
	Pulmonary veno-occlusive disease (PVOD)
	Pulmonary capillary haemangiomatosis (PCH)
	Persistent pulmonary hypertension of the newborn (PPHN)
Group II.	Pulmonary hypertension associated with left heart diseases
Group III.	Pulmonary hypertension associated with respiratory diseases and/or hypoxemia (including chronic obstructive pulmonary disease)
Group IV.	Pulmonary hypertension due to chronic thrombotic and/or embolic disease
Group V.	Miscellaneous group, e.g. sarcoidosis, histiocytosis X and lymphangiomatosis

Pulmonary hypertension is generally difficult to treat in the perioperative setting owing to the multiple factors that can exacerbate the tone of the pulmonary vasculature. Several hemodynamic factors have been identified as being associated with a worse prognosis: PAP> 85mmHg, RAP>20mmHg and CI <2L/min [1]. Also patients at the latter two stages of the NYHA classification at the time of diagnosis have a uniformly poorer prognosis. Pulmonary artery hypertension (PAH) by definition is defined as a mean pulmonary artery pressure greater than 25 mmHg at rest or 30 mmHg with exertion [2].

Over the years, there have multiple classes of drugs developed which act at multiple sites in the lung to treat PAH; however, no therapy aside from lung transplantation has been found to be totally curative. In this review, we will briefly review the current drugs available for intravenous use in the perioperative setting, followed by the inhaled drugs to treat PAH and the optimal combination of both therapies (Fig. **1**).

INTRAOPERATIVE MANAGEMENT OF PULMONARY HYPERTENSION

Pulmonary hypertension in the perioperative setting is common in the cardiac surgical population. For the anesthesiologist, the key symptoms elicited in the history are nonspecific and include chronic dyspnea on exertion or rest, chest pain which may or may not mimic angina and syncope as the severity progresses. Physical examination may vary depending on the severity of the disease, mild PAH exhibiting loud P2 heart sound on auscultation to the classic diastolic murmur. Severe PAH causing right heart failure may present hepatomegaly, peripheral edema and ascites.

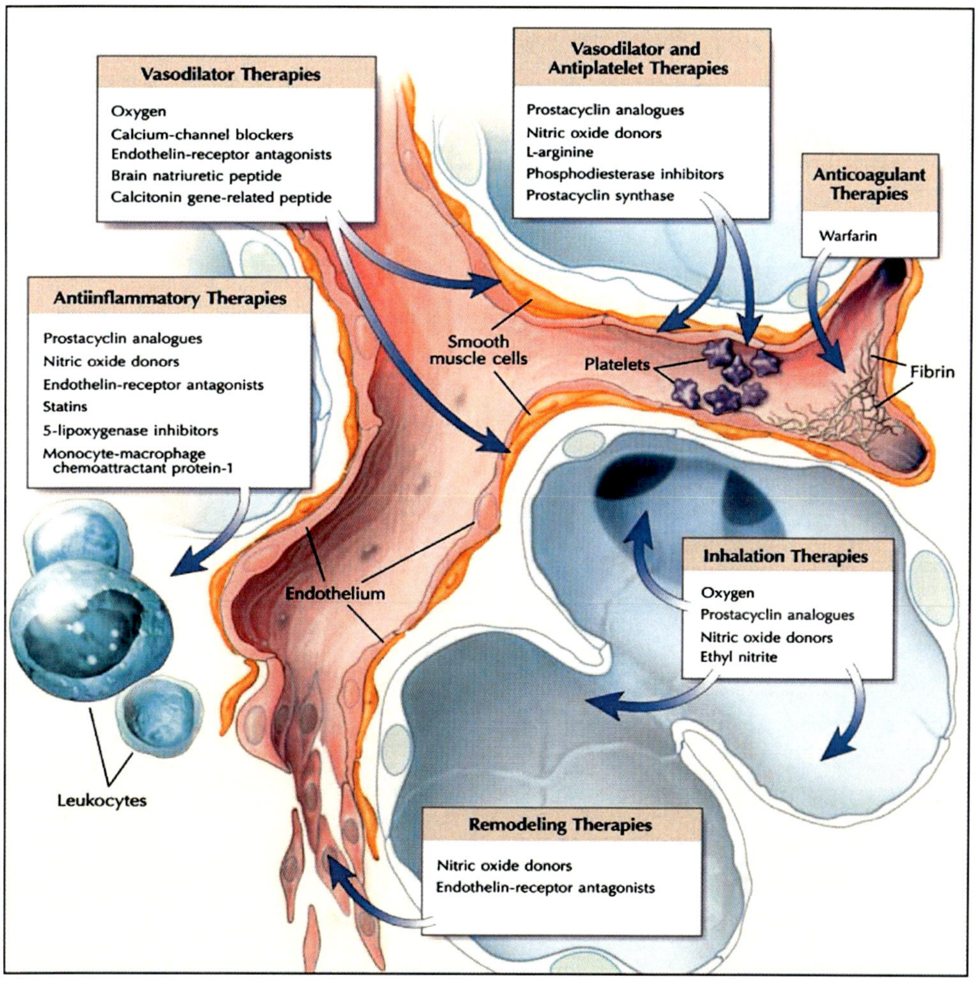

Fig. (1). Sites of action of drug modalities in the treatment of PAH, reprinted from NEJM 2004; 351: 16.

Chest x-ray may reveal enlargement of the main pulmonary artery and tapering of peripheral arteries. Echocardiographic findings in severe PAH have been well described and may include right ventricular hypertrophy, increased septal thickness and paradoxical septal motion. More severe cases may show a D-shaped left ventricle where the interventricular septum is shifted to the left, along with right atrial enlargement, tricuspid and pulmonary regurgitation. Pulmonary capillary wedge pressure is usually normal in the absence of heart disease. Transthoracic echocardiography is typically employed to estimate pulmonary artery pressures using the modified Bernoulli equation, the Doppler definition of PH is typically a tricuspid regurgitant jet velocity greater than 2.8m/sec. Using the right atrial pressure estimation of 5-15mmHg, this would estimate pulmonary artery systolic pressures of 36-46mmHg. A comprehensive echocardiogram also serves to evaluate for the presence of intracardiac defects and postcapillary causes of pulmonary hypertension and left sided heart

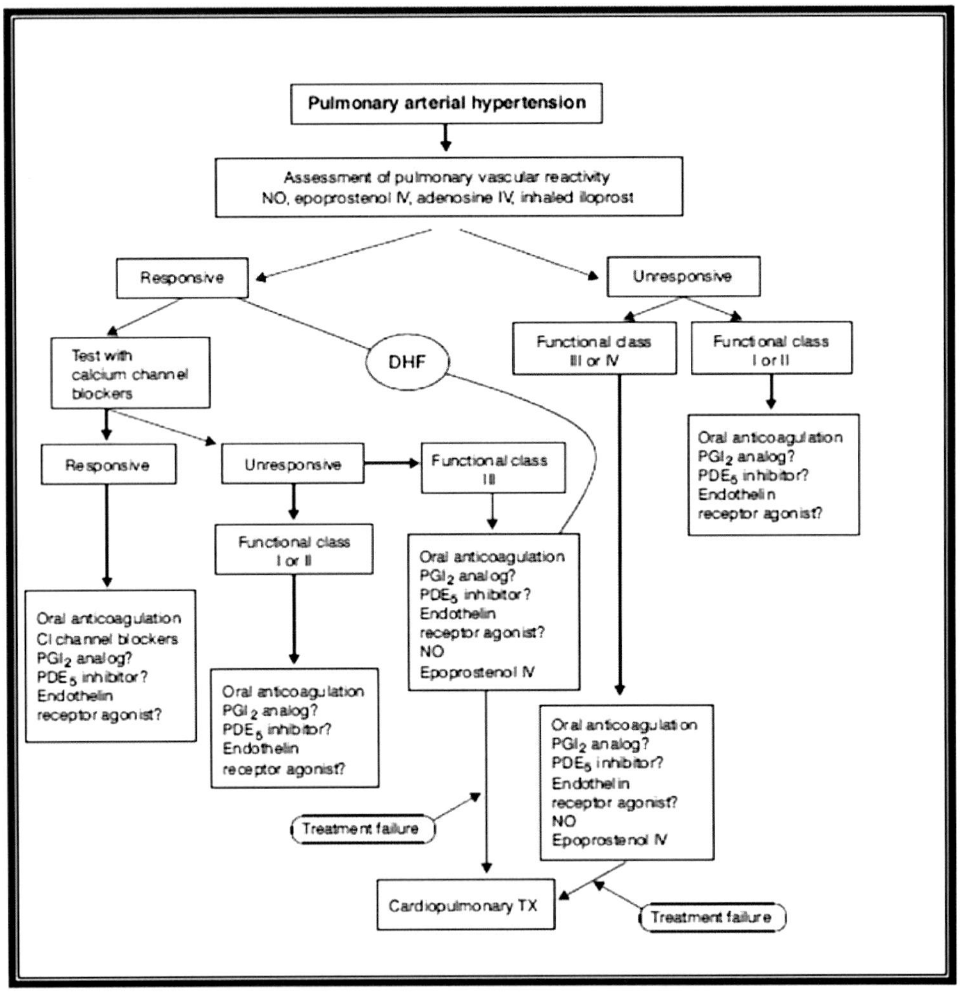

Ricachinevsky CP; J Pediatr (Rio J) 2006: 82; 153-65.

disease such as mitral valve disease, left ventricular dysfunction or diastolic dysfunction. For the final diagnosis, however it is the right heart catheterization that still remains the gold standard. It confirms the diagnosis of PH by demonstrating pulmonary artery pressure elevation in the presence of a normal pulmonary capillary wedge pressure (<15mmHg). In addition it also generates important data such as intracardiac pressures and cardiac index which serve to indicate prognosis. Importantly, vasodilator testing can be performed simultaneously with right heart catheterization; agents that are currently used include inhaled nitric oxide, intravenous prostacyclin and adenosine. Patients are labeled as responders if they exhibit a reduction of mean pulmonary artery pressure (MPAP) of at least 10mmHg to a value of 40mmHg or less with unchanged cardiac output. Finally, as part of the preoperative assessment the 6 minute walk test is frequently used, this strongly correlates with prognosis as well as being a means to assess the response to therapy either inpatient or outpatient. Ventilation/perfusion tomography, CT and MRI scanning are also important tools in the preoperative evaluation. Pulmonary angiography is less often used and is primarily indicated for patients with chronic thromboembolic pulmonary hypertension. It aids in locating the embolism and defining its extent.

The challenges of managing pulmonary hypertension vary in the two broad segments of patients that the anesthesiologist encounters. The first is the patient for cardiac surgery. For example in cardiac transplantation, elevated pulmonary vascular resistance (PVR) at the time of weaning from cardiopulmonary bypass contributes to immediate right ventricular failure and death. The key factor here is whether or not there is a reactive component to the PVR, which is directly responsive to the pulmonary capillary wedge pressure. Therefore, when the elevated PVR is primarily reactive, it will fall after transplantation. It is widely accepted that a PVR greater than about 5 Wood units unresponsive to pulmonary vasodilators and inotropes is a major contrain-dication to heart transplantation. In patients with elevated pulmonary arterial pressure (>50 mmHg) and little reactivity (mostly fixed pulmonary hypertension), the early mortality from cardiac graft failure is dramatically high. The transpulmonary gradient is used to categorize patients with PH. This is an index that is independent of pulmonary blood flow. This gradient is extrapolated by the difference between the mean pulmonary artery pressure and the pulmonary capillary wedge pressure. A gradient greater than 14 represents severe elevation of PVR. The key issue in the preoperative evaluation of these patients is the assessment of pulmonary vascular reactivity. As shown below, it defines the sequence of the investigations that follow.

Patients for non-cardiac surgery with severe pulmonary hypertension present an even greater challenge to the clinician in the operating room as there are multiple factors which can exacerbate the problem and it is usually an unanticipated issue. In these situations, a comprehensive plan from a multidisciplinary team is the most effective in management.

INITIAL NON-PHARMACOLOGIC MANAGEMENT

The first response of the clinician should be the maintenance and optimization of oxygenation and ventilation. The step involves the prevention and treatment of the classic predisposing factors which are known to exacerbate PAH: hypoxemia, hypercarbia, acidosis, hypothermia, and hypervolemia. Maintenance of deep anesthesia is critical as avoidance of sympathetic stimulation is one of the key factors that the anesthesiologist can control rapidly and effectively. Appropriate acid-based balance is also key to reducing pulmonary vascular resistance. In terms of hemodynamic monitoring, Swan- Ganz catheterization is recommended as is transesophageal echocardiography for continuous real time assessment of right and left ventricular function. Once the basic factors that can be controlled by the clinician are achieved, attention is given to right ventricular inotropes, particularly milrinone and dobutamine.

The final step in treating pulmonary hypertension is the use of selective pulmonary vasodilators initially through the intravenous route followed by inhaled pulmonary vasodilator therapy as needed.

INTRAVENOUS PULMONARY VASODILATORS

Nitroglycerin and Sodium Nitroprusside

These are the oldest pulmonary vasodilators used in the operating room. These are very effective as first line drugs and work through a cyclic GMP dependent mechanism. They are nitric oxide (NO) donors and in fact can be considered pro-drugs which release NO on metabolism. NO activates the soluble isoform of guanyl cyclase raising intracellular levels of cyclic GMP, dephosphorylation of the myosin light chains and reduction of the cytosolic calcium. The eventual result is relaxation of smooth muscle in a broad variety of tissues [3].

Years of research and experience with these nitrosovasodilators have suggested the existence of endogenous NO-modulated regulatory pathways. In the body, the generation of nitric oxide occurs *via* the action of the endogenous NO synthases. These oxidize the amino acid L-arginine to form NO, also rendering citrulline as a co-product [4].

A mitochondrial enzyme (aldehyde dehydrogenase) has been shown to play a key role in the biotransformation of the nitrates to NO [5].

Phosphodiesterase Inhibitors (PDE3)

The therapeutic usefulness of these drugs was first established in 1977 [6]. Since then, this group has had tremendous success in the management of multiple disease states in medicine. The primary substrate is the phosphodiesterase group of enzymes which are a superfamily of enzymes (11 groups) which degrade the phosphodiester group in the second messenger molecules cAMP and cGMP. These drugs therefore prolong the effects of physiological reactions that depend on cAMP and cGMP. In cardiopulmonary physio-logy, it is the phosphodiester groups 3 and 5 that are of prime importance. PDE5 has assumed greater scrutiny in pulmonary hypertension [7]. Increased PDE5 gene expression has been observed in PAH. Consequently, inhibition of this enzyme by specific PDE5 inhibitors increases the intracellular levels of cGMP, promoting the vasodilatory and antiproliferative effects protective in treating PAH. Sildenafil is a specific PDE5 inhibitor approved and highly effective for the management of pulmonary hypertension; however, it has no role in the intraoperative setting. In the operating room, the most commonly used agent in this class is milrinone, a PDE3 inhibitor. It is very effective to treat acute PAH, but has the important adverse effect of systemic vasodilatation along with the pulmonary vasodilatation it produces. Nebulized milrinone has been shown in some studies to avoid this adverse effect and will be discussed later. In cardiac surgery, milrinone has the added advantage of being an "inodilator" producing, aside from smooth muscle vasodilatation, an increase in cytosolic calcium and positive inotropy. The latter effect is independent of beta receptor stimulation.

B-type Natriuretic Peptide

Brain natriuretic peptide is a 32 amino acid polypeptide secreted by the ventricles of the heart (as opposed to atrial natriuretic peptide secreted by the atria). Both these endogenous hormones produce diuresis, natriuresis and vasodilation in response to volume overload. Recombinant human B-type natriuretic peptide binds to the particulate guanylate cyclase receptor of vascular smooth muscle and endothelial cells, leading to increased intracellular concentrations of guanosine 3'5'-cyclic monophosphate (cGMP) and smooth muscle cell relaxation. This results in arterial and venous dilation, evidenced by reductions in systemic vascular resistance, systemic arterial pressure, pulmonary capillary wedge pressure (PCWP), right atrial pressure, and mean pulmonary arterial pressure [8].

Infusion rates from 0.015 to 0.06 mcg/kg/min for 24 hours produces significant decreases in PCWP (27-39%), mean right atrial pressure and systemic vascular resistance (SVR); these effects are accompanied by increased cardiac index (CI) and stroke volume index (SVI) without an associated increase in heart rate [9]. In the operating room, it is typically started as a 2 ug/kg intravenous bolus followed by infusion of 0.01 ug/kg/minute. It has a half life of 18 minutes; tolerance has not been reported. This drug is used more often in the heart-lung transplant and ventricular-assist device population. It is currently the most selective and efficient intravenous pulmonary vasodilator without any significant systemic effects. It is being increasingly used to optimize high-risk patients with severe PAH for cardiac surgery.

Intravenous Prostaglandin Therapy (Prostaglandin I2)

Prostaglandins have been known for years to be potent endogenous vasodilators, in addition to inhibiting platelet aggregation. They also have been shown to have antiproliferative and cytoprotective properties [10]. In pulmonary hypertension, an important part of their therapeutic effect is associated with remodeling of the pulmonary vascular bed with subsequent reduction of endothelial cell injury and hypercoagulability [11]. There are two agents currently available: epoprostenol (Flolan) and iloprost. The former is inactivated in the circulation in 5 minutes. Iloprost is more potent than epoprostenol and has a half life of greater than 13 minutes [12]. Typical clinical indications include primary pulmonary hypertension, lung transplantation, adult respiratory distress syndrome, thromboembolic disease, shunts associated with congenital heart disease and portopulmonary hypertension [13]. Epoprostenol was approved for IV use in the treatment of primary pulmonary hypertension (PPH) by the FDA in December 1995.

The actions of epoprostenol, vasodilation of pulmonary and systemic arterial vascular beds, and platelet aggregation, are in direct opposition to thromboxane A_2, another prostaglandin. The inhibitory action of epoprostenol on platelet aggregation is mediated by the stimulation of adenylate cyclase and subsequent increase in cyclic adenosine monophosphate (AMP) in platelets. Hemodynamic effects of epoprostenol are due to increases in cyclic AMP in vascular smooth muscle and subsequent vasodilation. The hemodynamic effects of epoprostenol include decreased pulmonary vascular resistance, increased cardiac index, and increased oxygen delivery. The most significant side effects have been ascites and pulmonary edema from increased capillary permeability. Typical initial doses of epoprostanol and iloprost are 2 ng/kg/minute and 1 ng/kg/minute respectively; however, ultimately for acute use in the operating room, systemic hypotension limits the use of these drugs. Despite the known difficulties, epoprostenol is widely considered the long term intravenous therapy of choice for patients with advanced PH (functional class 4, right heart failure or more commonly as bridge to lung transplantation). The caveat to this, however is that patients requiring epoprostenol therapy be referred to experienced PH centers.

Calcium Channel Blockers

These are rarely the first line of drugs in the operating room, although they have been used to treat chronic pulmonary hypertension for the past few decades and have been shown in some studies to confer a survival advantage. Potential side effects include hypotension, pulmonary edema and RV failure.

Levosimendan

This is an inotrope which is a "calcium sensitizer." At therapeutic doses, levosimendan enhances myocardial contractility without increasing myocardial oxygen demand also producing coronary and systemic vasodilatation.

It increases cardiac tissue sensitivity to calcium without increasing tissue concentrations of calcium. Specifically the drug (a) inhibits phosphodiesterase III and (b) sensitizes troponin-C myofilaments to intracellular calcium ions. Animal pharmacology studies reveal that the drug stimulates cardiac potassium-ATP channels and glibenclamide inhibits this action. Clinically, levosimendan exhibits both inotropic and vasodilatory properties. The drug's mechanism purportedly minimizes the adverse effects associated with higher tissue concentrations of calcium which include cardiac arrhythmias and increased myocardial oxygen demand [14].

In comparison to dobutamine, a continuous 24-hour infusion of levosimendan decreased PCWP (Fig. **2**) [15], systemic vascular resistance, pulmonary vascular resistance (PVR) and pulmonary artery pressure (PAP) in patients with moderate to severe stable congestive heart failure. Dobutamine had no significant effect on these parameters.

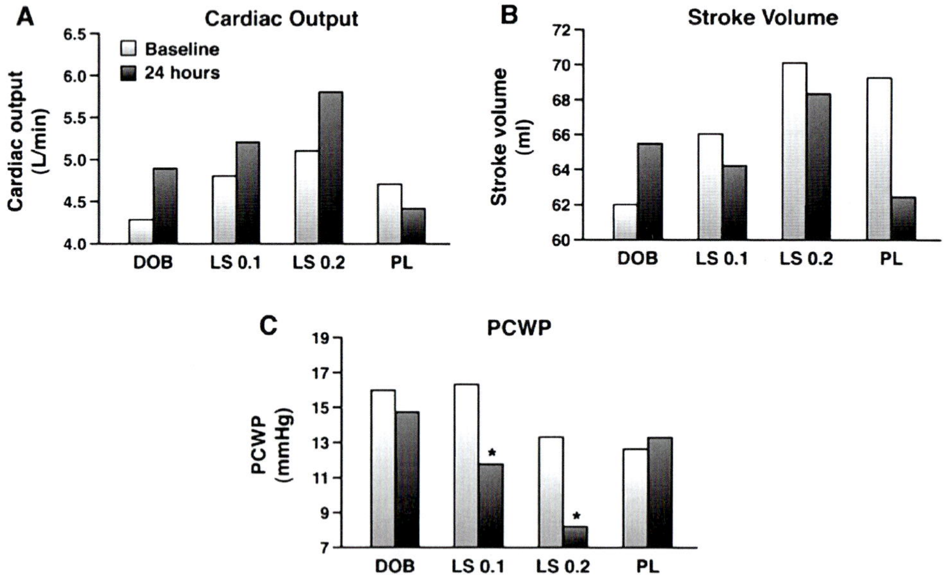

Fig. (2). Effects of levosimendan in heart failure patients, reprinted from J Am Coll Cardiol 2000; 36: 1903-1912.

The usual dosage of IV levosimendan used in clinical trials of patients with heart failure is 6 to 12 μg/kg loading dose over 10 minutes followed by 0.05 to 0.2 μg/kg/minute as a continuous infusion. Haemodynamic responses are generally observed within 5 minutes of commencement of infusion of the loading dose. Peak effects are observed within 10 to 30 minutes of infusion; the duration of action of levosimendan is about 1 to 2 hours [16].

The intraoperative use of levosimendan can be challenging owing to its concomitant vasodilatory effects. Consequently the administration of a vasopressor such as vasopressin is frequently necessary. The dose should be reduced in patients with severe renal insufficiency

INHALED SELECTIVE PULMONARY VASODILATORS

Inhaled Selective Pulmonary Vasodilators

Nitric oxide has long been the "gold standard" of inhaled pulmonary vasodilators and is the standard agent with which the other inhaled agents are compared. Since 1987 when it was first described as an important endothelium-derived relaxing factor, it has been extensively studied in both pediatric and adult patients as a key pulmonary vasodilator. It has been approved by the FDA to treat persistent pulmonary hypertension of the newborn since 1999. When inhaled, nitric oxide reacts with the iron in the heme portion of soluble guanylate cyclase, activating the enzyme. Activated guanylate cyclase produces cyclic guanosine 3',5'-monophosphate (cGMP), which then leads to vasodilation. Nitroglycerin and nitroprusside also stimulate cGMP formation, which results in smooth muscle relaxation. The common mechanism of action of these drugs is the release of nitric oxide. Inhaled nitric oxide appears to increase the partial pressure of arterial oxygen (PaO_2) by dilating pulmonary vessels in better ventilated areas of the lung and redistributing pulmonary blood flow away from lung regions with low ventilation/perfusion (V/Q) ratios toward regions with normal ratios [17].

In the body, nitric oxide is produced *via* synthesis from L-arginine by nitric oxide synthase (NOS) in a variety of tissues. Nitric oxide regulates many physiologic activities. Three NOS isoforms have been described: neuronal NOS, inducible NOS, a cytokine-inducible form, and endothelial NOS. It has been shown that all NOS isoforms can be induced or constitutively expressed. In addition, nitric oxide can be formed during reduced and acidotic conditions. Endothelial NOS is important in the regulation of systemic and pulmonary vascular tone and in lung development and disease. In cardiac endothelial cells, eNOS activity inhibits contractile tone and proliferation of smooth muscle cells, decreases platelet aggregation and monocyte adhesion, increases diastolic relaxation, and decreased the oxygen consumption by cardiac tissues. In addition, nitric oxide in cardiac myocytes opposes the inotropic action of catecholamines after muscarinic cholinergic or beta-adrenergic receptor stimulation. In the perioperative setting, nitric oxide is administered in a dose range of 5-40 parts per million *via* the inspiratory limb of the breathing circuit. Upon administration *via* the inhaled route nitric oxide is absorbed into the pulmonary vasculature, but systemic exposure is limited by rapid inactivation in blood cells. The half-life of nitric oxide is a few seconds. Methemoglobin and nitrate are the end products of nitric oxide metabolism present in the systemic circulation. Continuous monitoring of both nitric oxide and nitrogen dioxide levels is mandatory to avoid toxicity, and care should be taken not to exceed the recommended limit of 25 parts per million per 8 occupational hours. It is always mixed with a carrier gas in the operating room and intensive care unit. The typical nitric oxide cylinder contains up to 2200 parts per million mixed with nitrogen to prevent the formation of reactive metabolites [17]. The practical issues that determine the actual dose being administered are the fraction of inspired oxygen, the amount of the carrier gas and the ventilator settings. The general aim is to keep the levels of nitrogen dioxide below 2 parts per million. Nomograms are available to guide the clinician and aid accurate dosing. In the cardiovascular operating room, nitric oxide is the first agent used to treat pulmonary hypertension associated with cardiopulmonary bypass, acute right ventricular decompensation, lung and heart transplantation and in patients with cardiac assist devices. The efficacy and safety of nitric oxide in these conditions been extensively documented [18, 19] (Fig. **3**).

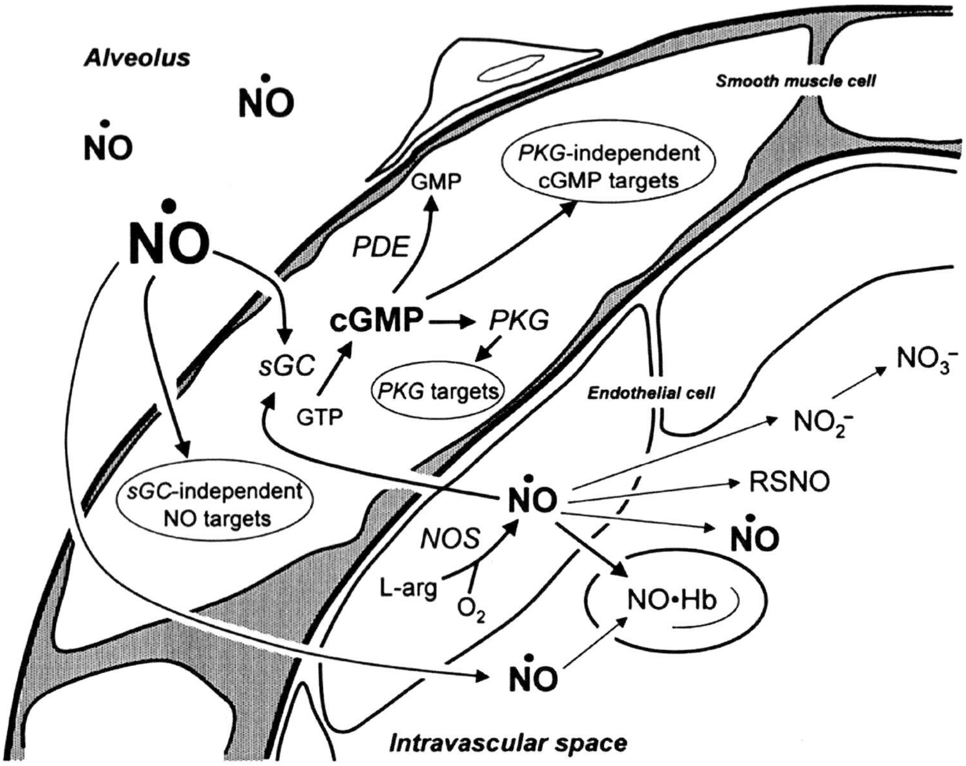

Fig. (3). No signaling pathway in the lung. PKG indicates cGMP-dependent protein kinases; NOS, NO synthase; L-arg, L-arginine; sGC, soluble guanylate cyclases; and RSNO, S-nitrosothiol. Reprinted from Zapol WM. Inhaled nitric oxide: A selective pulmonary vasodilator: Current uses and therapeutic potential. Circulation 2004; 109: 3106-3111.

LIMITATIONS OF NITRIC OXIDE

Nitric oxide has the potential to affect platelet function and has been shown in some studies to predispose bleeding; however, this is very rarely seen in clinical practice. In patients with impaired function of the left ventricle, NO has a potential to further impair left ventricular performance by dilating the pulmonary circulation and increasing the blood flow to the left ventricle, thereby increasing left atrial pressure and promoting pulmonary edema formation. Careful monitoring of cardiac output, left atrial pressure, or pulmonary capillary wedge pressure is important in this situation [17]. The development of methemoglobinemia is a significant complication of inhaled NO at higher concentrations, and rare deaths have been reported with overdoses of NO. The blood content of methemoglobin, however, generally will not increase to toxic levels with appropriate use of inhaled NO. Methemoglobin concentrations should be monitored intermittently during NO inhalation [17,20]. Rapid discontinuation of nitric oxide in a patient with pulmonary hypertension may trigger a rebound with hypoxemia and right ventricular failure. To reduce this risk, the withdrawal should be gradual with substitution of alternative agents. The nitrogen dioxide formed as a byproduct may trigger bronchospasm in susceptible patients. Lastly, cost is an issue with nitric oxide; it is very expensive. This became more apparent after FDA approval, and spawned the search for other agents that are nitric oxide donors. A brief review of the alternatives follows.

Inhaled Sodium Nitroprusside (SNP)

Inhaled SNP has little practical application in the operating room so far; however, there have been multiple animal studies to confirm its usefulness in treating reactive pulmonary vasculature. One study by Schutte H *et al.* showed that inhaled SNP produced dose-dependent pulmonary vasodilation in isolated perfused rabbit lungs with thromboxane-induced pulmonary hypertension [21]. In another study, Meadow *et al.* investigated the short-term effects of inhaled SNP (50 mg in 5 ml saline) in a porcine model of pH, induced by either hypoxia or group *B streptococci*. Inhaled SNP selectively decreased PAP in hypoxia-induced pH, which was sustained with continuous treatment for longer than 60 min. A reduced response was observed in *Streptococci* induced pH, and there was no associated improvement in oxygenation [22].

Nitroglycerin

There is very little reported in the literature on the use of inhaled nitroglycerin. Animal studies have reported some success; however, although nitroglycerin did produce dose-dependent pulmonary vasodilatation, it was significantly less efficacious than other agents including SNP. Gong *et al.* showed that aerosolized nitroglycerin produced a 31% decrease in PVR with no effect on systemic hemodynamics [23].

Phosphodiesterase Inhibitors

Nitric oxide exerts its vasodilative effect by increasing cellular concentrations of cyclic guanosine monophosphate. This is rapidly metabolized by phosphodiesterases which terminate its effect. The concept of using inhaled milrinone is not new. Haraldsson *et al.* in 2001 demonstrated that inhaled milrinone, a type 3 phosphodiesterase inhibitor that increases vascular smooth muscle adenosine-3,5-cyclicmonophosphate concentrations, caused selective pulmonary vasodilatation in cardiac surgical patients with postoperative pulmonary hypertension [24].

As of today, there have been greater than 70 randomized trials investigating the usefulness of milrinone in heart failure and pulmonary hypertension. Milrinone has been shown to improve both diastolic performance in patients with congestive heart failure and left ventricular compliance after cardiopulmonary bypass. There have been few studies so far, however investigating the effects of inhaled milrinone in the perioperative period.

Sablotzki A *et al.* in 2005 investigated the effects of inhaled milrinone in 18 heart transplant recipients. The mean pulmonary artery pressure (MPAP), transpulmonary gradient and pulmonary vascular resistance decreased only in patients with pulmonary hypertension, defined as a MPAP above 30mm Hg. With a dose of 2 mg inhaled through a nebulizer, no systemic side effects were seen. This was not an intraoperative study (Fig. **4**) [25].

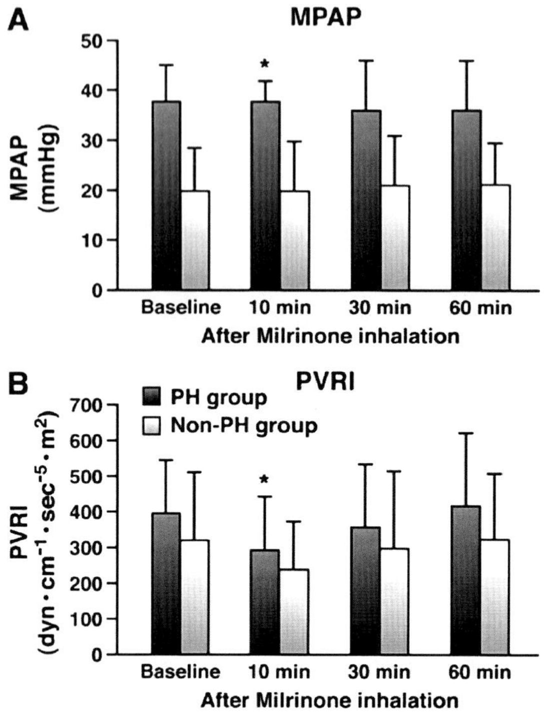

Fig. (4). *A*, Effect of milrinone-inhalation on mean pulmonary arterial pressure (MPAP) in patients with (n = 9) and without (n = 9) pulmonary hypertension; *P < .05 compared to baseline. *B*, Effect of milrinone-inhalation on pulmonary vascular resistance index (PVRI) in patients with (n = 9) and without (n = 9) pulmonary hypertension; *P < .05 compared to baseline. (With permission from Sablotzki A, Starzmann W, Scheubel R, *et al.* Selective pulmonary vasodilation with inhaled aerosolized milrinone in heart transplant candidates: *Can J Anaesth*. 2005; 52: 1076-1082.) © 2006.

In summary, inhaled milrinone presents a novel method of using a potent PDE3 inhibitor. It is cheaper than nitric oxide and less cumbersome to administer as compared to the other selective pulmonary venodilators, needing nothing more than an ultrasonic nebulizer that is connected to the inspiratory limb of the breathing circuit. A key aspect of using it in this fashion is that it can be started prior to cardiopulmonary bypass as an adjunct to therapy in the patient with anticipated right ventricular failure where it could prevent the post bypass reperfusion injury associated with severe pulmonary hypertension (Fig. **5**) [26].

Inhaled Prostaglandin I2 (Epoprostanol, Prostacyclin, Flolan)

The first clinical report of administration of inhaled PGI2 was described in 1978 [27]. PGI2 is a potent vasodilator and the most powerful inhibitor of platelet aggregation. It has been shown to promote the release of nitric oxide [28]. Nitric oxide in turn has been shown to enhance the production of PGI2 in human pulmonary endothelial cells [29]. PGI2 has a

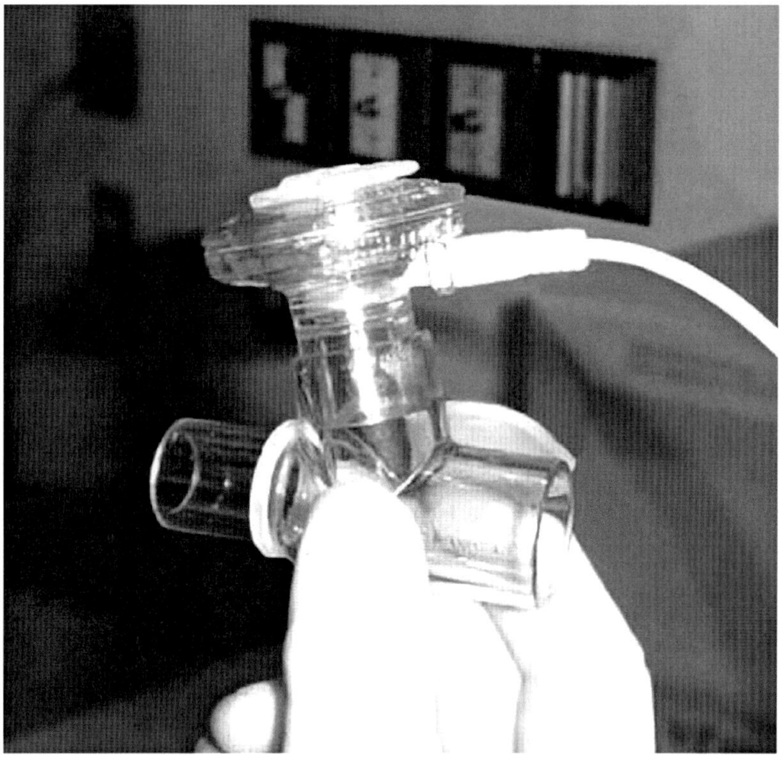

Fig. (5). Milrinone nebulizer.- from Y Denault, Seminars in Cardiothoracic and Vascular Anesthesia, Dec 2006: 3346-360.

short half life of 2.7. It is spontaneously hydrolyzed at neutral pH to inactive metabolites. PGI2 in its intravenous form has been in use for over 20 years for multiple indications and has been limited by its severe systemic side effects. In contrast, the inhaled form has no toxic effects or metabolites. It has emerged as a ready alternative to inhaled NO due to two huge advantages: its cost is one tenth that of NO and it bears no similar toxicity profile. It is also simpler to administer in that no monitoring of the drug or metabolites is required and unlike the titration of NO this drug is administered on a weight-based dose of 5-50 ng/kg/minute via a syringe pump connected to a nebulizer attached to the inspiratory limb of the breathing circuit. In trials, inhaled PGI2 has been proven to be equivalent to inhaled NO in multiple models of pulmonary hypertension, primary and thromboembolic, as well as that associated with LV failure, sepsis and post cardiac surgery [30]. In addition, because NO and PGI2 work through different pathways (cGMP and cAMP respectively) a synergistic effect is seen when administered together [31]. In the setting of lung transplantation, inhaled PGI2 has been shown to be particularly useful. In one study, 10 ng $\cdot$ kg^{-1} $\cdot min^{-1}$ of inhaled PGI2 produced an 11% decrease in mean PAP and a 25% decrease in intrapulmonary shunt [32].

Inhaled PGI2 is limited by a few largely theoretical complications. First, being a platelet inhibitor, there is always a concern for bleeding. This has not proven to be of clinical significance *in vivo*. Second, there have been some concerns with rebound pulmonary hypertension with abrupt discontinuation [33]. Iloprost, a stable derivative of PGI2 with similar vasodilator properties, has been proposed a possible alternative largely due to its longer half life of 30 minutes [34]. However, this is not approved for use in the United States. Tracheal and bronchial irritability with inhaled PGI2 is also a possibility, although clinically this is rare. JAK2-, Raf kinase and ACE inhibitors have been patented recently for the treatment of pulmonary arterial hypertension by Zisman [35] and Mitland [36] and Anker [37] respectively.

Prostaglandin E1 is another potential alternative via the inhaled route; however, further clinical studies are necessary as there is a lack of published data with this prostaglandin (Fig. **6**) [38]. Block has recently patented peptides for the treatment of hypertension [39]. Fong has also patented novel therapeutic agents for the treatment of arterial hypertension and angina [40].

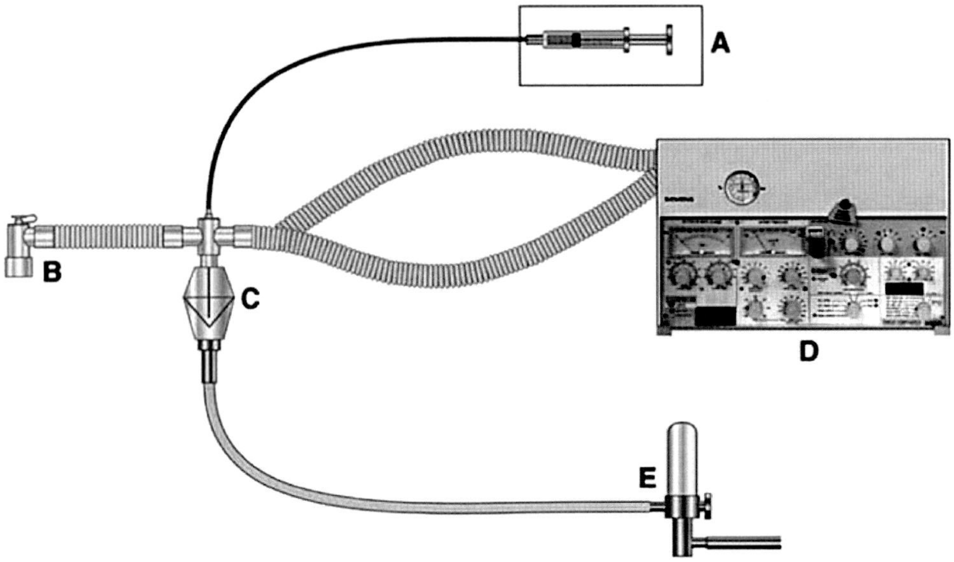

Fig. (6). A = syringe pump delivering epoprostenol solution; B = patient end of ventilator tubing; C = jet nebulizer; D = mechanical ventilator; E = nebulizer driving the gas at 6 L/min. From: van Heerden. Chest 2000; 117(3): 819-827.

CURRENT AND FUTURE DEVELOPMENTS

This review article has aimed at elucidating the newer options available to the acute care clinician in the operating room and intensive care unit in the management of perioperative pulmonary hypertension and right ventricular failure. In the clinical arena pulmonary hypertension, if left untreated, promptly can have very poor outcomes. Optimal management is multimodal and tiered from basic to more complex therapies. The first step in the approach is to create a favorable environment for pulmonary vasodilatation by optimizing ventilation: achieve hyperoxia, hypocapnea and alkalosis. The next step involves the use of appropriate ventricular inotropic support; this typically means the use of dobutamine, epinephrine and the PDE3 inhibitors, the best results often achieved with the synergistic combination of two or more of these drugs. Once these have been accomplished, attention is turned toward the use of the selective pulmonary vasodilators. The best practice is to use these along with intravenous adjuncts. At present, at most of the major medical centers in the USA, the key inhaled agents are nitric oxide and prostaglandin I2. Based on local practices and availability, inhaled agents may often be the first line of therapy, chosen over the intravenous agents. This is a decision made in the operating room or intensive care unit by the anesthesiologist/ intensivist and is primarily influenced by the clinical situation. In my practice which has a high proportion of critically ill heart-lung transplant patients I personally favor a more holistic approach toward the problem of pulmonary hypertension realizing that it is a complex clinical problem that needs multimodal therapy, reliance on one drug or modality often leads to failure.

Prostaglandin I2 has a better safety profile, is cheaper and more easily administered compared with Nitric oxide. The newer adjunctive agents include natriuretic peptide, endothelin antagonists and vasopressin which is the drug of choice in the setting of vasodilatory shock with pulmonary hypertension where it functions as a systemic vasoconstrictor and a mild pulmonary vasodilator. The clinician always has to keep in mind that the use of synergistic combinations of these agents is to be recommended in the management of this complex condition in order to improve perioperative outcomes. Recent trends in research in the field of PH seem to indicate that regression of established PH has been associated with a decrease of proliferation and induction of apoptosis in the wall of pulmonary arteries [41]. With this in mind two of the newer agents being trialed in some patients are listed below:

Simvastatin- caused benefit by inducing the apoptosis of neointimal smooth muscle cells.

Fluoxetine- this selective serotonin transporter inhibitor reversed the proliferation of pulmonary artery smooth muscle cells in a model of monocrotaline induced PH [42].

In conclusion, it seems that the most effective methods of combating pulmonary hypertension in the perioperative period would include preoperative optimization with endothelin antagonists such as Bosentan and Sitaxsentan to mitigate the vasoconstrictive and prolixferative effects in the pulmonary circulation in addition to the use of the Phosphodiesterase-5 inhibitors (such as sidenafil, vardenafil, tadalafil) which increase pulmonary cGMP promoting vasodilatory and antiproliferative effects. Successful outcomes in this highly challenging patient population mandate the former in addition to intraoperative management that emphasizes the utilization of basic anesthetic principles (maintainence of adequate oxygenation, ventilation and systemic perfusion), using a combination of intravenous and inhaled pulmonary vasodilators, left and right ventricular inotropes followed by comprehensive intensive care and long term follow up.

ABBREVIATIONS

PH = Pulmonary hypertension

PAH = Pulmonary artery hypertension

PVR = Pulmonary vascular resistance

GMP = Guanosine monophosphate

NO = Nitric oxide

PCWP = Pulmonary capillary wedge pressure

SVR = Systemic vascular resistance

CI = Cardiac index

SVI = Stroke volume index

PPH = Primary pulmonary hypertension

AMP = Adenosine monophosphate

PVR = Pulmonary vascular resistance

PAP = Pulmonary artery pressure

V/Q = Ventilation/perfusion

NOS = Nitric oxide synthase

SNP = Sodium nitroprusside

MPAP = Mean pulmonary artery pressure

REFERENCES

[1] D'Alonzo GE, Barst RJ, Ayres SM, *et al.* Survival in patients with primary pulmonary hypertension. Results from a national prospective registry. Ann Intern Med 1991; 115: 343-349.

[2] AACP Guidelines. Chest 2004; 126.

[3] Murad F. The Albert Lasker Medical Research Awards. Signal transduction using nitric oxide and cyclic guanosine mono-phosphate. JAMA 1996; 276: 1189-1192.

[4] Lowenstein CJ, Dinerman JL, Snyder SH. Nitric oxide: a physiologic messenger. Ann Inter Med 1994; 120: 227-237.

[5] Chen Z, Zhang J, Stamler JS. Identification of the enzymatic mechanism of nitroglycerin bioactivation. Proc Natl Acad Sci USA 2002; 99: 8306-8311.

[6] Weiss B, Hait WN. Selective cyclic nucleotide phosphodiesterase inhibitors as potential therapeutic agents. Ann Rev Pharmacol Toxicol 1977; 17: 441-477.

[7] Takimoto E, Champion HC, Li M, *et al.* Chronic inhibition of cyclic GMP phosphodiesterase 5A prevents and reverses cardiac hypertrophy. Nat Med 2005; 11: 214-222.

[8] Intravenous nesiritide *vs.* nitroglycerin for treatment of decompensated congestive heart failure: a randomized controlled trial. JAMA 2002; 287: 1531-1540.

[9] Mills RM, LeJemtel TH, Horton DP, *et al.* Sustained hemodynamic effects of an infusion of nesiritide (human b-type natriuretic peptide) in heart failure: a randomized, double-blind, placebo-controlled clinical trial. Natrecor Study Group. J Am College Cardiol 1999; 34: 155-162.

[10] Vane JR, Botting RM. Pharmacodynamic profile of prostacyclin. Am J Cardiol 1995; 75: 3A-10A.

[11] Friedman R, Mears JG, Barst RJ. Continuous infusion of prostacyclin normalizes plasma markers of endothelial cell injury and platelet aggregation in primary pulmonary hypertension. Circulation 1997; 96: 2782-2784.

[12] Haslam RJ, McClenaghan MD. Measurement of circulating prostacyclin. Nature 1981; 292: 364-366.

[13] Kuo PC, Johnson LB, Plotkin JS, Howell CD, Bartlett ST, Rubin LJ. Continuous intravenous infusion of epoprostenol for the treatment of portopulmonary hypertension. Transplantation 1997; 63: 604-606.

[14] Sandell EP, Hayha M, Antila S, *et al.* Pharmacokinetics of levosimendan in healthy volunteers and patients with congestive heart failure. J Cardiovas Pharmacol 1995; 26 Suppl 1: S57-62.

[15] Nieminen MS, Akkila J, Hasenfuss G, *et al.* Hemodynamic and neurohumoral effects of continuous infusion of levosimendan in patients with congestive heart failure. J Am College Cardiol 2000; 36: 1903-1912.

[16] Figgitt DP, Gillies PS, Goa KL. Levosimendan. Drugs 2001; 61: 613-627; discussion 628-619.

[17] Steudel W, Hurford WE, Zapol WM. Inhaled nitric oxide: basic biology and clinical applications. Anesthesiology 1999; 91: 1090-1121.

[18] Blaise G, Langleben D, Hubert B. Pulmonary arterial hypertension: pathophysiology and anesthetic approach. Anesthesiology 2003; 99: 1415-1432.

[19] Ichinose F, Roberts JD, Jr, Zapol WM. Inhaled nitric oxide: a selective pulmonary vasodilator: current uses and therapeutic potential. Circulation 2004; 109: 3106-3111.

[20] Haddad E, Millatt L, Johns R. Clinical applications of inhaled NO. In: Kadowitz P, ed. Lung Physiology. New York: Marcel Dekker, 2000.

[21] Schutte H, Grimminger F, Otterbein J, *et al.* Efficiency of aerosolized nitric oxide donor drugs to achieve sustained pulmonary vasodilation. J Pharmacol Exper Therapeut 1997; 282: 985-994.

[22] Meadow W, Rudinsky B, Bell A, Hipps R. Effects of nebulized nitroprusside on pulmonary and systemic hemodynamics during pulmonary hypertension in piglets. Pediat Res 1998; 44: 181-186.

[23] Gong F, Shiraishi H, Kikuchi Y, *et al.* Inhalation of nebulized nitroglycerin in dogs with experimental pulmonary hypertension induced by U46619. Pediatr Int 2000; 42: 255-258.

[24] Haraldsson A, Kieler-Jensen N, Ricksten SE. The additive pulmonary vasodilatory effects of inhaled prostacyclin and inhaled milrinone in postcardiac surgical patients with pulmonary hypertension. Anesth Analg 2001; 93: 1439-1445 (table of contents).

[25] Sablotzki A, Starzmann W, Scheubel R, Grond S, Czeslick EG. Selective pulmonary vasodilation with inhaled aerosolized milrinone in heart transplant candidates. Can J Anaesth 2005; 52: 1076-1082.

[26] Denault AY, Lamarche Y, Couture P, *et al.* Inhaled milrinone: a new alternative in cardiac surgery? Semin Cardiothor Vasc Anesth 2006; 10: 346-360.

[27] Szczeklik A, Gryglewski R, Nizankowska E, Nizankowski R, Musial J. Pulmonary and anti-platelet effects of intravenous and inhaled prostacyclin in man. Prostaglandins 1978; 16: 651-660.

[28] Shimokawa H, Flavahan NA, Lorenz RR, Vanhoutte PM. Prostacyclin releases endothelium-derived relaxing factor and potentiates its action in coronary arteries of the pig. Br J Pharmacol 1988; 95: 1197-1203.

[29] Wen F, Watanabe K, Yoshida M. Nitric oxide enhances PGI(2)production by human pulmonary artery smooth muscle cells. Prostaglandins Leuko Essent Fatty Acids 2000; 62: 369-378.

[30] Mikhail G, Gibbs J, Richardson M, *et al.* An evaluation of nebulized prostacyclin in patients with primary and secondary pulmonary hypertension. Eur Heart J 1997; 18: 1499-1504.

[31] Hill LL, Pearl RG. Combined inhaled nitric oxide and inhaled prostacyclin during experimental chronic pulmonary hypertension. J Appl Physiol 1999; 86: 1160-1164.

[32] Della Rocca G, Coccia C, Costa MG, *et al.* Inhaled areosolized prostacyclin and pulmonary hypertension during anesthesia for lung transplantation. Transplant Proc 2001; 33: 1634-1636.

[33] Miller OI, Tang SF, Keech A, Celermajer DS. Rebound pulmonary hypertension on withdrawal from inhaled nitric oxide. Lancet 1995; 346: 51-52.

[34] Grant SM, Goa KL. Iloprost. A review of its pharmacodynamic and pharmacokinetic properties, and therapeutic potential in peripheral vascular disease, myocardial ischaemia and extracorporeal circulation procedures. Drugs 1992; 43: 889-924.

[35] Zisman, LS: WO07101232 (**2007**).

[36] Maitland, MG, Ratain, M: WO07087575 (**2007**).

[37] Anker, S, Springer, J: WO07014586 (**2007**).

[38] van Heerden PV, Barden A, Michalopoulos N, Bulsara MK, Roberts BL. Dose-response to inhaled aerosolized prostacyclin for hypoxemia due to ARDS. Chest 2000; 117: 819-827.

[39] Block, L.Z.: EP1792915 (**2007**).

[40] Fong, B.: WO07050783 (**2007**).

[41] Archer, S.L., Michelakis, E.D.: Curr Opin Cardiol 2006; 21: 385-392.

[42] Chambers CD. NEJM 2006; 354: 579-87a.

The Role of Small, Dense LDL in Cardiovascular Risk: The Contributions of the Universities of Palermo and Zurich

Manfredi Rizzo*[,1] and Kaspar Berneis[2]

[1]*Department of Clinical Medicine and Emerging Diseases, University of Palermo, Via Maqueda, 175, 90133 Palermo, Italy*

[2]*Clinic for Endocrinology, Diabetes & Clinical Nutrition, University Hospital Zurich, Switzerland and Zurich Center for Integrative Human Physiology, University of Zurich, Switzerland*

Abstract: Low density lipoproteins (LDL) size seems to be an important predictor of cardiovascular events and progression of coronary artery disease and the predominance of small dense LDL has been accepted as an emerging cardiovascular risk factors by the National Cholesterol Education Program Adult Treatment Panel III. We recently showed increased LDL size or higher levels of small and dense LDL in different categories of patients at higher cardiovascular risk, such as those with coronary (including acute myocardial infarction) and non-coronary (including carotid disease, abdominal aortic aneurysm and peripheral arterial disease) forms of atherosclerosis or metabolic diseases (including type-II diabetes, polycystic ovary syndrome, growth hormone deficiency, gestational diabetes and the metabolic syndrome). Screening for the presence of small, dense LDL may potentially identify those with even higher risks and may contribute in directing specific treatments in order to prevent new cardiovascular events. This seems particularly true for statins and fibrates. Promising data are available for rosuvastatin, the latest statin molecule introduced in the market, and ezetimibe, a cholesterol absorption inhibitor.

Keywords: Small, dense LDL, cardiovascular risk, prevention.

INTRODUCTION

Low-density lipoproteins (LDL) comprise multiple subclasses with discrete size and density, different physicochemical composition and metabolic behaviour. Based on their characteristic appearance in analytical ultracentrifugation and gradient gel electrophoresis, up to seven distinct subclasses have been defined (Table **1**). It has been suggested that there are parallel metabolic channels within the delipidation cascade from very low density lipoprotein (VLDL) to LDL [1] and a metabolic relationship between large VLDL particles and small LDL particles has been demonstrated using stable isotopes in subjects with a predominance of small, dense LDL [2]. These studies have not yet identified the specific

*Corresponding author: Tel and Fax: +39 (091) 655-2945; E-mail: mrizzo@unipa.it

Atta-ur-Rahman / M. Iqbal Choudhary (Eds.)

precursors of individual LDL subclasses; however there are data from animal models suggesting that separate pathways may be responsible for the generation of distinct LDL particles [3]. Dietary intervention studies demonstrated inverse correlations between changes in large and small LDL, as well as between changes in medium sized and very small LDL which raise the possibility of precursor-product relationships between distinct LDL subclasses [4].

Table 1. Properties of LDL Subclasses (As Modified from 1)

LDL Subclasses	Peak Sf	Density Peak (g/mL)	Diameter (Å)
LDL-I	7-12	1.019-1.023	272-285
LDL-IIA	5-7	1.023-1.028	265-272
LDL-IIB	5-7	1.028-1.034	256-265
LDL-IIIA	3-5	1.034-1.041	247-256
LDL-IIIB	3-5	1.041-1.044	242-247
LDL-IVA	0-3	1.044-1.051	233-242
LDL-IVB	0-3	1.051-1.06	220-233

Activity of lipolytic enzymes is related to the size of LDL particles. A significant inverse relationship between postheparin lipoprotein lipase activity (LpL) and small, dense LDL has been demonstrated and induction of LpL by high fat diet was associated with an increase of large LDL and decrease of small and dense LDL. Reduced activity of LpL and increased activity of HL have been shown in subjects with a predominance of small and dense LDL particles [5]. HL has a higher affinity for LDL than LpL and is positively correlated with plasma TG, apolipoprotein B, mass of large VLDL and small, dense LDL, but not with the mass of large LDL [6], suggesting a central role for HL in the lipolytic conversion of these particles.

Triglyceridaemia seems to be the main determinant of LDL subclass distribution [7]. In fact, the formation of small, dense LDL particles is mostly observed in hypertriglyceridemic state, with an increased transfer of TG from TG-rich lipoproteins to LDL and HDL particles in exchange of cholesteryl esters through the action of CETP [8]. This phenomenon leads to the generation of VLDL particles enriched in cholesteryl esters and smaller TG-rich LDL particles that are good substrates for HL. As a consequence, predictive value of small and dense LDL is usually reduced when TG levels are taken into account [9]. For example, in a recently published analysis from the EPIC-Norfolk prospective population study, predictive power for cardiovascular events of LDL particle number and size was lost after adjustment for HDL-C and TG levels [10].

SMALL, DENSE LDL AND CARDIOVASCULAR RISK

Several reasons have been suggested to explain the enhanced atherogenicity of small, dense LDL. These particles are taken up more easily by arterial tissue than larger LDL [11], suggesting greater transendothelial transport. In addition, small, dense LDL have a decreased receptor-mediated uptake and an increased proteoglycan binding [12]. Sialic acid, due to its exposure at the LDL surface, plays a determinant role in the *in vitro* association of LDL with the polyanionic proteoglycans [13] and it has been shown that sialic acid content of LDL particles of subjects with the predominance of small and dense LDL is reduced. Further, oxidative susceptibility increases and antioxidant concentrations reduce with decreasing LDL size [14]. Altered properties of the surface lipid layer associated with reduced content of free cholesterol [15] and increased content of polyunsaturated fatty acids [16] might also contribute to enhanced oxidative susceptibility of small dense LDL.

To date, the association of LDL size with CVD has been tested in over fifty studies, including cross-sectional and prospective epidemiologic, as well as clinical intervention trials; these studies overall suggest that the quality of LDL exerts a direct influence on CVD risk. Due to previously described atherogenic properties, the predominance of small, dense LDL has been accepted as an emerging cardiovascular risk factor by the National Cholesterol Education Program Adult Treatment Panel III. It has also been shown that even small increases in the concentration of these particles may substantially contribute to the determination of total cardiovascular risk [17]. Other studies have investigated if the therapeutic modification of LDL size may be significantly associated with reduced cardiovascular risk. Such investigations used arteriographic changes as outcome variables and have reported that benefit was concentrated in patients with a predominance of small, dense LDL who received treatment that tend to reduce the amount of such particles [18-20].

These findings suggest that the therapeutic modification of LDL size may be significantly associated with reduced cardiovascular risk, even after multivariate adjustment for confounding factors. In addition, it has been reported [21], although not directly demonstrated, that the modulation of LDL size with fibrates probably contributed to the reduction of cardiovascular risk in large clinical trials [22-24]. Yet, it cannot be fully excluded that the increased CVD risk associated with smaller LDL size may also be a consequence of the broader pathophysiology of which small, dense LDL are a part (e.g. high TG, low HDL-C, increased LDL particle number, obesity, insulin resistance, diabetes, metabolic syndrome) [25-28].

WHICH SUBJECTS HAVE ELEVATED LEVELS OF SMALL, DENSE LDL?

With CAD or Type-2 Diabetes

It is well known that patients at very-high cardiovascular risk, such as those with CAD and type-II diabetes, have increased levels of atherogenic small dense LDL [1]. In addition, in recent years, it has been tested whether other categories of subjects at high cardiovascular risk may have increased levels of these particles too. Some authors have studied patients with vascular diseases; in fact, it has been stated by the NCEP ATP III that clinical forms of non-coronary atherosclerosis carry a risk for CAD equal to those with established CAD [29]. These conditions include carotid artery disease, peripheral arterial disease and abdominal aortic aneurysm.

With Carotid Artery Disease

Preliminarly, Landray *et al.* in 1998 [30] first showed an association between small, dense LDL and asymptomatic carotid atherosclerosis and this has been confirmed by other similar studies in healthy individuals [31-33]. Other authors found a significant relationship between LDL size and the occurrence of preclinical and clinical carotid atherosclerosis [34-38] and we recently demonstrated [39] that LDL size is significantly associated with carotid intima media thickness in patients with type 2 diabetes. Notably, in our study multivariate analysis revealed that LDL size was the strongest predictor of intima media thickness within all lipid parameters and the second strongest predictor (after smoking) among all traditional cardiovascular risk factors (Table **2**). Regarding clinical trials, Van Tits *et al.* [38] showed an association between intima media thickness regression and baseline LDL size (by statin therapy with atorvastatin and simvastatin) and this was confirmed by Wallenfeldt *et al.* [40] in a 3-year follow-up of 313 58-year-old subjects. These findings are consistent with a role of LDL size in modulating carotid atherosclerosis regression.

Table 2. Multivariate Analysis of Variance of 10 Cardiovascular Risk Factors for Coronary Heart Disease (CHD) and Intima Media Thickness (IMT) (as Modified from 39)

	Presence of IMT (MANOVA, p=)	Presence of CHD (MANOVA, p=)
Smoking (pack-years)	0.003	0.005
LDL size (angstrom)	0.03	0.002
LDL-cholesterol (mmol/L)	0.06	0.01
HDL-cholesterol (mmol/L)	0.06	0.01
Lipoprotein (a) (g/L)	0.06	0.5
Age (years)	0.2	0.9
Haemoglobin A1c (%)	0.3	0.5
C-reactive protein (mg/dL)	0.3	0.9
Systolic blood pressure (mm Hg)	0.6	0.2
Body Mass Index	0.8	0.2

With Peripheral Arterial Disease

Regarding subjects with peripheral arterial disease Lupattelli *et al.* [41] did not find any difference in LDL size between normolipemic non-diabetic patients with peripheral arterial disease and controls, matched for gender, age and body mass index; by contrast, O'Neal *et al.* [42] performed a similar study but on a larger sample-size and they found that smaller LDL size was associated with the presence of peripheral arterial disease in absence or presence of diabetes. These findings were confirmed by our recent study performed on patients with intermittent claudication [43]: in relation to age-BMI-matched controls, patients with peripheral arterial disease had lower LDL size with decreased larger subclasses and increased small and dense particles (Fig. **1**). Notably, multivariate analysis suggested an independent association between small, dense LDL and peripheral arterial disease, beyond which already established for smoking, diabetes and hypertension.

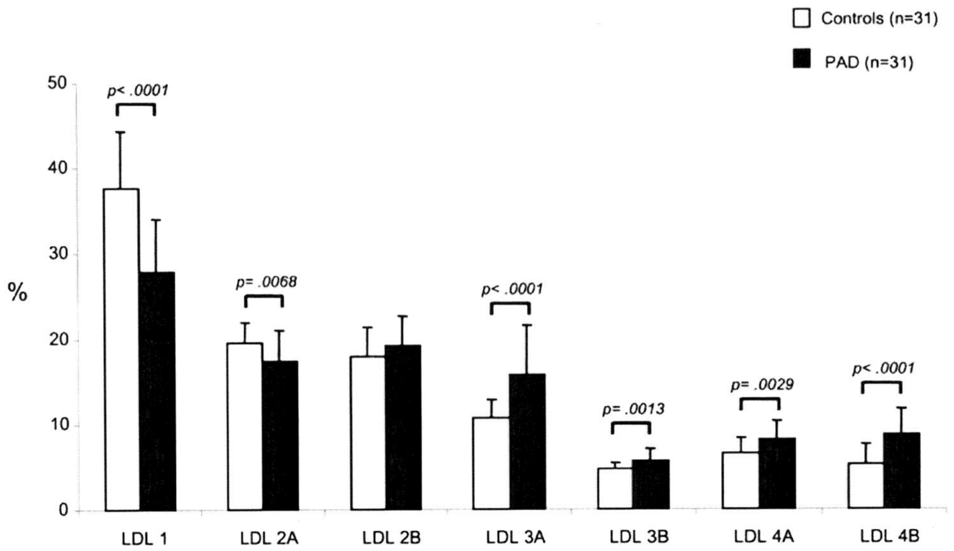

Fig. (1). LDL sublcasses in patients with PAD and controls [ref. 43].

With Abdominal Aortic Aneurysm

Limited data is available on cardiovascular risk factors in subjects with atherosclerotic abdominal aortic aneurysm. Gorter *et al.* [44] found an elevated prevalence of the metabolic syndrome (as defined by the NCEP ATP III) in patients with manifested atherosclerotic vascular diseases, including patients with abdominal aortic aneurysm. We have further recently shown that patients with abdominal aortic aneurysm have a smaller LDL size (Fig. **2**) and a different subclass distribution towards increased levels of small, dense LDL [45].

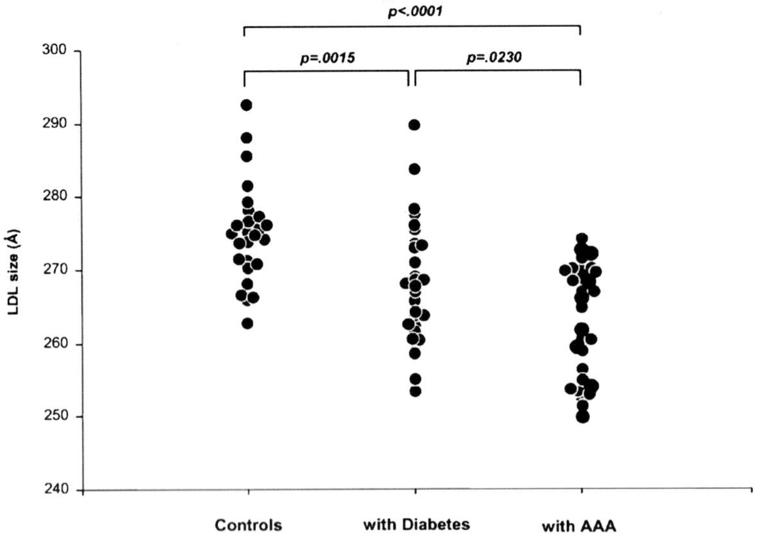

Fig. (2). LDL sublcasses in patients with AAA and controls [ref. 45].

With Metabolic Diseases

In addition to these findings from subjects with non-coronary forms of atherosclerosis, other recent studies showed elevated levels of small, dense LDL in patients with different metabolic diseases, including polycystic ovary syndrome (Fig. **3**) and growth hormone deficiency [46,47], and reduced LDL size in women with gestational diabetes [48], due to increased levels of small, dense LDL [49].

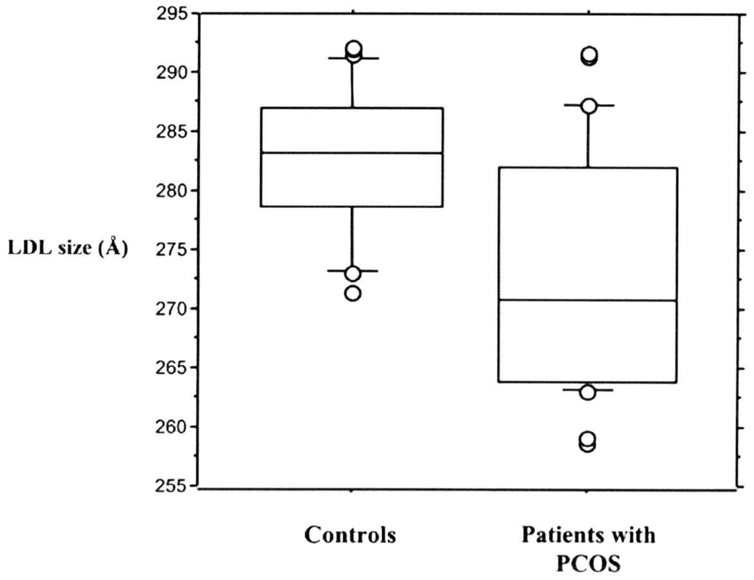

Fig. (3). Box plots of LDL size in patients with polycystic ovary syndrome (PCOS) and controls [ref. 46].

With the Metabolic Syndrome

Therefore, it cannot surprise that the predominance of small, dense LDL is a feature of the metabolic syndrome [50]. Haffner *et al.* already showed in 1995 that LDL size was decreased in subjects with multiple metabolic disorders [51]. Since no exact definition was available at that time regarding the metabolic syndrome, the authors examined in 488 non-diabetic subjects the association of LDL size with different clinical and biochemical variables (including insulin, proinsulin, increased triglycerides, decreased HDL-cholesterol, hypertension and impaired glucose tolerance). Hulthe *et al.* [34] assessed the prevalence of metabolic syndrome in a population-based sample of clinically 58 years old healthy men, using the WHO definition [52], showing that LDL size was significantly smaller in subjects with the metabolic syndrome. These findings were confirmed by a recent study performed on 105 patients with the metabolic syndrome [53], as assessed by the NCEP ATP III criteria: patients with the metabolic syndrome exhibited higher concentrations of small, dense LDL than individuals without it. The authors also showed that this increase was directly related to the number of components of the metabolic syndrome and mainly determined by triglyceride concentrations. In a recent study we have extended such observations, showing that small, dense LDL are strong predictors of cardio- and cerebrovascular events in subjects with the metabolic syndrome [54].

CONCLUSIONS

LDL size seems to be an important predictor of cardiovascular events and progression of coronary artery disease and the predominance of small dense LDL has been accepted as an emerging cardiovascular risk factor by the National Cholesterol Education Program Adult Treatment Panel III. We recently showed increased LDL size or higher levels of small and dense LDL in different categories of patients at higher cardiovascular risk, such as those with coronary (including acute myocardial infarction) and non-coronary (including carotid disease, abdominal aortic aneurysm and peripheral arterial disease) forms of atherosclerosis or metabolic diseases (including type-II diabetes, polycystic ovary syndrome, growth hormone deficiency, gestational diabetes and the metabolic syndrome). Screening of the presence of small, dense LDL may potentially identify the patients with even higher risk and may contribute in directing specific treatments in order to prevent new cardiovascular events.

REFERENCES

[1] Berneis KK, Krauss RM. Metabolic origins and clinical significance of LDL heterogeneity. J Lipid Res 2002; 43: 1363-1379.

[2] Krauss RM, Hellerstein MK, Neese RA, Blanche PJ, La Belle M, Shames DM. Altered metabolism of large low density lipoproteins in subjects with predominance of small low density lipoproteins. Circulation 1995; 92: 1-102.

[3] Rizzo M, Taylor JM, Barbagallo CM, Berneis K, Blanche PJ, Krauss RM. Effects on lipoprotein subclasses of combined expression of human hepatic lipase and human apoB in transgenic rabbits. Arterioscler Thromb Vasc Biol 2004; 24: 141-146.

[4] Krauss RM. Dietary and genetic probes of atherogenic dyslipidemia. Arterioscler Thromb Vasc Biol 2005; 25: 2265-2272.

[5] Jansen H, Hop W, van Tol A, Bruschke AV, Birkenhager JC. Hepatic lipase and lipoprotein lipase are not major determinants of the low density lipoprotein subclass pattern in human subjects with coronary heart disease. Atherosclerosis 1994; 107: 45-54.

[6] Campos H, Dreon DM, Krauss RM. Associations of hepatic and lipoprotein lipase activities with changes in dietary composition and low density lipoprotein subclasses. J Lipid Res 1995; 36: 462-472.

[7] Deckelbaum RJ, Granot E, Oschry Y, Rose L, Eisenberg S. Plasma triglyceride determines structure-composition in low and high density lipoproteins. Arteriosclerosis 1984; 4: 225-231.

[8] Guerin M, Le Goff W, Lassel TS, Van Tol A, Steiner G, Chapman MJ. Atherogenic role of elevated CE transfer from HDL to VLDL(1) and dense LDL in type 2 diabetes: impact of the degree of triglyceridemia. Arterioscler Thromb Vasc Biol 2001; 21: 282-288.

[9] Rizzo M, Berneis K. Who needs to care about small, dense low density lipoproteins? Int J Clin Pract 2007; 61:1949-1956.

[10] El Harchaoui K, van der Steeg WA, Stroes ES, *et al.* Value of low-density lipoprotein particle number and size as predictors of coronary artery disease in apparently healthy men and women: the EPIC-Norfolk Prospective Population Study. J Am Coll Cardiol 2007; 49: 547-553.

[11] Bjornheden T, Babyi A, Bondjers G, Wiklund O. Accumulation of lipoprotein fractions and subfractions in the arterial wall, determined in an in vitro perfusion system. Atherosclerosis 1996; 123: 43-56.

[12] Galeano NF, Al-Haideri M, Keyserman F, Rumsey SC, Deckelbaum RJ. Small dense low density lipoprotein has increased affinity for LDL receptor-independent cell surface binding sites: a potential mechanism for increased atherogenicity. J Lipid Res 1998; 39: 1263-1273.

[13] Camejo G, Lopez A, Lopez F, Quinones J. Interaction of low density lipoproteins with arterial proteoglycans. The role of charge and sialic acid content. Atherosclerosis 1985; 55: 93-105.

[14] Tribble DL, Rizzo M, Chait A, Lewis DM, Blanche PJ, Krauss RM. Enhanced oxidative susceptibility and reduced antioxidant content of metabolic precursors of small, dense low-density lipoproteins. Am J Med 2001; 110: 103-110.

[15] Tribble DL, Holl LG, Wood PD, Krauss RM. Variations in oxidative susceptibility among six low density lipoprotein subfractions of differing density and particle size. Atherosclerosis 1992; 93: 189-199.

[16] de Graaf J, Hak-Lemmers HL, Hectors MP, Demacker PN, Hendriks JC, Stalenhoef AF. Enhanced susceptibility to in vitro oxidation of the dense low density lipoprotein subfraction in healthy subjects. Arterioscler Thromb 1991; 11: 298-306.

[17] St Pierre AC, Cantin B, Dagenais GR, *et al.* Low-density lipoprotein subfractions and the longterm risk of ischemic heart disease in men: 13-year follow-up data from the Quebec Cardiovascular Study. Arterioscler Thromb Vasc Biol 2005; 25: 553-559.

[18] Rosenson RS, Otvos JD, Freedman DS. Relations of lipoprotein subclass levels and low-density lipoprotein size to progression of coronary artery disease in the Pravastatin Limitation of Atherosclerosis in the Coronary Arteries (PLAC-I) trial. Am J Cardiol 2002; 90(2): 89-94.

[19] Miller BD, Alderman EL, Haskell WL, Fair JM, Krauss RM. Predominance of dense low-density lipoprotein particles predicts angiographic benefit of therapy in the Stanford Coronary Risk Intervention Project. Circulation 1996; 94: 2146-2153.

[20] Zambon A, Hokanson JE, Brown BG, Brunzell JD. Evidence for a new pathophysiological mechanism for coronary artery disease regression: hepatic lipase-mediated changes in LDL density. Circulation 1999; 99: 1959-1964.

[21] Marais AD. Therapeutic modulation of low-density lipoprotein size. Curr Opin Lipidol 2000; 11: 597-602.

[22] Manninen V, Tenkanen L, Koskinen P, *et al.* Joint effects of serum triglyceride and LDL cholesterol and HDL cholesterol concentrations on coronary heart disease risk in the Helsinki Heart Study. Circulation 1992; 85: 37-45.

[23] Tenkanen L, Manttari M, Manninen V. Some coronary risk factors related to the insulin resistance syndrome and the treatment with gemfibrozil. Experience from the Helsinki Heart Study. Circulation 1995; 92:1779-1785.

[24] Rubins HB, Robins SJ, Collins D, *et al.* Gemfibrozil for the secondary prevention of coronary heart disease in men with low levels of high density lipoprotein cholesterol: Veterans Affairs High-density Lipoprotein Cholesterol Intervention Trials Study Group. N Engl J Med 1999; 341: 410-418.

[25] Sacks FM, Campos H. Low-Density Lipoprotein size and cardiovascular disease: a reappraisal. J Clin Endocr Metab 2003; 88: 4525-4532.

[26] Lamarche B, Lemieux I, Despres JP. The small, dense LDL phenotype and the risk of coronary heart disease: epidemiology, patho-physiology and therapeutic aspects. Diabet Metab 1999; 25: 199-211.

[27] Lada AT, Rudel LL. Associations of low density lipoprotein particle composition with atherogenicity. Curr Opin Lipidol 2004; 15: 19-24.

[28] Cromwell WC, Otvos JD. Low-density lipoprotein particle number and risk for cardiovascular disease. Curr Atheroscler Rep 2004; 6: 381-387.

[29] National Cholesterol Education Program (NCEP) Expert Panel on Detection, Evaluation, and Treatment of High Blood Cholesterol in Adults (Adult Treatment Panel III). Third Report of the National Cholesterol Education Program (NCEP) Expert Panel on Detection, Evaluation, and Treatment of High Blood Cholesterol in Adults (Adult Treatment Panel III) final report. Circulation 2002; 106: 3143-3421.

[30] Landray MJ, Sagar G, Muskin J, Murray S, Holder RL, Lip GYH. Association of atherogenic low-density lipoprotein subfractions with carotid atherosclerosis. QJM 1998; 91: 345-351.

[31] Skoglund-Andersson C, Tang R, Bond MG, de Faire U, Hamsten A, Karpe F. LDL particle size distribution is associated with carotid intima-media thickness in healthy 50-year-old men. Arterioscler Thromb Vasc Biol 1999; 19: 2422-2430.

[32] Bokemark L, Wikstrand J, Attvall S, Hulthe J, Wedel H, Fagerberg B. Insulin resistance and intima-media thickness in the carotid and femoral arteries of clinically healthy 58-year-old men. The Atherosclerosis and Insulin Resistance Study (AIR). J Intern Med 2001; 249: 59-67.

[33] Hallman DM, Brown SA, Ballantyne CM, Sharrett AR, Boerwinkle E. Relationship between low-density lipoprotein subclasses and asymptomatic atherosclerosis in subjects from the Atherosclerosis Risk in Communities (ARIC) Study. Biomarkers 2004; 9: 190-202.

[34] Hulthe J, Wiklund O, Olsson G, *et al.* Computerized measurement of LDL particle size in human serum. Reproducibility studies and evaluation of LDL particle size in relation to metabolic variables and the occurrence of atherosclerosis. Scand J Clin Lab Invest 1999; 59: 649-661.

[35] Hulthe J, Bokemark L, Wikstrand J, Fagerberg B. The metabolic syndrome, LDL particle size, and atherosclerosis: the Atherosclerosis and Insulin Resistance (AIR) study. Arterioscler Thromb Vasc Biol 2000; 20: 2140-2147.

[36] Liu ML, Ylitalo K, Nuotio I, Salonen R, Salonen JT, Taskinen MR. Association between carotid intima-media thickness and low-density lipoprotein size and susceptibility of low-density lipoprotein to oxidation in asymptomatic members of familial combined hyperlipidemia families. Stroke 2002; 33: 1255-1260.

[37] Watanabe T, Koba S, Kawamura M, *et al.* Small dense low-density lipoprotein and carotid atherosclerosis in relation to vascular dementia. Metabolism 2004; 53: 476-482.

[38] van Tits LJ, Smilde TJ, van Wissen S, de Graaf J, Kastelein JJ, Stalenhoef AF. Effects of atorvastatin and simvastatin on low-density lipoprotein subfraction profile, low-density lipoprotein oxidizability, and antibodies to oxidized low-density lipoprotein in relation to carotid intima media thickness in familial hypercholesterolemia. J Investig Med 2004; 52: 177-184.

[39] Berneis K, Jeanneret C, Muser J, Felix B, Miserez AR. Low-density lipoprotein size and subclasses are markers of clinically apparent and non-apparent atherosclerosis in type 2 diabetes. Metabolism 2005; 54: 227-234.

[40] Wallenfeldt K, Bokemark L, Wikstrand J, Hulthe J, Fagerberg B. Apolipoprotein B/apolipoprotein A-I in relation to the metabolic syndrome and change in carotid artery intima-media thickness during 3 years in middle-aged men. Stroke 2004; 35: 2248-2252.

[41] Lupattelli G, Pasqualini L, Siepi D, *et al.* Increased postprandial lipemia in patients with normolipemic peripheral arterial disease. Am Heart J 2002; 143: 733-738.

[42] O'Neal DN, Lewicki J, Ansari MZ, Matthews PG, Best JD. Lipid levels and peripheral vascular disease in diabetic and non-diabetic subjects. Atherosclerosis 1998; 136: 1-8.

[43] Rizzo M, Pernice V, Frasheri A, Berneis K. Atherogenic lipoprotein phenotype and LDL size and subclasses in patients with peripheral arterial disease. Atherosclerosis 2008; 197: 237-241.

[44] Gorter PM, Olijhoek JK, van der Graaf Y, *et al.* Prevalence of the metabolic syndrome in patients with coronary heart disease, cerebrovascular disease, peripheral arterial disease or abdominal aortic aneurysm. Atherosclerosis 2004; 173: 363-369.

[45] Rizzo M, Krayenbühl PA, Pernice V, Frasheri A, Rini GB, Berneis K. LDL size and subclasses in patients with abdominal aortic aneurysm. Int J Cardiol 2009; 134: 406-408.

[46] Berneis K, Rizzo M, Fruzzetti F, Lazzaroni V, Carmina E. Atherogenic lipoprotein phenotype and low-density lipoproteins size and subclasses in women with polycystic ovary syndrome. J Clin Endocrinol Metab 2007; 92: 186-189.

[47] Rizzo M, Trepp R, Berneis K, Christ ER. Atherogenic lipoprotein phenotype and LDL size and subclasses in patients with growth hormone deficiency before and after short-term replacement therapy. Eur J Endocr 2007; 156: 361-367.

[48] Qiu C, Rudra C, Austin MA, Williams MA. Association of gestational diabetes mellitus and low-density lipoprotein (LDL) particle size. Physiol Res 2007; 56(5): 571-578.

[49] Rizzo M, Berneis K, Altinova AE, *et al.* Atherogenic lipoprotein phenotype and LDL size and subclasses in women with gestational diabetes. Diabet Med 2008; 25: 1406-1411.

[50] Grundy SM, Cleeman JI, Daniels SR, *et al.* American Heart Association; National Heart, Lung, and Blood Institute. Diagnosis and management of the metabolic syndrome: an American Heart Association/National Heart, Lung, and Blood Institute Scientific Statement. Circulation 2005; 112: 2735-2752.

[51] Haffner SM, Mykkanen L, Robbins D, *et al.* A preponderance of small dense LDL is associated with specific insulin, proinsulin and the components of the insulin resistance syndrome in non-diabetic subjects. Diabetologia 1995; 38:1328-1336.

[52] World Health Organization. Definition, Diagnosis, and Classification of Diabetes Mellitus and its Complications: Report of a WHO Consultation. Geneva 1999.

[53] Gazi I, Tsimihodimos V, Filippatos T, Bairaktari E, Tselepis AD, Elisaf M. Concentration and relative distribution of low-density lipoprotein subfractions in patients with metabolic syndrome defined according to the National Cholesterol Education Program criteria. Metabolism 2006; 55:885-891.

[54] Rizzo M, Pernice V, Frasheri A, *et al.* Small, dense low-density lipoproteins are predictors of cardio- and cerebro-vascular events in subjects with the metabolic syndrome. Clin Endocr 2009; 70: 870-875.

Role of Omega-3 Fatty Acids in Cardiovascular Disease Prevention

GianLuca Colussi, Cristiana Catena, Elisa Nadalini, Alessandra Chiuch, Alessandro Di Fabio, Marica Valeri and Leonardo A. Sechi*

Division of Internal Medicine, Department of Experimental and Clinical Pathology and Medicine, University of Udine, Udine, Italy

Abstract: ω-3 and ω-6 Polyunsaturated fatty acids (PUFA) are the major families of PUFA that can be found as components of the human diet. After ingestion, both ω-3 and ω-6 PUFA are distributed to every cell in the body where they are involved in a myriad of physiological processes, including regulation of cardiovascular, immune, hormonal, metabolic, neuronal, and visual functions. At the cell level, these effects are mediated by changes in membrane phospholipids structure, interference with eicosanoid intracellular signaling, and regulation of gene expression. Two long-chain ω-3 PUFAs, the docosahexaenoic (DHA) and eicosapentaenoic (EPA) acid, are found in fatty fish and other marine sources and might be the putative dietary components thought to modify the cardiovascular risk in subjects consuming high amounts of such food. Evidence of an inverse relationship between fatty fish intake and cardiovascular risk has, in fact, emerged in studies performed more than twenty years ago in Eskimos and has been subsequently confirmed in other ethnic groups. The benefits of ω-3 PUFA might relate principally to prevention of coronary heart disease, coronary artery restenosis after angioplasty, and sudden arrhythmic death. In this brief review, we will cover the general biochemical aspects of ω-3 PUFA, summarize the evidence relating these fatty acids with control of cardiovascular risk factors and prevention of cardiovascular events, and overview the most recent and relevant patents that are related to these issues. More specifically, we will deal with the possibility to use PUFA in association with other molecules that can potentiate their antiinflammatory and antiatherogenic effects.

Keywords: ω-3 polyunsaturated fatty acids, ω-6 polyunsaturated fatty acids, docosahexaenoic acid, eicosapentaenoic acid, cardiovascular risk, atherosclerosis, inflammation, coronary heart disease, arrhythmia, aspirin, policosanols, statins.

INTRODUCTION

In the last decades, there has been a remarkable increase of public interest in ω-3 and ω-6 polyunsaturated fatty acids (PUFA) and their potential impact on human health. These fatty acids are not synthesized in the human body and are ingested as dietary components or oral supplements. ω-3 PUFA are found in appreciable amounts in fatty fish, such as sardines, salmon, and tuna, fish oil, walnuts, canola, and flaxseed oil and possess anti-

*Corresponding author: Tel: 39 0432 559804; E-mail: sechi@uniud.it

Atta-ur-Rahman / M. Iqbal Choudhary (Eds.)

inflammatory, anti-thrombotic, and anti-arrhythmic properties. Conversely, ω-6 PUFA are found in vegetable oils, such as corn, cottonseed, sunflower, safflower, and peanut oil and have proinflammatory and prothrombotic effects. Diets commonly eaten in the Western World contain an ω-3 to ω-6 PUFA ratio of 1:10 [1], that is much different from the ratio of 1:1 that was peculiar of the diets consumed by our ancestors.

A low incidence of cardiovascular death among traditionally living populations such as Eskimos and Alaskan Natives was reported in seminal papers [2-5] and was attributed to a lesser frequency of coronary atherosclerotic disease that could result from a high dietary intake of ω-3 PUFA from fatty fish or other fish-derived food. Many epidemiological studies have subsequently addressed the relation between the intake of ω-3 PUFA and cardiovascular disease and clinical trials have examined the effects of increased ω-3 PUFA consumption on cardiovascular events. This review will briefly cover the general biochemical aspects of ω-3 PUFA and summarize the evidence relating these fatty acids with control of cardiovascular risk factors and prevention of cardiovascular events.

BIOCHEMICAL BACKGROUND

ω-3 PUFA are fatty acids which the first double bond is placed three carbon atoms from the methyl terminal and this structural characteristic confers to them peculiar properties as compared to other PUFA, such as the ω-6 and ω-9 PUFA. The two most important bioactive ω-3 PUFA, the eicosapentaenoic acid (EPA) and docosahexaenoic acid (DHA), are generated from an essential precursor molecule, the α-linolenic acid. Humans do not have the biochemical pathways required to synthesize this essential precursor of PUFA and therefore these fatty acids must necessarily be obtained form external sources such as plants, for α-linolenic acid, or marine food, for EPA and DHA (Table **1**). In mammal species, α-linolenic acid enters cells via specific fatty acid carriers and is converted by acyl-CoA synthases in thioesters that are substrates for neutral and polar lipid synthesis in reactions of β-oxidation, elongation, and desaturation. A slow desaturation-elongation enzymatic process (rate of conversion of less than 1%) leads to formation of EPA (20 carbons) and DHA (22 carbons) that, in turn, are precursors of a family of eicosanoids that mediate the vasodilatory, anti-inflammatory, anti-thrombotic, and anti-arrhythmic effects of these molecules. The precursor of ω-6 PUFA is linoleic acid whose long-chain fatty acid derivative is arachidonic acid (20 carbons), the precursor of another family of eicosanoids that have pro-inflammatory and pro-thrombotic effects. α-linolenic and linoleic acid are competitors for the same enzymatic pathway that leads to the generation of their longer chain fatty acids whose tissue levels therefore depend very much from the amounts of the respective precursors. The ingestion of fish or fish oil provides directly ω-3 PUFA, thus avoiding the competition for enzymes in the convertion pathway.

The benefits of dietary ω-3 PUFA are attributed to their capacity to regulate specific cellular metabolic functions and gene expression [6]. ω-3 PUFA are incorporated into membrane phospholipids where they usually represent less than 10% of the total fatty acid amount. One of the targets for ω-3 PUFA effects on membrane function are lipid rafts that are cholesterol- and sphingolipid-rich regions of the outer layer of the plasma membrane [7]. These lipid rafts include proteins with multiple functions and contribute to determine the structure of many cell organelles and to modulate a number of membrane-related functions such as cellular transport, receptor function, and signal transduction. Experimental evidence indicates that lipid rafts are sensitive to changes of PUFA content *via* modifications occurring in both the phospholipid and protein compartments.

Table 1. Average Long-Chain ω-3 PUFA Contents of Some Types of Fish and Meat and of Some Supplemental Sources

Type of Food*	Combined EPA and DHA Content (g per 3-oz Serving)	Amount Required (oz) to Provide 1 g of EPA plus DHA Content
Fish		
Salmon	0.90-1.83	1.5-2.5
Sardines	0.98-1.70	2.0-3.0
Herring	1.71-1.81	2.0
Mackerel	0.34-1.57	2.0-8.5
Tuna	0.24-1.28	2.5-12.0
Halibut	0.4-1.0	3.0-7.5
Sole	0.42	7.0
Crab	0.35	8.5
Shrimp	0.27	11.0
Haddock	0.20	15.0
Catfish	0.15	20.0
Mussels	0.04	75.0
Meat		
Roast beef	0.02	150.0
Roast lamb	0.05	60.0
Roast pork	0.02	150.0
Chicken	0.04	75.0
Supplemental Source	**Combined EPA and DHA Content (g per Capsule)**	**Number of Capsules Required to Provide 1 g of EPA Plus DHA**
OMACOR® Reliant Pharmaceuticals, Inc., Liberty Corner, NJ	1	1
ESKIM® Sigma-Tau SpA, Rome, IT	1	1
ESAPENT® Pfizer Italia Srl, Rome, IT	1	1

EPA: eicosapentaenoic acid; DHA: docosahexaenoic acid.
*Contents indicated are approximated estimates because they can vary with species, season, diet in farmed fish, packaging methods, and cooking. Adapted from reference (1).

As already noted, ω-3 PUFA affect eicosanoid pathways leading to modulation of inflammatory responses. In fact, non-esterified PUFA released from membrane phospholipids can be substrates for both cyclooxygenases (COX) and lipooxygenases (LOX) whose activity leads to generation of prostanoid and thromboxanes on one side, and leukotrienes on the other. The products of COX are modulators of the haemostatic, inflammatory, and immune response, whereas the products of LOX have control of vasomotility and vascular extravasation [8,9]. In this context, it has been demonstrated that there is an interaction between more traditional anti-inflammatory drugs, such as aspirin, and ω-3 PUFA [10]. This interaction can be explained by the generation of specific compounds that can translate in prevention of inflammation associated with various diseases, including atherosclerosis. ω-3 PUFA have also well documented effects on gene expression and changes of mRNA levels for some lipogenic enzymes have been detected in animals fed ω-3 PUFA-enriched diets [11]. These effects appear to be mediated by activation of the peroxysome proliferator activating receptor-α (PPAR-α) that acts as a transcription factor [12] and modulates a group of genes that are involved in lipid metabolism.

ω-3 PUFA IN THE PREVENTION OF CORONARY HEART DISEASE

More than twenty years ago, epidemiological observations were reported indicating a low incidence of coronary death among native Alaskan and Greenland Eskimos who consumed a fish-rich diet [2,3]. The same observation was subsequently extended to other ethnic groups including Japanese and Pacific Islanders [13,14]. These observations led to the hypothesis that dietary fish consumption might decrease cardiovascular mortality. This hypothesis was tested in many prospective cohort studies that have used information obtained from food diaries and/or biologic markers to estimate dietary PUFA content. Results of these studies showed inconsistencies, since some studies confirmed the inverse relationship between dietary fish content and cardiovascular mortality rates [15-20] while others did not [21-27]. The relationship between fish intake and cardiovascular outcome was explored also in case-control studies [28,29] and randomized trials [30] reporting lower overall mortality, cardiovascular events, and sudden death, but not stroke, after consumption of dietary supplements containing EPA and DHA.

The Diet and Reinfarction Trial (DART) [30] was the first large study to examine the effects of dietary intake of ω-3 PUFA on the secondary prevention of myocardial infarction. In this 2-year follow-up study, 1,015 men who consumed two servings of fatty fish per week were compared with 1,018 men who never ate fish. The subjects who consumed fish had a 29% lower mortality but no difference in the incidence of myocardial infarction. The Lyon Diet Heart Study [31] was a randomized, secondary prevention trial that was performed in 605 patients with previous myocardial infarction. This study compared the effects of a Mediterranean-type diet (poor in total and saturated fats and rich in marine or plant derived ω-3 PUFA, vegetables and fruit, legumes, high-fiber cereals, antioxidants, minerals, vegetable proteins, and group B vitamins) with an American-type diet (rich in cholesterol, saturated fat, and linoleic acid) on recurrences of infarction and cardiovascular death. The study was planned for a 5-year follow-up, but it was interrupted after 27 months because of significantly lower incidence of both recurrent infarction and cardiovascular death in patients consuming the Mediterranean diet. The protective effect of this diet was maintained up to 4 years after the first infarction [32]. To date, the largest randomized controlled trial on the cardiovascular effects of ω-3 PUFA is the GISSI-Prevenzione Trial [33]. This randomized trial included 11,324 patients with coronary heart disease who received either 300 mg/day of vitamin E, 850 mg/day of ω-3 PUFA, both, or neither. After a follow-up of 3.5 years, subjects taking ω-3 PUFA had 45% lower incidence of sudden death and 20% lower all-cause mortality. The U.S. Physicians Health Study demonstrated a significant inverse relationship between blood levels of ω-3 PUFA and the risk of sudden death in subjects without history of coronary heart disease [34] and another study showed that an intake of 5.5 g/month of ω-3 PUFA decreased by 50% the risk of cardiac arrest [29]. The EURAMIC study, however, showed that fish consumption did not protect against the risk of myocardial infarction [35].

Many meta-analyses and systematic reviews [36-43] (Table **2**) have approached the problem trying to provide a conclusive evidence on this controversial subject. A recent

Table 2. Summary of the Results of the Major Meta-Analyses on the Effects of ω-3 PUFA on Cardiovascular Events

Main Study's Author	Period of Data Collection	Type of Population	Number of Participants	Type of ω-3 PUFA Source	Outcomes	Relative Risk (95% CI)*	Probability
Whelton SP *et al.* [40]	1985-2003	Primary prevention	228,864	Dietary	Fatal CHD	0.83 (0.76-0.90)	<0.005
					Total CHD	0.86 (0.81-0.92)	<0.005
Yzebe D *et al.* [41]	1966-2003	Secondary prevention	14,727	Dietary or supplement	All cause of mortality	0.84 (0.76-0.94)	<0.001
					Fatal MI	0.76 (0.66-0.88)	<0.001
					Non fatal MI	1.03 (0.87-1.19)	NS
					Non fatal stroke	1.36 (0.87-2.29)	NS
					Angina pectoris	1.03 (0.85-1.20)	NS
Bucher H *et al.* [39]	1966-1999	Secondary prevention	15,806	Dietary or supplement	Non fatal MI	0.8 (0.5-1.2)	NS
					Fatal MI	0.7 (0.6-0.8)	<0.001
					Sudden death	0.7 (0.6-0.9)	<0.01
					Overall mortality	0.8 (0.7-0.9)	<0.001
Hooper L *et al.* [42]	<2002	Secondary prevention	36,913	Dietary and supplement	Total mortality	0.87 (0.73-1.03)	NS
					Combined cardiovascular event	0.95 (0.82-1.12)	NS

*Risk related to consumption vs. low or no consumption. CI, confidence interval. CHD, coronary heart disease. MI, myocardial infarction.

meta-analysis of prospective cohort studies [36] has examined a selection of 11 studies and 13 cohorts including 222,364 subjects with an average follow-up of 11.8 years. Subjects with a higher fish intake had lower coronary heart disease mortality than subjects who never consumed fish or ate fish less than once a month, with a relative risk of 0.77 for subjects who ate fish for 2 to 4 times per week. Each 20 g/day increase in fish consumption was associated with a 7% lower risk of cardiovascular death. In the same way Konig *et al.* [37] demonstrated a dose-response relationship between fish consumption and coronary heart disease mortality or myocardial infarction. Small amounts of dietary fish were associated with 17% reduction in coronary heart disease mortality with a further 3.9% risk reduction with each additional 100 g of fish per week. A meta-analysis of randomized clinical trials [38] has examined a selection of 14 studies testing the effects of fish oil or α-linolenic acid supplementation. This analysis concluded that fish oil containing EPA and DHA reduce significantly total mortality, coronary heart disease death, and sudden death. In a meta-analysis that included secondary prevention studies with an average follow-up of 20 months, Bucher *et al.* [39] demonstrated a significant reduction in fatal myocardial infarction and sudden death but could not detect any significant difference in the outcome when the analysis considered the specific sources of ω-3 PUFA. In a meta-analysis of observational studies, Whelton *et al.* [40] showed that eating fish reduced the relative risk of both total and fatal coronary heart disease. Similar findings were reported by Yzebe *et al.* [41] in their systematic review in which it was shown that daily intake of ω-3 PUFA for a mean duration of 37 months reduced fatal myocardial infarction by 24% and all cause mortality by 16%. Finally, the most recent Cochrane database review on the use of ω-3 PUFA in cardiovascular prevention [42] has concluded that there is no clear and definite evidence that these compounds decrease cardiovascular events, in particular when they are derived from natural sources.

Currently, no studies have evaluated the potential preventive role of ω–3 PUFA in another high risk condition for cardiovascular disease such as type 2 diabetes. Two ongoing trials will be published in the next couple of years [44, 45]. The first trial (ORIGIN) is a multi-center randomized and placebo controlled study that considers in one arm the efficacy of 1 g/day of ω–3 PUFA in high risk diabetic patients in terms of cardiovascular events and cardiovascular death [44]. The second trial (AFORRD) examines the impact of 1 year of statin or 2 g/day of ω–3 PUFA treatment on lipid profiles and estimated cardiovascular risk in patients with type 2 diabetes without known cardiovascular disease. The results of the first four months of the latter study were recently published and no differences were seen between ω–3 PUFA and placebo groups in terms of triglyceride levels and estimated cardiovascular risk reduction [45]. In conclusion we don't have, at this moment, solid evidence for beneficial effects of ω–3 PUFA in primary or secondary cardiovascular prevention of patients with type 2 diabetes.

In summary, despite important clinical studies support the role of ω-3 PUFA as protective factors toward cardiovascular disease leading the expert committees of some scientific societies to recommend their use in secondary cardiovascular prevention, some controversy on this matter still persists. Further research will be needed to better define whether, in which subjects, in which form, at which dosage, and for how long time these compounds should be used to effectively prevent the development of cardiovascular events.

USE OF ω–3 PUFA IN OTHER CARDIOVASCULAR DISORDERS

Following the evidence of beneficial effects of ω–3 PUFA in the context of cardiovascular disease, effects were tested also in different cardiovascular disorders.

The Italian GISSI group has published recently a study (GISSI-HF) showing small beneficial effects of ω–3 PUFA in patients with symptomatic heart failure [46]. In this multi-center, double-blind study approximately 7,000 patients with chronic heart failure of

New York Heart Association class II-IV were randomized to take 1 g/day of ω–3 PUFA or placebo. After a median follow-up of 3.9 years, the authors find an adjusted hazard ratio of 0.91 (CI 95.5% 0.833-0.998) and 0.92 (CI 99% 0.849-0.999), in favor of ω–3 PUFA, respectively for any-cause mortality and incidence of hospital admission for cardiovascular reasons. Decreased mortality could be explained by the lower frequency of fatal and non-fatal arrhythmic events [46]. Interestingly, other studies showed favorable hemodynamic effects of ω–3 PUFA in healthy populations and, more specifically, reduction of left ventricular diastolic filling [47] and vascular peripheral resistances [48], and improvement of stroke volume and cardiac output [49].

Little evidence supports the use of ω–3 PUFA in cerebrovascular disease prevention. A meta-analysis of 8 studies including 9 cohorts comprising approximately 200,000 participants who were followed for a mean of 12.8 years [50] and a dose-response analysis on 4 observational and 1 case-control studies comprising approximately 131,000 participants [51] showed an inverse relationship between fish intake and risk of stroke, particularly of ischemic origin. More recently, Tanaka *et al.* [52] in a sub-analysis of the JELIS trial demonstrated a preventive effect in stroke recurrence of highly purified EPA supplementation on top of a low-dose statin treatment compared to statin treatment alone in a cohort of hypercholesterolemic Japanese patients. A potential explanation for the beneficial effect of ω–3 PUFA in stroke prevention comes from a work of Thies *et al.* who demonstrated, in patients awaiting carotid endoarteriectomy, that atherosclerotic plaques may incorporate ω–3 PUFA from fish oil supplementation enhancing plaque stability [53]. Despite these positive observation, the lack of specifically designed randomized controlled trials and the conflicting findings of the GISSI-Prevenzione trial that reported an increased frequency of stroke in patients treated with ω–3 PUFA [33], make the possible use of these fatty acids in cerebrovascular prevention as a matter of debate.

Finally, other studies have evaluated the possible benefits of ω–3 PUFA supplementation in peripheral arterial disease. The most important of these studies were grouped in a recent meta-analysis reviewed in the Cochrane database that included 6 placebo controlled studies for a total of 313 patients affected by intermittent claudication and followed from 1 to 24 months [54]. This meta-analysis didn't show any improvement in quality of life, pain-free walking distance, maximal walking distance, ankle-brachial pressure index and angiographic findings [54].

MECHANISMS BY WHICH ω-3 PUFA AFFECT ATHEROSCLEROSIS

Beneficial effects of ω-3 PUFA on cardiovascular disease might result, at least in part, from specific actions on traditional and emergent cardiovascular risk factors [55] (Fig. **1**). First, ω-3 PUFA have demonstrated a dose-dependent hypotensive effect in hypertensive patients. In a randomized dietary-supplementation trial on hypertensive patients, Bonaa *et al.* [56] demonstrated that administration of 6 g/day of ω-3 PUFA decreased systolic and diastolic blood pressure by 4.6 and 3.0 mm Hg, respectively, whereas supplementation with 6 g/day of corn oil did not affect blood pressure values. Similar results were reported in two other studies [57, 58]. A meta-analysis of 31 controlled trials showed that each 5 g/day increase of fish oil consumption decreases systolic blood pressure by 3.4 mm Hg and diastolic blood pressure by 2.0 mm Hg [59]. In addition, plasma triglyceride levels are decreased by ω-3 PUFA in patients with hypertriglyceridemia, an effect that could be ascribed to inhibition of the synthesis of very low density lipoproteins [60]. Studies on the effects of ω-3 PUFA on plasma lipid fractions have been reviewed showing that a dose of 4 g/day decreases plasma triglycerides by approximately 25% but leaves unaffected total cholesterol levels [61]. Recent evidence also indicates the possibility to enhance the effects

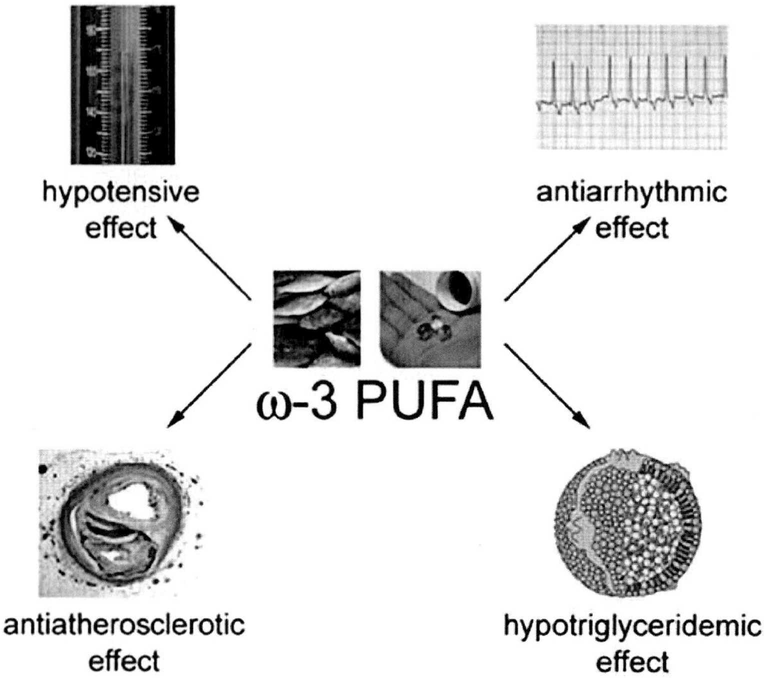

Fig. (1). Potential mechanisms likely to play a role in cardiovascular protection by ω-3 PUFA.

of drugs commonly used for the treatment of dyslipidemias, such as statins, with the co-administration of ω-3 PUFA [62]. In a randomized placebo controlled trial conducted in patients with coronary heart disease and patients with mixed dyslipidemia who were treated with statins, ω-3 PUFA (3 g/day) decreased high sensitive C reactive protein (CRP) by 38,5%, triglycerides by 31.1% and total cholesterol by 6,3% [63]. In this study, the reduction in CRP and triglycerides was significantly greater in patients who were taking both statins and ω-3 PUFA than in those who were taking statin alone. In a double-blind study conducted in high risk patients with combined hyperlipemia, Nordoy *et al.* [64] demonstrated that addition of 1.68 g/day of ω-3 PUFA to atorvastatin increases the effects on HDL-cholesterol and reduce systolic blood pressure. It has been shown also that ω-3 PUFA given in addition to simvastatin in patients with combined hyperlipemia may reduce the tissue factor pathway inhibitor, a potent blocker of tissue factor mediated activation of the haemostatic cascade that plays a role in atheromasic lesions, and reduce the prothrombotic activation present in the postprandial phase [65]. In summary, there is good evidence suggesting a favorable interaction between ω-3 PUFA and statins. Further studies will be necessary to elucidate the enhanced beneficial effect of the combined therapy with ω-3 PUFA and statins in cardiovascular disease primary and secondary prevention.

The impact of ω–3 PUFA supplementation on cardiovascular risk in type 2 diabetes has been recently evaluated in a systematic review of 24 randomized placebo controlled trials involving 1,533 participants [66]. The average ω–3 PUFA dose utilized and the duration of the treatment were respectively 2.4 g/day and 24 weeks. The analysis showed that ω–3 PUFA treatment reduced triglycerides and fibrinogen levels and platelet aggregation to ADP and collagen, increased the levels of LDL cholesterol, but had not effect on HDL-cholesterol, LDL particle size, glycemia, insulinemia, inflammatory biomarkers and blood pressure [66].

Beneficial effects of ω-3 PUFA-enriched diets have been demonstrated also on some emergent cardiovascular risk factors such as lipoprotein(a) and markers of a prothrombotic state, both factors that have been shown to contribute significantly to cardiovascular outcome [67]. We have evaluated the effects of ω-3 PUFA on lipoprotein(a) and haemostatic markers in two open protocols in which hypertensive patients with high baseline levels of these markers were treated with 4 g/day of ω-3 PUFA for 1 month or with 1 g/day for 6 months [68]. In the short term, blood pressure was significantly reduced (-10 mm Hg systolic; -7 mm Hg diastolic) by the administration of the high dose ω-3 PUFA, whereas no significant changes were observed in the long term. Total and LDL cholesterol were not significantly affected by ω-3 PUFA in both studies, whereas triglycerides were decreased by 23% with the high-dose. Plasma levels of lipoprotein(a) and D-dimer were significantly decreased by both ω-3 PUFA treatments (Fig. **2**), whereas fibrinogen was significantly reduced only by the low dose. ω-3 PUFA treatment did not modify significantly levels of homocysteine, plasminogen activator inhibitor-1, and prothrombin fragment 1+2. Other studies that aimed at exploring possible effects of ω-3 PUFA on prothrombotic markers and their potential relevance for cardiovascular outcomes are limited by the sample size and the appropriateness of the design and have shown contrasting results. Despite possible contribution of ω-3 PUFA induced changes in cardiovascular risk factors, available evidence does not indicate a sufficiently large benefit to explain the overall effect of these fatty acids on cardiovascular outcomes.

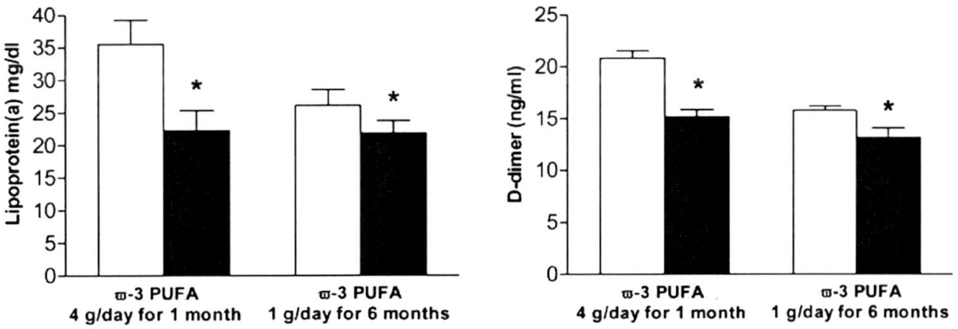

Fig. (2). Bar-graph showing mean (SE) values of lipoprotein(a) and D-dimer in hypertensive patients who were treated with ω-3 PUFA in two protocols with different dose and duration of treatment. Open bars, base time values; solid bars, values after treatment.
* $P<0.05$.

Detection of intermediate or "surrogate" cardiovascular endpoints is important in the prediction of future cardiovascular "hard" endpoints, such as myocardial infarction, stroke, sudden death, and congestive heart failure. Because beneficial effects of ω-3 PUFA on these intermediate endpoints might result in better cardiovascular protection, some studies have addressed the effects of these fatty acids on such endpoints and namely on the intimamedia thickness (IMT) of the carotid vessels. Carotid IMT is an imaging technique that evaluates the extent of subclinical atherosclerosis and provides important prognostic information [69]. A cross-sectional study compared the IMT in Japanese resident of a fishing village or a farming village and demonstrated that individuals with greater dietary intake of ω-3 PUFA had significantly thinner IMT than those with lower intake [70]. Similar evaluation was done in an American cohort where individuals were subdivided according to α-linolenic acid intake with evidence, in unadjusted analysis, of significantly thinner IMT in people consuming greater amounts of this fatty acid [71]. Only one randomized, controlled trial examined the effects of fish oil dietary supplementation on carotid preclinical atherosclerosis [72]. In this study, 223 patients with coronary artery disease were treated for 2 years with 1.65 g/day of ω-3 PUFA or placebo and B-mode ultrasound of carotid arteries was performed. Results showed that the degree of progression of carotid vascular disease was not significantly different in ω-3 PUFA (38%) and placebo (35%) treated individuals. Therefore, clear evidence of beneficial effects of ω-3 PUFA on IMT is lacking and so far, no studies have examined the effects of ω-3 PUFA on other intermediate cardiovascular endpoints.

In addition, the molecular mechanisms underlying the benefits of ω-3 PUFA on atherosclerosis have been extensively investigated in laboratory studies [73]. Long-chain ω-3 PUFA decrease adhesion molecule [74], vascular smooth muscle cell growth factor [75], and chemoattractant molecules [76] production and might therefore slow down the process of cell migration into the vessel wall intima that leads to atherosclerotic plaque formation. Moreover, there is some evidence suggesting that these fatty acids might have a vascular effect by protecting endothelium through inhibition of oxidative stress, an important player in the development and progression of atherosclerotic vascular lesions [77]. In one study, cultured endothelial cells were pretreated with fatty acids and subsequently exposed to either specific cytokines or lipopolysaccharide [78]. Pretreatment with DHA blunted the endothelial response to the pro-inflammatory stimulation in terms of vascular cell adhesion molecule-1 (VCAM-1) cellular expression or release of macrophage colony stimulating factor (M-CSF). These effects were associated with decreased production of reactive oxygen species (ROS) as shown by lower depletion of cellular reduced glutathione (GSH). Other studies demonstrated that pre-incubation with DHA decreases in a dose-dependent manner the cytokine-stimulated *in vitro* expression of VCAM-1 by endothelial cells [79] and decreases the adhesion of monocytes to endothelial cells [80]. Similar responses were observed also when cells were pretreated with EPA, although the magnitude of the effect was smaller [80]. These cellular mechanisms may contribute to explain some of the beneficial effects of ω-3 PUFA on the risk of cardiovascular disease.

USE OF ω-3 PUFA IN THE PREVENTION OF ARRHYTHMIA

Cardiac arrhythmias are an important cause of cardiac arrest and sudden death and both epidemiological studies and clinical trials have reported beneficial effects of fatty fish or fish oil intake on this specific cardiovascular endpoint. In particular, a decrease of sudden death in individuals with high fish oil consumption has been reported in the majority of randomized, controlled trials [81-84], in prospective cohort studies [17,26], and case-control studies [29]. This evidence has lead to hypothesize that long-chain ω-3 PUFA might in some way suppress life-threatening cardiac arrhythmias. The hypothesis has been tested in animal models of arrhythmia [85] and prospective, randomized, placebo-controlled trials in high risk patients (severe left ventricular hypertrophy, heart failure, and patients with implantable cardiac defibrillator) have been designed to address this problem [86-88]. Very preliminary results obtained in patients carrying implantable defibrillators for episodes of ventricular tachyarrhythmias demonstrated that recurrences of arrhythmia are more frequent in patients receiving fish oil supplements than those receiving a placebo [86]. A recent study, however, has shown a beneficial effect of ω-3 PUFA infusion on the induction of sustained ventricular tachycardia [89]. In this study, induction of sustained ventricular tachycardia was attempted in 10 patients who had implanted cardioverter defibrillators. Ventricular tachycardia was successfully induced in 7 of 10 patients; after infusion of ω-3 PUFA (3.8 g) tachycardia was still inducible in 2 patients, but not in the remaining 5 in whom the duration of the effective refractory period was increased. This is the first clinical study that directly demonstrates the antiarrhythmic properties of ω-3 PUFA, but is clearly limited by the sample size, absence of randomization, and absence of a control group. Another recent study performed in 160 patients after coronary artery by-pass grafting has demonstrated that administration of ω-3 PUFA at a dose of 2 g/day for a minimum of 5 days before surgical revascularization, decreases the rate of post-operative atrial fibrillation by 54.4% [90]. A recent systematic review of 12 controlled studies comprising approximately 33,000 patients with a follow-up range between 12 and 60 months has evaluated the effects of ω–3 PUFA on arrhythmias and mortality in patients with coronary artery disease or myocardial infarction. Analysis indicated that fish oil supplementation was responsible for a 20% reduction in cardiac cause mortality but did not have significant effects on the need of an implantable defribillator intervention, sudden cardiac death or all cause mortality [91]. An ongoing randomized, double-blind, and placebo controlled trial (FORomegaARD) will evaluate the efficacy of 1 g/day of ω–3 PUFA versus placebo on top of other specific medications, in patients with documented reversible atrial fibrillation episodes [92]. The trial, that plans to enroll approximately 1,400 patients, has as a primary endpoint the frequency of recurrence of atrial fibrillation and as secondary endpoints a composite of all-cause mortality, non-fatal stroke, non-fatal acute myocardial infarction, systemic embolism, heart failure development, and severe bleeding; all-cause hospitalization; survival free of thromboembolic events; and hospitalizations for cardiovascular reasons [92].

Important links between ω-3 PUFA and prevention of arrhythmias have been described also in studies conducted in experimental *in-vivo* and *in-vitro* models and have been reviewed recently [85]. Experiments using a variety of ischemic animal models [93], rats after coronary angioplasty [94], rats with transplanted heart [95], and studies performed with cultured cardiomyocytes [96] support the view that these long-chain fatty acids do have anti-arrhythmic properties. In fact, both feeding and infusion protocols have demonstrated in rats that the ω-3 PUFA have the ability to reduce both ventricular tachycardia and ventricular fibrillation [86].

The potential mechanisms responsible for the observed antiarrhythmic effect of EPA and DHA have yet to be fully clarified. Ingestion of ω-3 PUFA is followed by incorporation of these fatty acids into cardiac membrane phospholipids [97] where they increase membrane fluidity [98] and thereby modulate the function of transporters, receptors, and enzymes [99, 100]. Changes of COX and phospholipase included in membrane bilayers could affect the synthesis of some eicosanoids that modify the threshold to arrhythmia induction [101]. ω-3 PUFA directly affect electrophysiological properties of cardiomyocytes by modulating conductance and prolonging the persistence in the functional inactive state of both the fast sodium [102] and slow calcium [103] current.

PATENT REVIEW COVERAGE

Several patents on cardiovascular agents and drugs have been presented in the recent years and some of these patents have relevance to the topic of this review. The most important ones deal with the possibility to reinforce the anti-atherogenic, anti-inflammatory, and lipid-lowering effects of these molecules by co-administering them with other drugs with similar effects. For instance, it was unexpectedly discovered that there is an interaction between aspirin, cyclooxygenase II, and ω-3 PUFA [10]. This interaction occurs because of aspirin-driven formation of a family of at least 10 hydroxyl-compounds that have important anti-inflammatory properties on different tissues, and could be potentially employed in clinical conditions associated with inflammation, such as atherosclerosis [77]. Another recent finding is related to the possibility to combine ω-3 PUFA with inhibitors of 5-hydroxy-5-methyl-glutaryl-CoA (HMG-CoA) reductase or other cholesterol-lowering drugs such as policosanols [62, 104, 105].

CURRENT AND FUTURE DEVELOPMENTS

A large body of medical literature has evolved over the past decades evaluating the effects of ω-3 PUFA on cardiovascular disease. It is clear from the foregoing discussion that these long-chain fatty acids have been demonstrated to be effective in secondary prevention of myocardial infarction, with a particularly relevant effect on sudden death. This beneficial effect might be likely attributed to the antiarrhythmic properties of these fatty acids. Although additional research will be needed to better define precisely the role of these compounds in primary and secondary cardiovascular prevention, it would be wise to suggest oral supplementation of ω-3 PUFA in all post-MI patients and many scientific societies have now made recommendations relating the intake of fatty fish and long-chain ω-3 PUFA [106, 107].

Epidemiological evidence and studies on traditional and new cardiovascular risk factors suggest that long-chain ω-3 PUFA might play an important role also in primary cardiovascular prevention. Although this issue needs further investigation, consumption of long-chain ω-3 PUFA should be encouraged for all individuals and especially for those at a higher risk of cardiovascular disease. Potential benefit might derive from use of these molecules in appropriate combinations with other anti-inflammatory and lipid-lowering agents.

REFERENCES

[1] Kris-Etherton PM, Taylor DS, Yu-Poth S, *et al.* Polyunsaturated fatty acids in the food chain in the United States. Am J Clin Nutr 2000; 71: 179S-188.

[2] Bang HO, Dyerberg J, Hjoorne T. The composition of food consumed by Greenland Eskimos. Acta Med Scand 1976; 200: 69-73.

[3] Bang HO, Dyerberg J, Sinclair HM. The composition of the Eskimo food in north western Greenland. Am J Clin Nutr 1980; 33; 2657-2661.

[4] Middaugh JP. Cardiovascular deaths among Alaskan Natives, 1980-86. Am J Public Health 1990; 80: 282-285.

[5] Newman WP, Middaugh JP, Propst MT, Roger DR. Atherosclerosis in Alaska Natives and non-natives. Lancet 1993; 341: 1056-1057.

[6] Jump DB. The biochemistry of n-3 polyunsaturated fatty acids. J Biol Chem 2002; 277: 8755-8758.

[7] Ikonen E. Roles of lipid rafts in membrane transport. Curr Opin Cell Biol 2001; 13: 470-477.

[8] Hwang D. Fatty acids and immune responses-a new perspective in searching for clues to mechanisms. Annu Rev Nutr 2000; 20: 431-456.

[9] Sellmayer A, Hrboticky N, Weber PC. Lipids in vascular function. Lipids 1999; 34: S13- S18.

[10] Serhan, C.N., Clish, C.B.: US20067053230 (**2006**).

[11] Clarke SD, Jump DB. Regulation of gene transcription by polyunsaturated fatty acids. Prog Lipid Res 1993; 32: 139-149.

[12] Pan DA, Mater MK, Thelen AP, Peters JM, Gonzalez FJ, Jump DB. Evidence against the peroxisome proliferator-activated receptor alpha (PPARα) as the mediator for polyunsaturated fatty acid suppression of hepatic L-pyruvate kinase gene transcription. J Lipid Res 2000; 41: 742-751.

[13] Lindeberg S, Lundh B. Apparent absence of stroke and ischaemic heart disease in a traditional Melanesian island: a clinical study in Kitava. J Intern Med 1993; 233: 269-275.

[14] Hirai A, Terano T, Tamura Y, Yoshida S. Eicosapentaenoic acid and adult diseases in Japan: epidemiological and clinical aspects. J Intern Med 1989; 225: 69-75.

[15] Kromhout D, Bosschieter EB, de Lezenne Coulander C. The inverse relation between fish consumption and 20-year mortality from coronary heart disease. N Engl J Med 1985; 312: 1205-1209.

[16] Shekelle RB, Missel LV, Paul O, *et al.* Fish consumption and mortality from coronary heart disease. N Engl J Med 1985; 313: 820.

[17] Daviglus ML, Stamler J, Orencia AJ, *et al.* Fish consumption and the 30-year risk of fatal myocardial infarction. N Engl J Med 1997; 336: 1046-1053.

[18] Oomen CM, Feskens EJ, Rasanen L, *et al.* Fish consumption and coronary heart disease mortality in Finland, Italy, and the Netherlands. Am J Epidemiol 2000; 151: 999-1006.

[19] Hu FB, Bronner L, Willet WC, *et al.* Fish and omega-3 fatty acid intake and risk of coronary heart disease in women. JAMA 2002; 287: 1815-1821.

[20] Mozaffarian D, Lemaitre RN, Kuller LH, *et al.* Cardiac benefits of fish consumption may depend on the type of fish meal consumed: the Cardiovascular Health Study. Circulation 2003; 107: 1372-1377.

[21] Curb JD, Reed DM. Fish consumption and mortality from coronary heart disease. N Engl J Med 1985; 313: 821.

[22] Vollet Se, Heuch I, Bjelke E. Fish consumption and mortality from coronary heart disease. N Engl J Med 1985; 313: 820-821.

[23] Ascherio A, Rimm EB, Stampfer MJ, *et al.* Dietary intake of marine n-3 fatty acids, fish intake, and the risk of coronary disease among men. N Engl J Med 1995; 332: 977-982.

[24] Salonen JT, Nyyssonen K, Salonen R. Fish intake and the risk of coronary disease. N Engl J Med 1995; 333: 937.

[25] Rodriguez BL, Sharp DS, Abbot RD, *et al.* Fish intake may limit the increase in coronary heart disease morbidity and mortality among heavy smokers: the Honolulu Heart Program. Circulation 1996; 94: 952-956.

[26] Albert CM, Hennekens CH, O'Donnell CJ, *et al.* Fish consumption and risk of sudden cardiac death. JAMA 1998; 279: 23-28.

[27] Osler M, Andreasen AH, Hoidrup S. No inverse association between fish consumption and risk of death from all-causes, and incidence of coronary heart disease in middle-aged, Danish adults. J Clin Epidemiol 2003; 56: 274-279.

[28] Guallar E, Hennekens CH, Sacks FM, *et al.* A prospective study of plasma fish oil levels and incidence of myocardial infarction in US male physicians. J Am Coll Cardiol 1995; 25: 387-394.

[29] Siscovick DS, Raghunathan TE, King I, *et al.* Dietary intake and cell membrane levels of long-chain n-3 polyunsaturated fatty acids and the risk of primary cardiac arrest. JAMA 1995; 274: 1363-1367.

[30] Burr ML, Fehily AM, Gilbert JF, *et al.* Effects of changes in fat, fish, and fibre intakes on death and myocardial reinfarction: diet and reinfarction trial (DART). Lancet 1989; 2: 757-761.

[31] de Lorgeril M, Renaud S, Mamelle N, *et al.* Mediterranean alpha-linolenic acid-rich diet in secondary prevention of coronary heart disease. Lancet 1994; 343: 1454-1459.

[32] de Lorgeril M, Salen P, Martin JL, Monjaud I, Delaye J, Mamelle N. Mediterranean diet, traditional risk factors, and the rate of cardiovascular complications after myocardial infarction: final report of the Lyon Diet Heart Study. Circulation 1999; 99: 779-785.

[33] Dietary supplementation with n-3 polyunsaturated fatty acids and vitamin E after myocardial infarction: results of the GISSI-Prevenzione trial. Gruppo Italiano per lo Studio della Sopravvivenza nell'infarto miocardico. Lancet 1999; 354: 447-455.

[34] Albert CM, Campos H, Stampfer MJ, *et al.* Blood levels of long-chain n-3 fatty acids and the risk of sudden death. N Engl J Med 2002; 346: 1113-1118.

[35] Guallar A, Aro A, Jimenez FJ, Martin-Moreno JM, *et al.* Omega-3 fatty acids in adipose tissue and risk of myocardial infarction: the EURAMIC study. Arterioscler Thromb Vasc Biol 1999; 19: 1111-1118.

[36] He K, Song Y, Daviglus ML, *et al.* Accumulated evidence of fish oil consumption and coronary heart disease mortality: a meta-analysis of cohort studies. Circulation 2004; 109: 2705-11.

[37] Konig A, Bouzan C, Cohen JT, *et al.* A quantitative analysis of fish consumption and coronary heart disease mortality. Am J Prev Med 2005; 29: 335-346.

[38] Harper CR, Jacobson TA. Usefulness of omega-3 fatty acids and the prevention of coronary heart disease. Am J Cardiol 2005; 96: 1521-1529.

[39] Bucher HC, Hengstler P, Schindler C, *et al.* N-3 polyunstaurated fatty acids in coronary heart disease: a meta-analysis of randomized controlled trials. Am J Med 2002; 112: 298-304.

[40] Whelton SP, He J, Whelton PK, *et al.* Meta-analysis of observational studies on fish intake and coronary heart disease. Am J Cardiol 2004; 93: 1119-1123.

[41] Yzebe D and Lievre M. Fish oils in the care of coronary heart disease patients: a meta-analysis of randomized controlled trials. Fundam Clin Pharmacol 2004; 18: 581-592.

[42] Hooper L, Thompson RL, Harrison RA, *et al.* Omega 3 fatty acids for prevention and treatment of cardiovascular disease. Cochrane Database Syst Rev 2004; 4: CD003177.

[43] Covington MB. Omega-3 fatty acids. Am Fam Physician 2004; 70: 133-140.

[44] Origin Trial Investigators. Rationale, design, and baseline characteristics for a large international trial of cardiovascular disease prevention in people with dysglycemia: the ORIGIN trial (Outcome Reduction with an Initial Glargine Intervention). Am Heart J 2008; 155: 26-32.

[45] Holmann RR, Paul S, Farmer A, *et al.* Atorvastatin in factorial with Omega-3 EE90 risk reduction in diabetes (AFFORD): a randomized controlled trial. Diabetologia 2009; 52: 50-59.

[46] GISSI-HF Investigators. Effects of n-3 polyunsaturated fatty acids in patients with chronic heart failure (the GISSI-HF trial): a randomized, double-blind, placebo controlled trial. Lancet 2008; 372: 1223-1230.

[47] Grimsgaard S, Bonaa KH, Hansen JB, *et al.* Effects of highly purified eicosapentaenoic acid and docosahexaenoic acid on hemodynamics in humans. Am J Clin Nutr 1998; 68: 52-59

[48] Chin JP, Gust AP, Nestel PJ, *et al.* Marine oils dose-dependently inhibit vasoconstriction of forearm resistance vessels in humans. Hypertension 1993; 21: 22-28.

[49] Walser B, and Stebbins CL. Omega-3 fatty acid supplementation enhances stroke volume and cardiac output during dynamic exercise. Eur J Appl Physiol 2008; 104: 455-461.

[50] He K, Song Y, Daviglus ML, *et al.* Fish consumption and incidence of stroke: a meta-analysis of cohort studies. Stroke 2004; 35: 1538-1542.

[51] Bouzan C, Cohen JT, Connor WE, *et al.* A quantitative analysis of fish consumption and stroke risk. Am J Prev Med 2005; 29: 347-352.

[52] Tanaka K, Ishikawa Y, Yokoyama M, *et al.* Reduction in the recurrence of stroke by eicosapentaenoic acid for hypercholesterolemic patients: subanalysis of the JELIS trial. Stroke 2008; 27: 375-383.

[53] Thies F, Garry JM, Yaqoob P, *et al.* Association of n-3 polyunsaturated fatty acids with stability of atherosclerotic plaques: a randomized controlled trial. Lancet 2003; 361: 477-485.

[54] Sommerfield T, Price J, and Hiatt WR. Omega-3 fatty acids for intermittent claudication. Cochrane Database Syst Rev 2007; 4: CD003833.

[55] Howe PR. Dietary fats and hypertension. Focus on fish oil. Ann N Y Acad Sci 1997; 827: 339-352.

[56] Bonaa KH, Bjerve KS, Straume B, *et al.* Effect of eicosapentaenoic and docosahexaenoic acids on blood pressure in hypertension. A population-based intervention trial from the Tromso study. N Engl J Med 1990; 322: 795-801.

[57] Prisco D, Paniccia R, Bandinelli B, *et al.* Effect of medium-term supplementation with a moderate dose of n-3 polyunsaturated fatty acids on blood pressure in mild hypertensive patients. Thromb Res 1998; 91: 105-112.

[58] Knapp HR, FitzGerald GA. The antihypertensive effects of fish oil. A controlled study of polyunsaturated fatty acid supplements in essential hypertension. N Engl J Med 1989; 320: 1037-1043.

[59] Morris MC, Sacks F, Rosner B. Does fish oil lower blood pressure? A meta-analysis of controlled trials. Circulation 1993; 88: 523-533.

[60] Harris WS, Ginsberg HN, Arunakul N, *et al.* Safety and efficacy of Omacor in severe hypertriglyceridemia. J Cardiovasc Risk 1997; 4: 385-391.

[61] Harris WS. N-3 fatty acids and serum lipoproteins: human studies. Am J Clin Nutr 1997; 65: 1645-1654.

[62] Cavazza, C.: WO06013602A1 (**2006**).

[63] Hong H, Xu ZM, Pang BS, *et al.* Effects of simvastain combined with omega-3 fatty acids on high sensitive C-reactive protein, lipidemia, and fibrinolysis in patients with mixed dyslipidemia. Chin Med Sci J 2004; 19: 145-149.

[64] Nordoy A, Hansen JB, Brox J, *et al.* Effects of atorvastatin and omega-3 fatty acids on LDL subfractions and postprandial hyperlipemia in patients with combined hyperlipemia. Nutr Metab Cardiovasc Dis 2001; 11: 7-16.

[65] Nordoy A, Bonaa KH, Sandset PM, *et al.* Effect of omega-3 fatty acids and simvastatin on hemostatic risk factors and postprandial hyperlipemia in patients with combined hyperlipemia. Arterioscler Thromb Vasc Biol 2000; 20: 259-265.

[66] Hartweg J, Farmer AJ, Holman RR, *et al.* Potential impact of omega-3 treatment on cardiovascular disease in type 2 diabetes. Curr Opin Lipidol 2009; 20: 30-38.

[67] Catena C, Novello M, Lapenna R, *et al.* New risk factors for atherosclerosis in hypertension: focus on the prothrombotic state and lipoprotein(a). J Hypertens 2005; 23: 1617-1631.
[68] Colussi GL, Baroselli S, Sechi LA. ω-3 polyunsaturated fatty acids decrease plasma lipoprotein(a) levels in hypertensive subjects. Clin Nutr 2004; 23: 1246-1247.
[69] O'Leary DH, Polak JF, Kronmal RA, *et al.* Carotid-artery intima and media thickness as a risk factor for myocardial infarction and stroke in older adults. Cardiovascular Health Study Collaborative Research Group. N Engl J Med 1999; 340: 14-22.
[70] Yamada T, Malcom GT, Strong JP; *et al.* Difference in atherosclerosis between the populations of a fishing and a farming village in Japan. Ann NY Acad Sci 1997; 811: 412-419.
[71] Djoussé L, Folsom AR, Province MA, Hunt SC, Ellison RC. Dietary linolenic acid and carotid atherosclerosis : the National Heart, Lung, and Blood Institute Family Heart Study. Am J Clin Nutr 2003; 77: 819-825.
[72] Angerer P, Kothny W, Stork S, von Schacky C. Effect of dietary supplementation with omega-3 fatty acids on progression of atherosclerosis in carotid arteries. Cardiovasc Res 2002; 54: 183-190.
[73] De Caterina R, Madonna R, Massaro M. Effects of omega-3 fatty acids on cytokines and adhesion molecules. Curr Atheroscler Rep 2004; 6: 485-491.
[74] Miles EA, Thies F, Wallace FA, *et al.* Influence of age and dietary fish oil on plasmas soluble adhesion molecule concentrations. Clin Sci 2001; 100: 91-100.
[75] Baumann KH, Hessel F, Larass I, *et al.* Dietary ω-3, ω-6, and ω-9 unsaturated fatty acids and growth factor and cytokine gene expression in unstimulated and stimulated monocytes. Arterioscler Thromb Vasc Biol 1999; 19: 59-66.
[76] Sperling RI, Benincaso AI, Knoell CT, Larkin JK, Austen KF, Robinson DR. Dietary ω-3 polyunsaturated fatty acids inhibit phosphoinositide formation and chemotaxis in neutrophils. J Clin Invest 1993; 91: 651-660.
[77] Libby P. Inflammation in atherosclerosis. Nature 2002; 420: 868-874.
[78] Massaro M, Basta G, Lazzerini G, *et al.* Quenching of intracellular ROS generation as a mechanism for oleate-induced reduction of endothelial activation and early atherogenesis. Thromb Haemost 2002; 88: 335-344.
[79] De Caterina R, Cybulsky MI, Clinton SK, Gimbrone MA Jr, Libby P. The omega-3 fatty acid docosahexaenoate reduces cytokine-induced expression of proatherogenic and proinflammatory proteins in human endothelial cells. Arterioscler Thromb 1994; 14: 1829-1836.
[80] De Caterina R, Bernini W, Carluccio MA, Liao JK, Libby P. Structural requirements for inhibition of cytokine-induced endothelial activation by unsaturated fatty acids. J Lipid Res 1998; 39: 1062-1070.
[81] Marchioli R, Schweiger C, Tavazzi L, Valagussa F. Effect of ω-3 polyunsaturated fatty acids after myocardial infarction: results of GISSI-Prevenzione trial. Gruppo Italiano per lo Studio della Sopravvivenza nell'Infarto del Miocardio. Lipids 2001; 36: S119-S126.
[82] Singh RB, Niaz MA, Sharma JP, Kumar R, Rastogi V, Moshiri M. Randomized, double-blind, placebo-controlled trial of fish oil and mustard oil in patients with suspected acute myocardial infarction: the Indian experiment of infarct survival-4. Cardiovasc Drugs Ther 1997; 11: 485-491.
[83] Singh RB, Dubnov G, Niaz MA, *et al.* Effect of Indo-Mediterranean diet on progression of coronary artery disease in high-risk patients (Indo-Mediterranean Diet Heart Study): a randomized single-blind trial. Lancet 2002; 360: 1455-1461.
[84] Marchioli R, Barzi F, Bomba E, *et al.* Early protection against sudden cardiac death by n-3 polyunsaturated fatty acids after myocardial infarction. Circulation 2002; 105: 1897-1903.
[85] Matthan NR, Jordan H, Chung M, Lichtenstein AH, Lathrop DA, Lau J. A systematic review meta-analysis of the impact of ω-3 fatty acids on selected arrhythmia outcomes in animal models. Metabolism 2005; 54: 1557-1565.
[86] Raitt M, Conner W, Morris C, *et al.* Antiarrhythmic effects of n-3 polyunsaturated fatty acids in survivors of ventricular tachyarrhythmias. Circulation 2003; 108: 2723.
[87] Maggioni AP, Tavazzi L, Marchioli R, Tognoni G, Avanzini F, Roncaglioni MG. Perspectives on n-3 PUFAs: primary prevention, antiarrhythmic effects, congestive heart failure. Eur Heart J 2002; 3: D106-109.
[88] Brower IA, Zock PL, Wever EFD, *et al.* Rationale and design of randomized controlled clinical trial on supplemental intake of n-3 fatty acids and incidence of cardiac arrhythmia: SOFA. Eur J Clin Nutr 2003; 57: 1323-1330.
[89] Schrepf R, Limmert T, Weber PC, Theisen K, Sellmayer A. Immediate effects of n-3 fatty acid infusion on the induction of sustained ventricular tachycardia. Lancet 2004; 363: 1441-1442.
[90] Calò L, Bianconi L, Colivicchi F, *et al.* N-3 fatty acids for the prevention of atrial fibrillation after coronary artery bypass surgery: a randomized, controlled trial. J Am Coll Cardiol 2005; 45: 1723-1728.
[91] Leòn H, Shibata MC, Sivakumaran S, *et al.* Effect of fish oil on arrhythmias and mortality: systematic review. BMJ 2008; 337: a2931

[92] Macchia A, Varini S, Grancelli H, *et al.* The rationale and design of the FORomegaARD trial: A randomized, double-blind, placebo controller, independent study to test the efficacy of n-3 PUFA for the maintenance of normal sinus rhythm in patients with previous atrial fibrillation. Am Heart J 2009; 157: 423-427.

[93] McLennan PL, Abeywardena MY, Charnock JS. Dietary fish oil prevents ventricular fibrillation following coronary artery occlusion and reperfusion. Am Heart J 1988; 116: 709-717.

[94] Leaf A, Jorgensen MB, Jacobs AK, *et al.* Do fish oil prevent restenosis after coronary angioplasty? Circulation 1994; 90: 2248-2257.

[95] Grimminger F, Grimm H, Fuhrer D, *et al.* Omega-3 lipid infusion in a heart allotransplant model: shift in fatty acid and lipid mediator profiles and prolongation of transplant survival. Circulation 1996; 93: 365-371.

[96] Kang JX, Leaf A. Effects of long-chain poyunsaturated fatty acids on the contraction of neonatal rat cardiac myocytes. Proc Natl Acad Sci USA 1994; 91: 9886-9890.

[97] McLennan PL. Myocardial membrane fatty acids and the antiarrhythmic actions of dietary fish oil in animal models. Lipids 2001; 36: S111-114.

[98] Leifert WR, Jahangiri A, McMurchie EJ. Membrane fluidity changes are associated with antiarrhythmic effects of docosa-hexaenoic acid in adult rat cardiomyocytes. J Nutr Biochem 2000; 11: 38-44.

[99] Grynberg A, Fournier A, Sergiel JP, Athias P. Membrane docosahexaenoic acid vs. eicosapentaenoic acid and the beating function of the cardiomyocyte and its regulation through the adrenergic receptors. Lipids 1996; 31: 205-210.

[100] Dai J, Williams SA, Zeighelhoffer A. Structure-activity relationship of the effect of dietary supplementation of fish oil on experimental myocardial infarction. Circ Res 1995; 52: 167-171.

[101] Charnock JS. Omega-3 polyunsaturated fatty acids and ventricular fibrillation: the possible involvement of eicosanoids. Prostaglandins Leukot Essent Fatty Acids 1999; 61: 243-247.

[102] Xiao YF, Kang JX, Morgan JP, Leaf A. Blocking affects of polyunsaturated fatty acids on Na^+ channels of neonatal rat ventricular myocytes. Proc Natl Acad Sci USA 1995; 92: 11000-11004.

[103] Xiao YF, Gomez AM, Morgan JP, Lederer WJ, Leaf A. Suppression of voltage-gated L-type Ca^{2+} currents by polyunsaturated fatty acids in adult and neonatal rat ventricular myocytes. Proc Natl Acad Sci USA 1997; 94: 4182-4187.

[104] Berlin, R.: US20060020031A1 (**2006**).

[105] Berlin, R.: WO06014790A2 (**2006**).

[106] Kris-Etherton PM, Harris WS, Appel LJ. Fish consumption, fish oil, omega-3 fatty acids, and cardiovascular disease. American Heart Association Nutrition Committee. Circulation 2002; 106: 2747-2757.

[107] Van de Werf F, Ardissino D, Betriu A, *et al.* Management of acute myocardial infarction in patients presenting with ST-segment elevation. Eur Heart J 2003; 24: 26-66.

Chronic Diabetic Complications: Endothelial Cells at the Frontline

Zia A. Khan[1,2] and Subrata Chakrabarti[*,1,2,3]

[1]*Department of Pathology, University of Western Ontario, London, Ontario N6G 2V4, Canada*

[2]*Metabolism and Diabetes Research Program, Lawson Health Research Institute, London, Ontario N6G 2V4, Canada*

[3]*Department of Microbiology and Immunology, University of Western Ontario, London, Ontario N6G 2V4, Canada*

Abstract: We are approaching the 100-year anniversary of Dr. Frederick Banting's discovery of insulin for the treatment of diabetes. The population of patients with diabetes is ever-increasing. However, with the availability of insulin, the cause of mortality has shifted from diabetic coma and ketoacidosis to chronic secondary complications. Dysfunction and failure of selected organs is now the most prominent cause of morbidity and mortality. These 'target' organs include the eyes, kidneys, heart, lower limbs, and the nervous system. A common feature of these complications is the aberration in the vasculature of the target organs. Studies over the past few decades have shown that dysfunction of the vascular endothelial cells may be the key to the development and progression of the chronic diabetic complications. We present the hypothesis and supporting evidence that preservation and restoration of the endothelial cell function may potentially be the most efficient means of targeting the adverse effects of diabetes.

Keywords: Endothelial cells, diabetes, microangiopathy, macroangiopathy, basement membrane, extracellular matrix, fibronectin, oxidative stress, protein kinase c, aldose reductase, nitric oxide, endothelin, vasoactive factors, cardiomyopathy, advanced glycosylation end products, metabolic distress, glucose.

INTRODUCTION

According to the most recent estimates, diabetes affects over 6% of the world and 9% of the North American population [1]. This equates to an enormous economic burden [1]. Because of our lifestyle and yet to be untangled genetic determinants, a possible plateau or a decrease in this upward trend is nowhere in sight. The use of insulin has significantly lowered the high rate of mortality due to diabetic coma and ketoacidosis. Unfortunately, we have also witnessed a shift in the cause the diabetes-associated morbidity and mortality due to chronic secondary complications. These complications target selected organs and

*Corresponding author: Tel: 519-685-8500, Ext. 36350; Fax: 519-661-3370; E-mail: subrata.chakrabarti@schulich.uwo.ca

Atta-ur-Rahman / M. Iqbal Choudhary (Eds.)

manifest as angiopathy involving both the micro- (retinopathy, nephropathy, neuropathy, and cardiomyopathy) and macro- (accelerated atherosclerosis) vascular systems[2, 3]. Macroangiopathic changes may also affect the coronary artery, the carotid artery, as well as peripheral arteries. Identification of the underlying cause of these secondary complications is warranted and ever so timely. The first indication as to the potential cause comes from clinical studies conducted in the 1990s [4, 5]. The seminal findings of these studies pointed to hyperglycemia as the key mediator of target organ dysfunction in diabetes [4, 5]. There may be other factors that potentiate and contribute to the adverse effects of hyperglycemia such as hyperlipidemia and hyperinsulinemia. However, if we can achieve a tight glucose control, which is a daunting task in itself, we can prevent the development and progression of the complications [4,5]. This chapter will explore the hypothesis that vascular endothelial cell dysfunction is the origin of chronic diabetic complications and may very well be the most important therapeutic target.

ENDOTHELIAL CELLS – THE PRIMARY TARGET OF HYPERGLYCEMIC DAMAGE

Endothelial cells (ECs) line the blood vessels and are critical for the function and integrity of the vascular unit. ECs were first considered to be merely a non-thrombogenic cellular barrier. However, Florey and colleagues (1966) suggested that EC lining is dynamic, metabolically relevant for tissue function, and represents more than an inert cell sheet [6]. Soon after, the first successful *in vitro* EC culture was established [7]. This paved the path to the greater understanding of the role of ECs in the vascular system. We can now appreciate the important role ECs play in regulating vascular tone (blood flow and pressure), permeability, blood fluidity, thrombotic/fibrinolytic balance, and leukocyte traffic [8].

Due to the anatomical location and barrier function, ECs are the first cells to encounter circulating glucose. ECs incorporate glucose via facilitative diffusion [9, 10] and changes in the level of glucose does not lead to altered expression of the primary EC glucose transporter, glucose transporter-1 (Glut1) [9, 10]. This is in contrast to the contractile cells (smooth muscle cells and pericytes) in which Glut1 levels decrease following exposure to high levels of glucose [9, 10]. Therefore, increased or decreased plasma glucose levels may have profound effects in the ECs. Under physiological conditions (glucose levels ~ 5 mM or 90 mg/dL), glucose is primarily metabolized by the glycolytic pathway with the hexose monophosphate pathway and Krebs cycle accounting for less than 2% combined [11]. However, the oxidation of glucose through the Krebs cycle can be increased when glucose levels drop below 1 mM (18 mg/dL) [11]. The same holds true when glucose reaches supraphysiological levels [12]. In addition, higher than physiological levels of glucose also activate alternative metabolic pathways such as the polyol and hexoseamine pathways (Fig. **1**) [12, 13]. High levels of glucose cause biochemical changes in the ECs which are reminiscent of early molecular alterations in the target organs of diabetes [14-16]. *In vitro* studies have shown that exposure of EC to high glucose levels leads to activation of the EC which manifests as increased production of the extracellular matrix proteins (major proteins being collagen and fibronectin), procoagulant proteins (von Willebrand Factor; vWF), and altered cellular activities (proliferation and migration)[17-22]. Other factors, such as increased insulin levels, may also contribute to these factors [23-25]. Thus, all of the normal EC functional properties (summarized in Table **1**) may be affected by glucose and/or insulin in diabetes, making EC dysfunction a key pathological element in the development of chronic diabetic complications [26, 27].

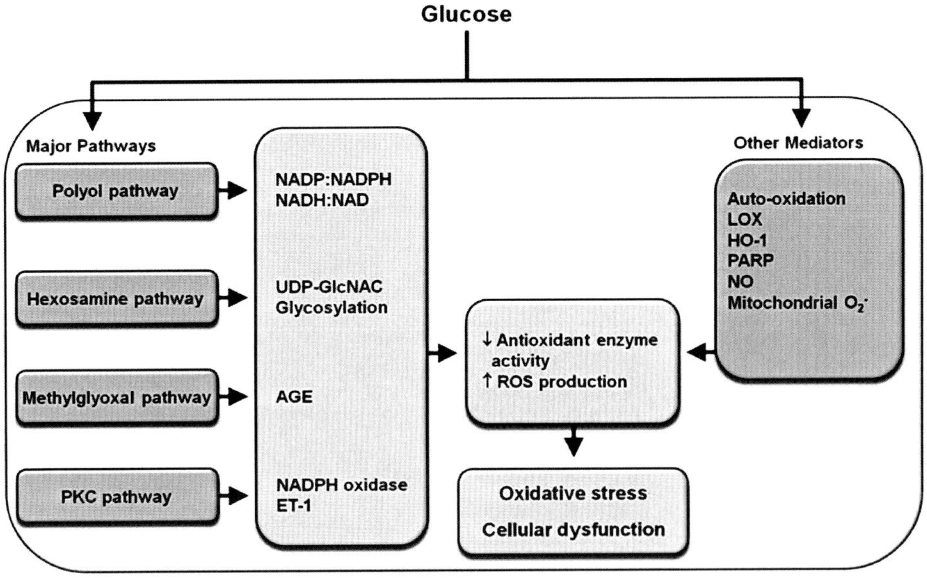

Fig. (1). Proposed mechanisms of glucose-induced biochemical changes in the ECs. High glucose levels lead to activation of polyol pathway, hexoseamine pathway, protein kinase C, AGE formation, and PARP activation. In addition, glucose may increase oxidative stress indirectly by activating lipoxygenase and heme oxygenase enzyme systems. These biochemical changes may culminate in increased ET-1 activity, reduced NO availability, oxidative stress and EC dysfunction [AGE = advanced glycation end product; ET-1 = endothelin-1; HOE-1 = heme oxygenase-1; LOX = lipoxygenase; NAD+ = nicotinamide adenine dinucleotide; NADH = nicotinamide adenine sinucleotide, reduced; NADP = nicotinamide adenine dinucleotide phosphate; NADPH = nicotinamide adenine dinucleotide phosphate, reduced; NO = nitric oxide; PARP = poly(ADP-ribose) polymerases; PKC = protein kinase C; ROS = reactive oxygen species; UDP-GlcNAC = UDP-N-acetylglucosamine].

Subsequent to EC dysfunction, the target tissues in diabetes exhibit poor blood flow and ischemia (Fig. **2**)[15, 16, 28]. This is brought upon by the combined effect of functional and structural alterations in the vasculature. The response of the target organs to reduced blood flow and ischemia, however, varies depending on the vascular bed. The retina (and possibly the kidney) responds to EC dysfunction and ischemia by enhancing new blood vessel formation [28]. Other target organs exhibit impaired vessel formation [29]. This suggests that the EC dysfunction may not be uniform in all organs in the patient with diabetes. The mechanism by which chronic diabetes leads to impairment of blood supply in some target organs while inducing unregulated angiogenesis in others remains undetermined. Selectivity in the target organs may suggest the importance of two key elements, the tissue microenvironment and the intrinsic properties of the targeted ECs. It is well known that ECs in the vasculature are heterogeneous [8] (as a product of both intrinsic and extrinsic properties). The variability in the ECs is evident at the level of cell size, cell shape, antigenicity, function, and susceptibility to pathological states. For example, Weible-Palade bodies (site of vWF storage in ECs) exhibit differential patterning in the vasculature being highest in number in the ECs close the heart as compared to other vascular beds [30-32].

Table 1. EC Function – and their Mediators Altered in Diabetes

EC Function	Mediators
Hemodynamic/Vascular Tone	*Vasoconstriction* Angiotensin II Endothelin-1 Thromboxane A_2 Prostaglandins H_2 and $F_{2\alpha}$ *Vasodilators* Bradykinin Nitrix Oxide Prostaglandin I_2
EC Growth and Proliferation	*Proliferation of ECs* Basic-Fibroblast Growth Factor Endothelin-1 Epidermal Growth Factor Hepatocyte Growth Factor Insulin-like Growth Factor (1 and 2) Nerve Growth Factor Oncofetal Fibronectin Platelet Derived Growth Factor Transforming Growth Factor-β Tumor Necrosis Factor-α Vascular Endothelial Growth Factor *Inhibition of EC proliferation* Angiostatin Endostatin Nitric Oxide Pigment Epithelium Derived Factor Prostaglandin I_2
Anti-thrombogenic/ -Fibrinolytic	*Pro-thrombogenic/fibrinolytic* Plasminogen Activator Inhibitor-1 von Willebrand Factor *Anti-thrombogenic/fibrinolytic* Nitric Oxide Tissue type-Plasminogen Activator Thrombomodulin
Inflammation	*Pro-inflammatory* E-selectin Intracellular Adhesion Molecules-1 Vascular Adhesion Molecule-1 *Anti-inflammatory* Nitric Oxide

The microenvironment may also change the EC phenotype. When aortic ECs are cultured on lung-derived extracellular matrix substrate, the cells begin to express lung endothelial cell adhesion molecule-1 (Lu-ECAM-1) [33], a marker specific to lung endothelium. The same is true for other organ extracellular matrix proteins. Culturing of bovine adrenal cortex ECs on kidney cell-derived matrix has been shown to cause fenestrae formation in the ECs [34].

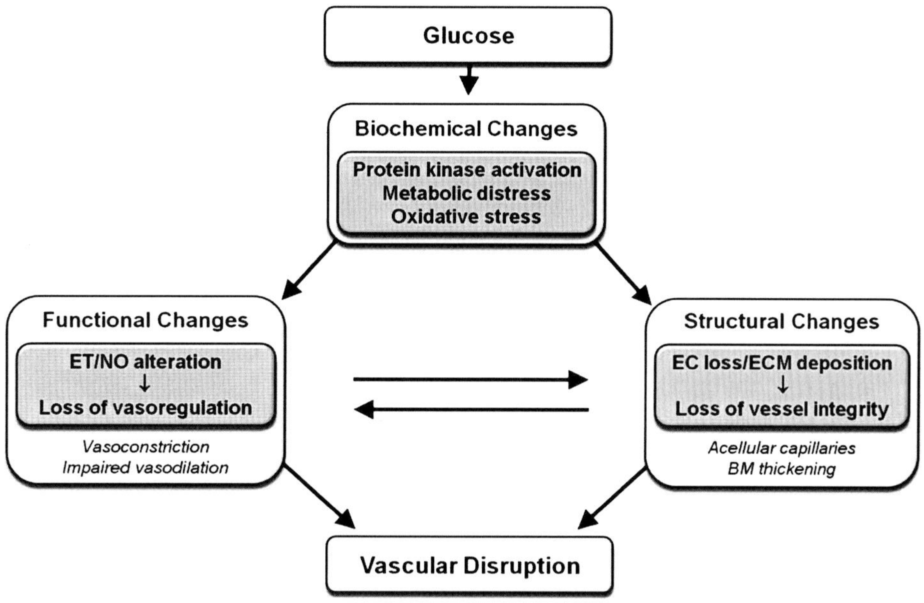

Fig. (2). Proposed mechanisms leading to vascular disruption in diabetes. High circulating glucose levels lead to biochemical dysfunction in the target organ vascular ECs. These biochemical changes include protein kinase activation, metabolic changes, and increased oxidative stress. As a result, both structural and functional aspects of the blood vessels are altered. Impaired vasoregulation, increased permeability, extracellular matrix expansion, and dysfunction of the vascular cells causes reduced blood flow in the target organ [BM = basement membrane; EC = endothelial cell; ECM = extracellular matrix; ET = endothelin; NO = nitric oxide].

Numerous biochemical and molecular changes within the vascular ECs lead to functional and structural alterations of the target organ vascular bed. There are three distinct events, analogous to a 3-act play that orchestrates the complex pathology of the vasculature in diabetes. These include a) damage, b) response, and c) remembering the unforgettable.

ACT 1: ALTERED VASOACTIVE FACTORS & REDUCED BLOOD FLOW IN TARGET ORGANS

EC dysfunction in the microvascular complications of diabetes is well established [16]. Even macrovascular atherogenesis exhibits an important EC component [35, 36]. ECs are important for the initiation and perpetuation of atherosclerotic process [37-39]. The initial events may include increased antiginicity and permeability whereas the later events may encompass the retention of atherogenic proteins as well as leukocytes. EC dysfunction has traditionally been defined as an impairment of endothelium-dependent vasodilation (EDV) in diabetes [40-42]. This is one of the earliest functional changes and it has been shown to precede the structural changes in the vasculature [43-48]. Studies have reported that acute exposure to high levels of glucose in healthy individuals results in impaired EDV [49, 50]. The underlying mechanism follows a two-hit model: an increase in expression/activity of vasoconstrictors and a concurrent decrease in expression/activity of vasodilators. The major vasoactive factor that is altered in diabetes is endothelin-1 (ET-1). ET-1, the most potent endogenous vasoconstrictor, is a short peptide that is primarily produced by the ECs [51, 52]. Dysfunction and/or activation of the ECs is, therefore, expected to alter the levels of ET-1 production. Augmented ET-1 levels have been reported in diabetes and have been shown to mediate vasoconstriction and reduced blood flow [14]. Increased activity of ETs has also been shown in the resistance arteries of diabetic patients [53]. Moreover, administration of exogenous ET-1 in humans reduces coronary and renal blood flow and increases vasoconstriction [54-56]. This suggests that inhibiting ET-1 may alleviate impaired EDV in diabetes. Improvement of the vasodilator responses have been noted in diabetic patients administered an ET antagonist (selective ETA receptor blocker BQ-123) [53]. ETA receptors are the main receptors present on the perivascular cells that mediate ET-induced vasoconstriction [14]. We have also reported that diabetes-induced retinal capillary vasoconstriction in experimental diabetes is normalized with a dual ET receptor antagonist (Bosentan/ dual ETA and ETB receptor blocker) [57].

As mentioned above, a concurrent alteration in the vasodilators may be required for EDV impairment in diabetes. Acetylcholine-induced paradoxical vasoconstriction in atheroscelerotic coronary arteries have suggested an important role of nitric oxide synthase (NOS) enzymes [58]. NOS are a family of enzymes that produce the vasodilator, nitric oxide (NO). There are three members of the family: neuronal NOS (type I), inducible NOS (type II), and endothelial NOS (type III). Acute exposure of ECs to glucose decreases NO generation by agonists such as bradykinin and A23187 [59]. Purified endothelial NOS when assayed in the presence of glucose also shows significantly lower level of NO production [59]. In addition to reduced generation, NO may also be sequestered by glucose-induced oxidative stress [14-16]. This creates an imbalance in the counter-activity of ETs and NO. Therefore, similar to the approach of inhibiting ET-1, we could potentially increase NO production to normalize EDV impairment. In support of this as a potential therapeutic approach, we have previously shown that treatment of diabetic animals with a NO donor, molsidomine, prevents diabetes-induced vasoconstriction in the retina [60]. Recent studies have also documented restoration of EC function by overexpression of endothelial NOS [61,62].

The mechanism of vasoactive factor alteration and scavenging is intimately related to increased oxidative stress. Increased glucose-induced oxidative stress is an early change in the ECs. The pathways which increase oxidative stress are multifactorial (Fig. **1**). Acute exposure to high ambient glucose causes glucose auto-oxidation [13]. A number of other pathways also induce oxidative stress including, protein kinase C activation, polyol and hexoseamine pathways, oxidized-low lipoprotein, and heme oxygenase pathway [63]. Oxidative stress, together with vasoactive factors, represents the major avenues that can be targeted to restore EC function (Table **2**). In fact, a number of patented dugs are available to achieve exactly that (Table **3**).

Table 2. Possible Pharmacological Targets for Restoration of EC Dysfunction in Diabetes

Targets	Effect
Vasoactive Factors	Vascular tone, cellular proliferation, ECM deposition
Angiotensin II	Vascular tone, growth factor expression
ET-1	
NO	
Oxidative Stress	
AGE/RAGE	
Aldose Reductase	
Heme Oxygenase	
Nuclear Factor-κB	
NADPH Oxidase	
PARP	
Protein Kinase C	
Others*	Cellular proliferation
ED-B⁺ Fibronectin	
MAPK	
Protein Kinase B	
SGK-1	
VEGF	

*Increase/decrease in cardiomyopathy/retinopathy. [AGE = advanced glycation end product; ED-B$^+$ FN = Extra domain-B containing fibronectin; ET-1 = endothelin-1; MAPK = mitogen activated protein kinase; NADPH oxidase = nicotinamide adenine dinucleotide phosphate-oxidase; NO = nitric oxide; PARP = poly (ADP-ribose) polymerase; RAGE = receptor for AGE; SGK-1 = serum- and gluococrticoid-regulated kinase-1; VEGF = vascular endothelial growth factor].

Table 3. Selective Agents for the Restoration of EC Dysfunction in Diabetes

Parameter/Targets	Agents	Patents [Reference]
Vascular Tone	Enalapril	US 4374829 [115]
ACE Inhibitors	Lisinopril	US 4374829 [115]
ET Antagonists	Quinapril	US 4344949 [116]
NO Prodrugs	Ramipril	US 4587258 [117]
	Perindopril	US 4508729 [118]
	Fosinoprol	US 4337201 [119]
	Benazapril	US 4410520 [120]
	A127722	US 6573285 [121]
	ABT 627	US 20050042172 [122]
	Bosentan	US 20030176356 [123]
	BQ123	US 6573285 [121]
	BQ 610	US 20030176356 [123]
	BQ788	US 20030176356 [123]
	FR 139317	US 20030176356 [123]
	LU 135252	US 20030176356 [123]

Parameter/Targets	Agents	Patents [Reference]
	PD 142893	US 20030176356 [123]
	PD 14565	US 20030176356 [123]
	PD 156707	US 6573285 [121]
	RES 701-1	US 6855701 [124]
	SB 209670	US 6573285 [121]
	TAK 044	US 6573285 [121]
	AcOM-DEA/NO	US 5366997 [125]
	DETA/NO (NOC-18)	US 5155137 [126]
	DPTA/NO (NOC-19)	US 5155137 [126]
	MAHMA/NO (NOC-9)	US 5155137 [126]
	PAPA/NO (NOC-15)	US 5155137 [126]
	PROLI/NO	US 6379660 [127]
	SPER/NO	US 5155137 [126]
	V-PYRRO/NO	US 5366997 [125]
Oxidative Stress	Benfotiamine	US 3064000 [128]
AGE Blockers/Breakers	ALT-711	US 6790859 [129]
ARI	Thiazolium compounds	US 6849629 [130]
PKCβ Inhibitor	Pyridazinone	To be filed
NADPH Oxidase	Arxxant	US 5902831 [131]
PARP	Apocynin	US 5990137 [132]
	Diapocynin	WO 9307868A1 [133]
	3-AB	WO 9307868A1 [133]
	NU 1025	WO 9911624A1 [134]
	6-(5H)-phenanthridinones	WO 9911624A1 [134]
	4-iodo-3-nitrobenzamide	WO 9911645A1 [135]
	GPI-6150	WO 991649A2 [136]
	DPQ	WO 9704771A1 [137]
	Benzimidazole-4-carboxamides	WO 0026192A1 [138]
	2-aryl-1H-benzimidazole-4-carboxamides	WO 0236576A1 [139]
	4-aryl-phthalazones PJ34	WO 0142219A2 [140]

[ACE = angiotensin-converting enzyme; AGE = advanced glycation end product; ARI = aldose reductase inhibitors; ET-1 = endothelin-1; NADPH oxidase = nicotinamide adenine dinucleotide phosphate-oxidase; NO = nitric oxide; PARP = poly (ADP-ribose) polymerase; PKCβ = protein kinase C isoform β].

ACT 2: GROWTH FACTORS AND MATRIX PROTEINS REGULATE THE BALANCE BETWEEN FIBROSIS & NEOVASCULARIZATION

We have recently proposed that a balance exists between fibrosis and neovascularization in diabetic complications [16]. The balance is shifted towards EC proliferation and neovascularization in diabetic retinopathy (and possible nephropathy) and towards scar formation/ fibrosis in diabetic cardiomyopathy and neuropathy. This balance was recently highlighted in diabetic retinopathy [64]. Understanding the differences between such contrasting effects of diabetes on the target organs is critical. Tissue microenvironment, intrinsic EC differences, as well as presence of other risk factors (hyperlipidemia, hyperinsulinemia) may be involved in the process. Current molecular understanding of the changes in the target organs shows the involvement of the same players such as metabolic distress, oxidative stress, and protein kinase C.

In retinopathy, the oxygenation state regulates various growth factors that promote angiogenesis in order to counter the effects of reduced blood flow and non-perfusion from altered vasoactive factors and cellular loss [65]. However, it is believed that unregulated expression of these growth factors leads to uncontrolled retinal neovascularization and blindness in the diabetic patients. These growth factors may also initiate elaboration of the mediators that are not necessarily regulated by tissue oxygenation. Similar to the retina, structural changes in the kidney in diabetes may also include increased angiogenesis. An increased glomerular filtration rate which may, in part, be due to an increased surface area has been reported in experimental diabetes [66]. This study has shown a 30-50% in surface area per glomerulus and 20-30% increase in the number of capillaries in that diabetic rat kidneys[66]. However, in contrast to the retina [16, 28] and possible kidney [66], diabetes leads to impairment in the neovascularization of the heart. It has been reported that diabetes causes reduced expression of vascular endothelial growth factor (VEGF) and its receptors in the myocardium [67]. VEGF is an EC-specific mitogen and has been demonstrated to cause angiogenesis in a number of disease models. The reduced VEGF expression in the heart is in contrast to the retina where high levels of VEGF have been shown [28]. In addition, collateral vessel formation has also been reported to be impaired in the hearts in diabetes [68-70]. One possible explanation could underlie defective VEGF signaling in monocytes which are important for the process of arteriogenesis [69]. Activated monocytes have been shown in ischemic tissues [71, 72]. Monocytes migrate in response to VEGF through the activation of VEGFR1 (also known as Flt-1). *In vitro* assays have shown that monocytes isolated from diabetic patients fail to migrate in response to VEGF [73]. Taken together, these findings suggest that reduced expression of growth factors and growth factor receptors and impaired signaling may in concert lead to inadequate neovascularization in the myocardium. Further studies investigating the contribution of 'angiogenesis' and 'arteriogenesis' in the heart are required before diabetic cardiomypathy may be adequately targeted.

Another mechanism of differential effects of high glucose levels could be the change in the microenvironment of the vascular cells. The vascular unit comprises two major cellular components (ECs and the perivascular cells) and the surrounding scaffolding proteins, extracellular matrix (ECM). The role of ECM in EC biology spans from proliferation, migration, and stabilization. Binding of the EC surface integrins to the ECM regulates cell survival/apoptosis, growth, as well as cytoskeletal changes [74]. The heterogeneity in the ECM, therefore, is important in EC function. Growth factor-induced changes in the ECs are also matrix-dependent [75]. Moreover, the neutralizing effect of angiostatic proteins (thrombospondin, endostatin, etc.) on growth factor-induced proliferation and migration also depends on the ECM [76].

ECM changes during tumorigenesis, which is believed to promote neovascularization, include increased expression of fibronectin (FN), collagen, and tenascin-C [77-79]. Whereas, laminin and collagen (IV) levels are decreased. These selective ECM protein changes are thought to invoke a proliferative response in the vascular ECs during angiogenesis [75]. A similar scenario is evident in the retinal vascular development [77]. In the retina, FN has been reported to be expressed in the active zones of vascularization [77]. Moreover, pericytes and laminin in the basement membranes (BM) appear with EC differentiation and vessel maturation. Could differential temporal/spatial expression of FN and laminin dictate increased angiogenesis in the retina while causing impaired vessel formation in the heart? Retinal BMs of diabetic animals have been shown to contain increased collagen α1 (IV), β1 and γ chains of laminin, and FN [80]. These changes are brought upon as early as 8 weeks following onset of diabetes [80]. In addition, upregulation of tenascin has been reported in retinal vessels of diabetic patients and animals [81, 82]. Other BMs in diabetic patients exhibit somewhat similar ECM protein profile [83-86]. In the rat myocardium, diabetes increases laminin expression at 2 months following onset [87]. Two simplistic theories can be formulated to explain these findings, a) proliferating ECM proteins outweigh differentiating ECM proteins, and b) differential proteolytic processing of ECM proteins may produce fragments which confer an 'angiogenic' phenotype in the ECs. In support of such a notion, we have recently shown increased expression of an embryonic splice variant of FN (ED-B^+ FN) in the vitreous samples of proliferative diabetic retinopathy [88]. Targeted inhibition of ED-B^+ FN is associated with decreased EC proliferation and tube morphogenesis [89]. It is also plausible that FN, which undergoes extensive proteolytic processing [90], produces angiogenic fragments [91, 92].

Lastly, in terms of the microenvironment, the presence of abundant cardiac fibroblasts may contribute to impaired vessel formation. In the heart, cardiomyocytes constitute about 70% of the volume but only 30% in terms of cell number [93, 94]. ECs outnumber the cardiomyocytes by a ratio of 3:1 [93, 94]. A significant number of cardiac fibroblasts are also present in the heart which may be responsible for the cardiac ECM deposition in addition to the cardiac ECs. Angiotensin II is able to cause cardiac fibroblast proliferation and collagen deposition [95, 96]. Studies have also indicated that angiotensin II exerts the action on cardiac fibroblasts through the induction of ET-1 [97, 98]. In addition to ECs, fibroblasts also express ET receptors [99]. *In vitro* studies reveal that isolated rat fibroblasts increase production of ECM components upon ET administration [99-101]. These changes can be readily blocked by ET antagonists. It has further been shown that endocardial capillary ECs (in culture) show a 25% higher growth index as compared to other vascular ECs. These findings indicate that tissue micrenvironment is an important regulator of impaired angiogenic response in the heart which could be mediated by increased ECM deposition. In clinical trials, ET antagonists have shown promise in short-term studies as indexed by improved cardiac index and pulmonary capillary pressure [102, 103]. However, long-term studies have yet to show beneficial effects [104].

An important unresolved question is why do the ECs of new blood vessels (in the retina for example) not susceptible to the glucose-induced damage? Part of the answer may lie in the protein that transports glucose to the ECs. A recent study of the human diabetic retina has shown that Glut1 is expressed in the nerve fiber layer, Muller cells, ganglion and the photoreceptors, the retinal capillaries and the retinal pigment epithelium [105]. Comparing these results to the retina specimens of non-diabetic subjects, it becomes evident that there is no significant change in the pattern or level of Glut1 expression. However, ECs of the neovascular membranes in advanced retinopathy (which entails increased EC proliferation and angiogenesis) did not show expression of Glut1 [105]. This implies that the mechanism by which the new blood vessels escape glucose-induced damage and cellular loss may involve reduced glucose transport and accumulation in the ECs.

ACT 3: THE LASTING MEMORY

A fascinating aspect of molecular changes that mediate the adverse effects of high glucose levels is that the phenotypic changes produced in the vascular cells are long-term. This is dubbed diabetic or hyperglycemic memory [106]. Recent studies attribute this memory to chromatin remodeling. According to this postulate, glucose-induced alteration of enzymes regulating methylation/demethylation causes long-term increases or decreases in target gene expression. Most recently, smooth muscle cells isolated from diabetic animals showed increased monocyte chemotactic protein-1 and interleukin expression which was mediated by methylation of histone-3 lysine-4 near the nuclear factor-κB (NF-κB) response element [107] and reduced histone-3 lysine-9 tri-methylation at the promoter region of these target genes [108]. A similar phenomenon is also seen in the ECs [109, 110]. A brief exposure of aortic ECs to high glucose levels was associated with increased NF-κB p65 expression and histone-3 lysine-4 monomethylation at the NF-κB p65 promoter region [110].

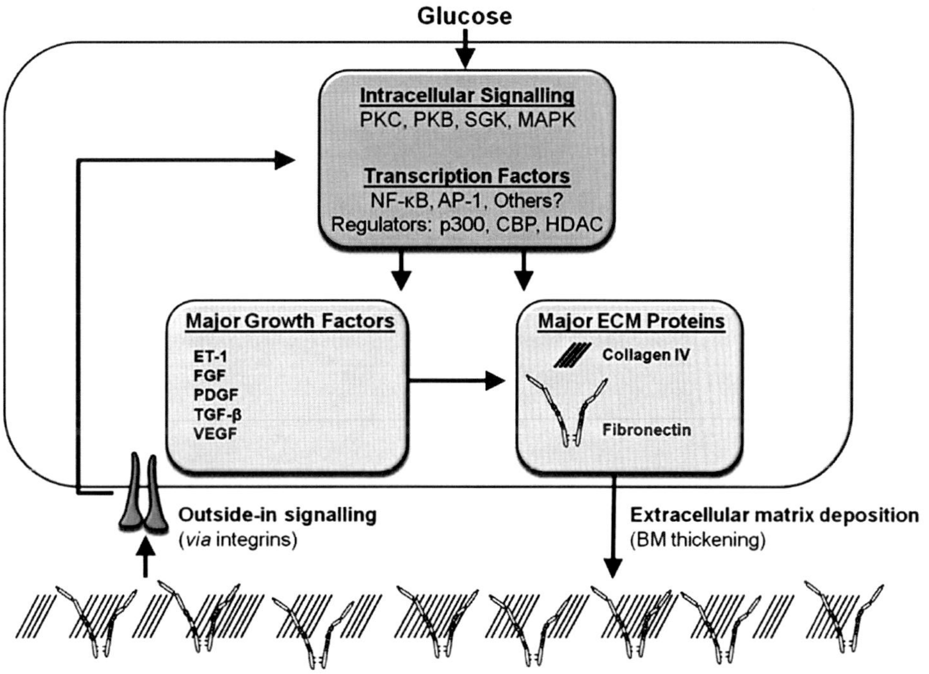

Fig. (3). Effect of glucose on growth factor and ECM protein expression. High levels of glucose increase expression of various growth factors which alter the ECs and cause increased ECM protein expression. Upregulated ECM proteins then signal to the ECs via ECM receptors, integrins. This may represent a feedback loop that mediates continuous adverse effects of hyperglycemia [AP-1 = activating protein-1; BM = basement membrane; bFGF = basic-fibroblast growth factor; CBP = CREB binding protein (CREB = cAMP-response element binding protein); ET-1 = endothelin-1; HDAC = histone deacetylase; MAPK = mitogen-activated protein kinase; NF-κB = nuclear factor-κB; PDGF = platelet-derived growth factor; PKB = protein kinase B; PKC = protein kinase C; SGK = serum- and glucocorticoid- regulated kinase; TGF-β = transforming growth factor-β; VEGF = vascular endothelial growth factor].

Modification of ECM proteins may also represent an important event in chronic stimulation of biochemical pathways such as protein kinase C and NF-κB (Fig. **3**). One consistent and continual structural change that accompanies diabetes *in vivo* and exposure to glucose *in vitro* is ECM protein deposition. Experimental evidence shows that the amount and the composition (type of ECM proteins) of ECM changes in diabetes. This matrix serves as a reservoir of growth factors and other signalling proteins. With continued exposure to high levels of glucose, the ECs may accumulate growth factors and other mitogens in the matrix. These accumulated factors may provide continual signaling to the ECs. In fact, ECs exposed to glucose for more than 72 hours have been shown to increase protein levels of VEGF [111]. We have also shown that the mRNA of VEGF is upregulated as early as 24 hours following exposure to high levels of glucose [89]. In addition to providing growth factors itself as a reservoir, the changing matrix may also regulate how ECs perceive and respond to the growth factors [75].

Finally, the ECM may also be modified by glycation. Glycation may decrease the turnover rate of the proteins and thus provide an efficient means of chronic signaling to the vascular ECs. Glucose reacts with proteins *via* Maillard reaction to produce advanced glycation end products (AGEs) [112] (Fig. **1**). AGE products have also been reported to cause NO scavenging [113]. Furthermore, AGE may interact with cell surface receptors (RAGEs) to increase cytokine/growth factor expression [114]. These findings support the notion that ECM is equally if not more important than growth factor alteration and may provide a more sustained signaling environment.

KEY CONCEPTS AND FUTURE DIRECTIONS

The hypothesis that diabetic complications arise as a result of EC dysfunction is increasing being acclaimed. A number of biochemical variables are involved which dictate tailored therapy for the prevention as well as restoration of the EC function in diabetes. Acute effects of hyperglycemia may be solely mediated by metabolic changes (polyol pathway, hexoseamine pathway), vascular tone (vasoactive factors), and oxidative stress. Patented agents targeting some of these altered pathways have shown promise in terms of delaying the progression of the complications. However, the key elements which still require clarification are: a) the factors involved in the late stages of the disease, b) the mechanisms underlying the promotion of blood vessels in some target organs while suppressing the process in other organs, and c) the molecular signature of diabetic complication. Deciphering these key concepts may provide the best therapeutic targets. Towards this aim, studies currently being undertaken will highlight the the precise role of ECM/BM changes (tissue environment), response of accessory cells, vasoactive factors, and oxidative stress in EC biology and diabetic complications. The restoration of the EC function may well become a pre-requisite for therapy development (please see Tables **2** and **3**). A possible avenue, which still requires investigation, may be the use of combinatorial therapy. For example, use of ET receptor antagonists (bosentan), NO donors (molsidomine or other prodrugs), and oxidative stress inhibitors (may comprise of PKC, NADPH oxidase, AGE breakers, and PARP inhibitors) together may provide defense against both early and late phases of the vascular disease. We believe that targeting the EC lining in the target organs would provide the most efficient therapeutic tool for the treatment of chronic diabetic complications.

ACKNOWLEDGEMENTS

The authors acknowledge grant supports from the Canadian Diabetes Association, the Canadian Institutes of Health Research, and the Lawson Health Research Institute.

REFERENCES

[1] International Diabetes Federation (IDF), Diabetes Atlas 3rd ed. Brussels 2006.

[2] Engerman R, Bloodworth JM, Jr., Nelson S. Relationship of microvascular disease in diabetes to metabolic control. Diabetes 1977; 26: 760-769.

[3] Strojek K. Features of macrovascular complications in type 2 diabetic patients. Acta Diabetol 2003; 40 (Suppl 2): S334-337.

[4] The Diabetes Control and Complications Trial Research Group. The effect of intensive treatment of diabetes on the development and progression of long-term complications in insulin-dependent diabetes mellitus. N Engl J Med 1993; 329: 977-986.

[5] United Kingdom Prospective Diabetes Study (UKPDS). 13: Relative efficacy of randomly allocated diet, sulphonylurea, insulin, or metformin in patients with newly diagnosed non-insulin dependent diabetes followed for three years. Br Med J 1995; 310: 83-88.

[6] Florey. The endothelial cell. Br Med J 1966; 5512: 487-490.

[7] Jaffe EA, Nachman RL, Becker CG, Minick CR. Culture of human endothelial cells derived from umbilical veins. Identification by morphologic and immunologic criteria. J Clin Invest 1973; 52: 2745-2756.

[8] Cines DB, Pollak ES, Buck CA, *et al.* Endothelial cells in physiology and in the pathophysiology of vascular disorders. Blood 1998; 91: 3527-3561.

[9] Mandarino LJ, Finlayson J, Hassell JR. High glucose downregulates glucose transport activity in retinal capillary pericytes but not endothelial cells. Invest Ophthalmol Vis Sci 1994; 35: 964-972.

[10] Kaiser N, Sasson S, Feener EP, *et al.* Differential regulation of glucose transport and transporters by glucose in vascular endothelial and smooth muscle cells. Diabetes 1993; 42: 80-89.

[11] Krutzfeldt A, Spahr R, Mertens S, Siegmund B, Piper HM. Metabolism of exogenous substrates by coronary endothelial cells in culture. J Mol Cell Cardiol 1990; 22: 1393-1404.

[12] Nishikawa T, Edelstein D, Du XL, *et al.* Normalizing mitochondrial superoxide production blocks three pathways of hyperglycaemic damage. Nature 2000; 404: 787-790.

[13] Brownlee M. Biochemistry and molecular cell biology of diabetic complications. Nature 2001; 414: 813-820.

[14] Khan ZA, Chakrabarti S. Endothelins in chronic diabetic complications. Can J Physiol Pharmacol 2003; 81: 622-634.

[15] Khan ZA, Chakrabarti S. Therapeutic targeting of endothelial dysfunction in chronic diabetic complications. Recent Pat Cardiovasc Drug Discov 2006; 1: 167-175.

[16] Khan ZA, Farhangkhoee H, Chakrabarti S. Towards newer molecular targets for chronic diabetic complications. Curr Vasc Pharmacol 2006; 4: 45-57.

[17] Baumgartner-Parzer SM, Wagner L, Pettermann M, *et al.* High-glucose--triggered apoptosis in cultured endothelial cells. Diabetes 1995; 44: 1323-1327.

[18] Boeri D, Almus FE, Maiello M, *et al.* Modification of tissue-factor mRNA and protein response to thrombin and interleukin 1 by high glucose in cultured human endothelial cells. Diabetes 1989; 38: 212-218.

[19] Cagliero E, Maiello M, Boeri D, Roy S, Lorenzi M. Increased expression of basement membrane components in human endothelial cells cultured in high glucose. J Clin Invest 1988; 82: 735-738.

[20] Graier WF, Grubenthal I, Dittrich P, Wascher TC, Kostner GM. Intracellular mechanism of high D-glucose-induced modulation of vascular cell proliferation. Eur J Pharmacol 1995; 294: 221-229.

[21] Maiello M, Boeri D, Podesta F, *et al.* Increased expression of tissue plasminogen activator and its inhibitor and reduced fibrinolytic potential of human endothelial cells cultured in elevated glucose. Diabetes 1992; 41: 1009-1015.

[22] McGinn S, Saad S, Poronnik P, Pollock CA. High glucose-mediated effects on endothelial cell proliferation occur via p38 MAP kinase. Am J Physiol Endocrinol Metab 2003; 285: E708-717.

[23] Arcaro G, Cretti A, Balzano S, *et al.* Insulin causes endothelial dysfunction in humans: sites and mechanisms. Circulation 2002; 105: 576-582.

[24] Campia U, Sullivan G, Bryant MB, *et al.* Insulin impairs endothelium-dependent vasodilation independent of insulin sensitivity or lipid profile. Am J Physiol Heart Circ Physiol 2004; 286: H76-82.

[25] Hopfner RL, Hasnadka RV, Wilson TW, McNeill JR, Gopalakrishnan V. Insulin increases endothelin-1-evoked intracellular free calcium responses by increased ET(A) receptor expression in rat aortic smooth muscle cells. Diabetes 1998; 47: 937-944.

[26] De Caterina R. Endothelial dysfunctions: common denominators in vascular disease. Curr Opin Clin Nutr Metab Care 2000; 3: 453-467.

[27] Stehouwer CD, Lambert J, Donker AJ, van Hinsbergh VW. Endothelial dysfunction and pathogenesis of diabetic angiopathy. Cardiovasc Res 1997; 34: 55-68.

[28] Khan ZA, Chakrabarti S. Growth factors in proliferative diabetic retinopathy. Exp Diabes Res 2003; 4: 287-301.

[29] Khan ZA, Farhangkhoee H, Mahon JL, *et al.* Endothelins: regulators of extracellular matrix protein production in diabetes. Exp Biol Med (Maywood) 2006; 231: 1022-1029.

[30] Hibbs RG, Burch GE, Phillips JH. The fine structure of the small blood vessels of normal human dermis and subcutis. Am Heart J 1958; 56: 662-670.

[31] Simionescu M, Simionescu N. The cardiovascular system. In: Weiss L, Greep, R, Eds. Histology. New York: McGraw Hill 1977; pp. 373-431.

[32] Weibel ER, Palade GE. New cytoplasmic components in arterial endothelia. J Cell Biol 1964; 23: 101-112.

[33] Zhu DZ, Cheng CF, Pauli BU. Mediation of lung metastasis of murine melanomas by a lung-specific endothelial cell adhesion molecule. Proc Natl Acad Sci USA 1991; 88: 9568-9572.

[34] Milici AJ, Furie MB, Carley WW. The formation of fenestrations and channels by capillary endothelium *in vitro*. Proc Natl Acad Sci USA 1985; 82: 6181-6185.

[35] Busse R, Fleming I. Endothelial dysfunction in atherosclerosis. J Vasc Res 1996; 33: 181-194.

[36] Vanhoutte PM. Endothelial dysfunction and atherosclerosis. Eur Heart J 1997; 18 (Suppl E): E19-29.

[37] Ross R. The pathogenesis of atherosclerosis: a perspective for the 1990s. Nature 1993; 362: 801-809.

[38] Williams KJ, Tabas I. The response-to-retention hypothesis of early atherogenesis. Arterioscler Thromb Vasc Biol 1995; 15: 551-561.

[39] Williams KJ, Tabas I. The response-to-retention hypothesis of atherogenesis reinforced. Curr Opin Lipidol 1998; 9: 471-474.

[40] Craven PA, DeRubertis FR, Melhem M. Nitric oxide in diabetic nephropathy. Kidney Int Suppl 1997; 60: S46-53.

[41] Kalfa TA, Gerritsen ME, Carlson EC, Binstock AJ, Tsilibary EC. Altered proliferation of retinal microvascular cells on glycated matrix. Invest Ophthalmol Vis Sci 1995; 36: 2358-2367.

[42] Yamagishi S, Fujimori H, Yonekura H, Yamamoto Y, Yamamoto H. Advanced glycation endproducts inhibit prostacyclin production and induce plasminogen activator inhibitor-1 in human microvascular endothelial cells. Diabetologia 1998; 41: 1435-1441.

[43] Johnstone MT, Creager SJ, Scales KM, *et al.* Impaired endothelium-dependent vasodilation in patients with insulin-dependent diabetes mellitus. Circulation 1993; 88: 2510-2516.

[44] McVeigh GE, Brennan GM, Johnston GD, *et al.* Impaired endothelium-dependent and independent vasodilation in patients with type 2 (non-insulin-dependent) diabetes mellitus. Diabetologia 1992; 35: 771-776.

[45] Nitenberg A, Valensi P, Sachs R, *et al.* Impairment of coronary vascular reserve and ACh-induced coronary vasodilation in diabetic patients with angiographically normal coronary arteries and normal left ventricular systolic function. Diabetes 1993; 42: 1017-1025.

[46] Saenz de Tejada I, Goldstein I, Azadzoi K, Krane RJ, Cohen RA. Impaired neurogenic and endothelium-mediated relaxation of penile smooth muscle from diabetic men with impotence. N Engl J Med 1989; 320: 1025-1030.

[47] Steinberg HO, Chaker H, Leaming R, *et al.* Obesity/insulin resistance is associated with endothelial dysfunction. Implications for the syndrome of insulin resistance. J Clin Invest 1996; 97: 2601-2610.

[48] Ting HH, Timimi FK, Boles KS, *et al.* Vitamin C improves endothelium-dependent vasodilation in patients with non-insulin-dependent diabetes mellitus. J Clin Invest 1996; 97: 22-28.

[49] Beckman JA, Goldfine AB, Gordon MB, Garrett LA, Creager MA. Inhibition of protein kinase Cbeta prevents impaired endothelium-dependent vasodilation caused by hyperglycemia in humans. Circ Res 2002; 90: 107-111.

[50] Williams SB, Goldfine AB, Timimi FK, *et al.* Acute hyperglycemia attenuates endothelium-dependent vasodilation in humans *in vivo*. Circulation 1998; 97: 1695-1701.

[51] Yanagisawa M, Kurihara H, Kimura S, *et al.* A novel potent vasoconstrictor peptide produced by vascular endothelial cells. Nature 1988; 332: 411-415.

[52] Inoue A, Yanagisawa M, Kimura S, *et al.* The human endothelin family: three structurally and pharmacologically distinct isopeptides predicted by three separate genes. Proc Natl Acad Sci USA 1989; 86: 2863-2867.

[53] Cardillo C, Campia U, Bryant MB, Panza JA. Increased activity of endogenous endothelin in patients with type II diabetes mellitus. Circulation 2002; 106: 1783-1787.

[54] Ahlborg G, Ottosson-Seeberger A, Hemsen A, Lundberg JM. Big ET-1 infusion in man causes renal ET-1 release, renal and splanchnic vasoconstriction, and increased mean arterial blood pressure. Cardiovasc Res 1994; 28: 1559-1563.

[55] Ahlborg G, Weitzberg E, Lundberg JM. Circulating endothelin-1 reduces splanchnic and renal blood flow and splanchnic glucose production in humans. J Appl Physiol 1995; 79: 141-145.

[56] Pernow J, Kaijser L, Lundberg JM, Ahlborg G. Comparable potent coronary constrictor effects of endothelin-1 and big endothelin-1 in humans. Circulation 1996; 94: 2077-2082.

[57] Deng D, Evans T, Mukherjee K, Downey D, Chakrabarti S. Diabetes-induced vascular dysfunction in the retina: role of endothelins. Diabetologia 1999; 42: 1228-1234.

[58] Ludmer PL, Selwyn AP, Shook TL, *et al.* Paradoxical vasoconstriction induced by acetylcholine in atherosclerotic coronary arteries. N Engl J Med 1986; 315: 1046-1051.

[59] Giugliano D, Marfella R, Coppola L, *et al.* Vascular effects of acute hyperglycemia in humans are reversed by L-arginine. Evidence for reduced availability of nitric oxide during hyperglycemia. Circulation 1997; 95: 1783-1790.

[60] Cukiernik M, Mukherjee S, Downey D, Chakabarti S. Heme oxygenase in the retina in diabetes. Curr Eye Res 2003; 27: 301-308.

[61] Lund DD, Faraci FM, Miller FJ, Jr., Heistad DD. Gene transfer of endothelial nitric oxide synthase improves relaxation of carotid arteries from diabetic rabbits. Circulation 2000; 101: 1027-1033.

[62] Zanetti M, Sato J, Katusic ZS, O'Brien T. Gene transfer of endothelial nitric oxide synthase alters endothelium-dependent relaxations in aortas from diabetic rabbits. Diabetologia 2000; 43: 340-347.

[63] Farhangkhoee H, Khan ZA, Kaur H, *et al.* Vascular endothelial dysfunction in diabetic cardiomyopathy: pathogenesis and potential treatment targets. Pharmacol Ther 2006; 111(2): 384-399.

[64] Kuiper EJ, Van Nieuwenhoven FA, de Smet MD, *et al.* The angio-fibrotic switch of VEGF and CTGF in proliferative diabetic retinopathy. PLoS One 2008; 3: e2675.

[65] Patz A. Clinical and experimental studies on retinal neovascularization. XXXIX Edward Jackson Memorial Lecture. Am J Ophthalmol 1982; 94: 715-743.

[66] Nyengaard JR, Flyvbjerg A, Rasch R. The impact of renal growth, regression and regrowth in experimental diabetes mellitus on number and size of proximal and distal tubular cells in the rat kidney. Diabetologia 1993; 36: 1126-1131.

[67] Chou E, Suzuma I, Way KJ, *et al.* Decreased cardiac expression of vascular endothelial growth factor and its receptors in insulin-resistant and diabetic States: a possible explanation for impaired collateral formation in cardiac tissue. Circulation 2002; 105: 373-379.

[68] Abaci A, Oguzhan A, Kahraman S, *et al.* Effect of diabetes mellitus on formation of coronary collateral vessels. Circulation 1999; 99: 2239-2242.

[69] Waltenberger J. Impaired collateral vessel development in diabetes: potential cellular mechanisms and therapeutic implications. Cardiovasc Res 2001; 49: 554-560.

[70] Weihrauch D, Lohr NL, Mraovic B, *et al.* Chronic hyperglycemia attenuates coronary collateral development and impairs proliferative properties of myocardial interstitial fluid by production of angiostatin. Circulation 2004; 109: 2343-2348.

[71] Arras M, Ito WD, Scholz D, *et al.* Monocyte activation in angiogenesis and collateral growth in the rabbit hindlimb. J Clin Invest 1998; 101: 40-50.

[72] Ito WD, Arras M, Winkler B, *et al.* Monocyte chemotactic protein-1 increases collateral and peripheral conductance after femoral artery occlusion. Circ Res 1997; 80: 829-837.

[73] Waltenberger J, Lange J, Kranz A. Vascular endothelial growth factor-A-induced chemotaxis of monocytes is attenuated in patients with diabetes mellitus: A potential predictor for the individual capacity to develop collaterals. Circulation 2000; 102: 185-190.

[74] Boudreau NJ, Jones PL. Extracellular matrix and integrin signalling: the shape of things to come. Biochem J 1999; 339(Pt 3): 481-488.

[75] Davis GE, Senger DR. Endothelial extracellular matrix: biosynthesis, remodeling, and functions during vascular morphogenesis and neovessel stabilization. Circ Res 2005; 97: 1093-1107.

[76] Addison CL, Nor JE, Zhao H, *et al.* The response of VEGF-stimulated endothelial cells to angiostatic molecules is substrate-dependent. BMC Cell Biol 2005; 6: 38.

[77] Jiang B, Liou GI, Behzadian MA, Caldwell RB. Astrocytes modulate retinal vasculogenesis: effects on fibronectin expression. J Cell Sci 1994; 107(Pt 9): 2499-2508.

[78] Lochter A, Bissell MJ. Involvement of extracellular matrix constituents in breast cancer. Semin Cancer Biol 1995; 6: 165-173.

[79] Noel A, Kebers F, Maquoi E, Foidart JM. Cell-cell and cell-matrix interactions during breast cancer progression. Curr Top Pathol 1999; 93: 183-193.

[80] Nishikawa T, Giardino I, Edelstein D, Brownlee M. Changes in diabetic retinal matrix protein mRNA levels in a common transgenic mouse strain. Curr Eye Res 2000; 21: 581-587.
[81] Ljubimov AV, Burgeson RE, Butkowski RJ, *et al.* Basement membrane abnormalities in human eyes with diabetic retinopathy. J Histochem Cytochem 1996; 44: 1469-1479.
[82] Spirin KS, Saghizadeh M, Lewin SL, *et al.* Basement membrane and growth factor gene expression in normal and diabetic human retinas. Curr Eye Res 1999; 18: 490-499.
[83] Silver MD, Huckell VF, Lorber M. Basement membranes of small cardiac vessels in patients with diabetes and myxoedema: preliminary observations. Pathology 1977; 9: 213-220.
[84] Sternberg M, Cohen-Forterre L, Peyroux J. Connective tissue in diabetes mellitus: biochemical alterations of the intercellular matrix with special reference to proteoglycans, collagens and basement membranes. Diabete Metab 1985; 11: 27-50.
[85] Tsilibary EC. Microvascular basement membranes in diabetes mellitus. J Pathol 2003; 200: 537-546.
[86] Williamson JR, Kilo C. Capillary basement membranes in diabetes. Diabetes 1983; 32(Suppl 2): 96-100.
[87] Fredersdorf S, Thumann C, Ulucan C, *et al.* Myocardial hypertrophy and enhanced left ventricular contractility in Zucker diabetic fatty rats. Cardiovasc Pathol 2004; 13: 11-19.
[88] Khan ZA, Cukiernik M, Gonder JR, Chakrabarti S. Oncofetal fibronectin in diabetic retinopathy. Invest Ophthalmol Vis Sci 2004; 45: 287-295.
[89] Khan ZA, Chan BM, Uniyal S, *et al.* EDB fibronectin and angiogenesis - a novel mechanistic pathway. Angiogenesis 2005; 8: 183-196.
[90] Pankov R, Yamada KM. Fibronectin at a glance. J Cell Sci 2002; 115: 3861-3863.
[91] Grant MB, Caballero S, Bush DM, Spoerri PE. Fibronectin fragments modulate human retinal capillary cell proliferation and migration. Diabetes 1998; 47: 1335-1340.
[92] Wilson SH, Ljubimov AV, Morla AO, *et al.* Fibronectin fragments promote human retinal endothelial cell adhesion and proliferation and ERK activation through alpha5beta1 integrin and PI 3-kinase. Invest Ophthalmol Vis Sci 2003; 44: 1704-1715.
[93] Jugdutt BI. Ventricular remodeling after infarction and the extracellular collagen matrix: when is enough enough? Circulation 2003; 108: 1395-1403.
[94] Weber KT. Cardiac interstitium in health and disease: the fibrillar collagen network. J Am Coll Cardiol 1989; 13: 1637-1652.
[95] Weber KT, Sun Y, Katwa LC, Cleutjens JP. Connective tissue: a metabolic entity? J Mol Cell Cardiol 1995; 27: 107-120.
[96] Weber KT, Sun Y, Tyagi SC, Cleutjens JP. Collagen network of the myocardium: function, structural remodeling and regulatory mechanisms. J Mol Cell Cardiol 1994; 26: 279-292.
[97] Alexander BT, Cockrell KL, Rinewalt AN, Herrington JN, Granger JP. Enhanced renal expression of preproendothelin mRNA during chronic angiotensin II hypertension. Am J Physiol Regul Integr Comp Physiol 2001; 280: R1388-1392.
[98] Bohlender J, Gerbaulet S, Kramer J, *et al.* Synergistic effects of AT(1) and ET(A) receptor blockade in a transgenic, angiotensin II-dependent, rat model. Hypertension 2000; 35: 992-997.
[99] Katwa LC, Guarda E, Weber KT. Endothelin receptors in cultured adult rat cardiac fibroblasts. Cardiovasc Res 1993; 27: 2125-2129.
[100] Guarda E, Katwa LC, Myers PR, Tyagi SC, Weber KT. Effects of endothelins on collagen turnover in cardiac fibroblasts. Cardiovasc Res 1993; 27: 2130-2134.
[101] Harada M, Itoh H, Nakagawa O, *et al.* Significance of ventricular myocytes and nonmyocytes interaction during cardiocyte hypertrophy: evidence for endothelin-1 as a paracrine hypertrophic factor from cardiac nonmyocytes. Circulation 1997; 96: 3737-3744.
[102] Luscher TF, Enseleit F, Pacher R, *et al.* Hemodynamic and neurohumoral effects of selective endothelin A (ET(A)) receptor blockade in chronic heart failure: the heart failure ET(A) receptor blockade trial (HEAT). Circulation 2002; 106: 2666-2672.
[103] Torre-Amione G, Young JB, Colucci WS, *et al.* Hemodynamic and clinical effects of tezosentan, an intravenous dual endothelin receptor antagonist, in patients hospitalized for acute decompensated heart failure. J Am Coll Cardiol 2003; 42: 140-147.
[104] Kalra PR, Moon JC, Coats AJ. Do results of the ENABLE (Endothelin Antagonist Bosentan for Lowering Cardiac Events in Heart Failure) study spell the end for non-selective endothelin antagonism in heart failure? Int J Cardiol 2002; 85: 195-197.
[105] Kumagai AK, Glasgow BJ, Pardridge WM. GLUT1 glucose transporter expression in the diabetic and nondiabetic human eye. Invest Ophthalmol Vis Sci 1994; 35: 2887-2894.
[106] Engerman RL, Kern TS. Progression of incipient diabetic retinopathy during good glycemic control. Diabetes 1987; 36: 808-812.
[107] Reddy MA, Villeneuve LM, Wang M, Lanting L, Natarajan R. Role of the lysine-specific demethylase 1 in the proinflammatory phenotype of vascular smooth muscle cells of diabetic mice. Circ Res 2008; 103: 615-623.

[108] Villeneuve LM, Reddy MA, Lanting LL, *et al.* Epigenetic histone H3 lysine 9 methylation in metabolic memory and inflammatory phenotype of vascular smooth muscle cells in diabetes. Proc Natl Acad Sci USA 2008; 105: 9047-9052.

[109] Brasacchio D, Okabe J, Tikellis C, *et al.* Hyperglycemia induces a dynamic cooperativity of histone methylase and demethylase enzymes associated with gene-activating epigenetic marks that coexist on the lysine tail. Diabetes 2009; 58: 1229-1236.

[110] El-Osta A, Brasacchio D, Yao D, *et al.* Transient high glucose causes persistent epigenetic changes and altered gene expression during subsequent normoglycemia. J Exp Med 2008; 205: 2409-2417.

[111] Hsu CC, Yin MC, Tian R. Ascorbic acid and uric acid suppress glucose-induced fibronectin and vascular endothelial growth factor production in human endothelial cells. J Diabetes Complications 2005; 19: 96-100.

[112] John WG, Lamb EJ. The Maillard or browning reaction in diabetes. Eye 1993; 7(Pt 2): 230-237.

[113] Bucala R, Tracey KJ, Cerami A. Advanced glycosylation products quench nitric oxide and mediate defective endothelium-dependent vasodilatation in experimental diabetes. J Clin Invest 1991; 87: 432-438.

[114] Thornalley PJ. Cell activation by glycated proteins. AGE receptors, receptor recognition factors and functional classification of AGEs. Cell Mol Biol (Noisy-le-grand) 1998; 44: 1013-1023.

[115] Harris, E.E.; Patchett, A.A.; Tristram, E.W.; Wyvratt, M.J.: US4374829 **(1983).**

[116] Hoefle, M.L.; Klutchko, S.: US4344949 **(1982).**

[117] Gold, E.H.; Neustadt, B.R.; Smith, E.M.: US4587258 **(1986).**

[118] Vincent, M.; Remond, G.; Laubie, M.: US4508729 **(1985).**

[119] Petrillo, E.W.J.: US4337201 **(1982).**

[120] Watthey, J.W.H.: US4410520 **(1983).**

[121] Lebwohl, D.E.: US6573285 **(2003).**

[122] Whittle, B.A.: US20050042172 **(2005).**

[123] Yorio, T.; Prasanna, G.; Dibas, A.; Stokely, M.E.: US20030176356 **(2003).**

[124] Lawrence III, J.l.; Donahue, J.K.: US6855701 **(2005).**

[125] Keefer, L.K.; Dunams, T.M.; Saavedra, J.E.: US5366997 **(1994).**

[126] Keefer, L.K., Hrabie, J.A.: US5155137 **(1992).**

[127] Saavedra, J.E.; Keefer, L.K.; Roller, P.P.; Akamatsu, M.: US6379660 **(2002).**

[128] Ito, A.; Hamanaka, W.; Takagi, H.; Wada, T.; Kawada, K.: US3064000 **(1962).**

[129] Ulrich, P.; Vasan, S.; Wagle, D.R.; Fang, S.-D.; Rho, T.; Egan, J.J.; Cerami, A.: US6790859 **(2004).**

[130] Mylari, B.L.: US6849629 **(2005).**

[131] Johnson, D.K.; Holland, J.A.: US5902831 **(1999).**

[132] Karanewsky, D.S.; Valentino, K.L.; Ternansky, R.J.: US5990137 **(1999).**

[133] Kun, E.; Mendeleyev, J.; Rice, W.G.: WO9307868A1 **(1993).**

[134] Li, J.H.; Tays, K.L.; Zhang, J.: WO9911624A1 **(1999).**

[135] Li, J.-H.; Zhang, J.; Jackson, P.F.; Maclin, K.M.: WO9911645A1 **(1999).**

[136] Jackson, P.F.; Li, J.-H.; Maclin, K.M.; Zhang, J.: WO0026192A1 **(1999).**

[137] Griffin, R.J.; Calvert, A.H.; Curtin, N.J.; Newell, D.R.; Golding, B.T.: WO9704771A1 **(1997).**

[138] Lubisch, W.; Kock, M.; Hoger, T.: WO0026192A1 **(2000).**

[139] Martin, N.M.B.; Smith, G.C.M.; White, C.R.; Newton, R.F.; Douglas, D.G.; Eversley, P.J.; Vile, J.: WO0236576A1 **(2002).**

[140] Szabo, C.; Jagtap, P.; Southan, G.; Salzman, A.L.: WO0142219A3 and WO0142219A2 **(2001).**

Oxidative Stress in Cardiovascular Disease: A New Avenue Toward Future Therapeutic Approaches

Reiko Inagi*

Division of Nephrology and Endocrinology, University of Tokyo, School of Medicine, Hongo, Bunkyo-ku, Tokyo 113-8655, Japan

Abstract: Oxidative stress is a common denominator in many aspects of the pathogenesis of atherosclerosis and cardiovascular diseases. Some drugs, such as vitamin C, vitamin E, and a free radical scavenger, edaravone, are prescribed with oxidative stress as their main target. Furthermore, the drugs in current clinical use, such as anti-hypertension reagents including angiotensin-converting enzyme (ACE) inhibitors and angiotensin receptor blockers (ARB), and anti-hyperlipidemic reagents like statins, protect various organs, e.g., vessel, brain, heart, and kidney, via anti-oxidative stress effects in addition to their original pharmacological properties. While results of clinical trials of anti-oxidative stress reagents in patients with cardiovascular disease are contradictory to date, this may be explained by a variety of reasons such as an inadequate study design. More competent anti-oxidative reagents are awaited, and superoxide dismutase mimetics, thiols, xanthine oxidase and NAD(P)H oxidase inhibitors, which regulate intracellular redox reaction and subsequently inhibit oxidative stress, are among promising candidates of future drug developments currently receiving much interest. In this review, the current advances will be highlighted in development of novel anti-oxidative therapeutic approaches against cardiovascular diseases.

Keywords: Angiotensin-converting enzyme (ACE) inhibitor, angiotensin receptor blocker (ARB), diabetes mellitus, endothelium, hypertension, ischemic heart disease, kidney failure, NAD(P)H oxidase, nitric oxide (NO), reactive oxygen species (ROS), redox, reduced glutathione (GSH), superoxide dismutase (SOD), thiol, xanthine oxidase.

INTRODUCTION

"Oxidative stress" is a condition with the presence of free radicals or radical-generating agents that overwhelm natural radical-blocking or radical-scavenging mechanisms. Oxidative stress can cause oxidative damage to DNA, proteins, and lipids, leading to various kinds of tissue injury. An increasing body of evidence suggests that oxidative stress is involved in the pathogenesis and progression of a wide range of cardiovascular diseases, including atherosclerosis, hypertension, type II diabetes, and hypercholesterolemia.

Vascular endothelial cells play a major role in oxidative stress of cardiovascular diseases by producing large amounts of reactive oxygen species (ROS). ROS include various molecules such as the superoxide anion (O_2^-), H_2O_2, the hydroxyl radical and a range of

*Corresponding author: E-mail: inagi-npr@umin.ac.jp

Atta-ur-Rahman / M. Iqbal Choudhary (Eds.)

lipid radicals. O_2^- is the key molecule among these, as many other ROS are formed as a consequence of reactions involving O_2^-. O_2^- and other radicals may react with nitric oxide (NO) causing nitrosative stress and endothelial dysfunction. The reaction of O_2^- with NO leads to production of peroxynitrite. Peroxynitrite per se is also a potent oxidant which can induce oxidation of proteins, lipids and DNA. In addition, ROS can stimulate vascular smooth muscle cell hypertrophy and hyperplasia, or initiate development of a vascular proinflammatory state *via* a variety of mechanisms. This pro-inflammatory state may be promoted *via* activation of redox-sensitive transcription factors, such as nuclear factor-kappaB (NF-κB) and leukocyte adhesion molecule, vascular cell adhesion molecule-1 (VCAM-1), by reduction in levels of NO or by angiotensin II (Ang-II)-dependent pathways.

The principle sources of ROS in the vasculature include NAD(P)H oxidase, xanthine oxidase, uncoupled endothelial nitric oxide synthase (eNOS), and the mitochondrial respiratory chain.

NAD(P)H oxidase is a membrane-bound enzyme complex and represents a major source of O_2^- in the vasculature [1, 2]. It is composed of electron transfer groups (gp91phox, nox1 or nox4), p22phox, and regulatory subunits (p47phox, p67phox, and rac1). In quiescent cells, NAD(P)H oxidase exists in an unassembled state. A number of pro-atherogenic stimuli, including low-density lipoprotein (LDL) and Ang-II, activate NAD(P)H oxidase by translocating p47phox and p67phox to the membrane and converting the oxidase into an assembled form.

Xanthine oxidase is an iron sulfur molybdenum flavo-protein with multiple functions. Xanthine oxidase is present in high concentrations in endothelial cells and serves as a source of ROS. It generates extracellular superoxide and peroxide moieties and metabolizes hypoxanthine, xanthine, and NADH to form O_2^- and H_2O_2. The role of xanthine oxidase in the cellular production of O_2^- is well established in the setting of ischemia reperfusion [3].

Because excessive ROS is extremely noxious, host cells are endowed with a number of scavenging systems to limit ROS levels. O_2^- may be dismutated by a family of SODs (superoxide dismutases) to H_2O_2. While MnSOD (SOD2) is located in the mitochondria, two isoforms of Cu/ZnSOD are located either intracellularly (SOD1) or extracellularly (ECSOD, SOD3). H_2O_2 can be scavenged to water by catalase (CAT) or by glutathione peroxidase (GPx) in the presence of reduced glutathione (GSH).

As discussed below, a multitude of studies in experimental animals, together with clinical data, suggest that oxidative stress is a common denominator in many aspects of the pathogenesis and progression of atherosclerosis and cardio-vascular diseases and serves as a promising target of therapeutic approaches [4, 5].

OXIDATIVE STRESS IN VARIOUS CARDIOVASCU-LAR DISEASES

Hypertension

Endothelial dysfunction and the accompanying increase in vascular ROS is observed in most rat models of hypertension. Treatment with anti-oxidants and SOD mimetics attenuates endothelial dysfunction and lowered blood pressure in a number of hypertension models, suggesting that increased ROS production is pathogenic. Furthermore, an increase in oxidative stress by GSH depletion can cause hypertension [6]. In the hypertensive rat, eNOS and NAD(P)H oxidase were identified as the principle sources of O_2^- [7-9]. Microarray gene expression analysis of SHRSP (spontaneously hypertensive stroke-prone) and Wistar Kyoto (WKY) rats identified glutathione S-transferase (GSTM1) as a candidate gene for hypertension [10].

Elevation of oxidative stress by-products as well as a decrease in anti-oxidant systems have been demonstrated in hypertensive human subjects [11-14]. Moreover, many of the adverse effects of hypertension on endothelial function may be reversed by intra-arterial infusion of anti-oxidants, such as vitamin C [15, 16].

Diabetes

Diabetes and insulin resistance can greatly increase the risk of cardiovascular disease. Many previous studies focused on the role of advanced glycation end-products (AGEs) in diabetes-related vascular complications. Wagle *et al.* filed a patent of the compositions comprising agents for inhibiting the formation of and reversing the pre-formed AGEs and breaking the subsequent cross-links [17]. Certain of the agents useful in the present invention are members of the class of compounds known as thiazoles, others are imidazoles or oxazoles. These compounds react with an early glycosylation product thereby preventing formation of the later AGEs that lead to cross-links, and thereby, to molecular or protein aging and other adverse molecular consequences. Additionally, they react with already formed AGEs to reduce the amount of such products.

Oxidative stress is also one of the main metabolic abnormalities causing microvascular complications such as retinopathy, nephropathy, and neuropathy in this disorder [18]. Increased oxidant production is a result of abnormal metabolism of glucose, free fatty acids, and other reactive metabolites in both insulin-deficient and insulin-resistant states [19-22]. Many biochemical pathways associated with hyperglycemia (glucose auto-oxidation, polyol pathway, prostanoid synthesis, and protein glycation) can increase the production of free radicals [23, 24]. Furthermore, exposure of endothelial cells to high glucose leads to augmented production of O_2^- [25, 26]. Mechanisms of increased O_2^- production in vascular tissue include uncoupling of eNOS and increased NAD(P)H oxidase activity [27, 28]. Levels of MnSOD are also decreased in streptozotocin diabetic rats [29]. Levels of O_2^- are also increased in hyperinsulinemic rats, which is believed to be related to activation of NAD(P)H oxidase [30].

Measurement of the lipid peroxide level and activities of antioxidant enzymes in aorta, heart and blood of streptozotocin-induced diabetic rats indicated that oxidative stress starts at an early stage of diabetes mellitus and increases progressively [31]. We recently established a novel model of mouse diabetic nephropathy which develops nodule-like glomerular lesions [32]. These mice were also associated with increased oxidative stress by-products. To support this notion, we demonstrated accumulation of carbonyl derivatives of proteins (protein carbonyl) as a biomarker of oxidative protein damage in human diabetic arteriosclerotic tissues [33]. Reduced antioxidant activity and increased oxidative stress occur early after the diagnosis of diabetes in human patients [34].

A role for ROS in the endothelial dysfunction associated with diabetes was proposed in the early 1990s [35]. Normalizing mitochondrial O_2^- has been shown to block pathways involved in hyperglycemic damage [36], and treatment with SOD improved vasodilation in isolated aortic rings from streptozotocin-induced diabetic rats [37]. Many of the adverse effects of high glucose on endothelial function, such as reduced endothelial-dependent relaxation and delayed cell replication, were also reversed by anti-oxidants in human diabetic patients [38, 39].

Hypercholesterolemia

Hypercholesterolemia increases endothelial O_2^- production and vascular oxidative stress, which may in turn contribute to endothelial damage and atherogenesis [26]. WHHL (Watanabe heritable hyperlipidemic) rabbits also show an increase in O2- levels [40].

Multiple mechanisms are involved in O2- production observed in hypercholesterolemia, including eNOS-, xanthine-oxidase- and NAD(P)H-oxidase-dependent mechanisms [41-43]. Endothelial cells, smooth muscle cells, neutrophils and monocytes all can oxidatively modify LDL to generate lipid peroxidation products and ROS. Subsequently, oxidized LDLs may recruit monocytes and favor their transformation into foam cells through a receptor-mediated intake (scavenger pathway). Moreover, oxidized LDLs show cytotoxic potential which is probably responsible for endothelial cell damage and macrophage degeneration in the atherosclerotic human plaque.

Increased levels of O2- generation and attenuated NO mediated responses were demonstrated in aortic rings from cholesterol-fed rabbits [44, 45]. Treatment of the animals with polyethylene glycolated SODs improved endothelium-dependent vasodilation [46, 47]. Supplementation with L-arginine has also been shown to reduce O_2^- levels and restore NO-mediated responses in cholesterol-fed animals [48].

An increase of oxidative stress in human hypercholesterolemic patients was also demonstrated [49].

Heart Failure

Heart failure is a state characterized by a number of processes that may promote ROS generation *in vivo*. These pro-oxidant pathways include cytokine activation, mitochondrial dysfunction, recurrent hypoxia reperfusion, and activation of the renin-angiotensin system. It has recently been shown that patients with heart failure may have increased leukocyte O_2^- production, which is related to severity of disease [50]. Increased activity of myocardial NAD(P)H oxidase has also been reported in heart failure [51].

In animal models of heart failure, levels of ROS are elevated and cardiac protection is observed with antioxidant treatment. The increase in ROS associated with left ventricular hypertrophy appears to be NAD(P)H oxidase-dependent. Myocardial NAD(P)H oxidase activity is elevated and expression of p22phox, gp91phox, p67phox and p47phox is increased in left ventricular tissue from guinea-pigs after aortic banding [52]. The gp91phox containing NAD(P)H oxidase has been shown to play an important role in the cardiac hypertrophic response to Ang II in mice [53]. Increased production of ROS, decreased endothelium-dependent relaxation and NO bio-availability have also been observed in the vasculature of rats after myocardial infarction [54, 55].

Studies by McMurray *et al.* confirmed that ROS activity was increased in plasma of patients with heart failure secondary to coronary artery disease, compared with controls [56]. Plasma malondialdehyde, a marker of lipid peroxidation, is elevated in these patients [57] and is related to exercise intolerance [58]. In other studies, increased concentrations of malondialdehyde and decreased concentrations of GSH, vitamins C and E were correlated with both NYHA (New York Heart Association) functional class [59]. Lower levels of EC-SOD have also been reported in subjects with coronary artery disease [60].

PHARMACOLOGICAL APPROACHES TO LOWER OXIDATIVE STRESS

Natural antioxidants are divided into three major categories of molecules.

1) Antioxidant proteins that reduce the hydroxyl radical production by binding metal ions.

2) Intracellular antioxidant enzymes responsible for the trapping of free radicals produced in situ, as by-products of cellular metabolism. Superoxide dismutase, catalase and GPx belong to this group.

3) Extracellular antioxidant substances such as alpha-tocopherol, β-carotene, vitamin C and others. These molecules protect lipoproteins from oxidative modification in the extracellular fluid.

Beyond these natural antioxidants, there are also a large number of pharmaceutical antioxidant agents.

While many *in vitro* and animal studies suggest a beneficial effect of antioxidants in preventing cardiovascular morbidity and mortality, results of large-scale clinical human trials have been controversial. This discrepancy can be explained by several reasons. We do not have a sensitive and accurate test for oxidative burden. Therefore, a target population of antioxidant therapy may be inadequate, and there may be a subset of patients who would be in a "more oxidized state" and thus show greater improvement with antioxidant therapy. Lack of a good estimation of oxidative stress also makes it difficult to interpret outcomes of the trials because we do not know whether the anti-oxidative therapy really reduced oxidative stress in the patients. Recently Kinkade Jr. *et al.* filed a patent of methods of detecting and quantifying biomarkers of oxidative stress in proteins [61]. The biomarker in this invention may be any amino acid that has undergone oxidation (or other modification, e.g., chloro-tyrosine, dityrosine) with emphasis on oxidized sulfur- or selenium-containing amino acids. The biomarker of oxidative stress in proteins may be detected with an antibody that binds to oxidized amino acids, specifically oxidized sulfur- or selenium-containing amino acids.

By all means, it is necessary to develop an appropriate methodology to evaluate oxidative stress in human subjects as well as a powerful antioxidant for the treatment of cardiovascular diseases.

NAD(P)H Oxidase Inhibition

Recently several pharmacological and molecular approaches to directly target the NAD(P)H oxidase enzyme have been proposed. Apocynin, a methoxysubstituted catechol, has been used by Peruvian Indians as an anti-inflammatory agent. It acts by blocking the assembly of p47phox into the membrane complex [62]. Apocynin decreases O_2^- production in rat and human vascular rings, increases NO production in cultured human endothelial cells, and improves endothelial function *ex vivo* in rats and humans [63]. Administration *in vivo* of apocynin to deoxycorticosteroneacetate-salt hypertensive rats decreased both vascular O_2^- production and blood pressure [64]. Although apocynin appears to be an effective NAD(P)H oxidase inhibitor in vascular tissue from both rats and man, it needs to be present in relatively high concentrations to be effective.

Rey *et al.* have also considered disruption of the active NAD(P)H oxidase complex as a means of reducing oxidative stress [65]. They used a chimeric peptide (gp91ds-tat) designed to cross cell membranes and then inhibit p47phox association with gp91phox. Infusion of this peptide into mice significantly inhibited hypertension and vascular O_2^- production induced by Ang-II.

Another recently developed compound, S17834, a benzo(b)pyran-4-one, has been shown to inhibit NAD(P)H oxidase activity, O_2^- production and attenuate atherosclerotic lesions in apolipoprotein-E deficient mice [66]. However, its exact mechanism of action remains to be elucidated.

Several studies have suggested 3-hydroxy-3-methylglu-taryl-CoA reductase inhibitors (statins) have NAD(P)H oxidase inhibition. Both O_2^- and H_2O_2 production by vascular tissue and leucocytes are inhibited by simvastatin in Ang-II-infused rats [67]. Prevention of O_2^- production by statins may be linked to prenylation-dependent Rac translocation and NAD(P)H oxidase inhibition [68].

Free Radical Scavenger

Edaravone (3-methyl-1-phenyl-2-pyrazolin-5-one, MCI-186), a synthetic antioxidant, is a ubiquitously acting direct free radical scavenger. Edaravone showed inhibitory effects on both water-soluble and lipid-soluble peroxyl radical-induced peroxidation systems, which are different from the inhibitory effects of vitamins C and E in each system, respectively.

Many experimental studies demonstrated beneficial effects of edaravone in situations associated with oxidative stress. Edaravone has been clinically prescribed in Japan since 2001 to treat patients with cerebral ischemia. For more details about edaravone, readers are recommended to read the recent review by Higashi and colleagues [69].

Inhibition of the Renin-Angiotensin System

Ang-II has been shown to be a potent stimulation of NAD(P)H oxidase activity in vascular smooth muscle, fibroblasts and endothelial cells and cardiomyocytes [26, 70-73]. Thus it is not surprising that angiotensin-converting enzyme (ACE) inhibition and Ang-II-receptor blocker (ARB) may play a key role in reducing levels of oxidative stress. Furthermore, we recently found that ACE inhibitors and ARB also reduce oxidative stress by chelating transition metals and inhibiting various oxidative steps, including carbon-centered and hydroxyl radicals [74, 75].

The Heart Outcomes Prevention Evaluation (HOPE) Study suggested that some of the beneficial effects of ACE inhibitors are independent of their effect on blood pressure [76]. One of the important mechanisms for this is inhibition of the renin-angiotensin system as an anti-oxidant strategy. Consistent with this hypothesis, ACE inhibition has been shown to improve endothelial function in patients with coronary artery disease [77]. Additionally ARBs have been shown to be antioxidant and vasoprotective in patients with coronary artery disease, again downregulating vascular NAD(P)H oxidase expression [78]. Treatment with either an ACE inhibitor or an ARB resulted in lower levels of vascular O_2^- [79].

Wolf applied a patent of a method for treating a subject having oxidative stress with inhibitors of the renin-angiotensin system or statins [80].

Vitamins and Dietary Anti-Oxidants

Epidemiological studies suggested that a greater intake of anti-oxidant vitamins, such as vitamin E, vitamin C and beta carotene, are associated with a reduced risk of cardiovascular disease [81-83]. Experimental studies utilizing animal models also supported this hypothesis

[84-86]. The primary component of vitamin E, alpha-tocopherol, has been proposed as the most prevalent antioxidant in protecting LDL [87]. Vitamin E has been shown to decrease LDL oxidation [88, 89] and to improve endothelial function [90, 91]. The WHO/MONICA Study provided some of the first supportive evidence for the role of vitamin E in coronary artery disease, suggesting that an individual's vitamin E plasma concentration may be indicative of ischemic heart disease mortality [92]. Similarly vitamin C administration has been shown to improve endothelium-dependent vasodilation [16, 93, 94]. Long-term treatment of apolipoprotein-E-deficient mice with vitamin C resulted in a decrease in levels of 7,8-dihydrobiopterin (BH2), an oxidized form of BH4.

Despite strong evidence demonstrating anti-oxidant effects of vitamins C and E in these studies, prospective randomized clinical trials have produced contrasting results. While the Cambridge Heart Anti-oxidant Study [95] and the Anti-oxidant Supplementation in Atherosclerosis Prevention Study [96] reported benefit by anti-oxidant therapy, Gruppo Italiano per lo Studio della Sopravvivenza nell'Infarto miocardico [97], the Heart Outcomes Prevention Evaluation [76], the Heart Protection Study [98] and the Primary Prevention Project [99] failed to show positive results. Data from these trials have been elegantly summarized in an editorial by Jialal and Devaray [88]. Numerous explanations have been proposed for the lack of observed benefit in the majority of randomized trials. They include oxidant stress status of the participants and dose and combination of vitamins administered.

Petrus filed a patent of compositions for the treatment and prevention of endothelial dysfunction consisting of a non-steroidal anti-inflammatory drug (NSAID), such as acetylsalicylic acid, in combination with dietary supplements [100]. An amino sugar, such as glucosamine, is incorporated to enhance the glucoaminoglycan defense of the gastrointestinal tract, anti-inflammatory properties, and synergistic effect with NSAIDs. The compositions of dietary supplements included a variety of anti-oxidants such as alpha-lipoic acid, viamin C, vitamin E, and coenzyme Q10.

A patent of a delivery system for oral delivery of the antioxidants vitamin C and vitamin E was also filed [101]. Early studies showed that if vitamin E is mixed into the sustained release vitamin C matrix, vitamin E is not absorbed very well. This method allows a slow release of vitamin C and a plain release of vitamin E, enabling us to obtain high concentrations and a controlled ratio between vitamin C and vitamin E in blood plasma. The system of the invention provides a ratio of concentrations between vitamin C and vitamin E in the blood plasma from 1:5 to 5:1, preferably from 1:1 to 3:1. The amount of vitamin C is preferably higher than that of vitamin E, with the most preferred ratio of 2.2:1.

Alpha-tocopherol and γ-tocopherol differ structurally only by a methyl group substitution at the 5-position. They both are redox agents which act under certain circumstances as antioxidants. Wechter filed a patent of the therapeutic benefit of administering γ-tocopherol and its derivatives such as LLU-α [102]. LLU-α is the compound 6-hydroxy-2,7,8-trimethylchroman-2-propanoic acid, and its molecular formula of $C_{15}H_{20}O_4$. LLU-α may be in the racemic form or as the S enatiomer (also denoted as (S)-LLU-α). LLU-α is capable of increasing sodium excretion in the urine in mammals without a corresponding increase in potassium excretion, and does not cause a significant change in mean arterial pressure. The compound additionally acts as a cardio-selective free radical scavenger.

Pratt and colleagues applied a patent of compounds such as 5-pyrimidinol and 3-pyridinol derivatives [103, 104]. They act as effective chain breaking antioxidants in an analogous fashion to the natural vitamins E and C. Their synthesis precludes that they may be prepared easily as either of the lipid- or water-soluble variety. Furthermore, compounds of the invention are stable to air oxidation and may be significantly more reactive toward peroxyl radicals than the most potent form of vitamin E.

Lockwood *et al.* applied a patent of a method to administer an effective amount of a synthetic analog or derivative of a carotenoid as an antioxidant therapy [105]. The gap junction channel, and connexin 43 in particular, plays an important role in maintaining cardiac electrical stability. As connexin 43 is induced by carotenoids, the administration of water soluble analogs or derivatives of carotenoids to a subject may ameliorate cardiovascular diseases associated with cardiac arrhythmia, assisting in the maintenance of electrical stability in cardiac tissue. The composition of an injectable structural carotenoid analog or derivative of astaxanthin may be particularly useful in the therapeutic methods of this invention. Astaxanthin, as a xanthophyll carotenoid, is highly lipid soluble in natural form with a small size (597 Da). Therefore, an injectable astaxanthin structural analog or derivative has a low likelihood of immunogenecity, and is a particularly desirable compound for the current therapeutic indication.

Other antioxidants included in natural diet include polyphenol, anthrocyanin, bioflavonoid, proanthocyanidin, and xanthone. Koffas *et al.* applied a patent of methods and compositions for production of flavonoids in microbial hosts [106]. This invention provides compositions and methods for the production of flavonoids in a non-plant host cell by introducing a set of heterologous genes encoding for the enzymes required for conversion of the particular substrate to the desired flavonoid.

L-Arginine

Numerous studies in both experimental animals and man have shown acute and chronic administration of L-arginine improves vascular function in cardiovascular disease [48, 107, 108]. The availability of L-arginine for reaction with eNOS should not be rate limiting, as intracellular levels of L-arginine are in the millimolar range, whereas the Km for the substrate is in the micromolar range. This apparent discrepancy is frequently referred to as the L-arginine paradox. Explanations for this paradox include decreased O_2^- production, decreased transport of arginine into endothelial cells, increased levels of asymmetric dimethylarginine and increased insulin release [109]. Most recently it has been suggested that translational control of NOS expression by arginine can explain the arginine paradox, at least for iNOS (inducible NOS) [110].

Nitroxides and nitrones are stabilized forms of the biological messenger nitric oxide. They also have some unique properties, e.g., unlike other antioxidants, they generally neither act as proxidants, nor do they propagate free radical chain reactions. These agents also inhibit the reaction of superoxide and nitric oxide to produce peroxinitrite. Wang *et al.* applied a patent of novel *N*-methyl-D-aspartate (NMDA)-receptor antagonists with antioxidant properties, nitrone adamantane derivatives and nitroxide adamantane derivatives, as therapeutic agents [111]. Nitrone and nitroxides are cell permeable and stable free radicals. Nitrone reacts with free radicals to form nitroxide, which acts as superoxide dismutase and stimulates the catalase-like activity of hemeproteins, resulting in protection of cells from free radical mediated damage. Nitroxide has one additional advantage over other antioxidants. Its concentration remains the same before and after the reaction because it acts as a catalyst.

Tucker *et al.* applied a patent of nitric oxide donating derivatives for the treatment of cardiovascular disorder [112]. Compounds provided by the invention include analogues of resveratrol, other stilbenes, other polyphenols, and flavonoids, with attached moieties that are capable of releasing nitric oxide when administered to a patient. These novel compounds have the ability to donate nitric oxide concomitant and co-localized with the release of a free radical scavenging antioxidant molecule. These compounds simultaneously have the capability to induce the expression of apolipoprotein A1 (apoAl) and thereby increase the blood levels of HDL and lower blood levels of cholesterol. The combined multivariate effects of these compounds may be used to decrease endothelial dysfunction, decrease vascular oxidative stress and decrease hyperlipidemia, and thereby treat cardiovascular disorders such as atherosclerosis, hypertension, coronary artery disease, and cerebrovascular disease.

Thiol-Containing Compounds

Over the years a number of thiol-containing compounds have been used experimentally to inhibit LDL oxidation and reduce oxidative stress. In glucose-fed rats alpha-lipoic acid attenuated hypertension, insulin resistance and oxidative stress [113], and in another study was shown to lower blood pressure in spontaneously hypertensive rats [114]. In the man, the classical sulphydryl compound N-acetylcysteine reduced cardiovascular events in patients with end-stage renal failure [115].

Recently, a great deal of attention has been given to possible antioxidant functions for α-lipoic acid, and its reduced form, dihydrolipoic acid (DHLA). Lipoate, or its reduced form, DHLA, reacts with reactive oxygen species and protects membranes by interacting with vitamin C and GSH, which may in turn recycle vitamin E. α-Lipoic acid administration has been shown to be beneficial in a number of oxidative stress models such as ischemia-reperfussion injury. Byrd applied a patent of an oral formulation of an inositol compound and α-lipoic acid [116]. The α-Lipoic acid and the inositol compound are combined with excipient materials in such a way that those materials provide for an immediate release of a first portion of the active ingredients from the formulation followed by a gradual release of any remaining active ingredients. The formulation of the invention can be used treat a variety of complications of diabetics including macrovascular disease, diabetic neuropathy, and diabetic nephropathy.

Mimetics and Stimulators of Anti-Oxidative Enzymes

Endogenous O_2^- is dismutated to H_2O_2 by a family of SODs. A number of SOD mimetics are available that cross the membrane and decrease oxidative stress with improvement of endothelial function [117, 118].

Schauss *et al.* applied a patent of invention related to the identification of compositions of trunk tissue of palm trees, e.g., the African Oil Palm (*E. guineensis*), as having high oxygen radical absorbarce capacity scores and SOD-like activity [119]. According to this invention, the palm trunk, juice, dietary supplements, and other compositions derived from the palm tree can be used to treat, reverse, and/or protect against the deleterious effects of free radicals and oxidative stress.

Selenium (as selenocysteine) is an essential component of the active sites of the antioxidant enzyme, GPx. Majeed *et al.* issued patents of compositions and methods containing bioavailable Se-methyl-L-selenocysteine, promoting antioxidative activity of the enzyme [120]. The bioavailability is enhanced by the addition of black pepper extract.

Myhill *et al.* applied patents of compositions and methods for enhancing the activity of antioxidant enzymes which include, e.g., SOD, CAT, and GPX, and thereby decreasing the tissue level of pathologic free radical species [121, 122]. An antioxidant-promoting composition comprises Bacopa monniera extract; milk thistle extract, ashwagandha powder, green tea extract, Gotu kola powder, *Ginko biloba* leaf extract; *Aloe vera* powder; turmeric extract; and N-acetyl cysteine.

Oiry *et al.* also filed patents of novel compounds possessing anti-oxidant activity in the preparation of medicaments intended to increase the intracellular and/or extracellular level of GSH [123, 124].

Xanthine Oxidase Inhibition

Cardillo *et al.* reported that the xanthine oxidase inhibitor oxypurinol improved endothelial function in hypercholesterolemia [125]. Another xanthine oxidase inhibitor allopurinol has also been shown to improve endothelial function in type II diabetes, chronic heart failure, and cigarette smokers [126-128].

Coenzyme Q10 (Co Q10)

CoQ10 is a fat-soluble quinone that is structurally similar to vitamin K and commonly known as ubiquinone. CoQ10 is essential for the production of cellular energy. Furthermore, CoQ10 is an endogenous antioxidant found in most living organisms. Studies utilizing rats showed a reductive shift in plasma aminothiol status and a decrease in skeletal muscle mitochondrial protein carbonyls after 13 weeks of supplementation [129]. CoQ10 supplementation improved endothelial function of conduit arteries of the peripheral circulation in dyslipidaemic patients with type II diabetes *via* increased endothelial release and/or activity of NO due to improvement in vascular oxidative stress [130]. The limited data from well-designed trials of CoQ10 in patients with heart failure indicated that there may be some benefits with CoQ10 therapy in ejection fraction and end diastolic volume [131].

Fantuzzi and colleagues discovered that CoQ10 and an amino acid such as carnitine can be readily dissolved in varying concentrations in a monoterpene, and recently applied a patent of solubilized CoQ10 [132]. Use of monoterpenes as dissolving agents greatly increased the ability to incorporate greater amounts of bioactive CoQ10 in formulations, such as soft gel capsules, thereby providing increased bioavailability in delivery.

CURRENT & FUTURE DEVELOPMENTS

The clinical importance of antioxidant vitamin supplementation has not necessarily been confirmed by large controlled trials. To the practicing physician, the benefits of ACE inhibition and ARB have been clearly described and the elucidation that, in part, some of the benefit may be derived from optimizing the oxidant milieu leads to the pursuit of other drugs or indeed molecular therapies that act in the same way. The promise of the SOD mimetics, xanthine oxidase inhibitors, and NAD(P)H oxidase inhibitors may soon provide clinicians with additional therapeutic options in the treatment of cardiovascular disease which will lower oxidative stress.

Recently, accumulating evidence demonstrates that oxidative stress links to hypoxia and endoplasmic reticulum (ER) stress. Hypoxia contributes to progression of not only cardiovascular disease but also various diseases as a common pathogenesis [133-136]. ER stress, which represents the ER dysfunction such as loss of protein folding ability resulting in malfolded protein accumulation in the ER, is induced by various stimuli including oxidative stress [137, 138]. Therefore, its pathogenesis has received a lot of attention in recent years. Hypoxia and ER stress induce important cellular responses, the hypoxia inducible factor (HIF) pathway and the unfolded protein response (UPR), respectively. Activation of these pathways basically protect the cell from oxidative stress. On the other hand, overwhelming oxidative stress suppresses HIF activation and induces apoptotic but not adaptive UPR, thereby causing vicious cycle of an increase in oxidative stress and disease progression.

From the viewpoint of the crosstalk of oxidative stress, hypoxia, and ER stress, it is emphasized that enhancement of the HIF pathway and/or the adaptive UPR might be the potential benefits of reducing oxidative stress *via* breaking the vicious cycle of these pathogenic environments. In fact, recent reports demonstrated that the chemical compounds, which activate HIF and induce the expression of target genes that adapt the cells to hypoxia, ameliorated cardiovascular damages [139, 140]. Similarly, the chemical compounds, which activate adaptive UPR by enhancing the unfolded-protein refolding and translation shut down, showed the organ protective effects against oxidative stress-related diseases including ischemia/reperfusion injury, diabetes mellitus, and atherosclerosis as well as kidney diseases [137,138, 141-145]. Further investigation will open up interesting possibility for potent and beneficial therapeutic approaches targeting hypoxia and/or ER stress in oxidative stress-related damages including cardiovascular diseases.

REFERENCES

[1] Mohazzab KM, Wolin MS. Sites of superoxide anion production detected by lucigenin in calf pulmonary artery smooth muscle. Am J Physiol 1994; 267(6 Pt 1): L815-22.

[2] Pagano PJ, Ito Y, Tornheim K, Gallop PM, Tauber AI, Cohen RA. An NADPH oxidase superoxide-generating system in the rabbit aorta. Am J Physiol 1995; 268(6 Pt 2): H2274-80.

[3] McCord JM. Oxygen-derived free radicals in postischemic tissue injury. N Engl J Med 1985; 312(3): 159-163. Review.

[4] Stocker R, Keaney JF Jr. Role of oxidative modifications in atherosclerosis. Physiol Rev 2004; 84(4): 1381-1478. Review.

[5] Hamilton CA, Miller WH, Al-Benna S, *et al.* Strategies to reduce oxidative stress in cardiovascular disease. Clin Sci (Lond) 2004; 106(3): 219-234. Review.

[6] Vaziri ND, Wang XQ, Oveisi F, Rad B. Induction of oxidative stress by glutathione depletion causes severe hypertension in normal rats. Hypertension 2000; 36(1): 142-146.

[7] Kerr S, Brosnan MJ, McIntyre M, Reid JL, Dominiczak AF, Hamilton CA. Superoxide anion production is increased in a model of genetic hypertension: role of the endothelium. Hypertension 1999; 33(6): 1353-1358.

[8] Hamilton CA, Brosnan MJ, McIntyre M, Graham D, Dominiczak AF. Superoxide excess in hypertension and aging: a common cause of endothelialdysfunction. Hypertension 2001; 37(2 Part 2): 529-534.

[9] Zalba G, San Jose G, Moreno MU, *et al.* Oxidative stress in arterial hypertension: role of NAD(P)H oxidase. Hypertension 2001; 38(6): 1395-1399.

[10] McBride MW, Carr FJ, Graham D, *et al.* Microarray analysis of rat chromosome 2 congenic strains. Hypertension 2003; 41(3 Pt 2): 847-853.

[11] Orie NN, Zidek W, Tepel M, Reactive oxygen species in essential hypertension and non-insulin-dependent diabetes mellitus. Am J Hypertens 1999; 12: 1169-1174.

[12] Koska J, Syrova D, Blazicek P, Marko M, Grna JD, Kvetnansky R, Vigas M. Malondialdehyde, lipofuscin and activity of antioxidant enzymes during physical exercise in patients with essential hypertension. J Hypertens 1999; 17: 529-535.

[13] Yasunari K, Maeda K, Nakamura M, Yoshikawa J. Oxidative stress in leukocytes is a possible link between blood pressure, blood glucose, and C-reacting protein. Hypertension 2002; 39: 777-780.

[14] Redon J, Oliva MR, Tormos C, Giner V, Chaves J, Iradi A, Saez GT. Antioxidant activities and oxidative stress byproducts in human hypertension. Hypertension 2003; 41: 1096-1101.

[15] Solzbach U, H.B., Jeserich M, Just H. Vitamin C improves endothelial dysfunction of epicardial coronary arteries in hypertensive patients. Circulation 1997; 96: 1513-1519.

[16] Taddei S, Virdis A, Ghiadoni L, Magagna A, Salvetti A. Vitamin C improves endothelium-dependent vasodilation by restoring nitric oxide activity in essential hypertension. Circulation 1998; 97(22): 2222-2229.
[17] Wagle, D., Vasan, S., Egan, J.: US20056960605 **(2005)**.
[18] Inagi R, Nangaku M, Miyata T. Synergistic contributions of carbonyl stress and megsin in diabetic nephropathy. Ann N Y Acad Sci 2005; 1043: 605-608. Review.
[19] Giugliano D, Ceriello A, Paolisso G. Oxidative stress and diabetic vascular complications. Diabetes Care 1996; 19(3): 257-267. Review.
[20] Evans JL, Goldfine ID, Maddux BA, Grodsky GM. Are oxidative stress-activated signaling pathways mediators of insulin resistance and beta-cell dysfunction? Diabetes 2003; 52(1): 1-8. Review.
[21] Boden G, Shulman GI. Free fatty acids in obesity and type 2 diabetes: defining their role in the development of insulin resistance and beta-cell dysfunction. Eur J Clin Invest 2002; 32(Suppl 3): 14-23. Review.
[22] Itani SI, Ruderman NB, Schmieder F, Boden G. Lipid-induced insulin resistance in human muscle is associated with changes in diacylglycerol, protein kinase C, and IkappaB-alpha. Diabetes 2002; 51(7): 2005-2011.
[23] Abou-Seif MA, Youssef AA. Oxidative stress and male IGF-1, gonadotropin and related hormones in diabetic patients. Clin Chem Lab Med 2001; 39(7): 618-623.
[24] Ruiz C, Alegria A, Barbera R, Farre R, Lagarda MJ. Lipid peroxidation and antioxidant enzyme activities in patients with type 1 diabetes mellitus. Scand J Clin Lab Invest 1999; 59(2): 99-105.
[25] Christ M, Bauersachs J, Liebetrau C, Heck M, Gunther A, Wehling M. Glucose increases endothelial-dependent superoxide formation in coronary arteries by NAD(P)H oxidase activation: attenuation by the 3-hydroxy-3-methylglutaryl coenzyme A reductase inhibitor atorvastatin. Diabetes 2002; 51(8): 2648-2652.
[26] Guzik TJ, West NE, Black E, *et al.* Vascular superoxide production by NAD(P)H oxidase: association with endothelial dysfunction and clinical risk factors. Circ Res 2000; 86(9): E85-90.
[27] Hink U, Tsilimingas N, Wendt M, Munzel T. Mechanisms underlying endothelial dysfunction in diabetes mellitus: therapeutic implications. Treat Endocrinol 2003; 2(5): 293-304. Review.
[28] Kim YK, Lee MS, Son SM, *et al.* Vascular NADH oxidase is involved in impaired endothelium-dependent vasodilation in OLETF rats, a model of type 2 diabetes. Diabetes 2002; 51(2): 522-527.
[29] Kamata K, Kobayashi T. Changes in superoxide dismutase mRNA expression by streptozotocin-induced diabetes. Br J Pharmacol 1996; 119(3): 583-589.
[30] Kashiwagi A, Shinozaki K, Nishio Y, *et al.* Endothelium-specific activation of NAD(P)H oxidase in aortas of exogenously hyperinsulinemic rats. Am J Physiol 1999; 277(6 Pt 1): E976-83.
[31] Kakkar R, Mantha SV, Kalra J, Prasad K. Time course study of oxidative stress in aorta and heart of diabetic rat. Clin Sci (Lond) 1996; 91(4): 441-448.
[32] Inagi R, Yamamoto Y, Nangaku M, *et al.* A Severe Diabetic Nephropathy Model With Early Development of Nodule-Like Lesions Induced by Megsin Overexpression in RAGE/iNOS Transgenic Mice. Diabetes 2006; 55(2): 356-366.
[33] Horie K, Miyata T, Maeda K, *et al.* Immunohistochemical colocalization of glycoxidation products and lipid peroxidation products in diabetic renal glomerular lesions. Implication for glycoxidative stress in the pathogenesis of diabetic nephropathy. J Clin Invest 1997; 100(12): 2995-3004.
[34] Marra G, Cotroneo P, Pitocco D, *et al.* Early increase of oxidative stress and reduced antioxidant defenses in patients with uncomplicated type 1 diabetes: a case for gender difference. Diabetes Care 2002; 25(2): 370-375.
[35] Langenstroer P, Pieper GM. Regulation of spontaneous EDRF release in diabetic rat aorta by oxygen free radicals. Am J Physiol. 1992; 263(1 Pt 2): H257-65.
[36] Nishikawa T, Edelstein D, Du XL, *et al.* Normalizing mitochondrial superoxide production blocks three pathways of hyperglycaemic damage. Nature 2000; 404(6779): 787-790.
[37] Hattori Y, Kawasaki H, Abe K, Kanno M. Superoxide dismutase recovers altered endothelium-dependent relaxation in diabetic rat aorta. Am J Physiol 1991; 261(4 Pt 2): H1086-94.
[38] Ting HH, Timmi, F., Boles KS, Creager SJ, Ganz P, Creager MA. Vitamin C improves endothelium-dependent vasodilation in patients with non-insulin-dependent diabetes mellitus. J Clin Invest 1996; 97: p. 22-28.
[39] Ting HH, Timimi FK, Haley EA, Roddy MA, Ganz P, Creager MA. Vitamin C improves endothelium-dependent vasodilation in patients with insulin-dependent diabetes mellitus. J Am Coll Cardiol 1998; 31(3): 552-557.
[40] Miller FJ Jr., Gutterman DD, Rios CD, Heistad DD, Davidson BL. Superoxide production in vascular smooth muscle contributes to oxidative stress and impaired relaxation in atherosclerosis. Circ Res 1998; 82(12): 1298-1305.

[41] Stepp DW, Ou J, Ackerman AW, Welak S, Klick D, Pritchard KA Jr. Native LDL and minimally oxidized LDL differentially regulate superoxide anion in vascular endothelium in situ. Am J Physiol Heart Circ Physiol 2002; 283(2): H750-9.

[42] Warnholtz A, Nickenig G, Schulz E, *et al.* Increased NADH-oxidase-mediated superoxide production in the early stages of atherosclerosis: evidence for involvement of the renin-angiotensin system. Circulation 1999; 99(15): 2027-2033

[43] Hathaway CA, Heistad DD, Piegors DJ, Miller FJ Jr. Regression of atherosclerosis in monkeys reduces vascular superoxide levels. Circ Res 2002; 90(3): 277-283.

[44] Ohara Y, Peterson TE, Harrison DG. Hypercholesterolemia increases endothelial superoxide anion production. J Clin Invest 1993; 91(6): 2546-2551.

[45] Mugge A, Brandes RP, Boger RH, *et al.* Vascular release of superoxide radicals is enhanced in hypercholesterolemic rabbits. J Cardiovasc Pharmacol 1994; 24(6): 994-998.

[46] Mugge A, Elwell JH, Peterson TE, Hofmeyer TG, Heistad DD, Harrison DG. Chronic treatment with polyethylene-glycolated superoxide dismutase partially restores endothelium-dependent vascular relaxations in cholesterol-fed rabbits. Circ Res 1991; 69(5): 1293-1300.

[47] White CR, Brock TA, Chang LY, *et al.* Superoxide and peroxynitrite in atherosclerosis. Proc Natl Acad Sci USA 1994; 91(3): 1044-1048.

[48] Boger RH, Bode-Boger SM, Mugge A, *et al.* Supplementation of hypercholesterolaemic rabbits with L-arginine reduces the vascular release of superoxide anions and restores NO production. Atherosclerosis 1995; 117(2): 273-284.

[49] Nourooz-Zadeh J, Smith CC, Betteridge DJ. Measures of oxidative stress in heterozygous familial hypercholesterolaemia. Atherosclerosis 2001; 156(2): 435-441.

[50] Ellis GR, Anderson RA, Lang D, *et al.* Neutrophil superoxide anion-generating capacity, endothelial function and oxidative stress in chronic heart failure: effects of short- and long-term vitamin C therapy. J Am Coll Cardiol 2000; 36(5): 1474-1482.

[51] Heymes C, Bendall JK, Ratajczak P, *et al.* Increased myocardial NADPH oxidase activity in human heart failure. J Am Coll Cardiol 2003; 41(12): 2164-2171.

[52] Li JM, Gall NP, Grieve DJ, Chen M, Shah AM. Activation of NADPH oxidase during progression of cardiac hypertrophy to failure. Hypertension 2002; 40(4): 477-484.

[53] Bendall JK, Cave AC, Heymes C, Gall N, Shah AM. Pivotal role of a gp91(phox)-containing NADPH oxidase in angiotensin II-induced cardiac hypertrophy in mice. Circulation 2002; 105(3): 293-296.

[54] Wiemer G, Itter G, Malinski T, Linz W. Decreased nitric oxide availability in normotensive and hypertensive rats with failing hearts after myocardial infarction. Hypertension 2001; 38(6): 1367-1371.

[55] Bauersachs J, Bouloumie A, Fraccarollo D, Hu K, Busse R, Ertl G. Endothelial dysfunction in chronic myocardial infarction despite increased vascular endothelial nitric oxide synthase and soluble guanylate cyclase expression: role of enhanced vascular superoxide production. Circulation 1999; 100(3): 292-298.

[56] McMurray J, Chopra M, Abdullah I, Smith WE, Dargie HJ. Evidence of oxidative stress in chronic heart failure in humans. Eur Heart J 1993; 14(11): 1493-1498.

[57] Diaz-Velez CR, Garcia-Castineiras S, Mendoza-Ramos E, Hernandez-Lopez E. Increased malondialdehyde in peripheral blood of patients with congestive heart failure. Am Heart J 1996; 131(1): 146-152.

[58] Nishiyama Y, Ikeda H, Haramaki N, Yoshida N, Imaizumi T. Oxidative stress is related to exercise intolerance in patients with heart failure. Am Heart J 1998; 135(1): 115-120.

[59] Keith M, Geranmayegan A, Sole MJ, *et al.* Increased oxidative stress in patients with congestive heart failure. J Am Coll Cardiol 1998; 31(6): 1352-1356.

[60] Landmesser U, Merten R, Spiekermann S, Buttner K, Drexler H, Hornig B. Vascular extracellular superoxide dismutase activity in patients with coronary artery disease: relation to endothelium-dependent vasodilation. Circulation 2000; 101(19): 2264-2270.

[61] Kinkade Jr., J.M., Shapira, R., Jensen, P.E., Le, N-A., Pohl, J., Brown, W.V.: US20056953666 **(2005)**.

[62] Meyer JW, Holland JA, Ziegler LM, Chang MM, Beebe G, Schmitt ME. Identification of a functional leukocyte-type NADPH oxidase in human endothelial cells: a potential atherogenic source of reactive oxygen species. Endothelium 1999; 7(1): 11-22.

[63] Hamilton CA, Brosnan MJ, Al-Benna S, Berg G, Dominiczak AF. NAD(P)H oxidase inhibition improves endothelial function in rat and human blood vessels. Hypertension 2002; 40(5): 755-762.

[64] Beswick RA, Dorrance AM, Leite R, Webb RC. NADH/NADPH oxidase and enhanced superoxide production in the mineralocorticoid hypertensive rat. Hypertension 2001; 38(5): 1107-1111.

[65] Rey FE, Cifuentes ME, Kiarash A, Quinn MT, Pagano PJ. Novel competitive inhibitor of NAD(P)H oxidase assembly attenuates vascular O(2)(-) and systolic blood pressure in mice. Circ Res 2001; 89(5): 408-414.

[66] Cayatte AJ, Rupin A, Oliver-Krasinski J, *et al.* S17834, a new inhibitor of cell adhesion and atherosclerosis that targets nadph oxidase. Arterioscler Thromb Vasc Biol 2001; 21(10): 1577-1584.

[67] Delbosc S, Cristol JP, Descomps B, Mimran A, Jover B. Simvastatin prevents angiotensin II-induced cardiac alteration and oxidative stress. Hypertension 2002; 40(2): 142-147.

[68] Wassmann S, Laufs U, Baumer AT, *et al.* Inhibition of geranylgeranylation reduces angiotensin II-mediated free radical production in vascular smooth muscle cells: involvement of angiotensin AT1 receptor expression and Rac1 GTPase. Mol Pharmacol 2001; 59(3): 646-654.

[69] Higashi Y, Jitsuiki D, Chayama K, Yoshizumi M. Edaravone (3-Methyl-1-Phenyl-2-Pyrazolin-5-one), A novel free radical scavenger, for treatment of cardiovascular diseases. Recent Patents on Cardiovascular Drug Discovery 2006; 1: 85-93.

[70] Laursen JB, Rajagopalan S, Galis Z, Tarpey M, Freeman BA, Harrison DG. Role of superoxide in angiotensin II-induced but not catecholamine-induced hypertension. Circulation 1997; 95(3): 588-593.

[71] Cifuentes ME, Rey FE, Carretero OA, Pagano PJ. Upregulation of p67(phox) and gp91(phox) in aortas from angiotensin II-infused mice. Am J Physiol Heart Circ Physiol 2000; 279(5): H2234-40.

[72] Wang HD, Xu S, Johns DG, *et al.* Role of NADPH oxidase in the vascular hypertrophic and oxidative stress response to angiotensin II in mice. Circ Res 2001; 88(9): 947-953.

[73] Berry C, Hamilton CA, Brosnan MJ, *et al.* Investigation into the sources of superoxide in human blood vessels: angiotensin II increases superoxide production in human internal mammary arteries. Circulation 2000; 101(18): 2206-2212.

[74] Miyata T, van Ypersele de Strihou C, Ueda Y, *et al.* Angiotensin II receptor antagonists and angiotensin-converting enzyme inhibitors lower *in vitro* the formation of advanced glycation end products: biochemical mechanisms. J Am Soc Nephrol 2002; 13(10): 2478-2487.

[75] Izuhara Y, Nangaku M, Inagi R, *et al.* Renoprotective properties of angiotensin receptor blockers beyond blood pressure lowering. J Am Soc Nephrol 2005; 16(12): 3631-3641.

[76] Yusuf S, Sleight P, Pogue J, Bosch J, Davies R, Dagenais G. Effects of an angiotensin-converting-enzyme inhibitor, ramipril, on cardiovascular events in high-risk patients. The Heart Outcomes Prevention Evaluation Study Investigators. N Engl J Med 2000; 342(3): 145-153.

[77] Mancini GB, Henry GC, Macaya C, *et al.* Angiotensin-converting enzyme inhibition with quinapril improves endothelial vasomotor dysfunction in patients with coronary artery disease. The TREND (Trial on Reversing ENdothelial Dysfunction) Study. Circulation 1996; 94(3): 258-265.

[78] Rueckschloss U, Quinn MT, Holtz J, Morawietz H. Dose-dependent regulation of NAD(P)H oxidase expression by angiotensin II in human endothelial cells: protective effect of angiotensin II type 1 receptor blockade in patients with coronary artery disease. Arterioscler Thromb Vasc Biol 2002; 22(11): 1845-1851.

[79] Berry C, Anderson N, Kirk AJ, Dominiczak AF, McMurray JJ. Renin angiotensin system inhibition is associated with reduced free radical concentrations in arteries of patients with coronary heart disease. Heart 2001; 86(2): 217-220.

[80] Wolf, G.: US20050065184 **(2005)**.

[81] Rimm EB, Stampfer MJ. Antioxidants for vascular disease. Med Clin North Am 2000; 84(1): 239-249. Review.

[82] Stampfer MJ, Hennekens CH, Manson JE, Colditz GA, Rosner B, Willett WC. Vitamin E consumption and the risk of coronary disease in women. N Engl J Med 1993; 328(20): 1444-1449.

[83] Rimm EB, Stampfer MJ, Ascherio A, Giovannucci E, Colditz GA, Willett WC. Vitamin E consumption and the risk of coronary heart disease in men. N Engl J Med 1993; 328(20): 1450-1456.

[84] Crawford RS, Kirk EA, Rosenfeld ME, LeBoeuf RC, Chait A. Dietary antioxidants inhibit development of fatty streak lesions in the LDL receptor-deficient mouse. Arterioscler Thromb Vasc Biol 1998; 18(9): 1506-1513.

[85] Davidge ST, Ojimba J, McLaughlin MK. Vascular function in the vitamin E-deprived rat: an interaction between nitric oxide and superoxide anions. Hypertension 1998; 31(3): 830-835.

[86] Terasawa Y, Ladha Z, Leonard SW, *et al.* Increased atherosclerosis in hyperlipidemic mice deficient in alpha –tocopherol transfer protein and vitamin E. Proc Natl Acad Sci USA 2000; 97(25): 13830-13834.

[87] Spencer AP, Carson DS, Crouch MA. Vitamin E and coronary artery disease. Arch Intern Med 1999; 159(12): 1313-1320. Review.

[88] Jialal I, Devaraj S. Antioxidants and atherosclerosis: don't throw out the baby with the bath water. Circulation 2003; 107(7): 926-928.

[89] Gotoh N, Noguchi N, Tsuchiya J, *et al.* Inhibition of oxidation of low density lipoprotein by vitamin E and related compounds. Free Radic Res 1996; 24(2): 123-134.

[90] Green D, O'Driscoll G, Rankin JM, Maiorana AJ, Taylor RR. Beneficial effect of vitamin E administration on nitric oxide function in subjects with hypercholesterolaemia. Clin Sci (Lond) 1998; 95(3): 361-367.

[91] Heitzer T, Yla Herttuala S, Wild E, Luoma J, Drexler H. Effect of vitamin E on endothelial vasodilator function in patients with hypercholesterolemia, chronic smoking or both. J Am Coll Cardiol 1999; 33(2): 499-505.

[92] Gey KF, Puska P, Jordan P, Moser UK. Inverse correlation between plasma vitamin E and mortality from ischemic heart disease in cross-cultural epidemiology. Am J Clin Nutr 1991; 53(Suppl 1): 326S-334S.

[93] Hornig B, Arakawa N, Kohler C, Drexler H. Vitamin C improves endothelial function of conduit arteries in patients with chronic heart failure. Circulation 1998; 97(4): 363-368.

[94] Gokce N, Keaney JF Jr, Frei B, *et al.* Long-term ascorbic acid administration reverses endothelial vasomotor dysfunction in patients with coronary artery disease. Circulation 1999; 99(25): 3234-3240.

[95] Stephens NG, Parsons A, Schofield PM, Kelly F, Cheeseman K, Mitchinson MJ. Randomised controlled trial of vitamin E in patients with coronary disease: Cambridge Heart Antioxidant Study (CHAOS) Lancet 1996; 347(9004): 781-786.

[96] Salonen RM, Nyyssonen K, Kaikkonen J, *et al.* Antioxidant Supplementation in Atherosclerosis Prevention Study. Six-year effect of combined vitamin C and E supplementation on atherosclerotic progression: the Antioxidant Supplementation in Atherosclerosis Prevention (ASAP) Study. Circulation 2003; 107(7): 947-953.

[97] GISSI-Prevenzione Investigators (Gruppo Italiano per lo Studio della Sopravvivenza nell'Infarto miocardico) Dietary supplementation with n-3 polyunsaturated fatty acids and vitamin E after myocardial infarction: results of the GISSI-Prevenzione trial. Lancet 1999; 354(9177): 447-455.

[98] Heart Protection Study Collaborative Group. MRC/BHF Heart Protection Study of antioxidant vitamin supplementation in 20,536 high-risk individuals: a randomised placebo-controlled trial. Lancet 2002; 360(9326): 23-33.

[99] de Gaetano G, Collaborative Group of the Primary Prevention Project. Low-dose aspirin and vitamin E in people at cardiovascular risk: a randomized trial in general practice. Collaborative Group of the Primary Prevention Project. Lancet 2001; 357(9250): 89-95.

[100] Petrus, E.J.: US20056930099 (**2005**).

[101] H.o slashed.jgaard, B., Poulsen, H.E., Salonen, J.: US20046805880 (**2004**).

[102] Wechter, W.J.: US20056908943 (**2005**).

[103] Pratt, D.A., Valgimigli, L., DiLabio, G.A.: US20046835216 (**2004**).

[104] Pratt, D.A., Valgimigli, L., DiLabio, G.A.: US20050065174 (**2005**).

[105] Lockwood, S.F., O'Malley, S., Watumull, D.G., Hix, L.M., Jackson, H., Nadolski, G.: US20050143475 (**2005**).

[106] Koffas, M., Leonard, E., Yan, Y., Chemler, J.: US20060019334 (**2006**).

[107] Clarkson P, Adams MR, Powe AJ, *et al.* Oral L-arginine improves endothelium-dependent dilation in hypercholesterolemic young adults. J Clin Invest 1996; 97(8): 1989-1994.

[108] Tousoulis D, Davies G, Tentolouris C, Crake T, Toutouzas P. Coronary stenosis dilatation induced by L-arginine. Lancet 1997; 349(9068): 1812-1813.

[109] Loscalzo J. What we know and don't know about L-arginine and NO. Circulation 2000; 101(18): 2126-2129.

[110] Lee J, Ryu H, Ferrante RJ, Morris SM Jr., Ratan RR. Translational control of inducible nitric oxide synthase expression by arginine can explain the arginine paradox. Proc Natl Acad Sci USA 2003; 100(8): 4843-4848.

[111] Wang, Y., Larrick, J.W.: US20040186320 (**2004**).

[112] Tucker, J., McCaffrey, D., Wong, N.C.W.: US20050080024 (**2005**).

[113] El Midaoui A, de Champlain J. Prevention of hypertension, insulin resistance, and oxidative stress by alpha-lipoic acid. Hypertension 2002; 39(2): 303-307.

[114] Vasdev S, Ford CA, Parai S, Longerich L, Gadag V. Dietary alpha-lipoic acid supplementation lowers blood pressure in spontaneously hypertensive rats. J Hypertens 2000; 18(5): 567-573.

[115] Tepel M, van der Giet M, Statz M, Jankowski J, Zidek W. The antioxidant acetylcysteine reduces cardiovascular events in patients with end-stage renal failure: a randomized, controlled trial. Circulation 2003; 107(7): 992-995.

[116] Byrd, E.A.: US20060024367 (**2006**).

[117] Fontana L, McNeill KL, Ritter JM, Chowienczyk PJ. Effects of vitamin C and of a cell permeable superoxide dismutase mimetic on acute lipoprotein induced endothelial dysfunction in rabbit aortic rings. Br J Pharmacol 1999; 126(3): 730-734.

[118] Nakazono K, Watanabe N, Matsuno K, Sasaki J, Sato T, Inoue M. Does superoxide underlie the pathogenesis of hypertension? Proc Natl Acad Sci USA 1991; 88(22): 10045-10048.

[119] Schauss, A., Fong Kin Voon; W.: US20060024390 (**2006**).

[120] Majeed, M., Ananthanarayanan, N., Kalyanam, N., Rajendran, R., George, S., Prakash, S.: US20066982273 (**2006**).

[121] Myhill, P.R., Driscoll, W.J.: US20060008544 (**2006**).

[122] Myhill, P.R., Driscoll, W.J.: US20060008543 (**2006**).

[123] Oiry, J., Puy, J.-Y., Imbach, J.-L., Clayette, P., Fretier, P.: US20066989372 (**2006**).

[124] Oiry, J., Puy, J.-Y., Imbach, J.-L., Clayette, P., Fretier, P.: US20056979747 (**2005**).

[125] Cardillo C, Kilcoyne CM, Cannon RO 3rd, Quyyumi AA, Panza JA. Xanthine oxidase inhibition with oxypurinol improves endothelial vasodilator function in hypercholesterolemic but not in hypertensive patients. Hypertension 1997; 30(1 Pt 1): 57-63.

[126] Butler R, Morris AD, Belch JJ, Hill A, Struthers AD. Allopurinol normalizes endothelial dysfunction in type 2 diabetics with mild hypertension. Hypertension 2000; 35(3): 746-751.

[127] Farquharson CA, Butler R, Hill A, Belch JJ, Struthers AD. Allopurinol improves endothelial dysfunction in chronic heart failure. Circulation 2002; 106(2): 221-226.

[128] Guthikonda S, Sinkey C, Barenz T, Haynes WG. Xanthine oxidase inhibition reverses endothelial dysfunction in heavy smokers. Circulation 2003; 107(3): 416-421.

[129] Kwong LK, Kamzalov S, Rebrin I, *et al.* Effects of coenzyme Q(10) administration on its tissue concentrations, mitochondrial oxidant generation, and oxidative stress in the rat. Free Radic Biol Med 2002; 33(5): 627-638.

[130] Watts GF, Playford DA, Croft KD, Ward NC, Mori TA, Burke V. Coenzyme Q(10) improves endothelial dysfunction of the brachial artery in Type II diabetes mellitus. Diabetologia 2002; 45(3): 420-426.

[131] Weant KA, Smith KM. The role of coenzyme Q10 in heart failure. Ann Pharmacother 2005; 39(9): 1522-1526.

[132] Fantuzzi, M., Udell, R.G.: US20050079164 (**2005**).

[133] Nangaku M, Inagi R, Miyata T, Fujita T. Hypoxia and hypoxia-inducible factor in renal disease. Nephron Exp Nephrol 2008; 110(1): e1-7. Review.

[134] Hirota SA, Beck PL, MacDonald JA. Targeting hypoxia-inducible factor-1 (HIF-1) signaling in therapeutics: implications for the treatment of inflammatory bowel disease. Recent Pat Inflamm Allergy Drug Discov 2009; 3(1): 1-16.

[135] Muz B, Khan MN, Kiriakidis S, Paleolog EM. Hypoxia. The role of hypoxia and HIF-dependent signalling events in rheumatoid arthritis. Arthritis Res Ther 2009; 11(1): 201.

[136] Crawford TN, Alfaro DV 3rd, Kerrison JB, Jablon EP. Diabetic retinopathy and angiogenesis. Curr Diabetes Rev 2009; 5(1): 8-13.

[137] Kim I, Xu W, Reed JC. Cell death and endoplasmic reticulum stress: disease relevance and therapeutic opportunities. Nat Rev Drug Discov 2008; 7(12): 1013-1030.

[138] Inagi R. Endoplasmic reticulum stress in the kidney as a novel mediator of kidney injury. Nephron Exp Nephrol 2009; 112(1): e1-9. Review.

[139] Eckle T, Köhler D, Lehmann R, El Kasmi K, Eltzschig HK. Hypoxia-inducible factor-1 is central to cardioprotection: a new paradigm for ischemic preconditioning. Circulation. 2008; 118(2): 166-175.

[140] Raphael J, Zuo Z, Abedat S, Beeri R, Gozal Y. Isoflurane preconditioning decreases myocardial infarction in rabbits via up-regulation of hypoxia inducible factor 1 that is mediated by mammalian target of rapamycin. Anesthesiology 2008; 108(3): 415-425.

[141] Zhang K, Kaufman RJ. The unfolded protein response: A stress signaling pathway critical for health and disease. Neurology 2006; 66: S102-109.

[142] Oyadomari S, Mori M. Roles of CHOP/GADD153 in endoplasmic reticulum stress. Cell Death Differ 2004; 11: 381-389.

[143] Xu C, Bailly-Maitre B, Reed JC. Endoplasmic reticulum stress: Cell life and death decisions. J Clin Invest 2005; 115: 2656-2664.

[144] Ogawa S, Kitao Y, Hori O. Ischemia-induced neuronal cell death and stress response. Antioxid Redox Signal 2007; 9: 573-587.

[145] Inagi R, Kumagai T, Nishi H, Kawakami T, Miyata T, Fujita T, Nangaku M. Preconditioning with endoplasmic reticulum stress ameliorates mesangioproliferative glomerulonephritis. J Am Soc Nephrol 2008; 19: 915-922.

The Clinical Impact of Hyperphosphatemia in Chronic Kidney Disease Patients: The Role of Lanthanum Carbonate

Mario Cozzolino* and Diego Brancaccio

Renal Division, S. Paolo Hospital, University of Milan, Italy

Abstract: Vascular calcification is a very common event in patients affected by diabetes and chronic kidney disease (CKD). Recently, it has been well documented that abnormalities in mineral and bone metabolism in CKD patients associate with increased morbidity and mortality. Elevated serum phosphate and calcium-phosphate product levels play an important role in the pathogenesis of vascular mineralization in uremic patients and also appear to be associated with increased cardiovascular mortality. Together with classical passive precipitation of calcium-phosphate in soft tissues, during the last decade it has been demonstrated that inorganic phosphate may cause extraskeletal calcification directly through a real "ossification" of the tunica media in the vasculature of CKD patients. Therefore, control of phosphate retention is now an even more crucial target of treatment in patients affected by chronic kidney disease. The "classical" treatment of secondary hyperparathyroidism and hyperphosphatemia in CKD patients consists of either calcium or aluminium based phosphate-binders and calcitriol administration. Unfortunately, this "old generation" therapy is not free of complications. Lanthanum carbonate represents a novel phosphate binder used for the treatment of hyperphosphataemia in patients with renal failure. This new calcium- and aluminium-free phosphate binder can be used to treat hyperphosphatemia and secondary hyperparathyroidism, reduce atherosclerotic process, and prevent vascular calcification in CKD.

Keywords: Phosphate-binders, lanthanum carbonate, vascular calcification, secondary hyperparathyroidism, dialysis.

INTRODUCTION

Accelerated atherosclerosis and vascular calcifications play a key role in the pathogenesis of cardiovascular disease in chronic kidney disease (CKD) patients [1, 2]. In fact, these patients develop extensive medial calcification, which causes increased arterial stiffness and high morbidity and mortality due to cardiovascular events [3]. Calcification of soft tissues and blood vessel walls occurs frequently in dialyzed patients compared to the non-uremic population [4-6]. Mineral metabolism disorders and increased serum calcium-phosphate product, have been recently investigated as inducing factors on cardiovascular calcification. In fact, cardiovascular disease in renal failure appears greatly associated to

*Corresponding author: Tel: 02/81844723; Fax: 02/89129989; E-mail: mariocozzolino@hotmail.com

bone metabolism alterations [7, 8]. Recent *in vitro* evidence showed that vascular smooth muscle cells calcify in a high phosphate medium [9]. In addition, low levels of two inhibitory proteins, such as fetuin-A and MGP, seems to play an important role in calcium-phosphate deposition in extra-skeletal tissues.

In addition to these classic alterations in bone and mineral metabolism, an active process has been documented [9]. Enhanced serum phosphate levels have been recently investigated as inducing factors on extra-skeletal calcification in uremic population. In particular, elevated blood levels of phosphate are associated with ectopic calcifications and increased risk of calciphylaxis [10-12]. *in vitro* Studies demonstrated that human aortic smooth muscle cells calcify when incubated in a high phosphate medium, where calcium and calcitriol are not changed [13].

In the last decade, several studies defined calcification of atherosclerotic lesions as an active process similar to bone formation. Furthermore, vascular calcification was shown to involve not only a passive calcium-phosphate deposition on atherosclerotic vessels but also an active "ossification" of vascular structures.

Since vascular calcifications are predictive of higher morbidity and mortality, the control of serum phosphorus in CKD patients becomes crucial in preventing increases in calcium-phosphate product, secondary hyperparathyroidism, and so far vascular mineralization [14]. Recent studies have shown that new pharmacological tools may be useful to prevent vascular calcifications in animals and humans [15-17].

In this review, we analyzed the role of phosphate on inducing vascular mineralization and secondary hyperparathyroidism, and the efficacy of lanthanum carbonate, as a new potent phosphate binder, in the treatment of hyper-phosphatemia in CKD patients.

HYPERPHOSPHATEMIA AND VASCULAR CALCIFICATION

During the past 40 years, different studies have shown that phosphate retention not only induces secondary hyperparathyroidism but also accelerates kidney failure by inducing renal calcifications [18]. Clearly, Gimenez *et al.* [19] showed that patients with higher serum calcium-phosphate product, renal calcium content, and histologic calcium deposition were those with serum creatinine levels above 1.5 mg/dl. In experimental renal failure, high dietary phosphate-induced acceleration of kidney function deterioration is associated with renal calcium-phosphate deposition and tubular-interstitial damage [20].

Furthermore, several investigators have been deeply interested in studying the mechanisms of vascular mineralization. In fact, extraskeletal calcification seems to be characterized not only by a passive calcium-phosphate deposition in the vasculature, but also by an active transformation of arterial walls in bone structures regulated by genes associated with osteoblastic functions [7]. Moreover, recent studies demonstrated the phosphate regulation of vascular calcification and provide some insights into the mechanisms for phosphate-induction of metastatic calcifications. Jono *et al.* [13] showed that high phosphorus levels in the incubation media (2 mmol/l) increased human aortic smooth muscle cells (HSMCs) calcification. Phosphate-containing mineral deposition was predominant in the extracellular matrix [13]. However, new evidences are necessary to better understand pathogenic mechanisms of vascular calcification in chronic kidney disease, and the potential role of phosphate on controlling directly this disease.

The control of serum phosphorus levels is critical in preventing ectopic calcification in CKD. In humans, cardiovascular calcification often occurs with advanced age, atherosclerosis, and diabetes mellitus. Several studies showed a higher prevalence of coronary plaques in dialyzed patients compared to the non-uremic population [10, 21]. In addition, vascular alterations in CKD associate with accelerated atherosclerosis and vascular stiffening, and left ventricular hypertrophy, that are major causes of cardiovascular mortality in hemodialysis patients [3]. Both accelerated atherosclerosis and mineralization of arterial intima and media caused arterial stiffness, hypertension, and increased cardiovascular mortality [22].

Enhancements in serum phosphate and calcium-phosphate product levels associate with arterial calcification in renal failure. Ongoing evidence demonstrates that calcium-containing phosphate-binders can increase calcium load. A new non-invasive imaging technology, Electron Beam Computed Tomography (EBCT), demonstrated that both hyperphosphatemia and increased calcium-phosphate pro-duct cause a progressive increase in calcium deposition in the coronary arteries, mitral and aortic valves in patients with advanced renal failure [10]. A study of adolescents and young adults hemodialysis patients by Goodman *et al.* [11] noted a correlation between coronary artery calcification, detected by EBCT, duration of dialysis, serum phosphorus, calcium-phosphate product levels and more importantly the daily intake of calcium.

HYPERPHOSPHATEMIA AND SECONDARY HYPERPARATHYROIDISM

Hyperphosphatemia due to decreased glomerular filtration rate is an important factor in the pathogenesis of secondary hyperparathyroidism [23]. Elevated serum phosphate levels induce secondary hyperparathyroidism through indirect and direct mechanisms [24]. In addition, hyperphosphatemia inhibits calcitriol production [25], which consequent hypocalcemia. Therapeutic dosage of stabilized Lanthanum carbonate compositions are used for treatment hyperphosphataemia [26].

The direct effects of phosphorus have been demonstrated both *in vitro* and *in vivo* studies. In fact, a high phosphorus concentration stimulates PTH secretion in intact rat parathyroid glands [27]. Unfortunately, the *in vitro* effects of phosphorus on PTH secretion could be observed in intact parathyroid tissue preparations, but not in isolated dispersed parathyroid cells [28]. Recently, several studies have showed some mechanisms by which phosphorus may regulate parathyroid function. The regulation of PTH mRNA by phosphorus has been found to occur post-transcriptionally though binding of parathyroid cytosolic proteins to the 3′-UTR and in particular to the terminal 60 nucleotides of PTH-mRNA [29].

In 2 weeks after 5/6 nephrectomy in rats, uremia-induced mitotic activity is further enhanced by high dietary phosphate, but prevented by phosphorus restriction [24]. In contrast to the mitogenic effects of hyperphosphatemia, dietary phosphorus restriction appears to counteract the proliferative signals induced by uremia, thus preventing parathyroid cell replication and consequently, the increase in parathyroid gland size [30].

Recent studies on the opposing effects of high and low dietary phosphate on parathyroid gland growth demonstrated that the low phosphorus-induction of p21 (an inhibitor of kinases of the cell-cycle) mRNA and protein content in parathyroid glands contributes to the antiproliferative effects of phosphate restriction on uremia-induced parathyroid cell growth [31]. In this uremic rat model, a role of low-phosphate induction of p21 expression in the arrest of parathyroid hyperplasia is supported by the demonstration that temporal increases in p21 protein expression correlate inversely with parathyroid levels of a marker of mitotic activity proliferating nuclear cell antigen (PCNA) [31].

In the search for mitogenic stimuli triggered by high dietary phosphate, we next focused on transforming growth factor-α (TGFα). TGFα, known to promote growth not only in malignant transformation but also in normal tissues [32], is enhanced in hyperplastic and adenomatous human parathyroid glands [33]. The opposing effects of high and low dietary phosphate on uremia-induced parathyroid cell growth has been recently demonstrated. In fact, high phosphate diet worsens uremia-induced parathyroid hyperplasia by increasing parathyroid expression of TGFα The rapid return of parathyroid TGFα content to normal levels by phosphate restriction also suggests that low phosphorus may counteract uremia-induced parathyroid cell growth not only through induction of p21 expression, but also by preventing the enhancement of parathyroid TGFα [31, 34].

Increases in parathyroid TGFα could induce cell growth through autocrine and paracrine mechanisms upon activation of its receptor, the epidermal growth factor receptor (EGFR) [35]. In human parathyroid glands, Gogusev *et al.* [33] demonstrated the presence of EGFR protein in 4 out 5 adenomas, in 13 of 15 tissue samples of hyperplasia secondary to renal failure, and in most samples of normal parathyroid tissue. No differences in the expression patterns were observed among groups. However, studies in 104 human hyperplastic parathyroid glands, which failed to detect EGFR protein, showed higher EGFR mRNA expression in carcinoma and primary hyperplasia compared to adenomas and hyperplasia secondary to renal failure [36].

Furthermore, similar to the changes in TGFα expression, high dietary phosphate enhances parathyroid EGFR content to levels above normal, while phosphorus restriction prevented the increases in EGFR levels [37, 38].

PHOSPHATE BINDERS IN CKD PATIENTS

Serum phosphate levels in uremic patients can be controlled by the reduction of phosphate oral intake, an adequate dialysis schedule and the use of intestinal phosphate binders.

During homeostasis, almost 60% of the ingested phosphate is absorbed by the gut and this amount is increased by the oral assumption of vitamin D. In order to reduce the intestinal phosphate absorption, the main approach is to evaluate the phosphate dietary intake of each patient and to provide appropriate counselling. However, patients on CKD ingest a consistent dietary intake of phosphate (not less than 900-1000 mg/day) secondary to the dietary protein amount of 1.00-1.20 g /kg/ body weight in the recommended daily diet [39]. It is a common observation that dietary phosphorus restriction, in the long term, is rarely followed by the most of the patients.

Considering that intermittent hemodialysis, as currently performed thrice weekly, is usually unable to maintain phosphorus balance at acceptable levels, the use of P binders appears to be an essential treatment to control phosphate overload in CKD patients.

In 2003, the K/DOQI guidelines defined the targets [40] for serum phosphate, calcium, Ca x P, and PTH levels. However, only in a minority of patients the actual therapeutic strategies are able to achieve all these four K/DOQI guidelines.

THE CALCIUM SALTS

After the understanding of the tragic effects of aluminum accumulation in patients treated with aluminum hydroxyde, calcium salts became the most widely used class of phosphate binder during the end of the '80s and the following decade [41-43]. At that time, calcium carbonate was introduced as first choice drug, at high dosage (3.5 to 8.8 g / day), because there was a general consensus that, in addition to P binding, high serum calcium levels were helpful to ameliorate the control of PTH secretion. Many reports however indicate that this strategy was associated with persistent hypercalcemia [43, 44].

More specifically the prevalence of hypercalcemia in clinical trials with calcium carbonate ranged from 20 to 60 %. Furthermore, a simultaneous treatment with calcium carbonate and calcitriol may increase intestinal absorption of calcium and phosphorous leading to an over-suppression of PTH production and low-turnover bone disease [44].

Compared to calcium carbonate, more soluble calcium salts, as calcium acetate, decrease the serum phosphate level at a lower dose of elemental calcium, but without a concomitant reduction of hypercalcemic events. Also with calcium acetate, the risk of hypercalcemia still persist [45-47]. Clearly, hypercalcemia is a major concern in CKD patients. While on a previous report, Block *et al.* [48] did not observe an association between calcium levels and mortality, a more recent study in a larger cohort by the same Authors has shown that the risk of death in CKD is associated with serum calcium levels [47]. Consistently with these observations, in several studies conducted in CKD patients coronary calcification was related to serum phosphorus concentration, Ca x P product and the dose of calcium contained in the phosphate binders [11, 49].

These data indicate that calcium overload is associated with a greater prevalence and progression of vascular calcification and that normal serum calcium levels are not representative of a present or past exposure to calcium overload.

A CALCIUM- AND ALUMINUM-FREE PHOSPHATE BINDER: THE EXPERIENCE WITH SEVELAMER HYDROCHLORIDE

Sevelamer hydrochloride, is a 3rd generation phosphate binder. This compound is a quaternary amine anion exchange resin that binds phosphate ions and releases protons [50].

The "Treat-to-Goal" trial was the main study designed to investigate the efficacy, safety, and tolerability of sevelamer. This study was a prospective randomized control trial, designed to compare the efficacy of sevelamer and calcium carbonate to control serum P and Ca x P product levels as well as the progression of coronary and aortic calcification assessed by EBCT on 200 dialysis patients over 52 weeks of follow-up [14]. Although the average of serum calcium levels remained among a normal range in both sevelamer- and calcium-treated group, serum calcium levels and incidence of hypercalcemia were lower in sevelamer treated patients (calcium levels: 9.2 and 9.6 mg/dL in the sevelamer and in the calcium carbonate groups respectively, p=002. Incidence of hypercalcemia: 16% in calcium carbonate and 5% in the sevelamer group, p=0.04). Furthermore, sevelamer was associated with a lower median percent increase in coronary arteries (25% *vs.* 6%, p= 0.02) and aortic (28% *vs.* 5%, p=0.02) calcium scores compared to calcium carbonate.

In a recent post-hoc analysis of the "treat to goal" study in which bone calcium content was assessed in the two groups of patients., Raggi *et al.* [51] showed that patients randomized to receive calcium salts had a significant reduction in thoracic trabecular and cortical bone attenuation, in association with higher concentration of serum calcium, lower PTH levels and reduced total and bone-specific alkaline phosphatase. These data suggest that calcium salts might increase the progression of vascular calcification by a consistent calcium overload, as the main substrate for calcification, by at least two mechanisms: 1) direct calcium overload from phosphate-binding salts, 2) indirect reduction of calcium storage in skeletal tissue secondary to hyperparathyroidism.

In addition, sevelamer is able to bind phosphate in the gut, avoiding vascular effects related to calcium overload. Reduction in total serum cholesterol and low-density lipoprotein is a further, peculiar, advantage of this phosphate-binder [14, 50]. However the limited hypophosphatemic effect demanding the use of several pills in many patients hinders compliance thus making problematic the management of hyperphosphatemia in CKD patients.

LANTHANUM CARBONATE: A NEW POTENT PHOSPHATE BINDER

Lanthanum is a rare earth element whose atomic number is 57. In form of carbonate it is an aluminium and calcium-free salt whose binding capacity is very high, similar to that of aluminium hydroxide. One major issue of this new compound is its pharmacology.

In vitro Binding Effects

The phosphate-binding efficacy of lanthanum carbonate was compared with those of aluminum hydroxide, calcium carbonate and calcium acetate in an *in vitro* study at pH 3.5 and 7 [52]. At each pH, lanthanum carbonate showed good phosphate-binding efficacy, which was similar to that of aluminium hydroxide and superior to those of calcium carbonate and calcium acetate.

In vivo Phosphate Binding

In 5/6 nephrectomized rats lanthanum carbonate and aluminium hydroxide showed a greater reduction in urinary phosphorus excretion, compared to sevelamer and calcium carbonate [52]. Rare earth metal compounds are used in the treatment of hyperphosphatemia in mammals and to remove phosphate from the gastrointestinal tract [53-55].

Absorption and Distribution

Lanthanum is very poorly absorbed from gastrointestinal tract (0.0007% in rat and 0.00005% in dogs). In rats, lanthanum was largely excreted with the faeces within 7 days, the bulk being transported *via* biliary system. In healthy volunteers lanthanum was excreted by the kidney in extremely small amount (0.00003% of the administered oral dose). With a chronic daily dose of lanthanum carbonate up to 2000 mg/kg/day (a dose of one order of magnitude greater than that currently used in patients with chronic renal failure) the majority of tissues had concentration of less than 1 ug/g, while concentration in liver and bone were less than 10 ug/g.

Recent data by Lacour *et al.* in 5/6 nephrectomized rats [56] have shown that oral administration of lanthanum carbonate may cause substantial lanthanum accumulation in liver, lung and kidneys suggesting that uremia might increase the intestinal absorption of lanthanum.

Hutchison *et al.* [57] investigated the eventual hepatotoxicity of Lanthanum, excluding any adverse effect of oral administration on serum liver markers or on liver histology, with both single or multiple-dose models. By intravenous administration Lanthanum carbonate induced only mild liver inflammation in dogs at plasma lanthanum concentrations 20.000 times higher than those measured in lanthanum treated dialysis patients. These data suggest that, increased serum or tissue concentrations of Lanthanum do not necessarily imply toxicity.

Several studies demonstrated that Lanthanum carbonate is an efficacious phosphate binder in CKD patients. Lanthanum significantly reduced serum phosphorus levels when administered at doses between 2250 and 3000 mg per day over 4-6 weeks. The efficacy of lanthanum salts was also studied in double blind and randomised fashion by Finn [58]. In this study 145 patients were randomized to receive either lanthanum carbonate in daily dose of 225, 675, 1.350 or 2.250 mg *versus* placebo for 6 weeks. The intention to treat analysis showed a dose-dependent reduction of serum phosphorous level starting at a dose of 675 mg, documenting the efficacy of lanthanum carbonate across a wide range of doses.

Aluminum-like effects of Lanthanum on bone was specifically evaluated by D'Haese *et al.* [59] in a multicenter study which contemplated bone biopsies and the measurement of dynamic indexes of bone turnover. 98 patients on CKD were randomized to receive Lanthanum carbonate or calcium carbonate for one year. Repeated bone biopsies, performed in basal conditions and at the end of follow up, were available in 63 patients. In the Lanthanum group the number of patients with adynamic bone, osteomalacia or high turnover decreased from 36% at baseline to 18% while in the calcium carbonate group the number of patients with these alterations increased from 43% to 53%. Thus lanthanum carbonate treated patients do not evolve toward low bone turnover, nor present any aluminum-like effects on skeletal tissues [59]. Moreover, longer observations in a large cohort of patients treated for up to 3 years confirmed that the drug is safe and well tolerated [60]. Accordingly, no histological evidence of osteomalacia was observed in CKD patients treated with Lanthanum Carbonate for up to 5 years [61].

THE RECENT EXPERIENCE WITH LANTHANUM CARBONATE

In the last 5 years, new clinical data support the efficacy and safety of lanthanum carbonate on reducing hyperphosphatemia in CKD patients. Lanthanum carbonate is a promising new non-aluminium, calcium-free phosphate binder. Pre-clinical and clinical studies have demonstrated a good safety profile, and it appears well tolerated and effective in reducing phosphate levels in dialysis patients. Its identified adverse events are apparently mild to moderate in severity and mostly GI related. It appears to be effective as a mono-therapy, with a reduced pill burden, but like sevelamer, it is significantly more expensive than calcium-based binders. Data on its safety profile over 6 years of treatment are now available. In this recent publication, Hutchison et al [62] demonstrated that lanthanum carbonate was not associated with any adverse changes in transaminases or bilirubin. The incidence and nature of adverse events associated with the liver during lanthanum carbonate treatment was similar to that in the comparator groups. For patients who enrolled into the subsequent long-term follow-up study (up to 6 years of treatment), changes in transaminases were not clinically relevant and mean values were similar to those observed in the earlier trials. Overall, there was no increase in the incidence of adverse events associated with the liver reported after up to 6 years of treatment when compared with the results of the initial studies.

On the basis of its proven efficacy and safety profiles, it is justifiable to consider lanthanum carbonate as a first-line phosphate binder for dialysis patients. However, such decisions are rarely made on solely clinical grounds, and while it is clearly effective without evidence of toxicity, it is also expensive, with three 500 mg lanthanum tablets costing approximately the same as five 800 mg sevelamer pills. Furthermore the dose of lanthanum can be increased without increasing the number of tablets, since it is manufactured in different strengths – 500, 750, and 1000 mg – making it unique among phosphate binders. The reduced pill burden combined with palatability and tolerability may lead to improvement in patient adherence to therapy, and therefore better phosphate control, although adherence is not solely related to pill burden.

In a multicenter, open-label trial, patients on a stable dialysis regimen were screened while receiving phosphate-binder therapy, then entered into a washout phase [63]. Patients with serum phosphate >1.78 mmol/L after washout entered into the main 12-week treatment phase (N = 367), during which they were treated to target (K/DOQI: 1.13–1.78 mmol/L) with lanthanum carbonate monotherapy. Mean serum phosphate levels were significantly reduced after 12 weeks of lanthanum carbonate monotherapy vs previous phosphate-binder therapy. The mean number of phosphate-binder tablets being taken per day at screening was 7.6, but during treatment with lanthanum carbonate, most patients were taking doses of up to 3000 mg/day, achievable with 3 × 1000 mg tablets per day. These findings suggest that lanthanum carbonate monotherapy offers effective control of serum phosphate and, owing to a low tablet burden, may help to simplify the management of hyperphosphatemia in patients with CKD Stage 5.

CURRENT AND FUTURE DEVELOPMENTS

Several factors concur to determine cardiovascular complications and decrease life expectancy in CKD patients while bone disease still remains a major therapeutic challenge. To date hyperphosphatemia is one of the few risk factors which appears amenable to treatment to reduce the high cardiovascular burden of CKD and to limit bone disease in this population. Yet hyperphosphatemia and disordered calcium metabolism still remain a largely unexploited area for cardiovascular and bone disease prevention as well.

Aluminum salts are most potent phosphate binders but the use of these drugs on a long term basis is limited by multiple toxicities. Calcium carbonate and Calcium acetate are efficacious hypophosphatemic agents. However the risk of hypercalcemia and the attendant cardiovascular calcifications represents an objective limitation to the use of these drugs when needed at a high dosage.

Among the 3rd generation of P binders, sevelamer appears to be a weak binder and the fairly high number of pills often needed to control serum phosphate poses problems of compliance when this drug is used. Lanthanum carbonate is a much promising new opportunity for countering hyperphosphatemia in dialysis patients because this drug has an efficacious profile similar to aluminum salts with no apparent evidence of bone or organ toxicity.

REFERENCES

[1] Raggi P. Cardiovascular calcification in end stage renal disease. Contrib Nephrol 2005; 149: 272-278.

[2] Brancaccio D, Cozzolino M. The mechanism of calcium deposition in soft tissues. Contrib Nephrol 2005; 149: 279-286.

[3] London GM. Cardiovascular calcifications in uremic patients: clinical impact on cardiovascular function. J Am Soc Nephrol 2003; 14: S305-S309.

[4] Hruska KA, Mathew S, Saab G. Bone morphogenetic proteins in vascular calcification. Circ Res 2005; 97: 105-114.

[5] Ansari A, Kaupke CJ, Vaziri ND, *et al.* Cardiac pathology in patients with end-stage renal disease maintained on hemodialysis. Int J Artif Organs 1993; 16: 31-36.

[6] Schwartz U, Buzzello M, Ritz E, *et al.* Morphology of coronary atherosclerotic lesions in patients with end-stage renal failure. Nephrol Dial Transplant 2000; 15: 218-223.

[7] Cozzolino M, Dusso A, Slatopolsky E. Role of calcium - phosphate product and bone associated proteins on vascular calcification in renal failure. J Am Soc Nephrol 2001; 12: 2511-2516.

[8] Ganesh SK, Stack AG, Levin NW, *et al.* Association of elevated serum PO_4, Ca x PO_4 product, and parathyroid hormone with cardiac mortality risk in chronic hemodialysis patients. J Am Soc Nephrol 2001; 12: 2131-2138.

[9] Cozzolino M, Brancaccio D, Gallieni M, Slatoposlky E. Pathogenesis of vascular calcification in chronic kidney disease. Kidney Int 2005; 68(2): 429-436.

[10] Braun J, Oldendorf M, Moshage W, *et al.* Electron beam computed tomography in the evaluation of cardiac calcification in chronic dialysis patients. Am J Kidney Dis 1996; 27: 394-401.

[11] Goodman WG, Goldin J, Kuizon BD, *et al.* Coronary-artery calcification in young adults with end-stage renal disease who are undergoing dialysis. N Engl J Med 2000; 342: 1478-1483.

[12] London GM, Pannier B, Marchais SJ, Guerin AP. Calcification of the aortic valve in the dialyzed patient. J Am Soc Nephrol 2000; 11: 778-783.

[13] Jono S, McKee MD, Murry CE, *et al.* Phosphate regulation of vascular smooth muscle cell calcification. Circ Res 2000; 87(7): E10-17.

[14] Chertow GM, Burke SK, Raggi P, *et al.* Sevelamer attenuates the progression of coronary and aortic calcification in hemodialysis patients. Kidney Int 2002; 62: 245-252.

[15] Chertow GM, Burke SK, Dillon MA, Slatopolsky E. Long-term effects of sevelamer hydrochloride on the calcium x phosphate product and lipid profile of hemodialysis patients. Nephrol Dial Transplant 1999; 14: 2907-2914.

[16] Hergesell O, Ritz E. Stabilized polynuclear iron hydroxide is an efficient oral phosphate binder in uraemic patients. Nephrol Dial Transplant 1999; 14: 863-867.

[17] Hutchinson AJ. Calcitriol, lanthanum carbonate and other new phosphate binders in the management of renal osteodystrophy. Peri Dial Intern 1999; 19 (Suppl 2): S408-412.

[18] Loghman-Adham M. Role of phosphate retention in the progression of renal failure. J Lab Clin Med 1993; 122: 15-25.

[19] Gimenez LF, Solez K, Walker WG. Relation between renal calcium content and renal impairment in 246 human renal biopsies. Kidney Int 1987; 31: 93-99.

[20] Borle AB, Clark I. Effects of phosphate-induced hyperparathyroidism and parathyroidectomy on rat kidney calcium *in vivo*. Am J Physiol 1981; 241: E136-E141.

[21] Kajbaf S, Veinot JP, Ha A, Zimmerman D. Comparison of surgically removed cardiac valves of patients with ESRD with those of the general population. Am J Kidney Dis 2005; 46: 86-93.

[22] Blacher J, Safar ME, Guerin AP, *et al.* Aortic pulse wave velocity index and mortality in end-stage renal disease. Kidney Int 2003; 63(5): 1852-1860.

[23] Delmez JA, Slatopolsky E. Hyperphosphatemia: its conesquences and treatment in patients with chronic renal disease. Am J Kidney Dis 1992; 19: 303-317.

[24] Rodriguez M, Almaden Y, Hernandez A, Torres A. Effect of phosphate on the parathyroid gland: direct and indirect? Curr Opin Nephrol Hypertens 1996; 5: 321-328.

[25] Portale AA, Halloran BP, Morris RC, Jr. Physiologic regulation of the serum concentration of 1,25-dihydroxyvitamin D by phosphorus in normal men. J Clin Invest 1989; 83: 1494-1499.

[26] Ferdinando, J.C.; Davies, P.N. US0121127A1 (**2006**).

[27] Almaden Y, Canalejo A, Hernandez A, *et al.* Direct effect of phosphorus on PTH secretion from whole rat parathyroid glands *in vitro*. J Bone Miner Res 1996; 11: 970-976.

[28] Nielsen PK, Feldt-Rasmussen U, Olgaard K. A direct effect *in vitro* of phosphate on PTH release from bovine parathroid tissue slices but not from dispersed parathyroid cells. Nephrol Dial Transplant 1996; 11: 1762-1768.

[29] Moallem E, Kilav R, Silver J, Naveh-Many T. RNA-protein binding and post-transcriptional regulation of parathyroid hormone gene expression by calcium and phosphate. J Biol Chem 1998; 273: 5253-5259.

[30] Wang Q, Palnitkar S, Parfitt AM. Parathyroid cell proliferation in normal human parathyroid tissue: implications for the pathogenesis of hyperparathyroidism. Clin Endocrinol 1997; 46: 343-349.

[31] Dusso AS, Pavlopoulos T, Naumovich L, *et al.* p21^{waf1} and TGF-α mediate dietary phosphate-regulation of parathyroid cell growth. Kidney Int 2001; 59: 855-865.

[32] Kumar V, Bustiin SA, McKay IA. Transforming growth factor α. Cell Biol Int 1995; 19: 373-388.

[33] Gogusev J, Duchambon P, Soermann-Chopard C, *et al.* De novo expression of transforming growth factor-α in parathyroid gland tissue of patients with primary or secondary uraemic hyperparathyroidism. Nephrol Dial Transplant 1996; 11: 2155-2162.

[34] Cozzolino M, Lu Y, Finch J, *et al.* p21^{WAF1} and TGF-α mediate parathyroid growth arrest by vitamin D and high calcium. Kidney Int 2001; 60: 2109-2117.

[35] Wong ST, Winchell LF, McCune BK, *et al.* The TGF-α precursor expressed on the cell surface binds to the EGF receptor on adjacent cells, leading to signal transduction. Cell 1989; 56: 495-500.

[36] Sadler GP, Morgan JM, Jasani B, *et al.* Epidermal growth factor receptor status in hyperparathyroidism: immunocytochemical and *in situ* hybridization study. World J Surg 1996; 20: 736-743.

[37] Dusso A, Cozzolino M, Lu Y, *et al.* 1,25-Dihydroxyvitamin D downregulation of TGFα/EGFR expression and growth signaling: a mechanism for the antiproliferative actions of the sterol in parathyroid hyperplasia of renal failure. J Steroid Biochem Mol Biol 2004; 89-90: 507-511.

[38] Cozzolino M, Lu Y, Sato T, *et al.* A critical role for enhanced-TGFα and EGFR expression in the initiation of parathyroid hyperplasia in experimental renal disease. Am J Physiol Renal Physiol 2005; 289(5): F1096-F1102.

[39] Kopple JD. National Kidney Foundation K/DOQI clinical practice guidelines for nutrition in chronic renal failure. Am J Kidney Dis 2001; 37 (S2): S66-S70.

[40] Gonzales EA, Al-Aly Z, Martin KJ. Difficulties in achieving the K/DOQI practice guidelines for bone and mineral metabolism. Semin Dial 2005; 18: 171-174.

[41] Slatopolsky E, Weerts C, Lopez-hilker S, *et al.* Calcium carbonate as a phosphate binder in patients with chronic renal failure undergoing dialysis. N Engl J Med 1986; 315: 157-161.

[42] Taylor JE, Henderson IS, Stewart WK, Mactier RA. Calcium carbonate 1250 mg/1260 mg: an affective phosphate binder. Scott Med J 1990; 35: 45-47.

[43] Caravaca F, Santos I, Cubero JJ, *et al.* Calcium acetate *versus* calcium carbonate as phosphate binders in hemodialysis patients. Nephron 1992; 60: 423-427.

[44] Emmet M, Sirmon MD, Kirkpatrick WG, *et al.* Calcium acetate control of serum phosphorus in hemodialysis patients. Am J Kidney Dis 1991; 17: 544-550.

[45] Schaefer K, Scheer J, Asmus G, *et al.* The treatment of uraemic hyperphosphatemia with calcium acetate and calcium carbonate: a comparative study. Nephrol Dial Transplant 1991; 6: 170-175.

[46] Choy BY, Lo WK, Cheng IK. Effectiveness of calcium acetate as phosphate binder in patients undergoing continuous ambulatory peritoneal dialysis. Hong Kong Med J 1998; 4: 23-26.

[47] Almirall J, Veciana L, Llibre J. Calcium acetate *versus* calcium carbonate for the control of serum phosphorus in hemodialysis patients. Am J Nephrol 1994;14(3):192-196.

[48] Block GA, Hulbert-Shearon TE, Levin NW, Port FK. Association of serum phosphorus and calcium x phosphate product with mortality risk in chronic hemodialysis patients: a national study. Am J Kidney Dis 1998; 31: 607-617.

[49] Block GA, Klassen PS, Lazarus JM, *et al.* Mineral metabolism, mortality, and morbidity in maintenance hemodialysis. J Am Soc Nephrol 2004; 15: 2208-2218.

[50] Chertow GM, Burke SK, Lazarus JM, *et al.* Poly [allylamine hydrochloride] (Renagel): a noncalcemic phosphate binder for the treatment of hyperphosphatemia in chronic renal failure. Am J Kidney Dis 1997; 29: 66-71.

[51] Raggi P, James G, Burke SK, *et al.* Decrease in thoracic vertebral bone attenuation with calcium-based phosphate binders in hemodialysis. J Bone Miner Res 2005; 20: 764-72.

[52] Pennick M, Damment SJP, Gill M. The pharmacokinetics and tissue distribution of lanthanum carbonate (Fosrenol®) a novel non-aluminium, non-calcium phosphate binder. *Poster presented at the 36th Annual Meeting of the American Society of Nephrology*, San Diego, CA, 14-17 November (**2003**).

[53] Almirall J, Lopez T, Vallve M, Ruiz A, Llibre J, Betriu A. Safety and efficacy of sevelamer in the treatment of uncontrolled hyperphosphataemia of haemodialysis. Nephron Clin Pract 2004; 97(1): c17-c22.

[54] Moerck, R.E.; Spitler, T.M.; Schauer, E.A.; Prochazka, J. US20060083791A1 (**2006**).

[55] Murrer, B.A.; Powell, N.A. US5968976 (**1999**).

[56] Lacour B, Lucas A, Auchèere D, *et al.* Chronic renal failure is associated with increased tissue deposition of lanthanum after 28-day oral administration. Kidney Int 2005; 67: 1062-1069.

[57] Hutchison A. Analysis of liver function and hepatobiliary adverse event data from 2000 dialysis patients participating in clinical trials on the new phosphate binder, lanthanum carbonate. *Abstract presented at the EDTA-ERA Annual Meeting, Istanbul*, Turkey, June 4-7, (**2005**).

[58] Finn WF, Joy MS, Hladik and the Lanthanum Study Group. Efficacy and safety of lamthanum carbonate for reduction of serum phosphorus in patients with chronic renal failure receiving hemodialysis. Clin Nephrol 2004; 62: 193-201.

[59] D'Haese PC, Spasovski GB, Sikole A, *et al.* A multicenter study on the effects of lanthanum carbonate (Fosrenol TM) and calcium carbonate on renal bone disease in dialysis patients. Kidney Int 2003; 63 (Suppl 85): S73-S78.

[60] Hutchison A. Analysis of haematological data from over 2000 dialysis patients participating in clinical trials on the new phosphate binder, lanthanum carbonate. *Abstract presented at the EDTA-ERA Annual Meeting*, Istanbul, Turkey, June 4-7, (**2005**).

[61] Malluche HH, Freemont A, Denton J, *et al.* No evidence of osteomalacia in dialysis patients treated with lanthanum carbonate for up to 5 years. *Poster presented at the 37th Annual Meeting of the American Society of Nephrology*, St Louis, MO, USA. 29 oct-1 Nov, (**2004**).

[62] Hutchison AJ, Barnett ME, Krause RJ, Siami GA, Lanthanum Carbonate Study Group. Lanthanum carbonate treatment, for up to 6 years, is not associated with adverse effects on the liver in patients with chronic kidney disease Stage 5 receiving hemodialysis. Clin Nephrol 2009; 71(3): 286-295.

[63] Hutchison AJ, Laville M, on behalf of the SPD405–313 Lanthanum Study Group. Switching to lanthanum carbonate monotherapy provides effective phosphate control with a low tablet burden. Nephrol Dial Transplant 2008; 23(11): 3677-3684.

Myocardial Protection Against Ischemia-Reperfusion Injury: Novel Approaches in Maintaining Homeostatic Stability in Blood

Maqsood M. Elahi[1] and Bashir M. Matata[*,2]

[1]Department of Cardiothoracic Surgery, Faculty of Medicine and Surgery, PIC, Lahore, Pakistan, [2]Liverpool Heart and Chest Hospital NHS Trust, Thomas Drive, Liverpool, L14 3PE United Kingdom

Abstract: Homeostatic vascular response to complement activation in cardiac surgery patients requiring cardiopulmonary bypass results in mechanisms leading to ischemia-reperfusion injury and myocardial cell death. Various pro-inflammatory cytokines, released by the inflamed tissue, play an essential role in the activation of the complement system and co-localize with activated complement proteins within the circulating blood and the myocardium.

Throughout the past decade, much effort has thus been spent on deciphering the molecular signaling pathways mediating this pathophysiology. Basic and clinical investigations into many of the diverse aspects of cardiovascular drugs discovery employ varied approaches aimed at determining physiologic and pathophysiological efficiency of candidate agents for therapeutic utility. Identification of novel molecules regulating homeostatic dysfunction has offered the basis, with ultimate hope of identifying agents capable of exerting salutary influence upon cardiac and vascular tissue.

This review will provide detailed synopses on recent insights into the ischemia-reperfusion signaling and associated myocardial injury. In addition, we will consider current and emerging novel approaches in attenuating cardiopulmonary bypass mediated injury with ultimate goal to prevent or delay the onset of post pump modulated heart failure and sudden deaths in such patients. Careful examination of the literature on recent patented and non-patented publications has identified several agents shown to be effective and specific in modulating and abrogating ischemia-reperfusion injury with some suggestions of potential clinical use.

Keywords: Cytokines, reperfusion injury, protein kinase, macrophages, TNF-α, iNOS, ROS, oxidative stress, complement, pharmacological inhibition.

INTRODUCTION

The generation of reactive oxygen species (ROS) during the reintroduction of coronary blood flow by revascularization to a previously ischemic area is one of the main mechanisms underlying myocardial reperfusion injury [1]. Damage occurs when endogenous free

*Corresponding author: E-mail: matata_bashir@hotmail.com

Atta-ur-Rahman / M. Iqbal Choudhary (Eds.)

radicals scavenging mechanisms are overwhelmed or are themselves adversely affected by the ischemic insult [1]. This ability of ROS to alter myocardial function has already been shown *in vitro* and *in vivo* [2, 3] and the exposure of the heart to free radical generating systems or the addition of H_2O_2 to the perfusion medium is associated with alterations in cardiac function and biochemical changes similar to these observed in the damaged myocardium as a result of ischemia and reperfusion [4]. Therefore, it has been hypothesized that reperfusion, although necessary for the preservation of reversibly injured tissue, is associated with additional injury mediated largely by blood leukocytes [5, 6].

The existence of reperfusion injury as a separate entity is controversial, with some researchers suggesting that reperfusion exacerbates the cellular injury sustained during the ischemic period as evidenced by an extension in infarct size, following a fixed period of ischemia [7-9].

A few studies, on the other hand, indicate that oxidative stress and abrupt metabolic changes that accompany reperfusion can initiate cellular injury in the absence of ischemia [10, 11]. The only convincing means of demonstrating the existence of reperfusion injury in the context of ischaemic heart disease is by showing myocytes death in the regions affected and that this can be modified by interventions administered at the time of reperfusion.

Despite significant advances in the study of ischemia-reperfusion, patients with coronary reperfusion still have adverse clinical outcomes. It is suggested that this is in part due to the activation of inflammatory pathways by ROS that in turn regulate complement activation by direct effect on one of the complement's alternate pathway as evidenced by localization of various complement components within the ischemic tissue [12-14]. By using an experimental model of human endothelial cells, other reports involving the depletion of complement and its components have supported the above observations by establishing that the lectin pathway initiates complement activation after hypoxia-reoxygenation [15, 16]. These findings have expanded our ability to understand and recognize that the apparent differences in responses imparted by scavengers or inhibitors of ROS production may involve the regulation of important mechanisms such as auto-oxidation, nitration and phosphorylation of key redox-sensitive residues found in regulator molecules and release of antioxidant molecules from erythrocytes or an upregulation of activities of antioxidant enzymes [17, 18].

Some reports have suggested that antioxidant prophylaxis may reduce oxidative stress and systemic inflammatory reaction [19] and help in reducing complications associated with ischemic injury [20, 21]. However, despite the initial optimism almost all large randomized clinical trials for antioxidants have failed to demonstrate favorable outcomes in improving the quality of life of patients undergoing cardiopulmonary bypass operations [22-24]. Other authors have reported that it is the circulating activated leukocytes that act as the mediators of oxidative stress of which the antioxidant capacity can no longer be compensated even if supplemented exogenously, thereby not improving the clinical outcome [25]. This suggests that antioxidant supplementation in ischemia-reperfusion state may not be an effective treatment in view of the overwhelming levels of generated ROS in blood. Recently, a novel C5 complement monoclonal anti-body fragment has been developed to prevent the complement-mediated myocardial damage from ischemia and reperfusion; however, this has failed to demonstrate any substantial evidence [26, 27]. As new agents capable of modulating ischemia-reperfusion injury are being developed, we focused on signaling pathways that hold promise as potentially new therapeutic strategies in attenuating myocardial injury when applied. This approach involves the activation of specific signaling kinase cascades, which in turn, protect the heart from reperfusion-induced cell death by recruiting innate cellular anti-apoptotic pathways of survival.

SIGNIFICANCE OF OXIDANTS AND INFLAMMATORY MEDIATORS DURING CARDIAC SURGERY

Traditionally, oxidative stress has been viewed as a pathologic process that contributes to cell damage. However, we propose that ROS are widely used as second messengers that propagate the proinflammatory and growth stimulatory signals. The complex mechanisms involved in the response of blood to the stresses of the heart and lung bypass machine otherwise known as cardiopulmonary bypass (CPB) during "on-pump" cardiac surgery are still far from clear. However, there is some evidence to suggest that complications (morbidity) associated with CPB can in part be attributed to the generalized redox-driven inflammatory response that is known to be induced by the contact of blood with the internal surfaces of the materials that make up the bypass circuits. We have recently conducted studies that have led to the hypothesis that "oxidoreductase dysequilibrium" occurs during extracorporeal blood recirculation involving virtually every arm of the inflammatory response including complement activation, although conflicting data still exist [28]. Indeed, researchers are beginning to realize that oxidative stress and inflammation are related and perhaps inseparable and that a reduced cytokine response may be directly translated into changes in clinical outcomes. Furthermore, absolute perioperative values of inflammatory markers are probably less important than the balance between the oxidoinflammatory cascade and anti-inflammatory feedback mechanisms [28].

Substantial evidence [29] further suggests that the same response during CPB surgery is initiated in response to non-physiologic conditions. These material-dependent and -independent stimuli tip the balance between the processes of activation and inhibition of these systems, an event that may lead to altered redox status, upregulation of gene expression, transcriptional/translational activities, and changes in the signaling pathways. The complexity of this dysequilibrium means that the implementation of an effective anti-inflammatory strategy is a difficult challenge.

Our previous investigations have also suggested that NO donors can have protective effects against ischemia-reperfusion injury and may improve cardiac, gut, or renal function; however, the underlying mechanisms of endothelial dysfunction are not clear, in particular how diabetes affects the balance between NO production and inactivation [30] Hence, it is evident that NO production frequently accompanies inflammatory state, although it is still unclear whether it promotes, inhibits, or has no effect on the inflammatory process per se.

This may be explained by varying levels of NO in inflammation; however, when interpreting the results of such studies, it is important to keep in perspective the disease process being studied.

It is now known that at the heart of the mechanisms leading to capillary leak syndrome is the vascular endothelium that becomes increasingly permeable within minutes of any acute inflammatory stimulus. We studied the impact of inspired NO gas on physiological function and markers of inflammation-oxidative stress for subjects (n=15, age 62+4.5 and 12/3 M/F) scheduled for coronary artery bypass graft (CABG) operation. Outcomes from subjects that received 5 ppm and 20 ppm of inspired NO (n=5/group) were compared to those not given NO gas. Breath-to-breath measurement commenced at the start of intubation and continued up to 4h later. Indices of cardiovascular function, alveolar-capillary gas exchange and haematological parameters were not significantly different in outcomes for the inspired NO groups as compared with control. We observed a reduction in mean systemic arterial in all subjects at 30 min and 4h after bypass when compared with pre bypass values.

Markers of systemic inflammatory response and oxidative stress increased during CPB particularly at 4h and 24h after the initiation of bypass. In contrast, we observed a reduction in expired NO, at 24h after surgery in the groups given inspired NO. In addition, there was also a significant reduction in oxidative stress markers in blood at 24h after surgery for the groups given inspired NO as compared with the control group. In contrast, cytokines response remained similar in all the three groups at all time points. Our results suggested that inspired NO gas has an antioxidant property that reduces the levels of cell death, and is not associated with significantly worse-off physiological outcomes (Fig. **1**) [31].

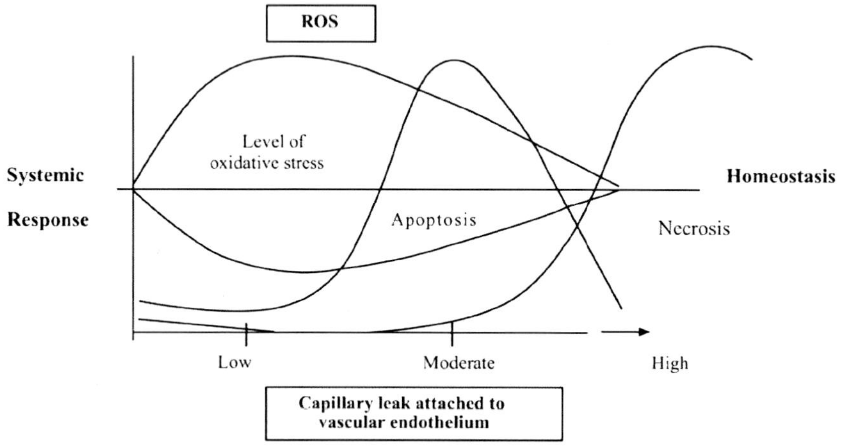

Fig. (1). Inflammatory signals stimulate an oxidative stress that has a dose-dependent effect on the disruption of cellular homeostasis [29].

THE CONTRIBUTION OF SIGNALING PATHWAYS TO ISCHEMIA REPERFUSION INJURY

In order to target the ischemia-reperfusion injury in cells, the activation of the existing innate cellular signaling pathways of survival may afford an opportunity for protecting the heart. Ischemia-reperfusion has been shown to activate the pro-survival kinase signalling cascades, phosphatidylinositol-3-OH kinase (PI3K)-Akt and p42/p44 extracellular signal-regulated kinases (Erk 1/2), both of which have been implicated in cellular survival, through their recruitment of anti-apoptotic pathways of protection [32]. There are of course several other kinases that have been implicated in the induction of ischemia-reperfusion injury through their effects on apoptotic pathways, such as p38 and JNK, MAPK, PKA, Rho kinase and JAK-STAT and are described in Fig. (**2**) and discussed further below.

Cyclic GMP/ PKG-1 Pathway

The cGMP/PKG-1 signaling pathways have recently emerged as a promising target for interventions. Cyclic GMP (cGMP) is the second messenger for membrane bound

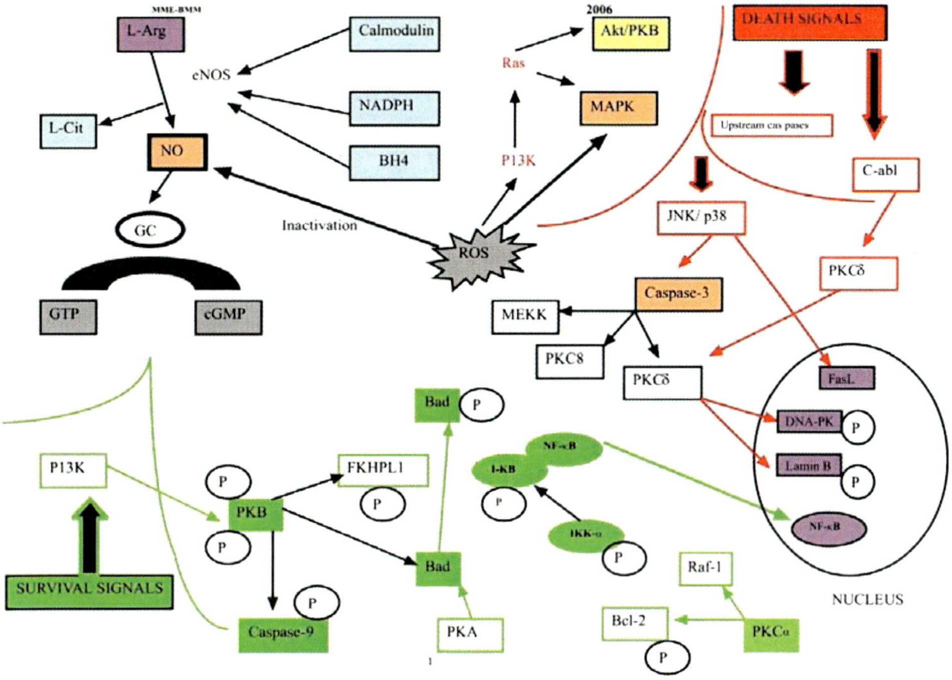

Fig. (2). Ischemia- reperfusion kinase signaling pathways involved directly in the regulation of survival and apoptotic cascades. Extracellular factors (shown in red) modulated by NO and ROS led mechanisms induce activation of JNK/ P38 MAPK and effector caspases. Activation of JNK leads to induction of pro-apoptotic genes leading Fas Ligands (FasL) death signals are also relayed via activation of c-abl leading to nuclear translocation of PKC and its targets. Signals of cell survival (shown in red) include activation of PKB, *via* P13K, which leads to phosphorylation and inactivation of Bad, caspase 9 and forkhead transcription factor (FKHRL1).

guanylate-cyclase receptors, as well as ubiquitous gas nitric oxide (NO) [33]. Nitric oxide (NO) stimulates cGMP formation *via* activation of soluble guanylyl cyclase. In experiments conducted in cultured cardiomyocytes, NO dependent cGMP formation has demonstrated antiapoptotic properties. Conversely transgenic mice lacking the endothelial form of NO-synthase display increased injury in response to ischemia-reperfusion [34]. A major down-stream effector of cGMP signaling in cardiomyocytes is the cGMP dependent protein kinase type-1 (PKG-1) [35]. PKG-1 mediates many of the effects of NO in different tissues, such as vascular smooth muscle cell dilation [36].

So what are the mechanisms that mediate the anti-ischaemic properties of PKG-1 in the heart? Recent studies demonstrated that cGMP-induced PKG-1 activation reduces NFAT (nuclear factor of activated T cells) translocation and transcriptional activity following phenylephrine (PE) stimulation of cardiomyocytes [37]. However, the molecular targets that mediates its inhibition by PKG-1 remains to be revealed. In this regard, several calcium regulating proteins have been identified as substrates for PKG-1 in the heart, including the L-type calcium channel and troponin I [33]. Further exploration of cGMP/PKG-1 signaling could reveal new therapeutic strategies to modulate cardiac ischemia-reperfusion injury. The underlying molecular mechanisms include deactivation of NFAT-P13k/Akt-, as well as ERK 1/ 2 signalling. Phosphoinositide 3-Kinase/AKT. The Phosphoinositide 3 kinase (P13K)-family of enzymes that display both protein and lipid kinase activity have been linked with signaling in many cellular functions such as growth, survival and proliferation [38]. A growing body of evidence suggests that PI3K-Akt signaling cascade is activated in response to the activation of a wide range of receptors, including those for growth factors and G-protein-coupled receptors [39]. Many stimuli have been shown to activate the serine/threonine kinase Akt, (also known as protein kinase B) and P13K-activation is an important common step in this process [40, 41]. Of the 3 Akt genes only Akt -1 and -2 are expressed at substantial levels in the heart. It is well established that transgenic over expression of Akt/ PKB is sufficient to induce significant myocytes injury in mice with or without affecting systolic function [42,43]. On one hand these findings reveal an important role for Akt signaling in ischemia-reperfusion injury, and could therefore be interesting targets for the prevention and/ or treatment of reperfusion injury.

What are the mediators of the P13K/ Akt signaling? There are opinions that suggest that P13K/Akt signaling activates other signaling pathways notably mTOR (mammalian target of rapamycin) activation [44]. Though the detailed mechanism underlying mTOR (mammalian target of rapamycin) activation by Akt/PKB remains the subject of controversy, the involvement of the tuberous sclerosis genes TSC-1 and TSC-2 in the process has been demonstrated in numerous studies [40]. Over-expression of TSC-1/2 impairs the regulation of the downstream mTOR targets [45]. TSC-2 is phosphorylated at least in two sites by Akt and its phosphorylation apparently alleviates the inhibitory effects of TSC 1/2 on mTOR signalling. The significance of mTOR in regulating this is established by its ability to inhibit protein synthesis *via* the translational effectors [46]. However, further studies will be necessary to determine if an effective treatment can be developed based on this idea.

In addition to the mTOR, another downstream target of PI3K signaling is Glycogen synthase kinase-3β (GSK-3β), a widely expressed kinase that phosphorylates transcription factors of the NFAT family, thereby promoting their translocation to the cytoplasm where they are inactive [47]. The activity of GSK-3β is controlled by the phosphorylation status of serine-9. Various *in vitro* and *in vivo* studies have indicated that GSK-3β is a central endogenous negative regulator of this phenomenon in response to many stress stimuli, like endothelin-1 (ET-1), phenylephrine (PE), and Fas signalling [48, 49].

In contrast to other kinases, GSK-3β is highly active in unstimulated cells and negatively regulates most of its targets. NFAT family of transcription factors involved in the hypertrophic response that are phosphorylated by GSK-3β include GATA-4 [49] and eukaryotic initiation factor (EIF) [50]. Given that GSK-3β phosphorylates and inactivates NFAT, it is tempting to refer to the protein kinase GSK-3β as the opponent of the central phosphates that regulates the reperfusion injury. Another issue to be addressed is the direct effect of GSK-3β on cardiac function, in that signaling through GSK-3β can confer protection against ischemia- reperfusion injury by downregulating the sarcoplasmic reticulum calcium ATPase (SERCA2a) [51]. These findings have to be taken into consideration when new therapeutic strategies that modulate GSK-3β signaling are in the process of development. Further explorations of the effects of GSK-3 β on cardiac function could help to identify ways to inhibit ischemia reperfusion without negatively affecting remodeling of the heart and systolic or diastolic function.

G-PROTEIN COUPLED RECEPTORS- G_Q/G_{11}-SIGNALING

Myocardial G-protein coupled receptors (GPCRs) [52] represent a group of seven transmembrane spanning-domain receptors, which play an important role in the regulation of acute hemodynamic effects within the cardiovascular system [53]. What are the downstream effectors of Gq signaling in the heart? A well-established target triggered by Gq/G11 is the activation of Phospholipase-Cβ (PLCβ), which leads to generation of diacylglycerols *via* an inositol 1,4,5-trisphosphate (IP3)-mediated increase in cytosolic $[Ca^{2+}]$. Another mediator of Gq-signaling that has become the focus of recent investigations is the protein kinase C (PKC family) that is comprised of at least 12 members. PKC activation results in translocation of these enzymes to isoform-specific intracellular locations [53] and binding to isoform-specific anchoring proteins labeled as receptors for activated C kinases (RACKs) [54]. Although multiple studies implicate the various PKC isoforms in the pathogenesis of ischemia reperfusion injury, the definite role of each isoform has not been fully elucidated. Reports based on *in vitro* studies have demonstrated that PKC-α and PKC-ε are involved in the ischemic preconditioning of the human myocardium with PKC-ε upstream and PKC-α downstream of mitochondrial potassium sensitive ATP (mitoKATP) channels [55]. Studies employing genetic ablation of single PKC-isoforms are likely to be limited by isoforms crosstalk and overlapping functions, whereas effects of genetic over-expression of individual isoforms may be perturbed by altered intracellular locations compared to endogenous proteins. Thus targeting of intracellular PKC-docking sites seems to be a promising approach for the investigation of specific PKC isoforms.

Consistent with these findings, over-expression of muscle ring finger protein-1 (MURF-1) as well as dominant negative inhibition of focal adhesion kinase (FAK), blunt adrenergic ERK1/ 2 activation and ERK dependent reperfusion injury. Another downstream target of PKC-ε is protein kinase D1 (PKD-1) [56]. Upon stimulation of GPCR agonist PKD-1 is activated by PKCε. Besides modifying PKC signaling Gq/ G11 proteins also modulate the P13K/Akt signaling pathway via interaction with the catalytic P13K subunit p110Y [57, 58]. P110Y was shown to participate in two distinct signalling pathways (1) a kinase dependent pathway that controls PKB/Akt as well as MAPK phosphorylation, and seems to be bene-ficial in the ischemia-induced injury [59] and (2) a kinase-independent activity that negatively modulates cardiac contractility. Specific inhibition of this maladaptive conse-quence of P110Y activation could be a promising goal of future therapeutic strategies to prevent the transition from ischemic injury to heart failure. In summary, these data demons-trate a crucial role of G_q/G_{11} in mediating maladaptive cardiac response to pathological stress stimuli.

Phosphorylation and Inactivation of the Pro-Apoptotic Proteins

Activation of the PI3K-Akt or the MEK 1/2-Erk 1/2 cascades phosphorylates the pro-apoptotic protein BAD, either directly [60] or indirectly *via* the recruitment of distal signaling moieties such as the 70-kDA ribosomal protein S6 kinase (p70S6K) [61] or the p90 ribosomal S6 kinase (p90RSK) [62]. Phosphorylation of BAD results in its binding to 14-3-3 protein family which sequesters it from its mitochondrial target, thereby preventing apoptosis [63]. In response to an apoptotic stimulus, the pro-apoptotic protein, Bax, under-goes a conformational change that allows it to translocate to the mitochondria [64, 65], where it induces mitochondrial cytochrome *c* release by either forming a pore in the outer mitochondrial membrane itself or by interacting with and opening the mitochondrial permeability transition pore (mPTP) [66]. Activation of either the PI3K-Akt or the Erk 1/2 pathway inhibits the conformational change in BAX required for its translocation to the mitochondria, therefore preventing apoptosis [64, 65, 67]. Withdrawal of survival factors results in the expression de novo of the pro-apoptotic protein, BIM [67]. Weston and coworkers [67] demonstrated that the inhibition of either the PI3K-Akt or the Erk 1/2 pathways resulted in an increase in BIM expression, implying that these pathways may exert an inhibitory influence on BIM. By phosphorylating Mdm2, activation of the PI3K-Akt pathway targets the pro-apoptotic protein, p53, for degradation, thereby preventing apoptosis [68].

Inhibiting Mitochondrial Cytochrome-c Release, Phosphorylating and Inactivating Caspases

Kennedy and associates [69] found that Akt was able to inhibit mitochondrial cytochrome *c* release and maintain mitochondrial membrane potential, independent of BAD. One potential route for mitochondrial cytochrome *c* release into the cytosol is through the opening of the mPTP [70]. Based on this observation, it would be reasonable to postulate that Akt may actually suppress cytochrome *c*-induced apoptosis by inhibiting opening of the mPTP, thereby retaining cytochrome *c* within the mitochondrial inter-membranous space.

Given that mitochondrial cytochrome *c* is required to activate caspases, the findings of this study suggest that Erk 1/2 activation is able to inhibit cytochrome *c*-induced caspase activation. A potential explanation for this may be that up-regulation of the Erk 1/2 cascade inactivates one component of the caspase cascade, a proposition which is supported by the finding that Erk 1/2 kinase activation has been shown to inhibit apoptosis, by inhibiting caspase 3 activation in haematopoietic cells [71]. Furthermore, by phosphorylating and inactivating pro-caspase 9, Akt activation can suppress the mitochondrial apoptotic death pathway [72]. In addition to influencing components of the apoptotic signaling pathway, activation of these kinase cascades may also induce cellular protection through the phosphorylation and activation of non-apoptotic proteins.

Transcriptional Regulation by ROS

We have previously demonstrated during blood recirculation that there is an increased production of superoxide ($O_2^{\cdot}$) and peroxynitrite ($ONOO^{-}$) that were associated with a reduction in antioxidant capacity, proinflammatory cytokines and attenuation of complement activity in ischemic blood [17,18]. It was further reported that blockade of NO attenuated TNF-α, but enhanced IL-6 turnover, suggesting a possible post-transcriptional regulation by these oxidant species. These results contribute to the understanding of the mechanism of extracorporeal blood circulation-induced tissue damage and may represent a potential therapeutic target for the inflammatory process induced by ischemia-reperfusion [73].

FUNCTIONAL ADAPTATION TO OXIDATIVE STRESS BY MEMORY T CELLS

Although the pathogenic role of T cells in cardiovascular diseases is well established, the complex function of the various T cell subsets in these disorders is far from clear. Available evidence suggests that the release of ROS by T cells may serve as an anti-atherogenic process [74, 75]. In contrast, evidence suggests that the activation of the inflammatory

CD4+CD28− T cell subsets may propagate ischaemia reperfusion injury [74, 75]. The dynamics of T cell response within the plaque are still poorly understood, with both antigen-dependent (e.g., heat shock proteins, oxidized lipoproteins, different microbial antigens) and antigen-independent (e.g., IL-7 and -15) stimuli being involved. Interestingly, T cell subsets that produce the inflammatory cytokine CCR7 potentially play a role in the promotion of T cell infiltration and inflammation within the atherosclerotic lesion [74-76].

We thus suggest that the balance between antioxidant and oxidant molecules may be critical in conferring sensitivity, or resistance, to myocardial protection as a feature that may be driven by oxidative stress [77]. Further studies are however, needed to expand our understanding of how oxidative stress impacts on the T cells signalling pathways. It would be very exciting and informative if we could understand how the critical components of the signalling pathways are genetically manipulated probably by deletion or other types of mutations.

PHOSPHORYLATION OF FACTORS CONCERNED WITH THE REGULATION OF GENE EXPRESSION

Akt phosphorylates and activates IKK-α, which leads to the activation and translocation of NF-κB to the nucleus, where it acts as a transcription factor for a variety of survival pathways [78]. The contribution of NF-κB to apoptotic cell death during the reperfusion phase is inconclusive; with studies showing it to be anti-apoptotic [79], while others suggesting that it has a pro-apoptotic action [80]. In parallel to this the emerging concept of the contribution of NO to systemic inflammatory response and its effect is regulated by the downstream redox-sensitive transcription signaling pathway has opened a new venue. In this context, we recently reported that the inflammatory response to extracorporeal circulation of blood is mainly mediated by NO through a mechanism that involves the activation of the transcription factor NF-κB [81]. Therefore, the modulation of NO production and the downstream signaling pathway *via* NF-κB may represent new therapeutic targets for reducing inflammation during CPB and the derived cardiac and systemic complications.

Activation of Complement Dependent Pathways

The complement system is a major constituent of the humoral branch of the immune system and is a complex cascade of protein that are activated in 3 distinct ways, designated the classical, alternative and lectin pathways. Activation of classical pathway is initiated by C1q binding to antigen-antibody complexes, whereas activation of the alternative or lectin pathway is antibody independent [82]. The alternative pathway is activated by spontaneously cleaved C3 or by C3b generated by one of the other pathways [83]. The lectin pathway is activated by mannose binding lectin (MBL) interacting with its ligand leading to activation of two MBL-associated serine proteases (MASPs) [84, 85].

As well as its purpose in complement activation, MBL also functions to promote opsono-phagocytosis, control of inflammatory response (by modulating cytokine release from monocytes), and promotion of apoptosis (demonstrated by its binding to apoptotic T-cells) [86]. In complement activation MBL acts together with MASPs in a similar fashion to the C1q, C1r and C1s components of the classical pathway [87]. To date three MASPs have been identified; MASP-1, MASP-2 and MASP-3 as well as a non-enzymatic protein known as the MBL-associated protein of 19 kDa (MAp19). Of these four proteins it is MASP-2 that has been identified as combining with MBL to play a role in the activation of complement components C4 and C2 in ischemia reperfusion mechanism [88].

There is evidence that the complement system is activated after ischaemia-reperfusion where studies have shown localization of various complement components within the ischemic tissue and that protection from ischemia-reperfusion injury can be achieved by complement depletion [89]. Moreover it has also been demonstrated that blocking the MBL pathway by using monoclonal antibodies against MBL protects the heart against ischemia-reperfusion injury [90]. Other more recent studies involving MBL depletion have supported the above observations by establishing that the lectin pathway also initiates complement activation after hypoxia-reoxygenation in an experimental model using human endothelial cells [91]. Despite this evidence it is still not clear whether ROS and components of the blood complement pathways interact during ischemia-reperfusion injury. We have recently reported that there is some specific role of ROS in generating molecular modifications in the key components of the pathways of complement activation that may affect overall complement reactivity [12]. This may suggest that ROS plays an important role in regulating complement activation independently of the classical and MBL pathways and that increased activities may be attributable to a direct effect on the alternate pathway, a feature that can have implications on the overall therapeutic strategy.

PROTECTING THE HEART AGAINST ISCHEMIA REPERFUSION INJURY

Careful examination of the literature has identified reported patents (Table **1**) that could be effective and specific in reducing/ mediating the ischemia-reperfusion injury for future clinical use. This includes several agents that may modulate complement-mediated inflammation exacerbated by tissue injury *via* ischemic necrosis. Others have been hypothesized to attenuate reperfusion-induced cell death *via* the various anti-apoptotic mechanisms listed previously and may operate via the activation of the pro-survival kinase cascades, during the first few minutes of reperfusion, following a lethal ischemic insult [92]. The activation of these pro-survival kinase pathways *via* the PI3K-Akt and Erk 1/2 cascades at the time of reperfusion appears to be sufficient stimuli to induce a cardio-protective response. We focus therefore in this review on those therapeutic strategies that have been shown to protect the heart when given during the reperfusion phase, and whose mechanism of protection has been linked to activation of the pro-survival kinase cascades.

Table 1. Published Patents of Compounds Useful in Reducing Ischaemia-Reperfusion Injury in Ischemic Heart Disease

Compound	Effect	Inventors	US Patent	Publication Date
Thrombopoietin	Therapeutic or prophylactic treatment method of ischemia, such as due to myocardial infarction, by administering thrombopoietin, alone or in combination with other drugs, to a patient suffering from or at risk of cardiac injury, such as myocardial ischemia. The thrombopoietin is administered in a concentration such that the subject's platelet count or production of platelets is not significantly affected.	Baker JE, Yang S [148]	20070173449	2007-07-26

Compound	**Effect**	**Inventors**	**US Patent**	**Publica-tion Date**
Seventeen amino acid peptide (Peptide P)	Peptide P, having the amino acid sequence Tyr-D-Ala-Phe-Ala-Asp-Val-Ala-Ser-Thr-Ile-Gly-Asp-Phe-His-Ser-Ile-NH2-SEQ ID NO: 1, is useful to treat ischemia.	Oeltgen PR, Kindy MS. [149]	6967192	2005-11-22
Botulinum toxin	The methods include a step of administering an effective amount of a botulinum toxin directly to a blood vessel of a mammal thereby treating a cardiovascular disease.	Brooks GF, Donovan S. [150]	6767544	2004-07-27
Adenosine receptor agonists and antagonists	This comprises the simultaneous administration of specific A3/A1 receptor agonists, to patients suffering from ischemic damage or at risk for the same. In yet another embodiment of the invention, a binary conjugate which acts as an agonist for the A3 receptor and an antagonist at the A2a receptor, is administered to reduce or prevent ischemic damage to the heart.	Liang BT, Jacobson KA. [151]	6586413	2003-07-01
Peptide dimers as agonists of the erythropoietin (EPO) receptor	Peptide dimers as agonists of the erythropoietin (EPO) receptor, and associated methods of synthesis and use	Balu P [152]	6703480	2004-03-09
Orally active A1 adenosine receptor agonists	Esters of N^6 -oxa, thia, thioxa and azacycloalkyl substituted adenosine derivatives, selective for adenosine type 1 receptor agonists that are useful for the treatment cardiovascular diseases.	Blackburn B K, Melville C, Zablocki JA, Palle VP, Elzein EO, Wang L. [153]	6576619	2003-06-10
Nitroxyl Anion Donors	The present invention relates to the administration of a nitroxyl anion donating compound prior to ischemia to attenuate ische-mia/reperfusion injury. Accordingly, nitroxyl anion donating compounds such as Angeli's salt would be useful treatment agents to prevent or protect against such adverse conditions.	Wink DA, Feelisch M, Pagliaro P, Kass DA, Paolocci N, Miranda KM, Fukuto JM. [154]	0038947A1	2003-06-16
Deltorphins	The invention relates to the use of deltorphins to treat cerebral ischemia and ischemic heart disease	Oeltgen PR, Kindy MS, Bishop PD [155]	6294519B1	2001-09-25
Method for the prevention of apoptosis	Heparin reduces ischemia-reperfusion injury to myocardium by disrupting multiple levels of the inflammatory cascade, including the novel obser-vation that heparins inhibit activation of the pro-inflammatory transcription factor NF-kappa B.	Kennedy TP. [156]	6489311	2000-05-02
NO donors	Disclosed herein are compositions containing NO donors, inhibitors of iNOS induction, and endopeptidase inhibitors, and methods for their use for combating injury induced by ischemia and reperfusion following ischemic episodes.	Singh I. [157]	5912019	1999-06-15

Compound	Effect	Inventors	US Patent	Publication Date
Adenosine agonists	Useful as antihypertensive, cardioprotective, anti-ischemic, and anti-lipolytic agents, pharmaceutical compositions including such compounds, and their use in treating hypertension, myocardial ischemia, ameliorating ischemic injury and myocardial infarct size consequent to myocardial ischemia, hyperlipidemia and hypercholesterolemia are claimed.	Spada AP, Fink CA, Myers MR. [158]	5736554	1998-04-07
2, N^6-disubstituted adenosines, tri-O-ester derivatives	The compounds have been found useful for treating cardiovascular ischaemia.	Lau J, Knutsen LJS, Sheardown M, Hansen AJ. [159]	5484774	1996-01-16
Compound for reducing myocardial reperfusion injury	This invention relates to a method to treat a heart attack victim to reduce heart muscle damage. In particular, the invention relates to a met Grant Statement This research was supported in part by the National Institute of Health, Grant R01 HL40892-01.	Forman MB, Jackson EK. [160]	5206222	1993-04-27
Composition for treatment of ischemic disorder in organs	The present invention relates to a pharmaceutical composition for the prophylaxis and treatment of ischemic disorder in mammalian organs which contains, as an ingredient, a compound of the formula: ##STR1## wherein R_1, R_2 and R_3 are independently the methyl group or a hydrogen atom, or a salt thereof.	Shimamoto N, Ogata K. [161]	4948786	1990-08-14
Complement inhibitors	Inulin poly(H-sulfate) and salts therefore useful as complement inhibitors.	Nair VG, Joseph JP, Bernstein S. [162]	4021545	1977-05-03

Protection by Activation of the PI3K-Akt and Erk 1/2 Pathways

Jonassen and coworkers [93] demonstrated a reduction in infarct size associated with the administration of glucose- insulin-potassium (GIK) at the time of reperfusion, and in studies using cardiomyocytes subjected to hypoxia, the authors further demonstrated that insulin given, at the time of reoxygenation, attenuated the apoptotic and necrotic components of cell death [94]. Insulin-mediated cardioprotection was also shown to correlate with phosphorylation of Akt and BAD, with insulin inducing phosphorylation of Akt and BAD to a level greater than that observed in control hearts [95]. Early reperfusion of insulin was reported to limit infarct size, an effect that was abrogated in the presence of both wortmannin (the PI3K inhibitor) and rapamycin (the mTOR-p70S6K inhibitor). In this study it was also shown that 15 min administration of insulin was sufficient to induce protection. Furthermore, early reperfusion of insulin was essential, as delaying its administration to 15 min after the onset of reperfusion, was not associated with protection. The fact that insulin has to be present in the first few minutes of reperfusion to induce protection lends support to the hypothesis that insulin protects at reperfusion by inhibiting opening of the mPTP, as opening of the latter has been shown to mediate cell death in the first few minutes of reperfusion [95]. A study by Gao *et al.* [96] has also implicated eNOS, another downstream target of Akt phosphorylation, in insulin-mediated cardio-protection at reperfusion.

In the isolated perfused rat heart, the administration of insulin like growth factor-1 (IGF-1) at reperfusion induced cardio-protection that was sensitive to wortmannin [97]. Studies in transgenic mice over-expressing IGF-1 were found to have a higher basal activation of Akt and, at reperfusion, the level of Akt activation was amplified even further [98].

In these mice, the increased levels of Akt activation were demonstrated to correlate with protection and were also shown to be wortmannin-sensitive [98]. Downstream of these kinase cascades, BAD [99], Bax, caspase 3 [100] and p70S6K have been implicated in IGF-1-induced cellular protection.

Protection by Recruiting PI3K-Akt and Erk 1/2 Signaling Cascades

Transforming growth factor-β1 (TGF-β1) is a cytokine that regulates cell growth and differentiation and modulates apoptosis in many cell types. The cardio-protective properties of TGF-β1 were first investigated in the early 1990s by Lefer *et al.* [101] who demonstrated protection against ischaemia-reperfusion injury in the rat heart *ex vivo* and *in vivo* and that TGF-β1-induced protection was demonstrated to be dependent on the Erk 1/2 cascade [102]. Similarly, cardiotrophin-1 (CT-1) is a member of the interleukin-6 (IL-6) family of cytokines and has been shown to be cardio-protective, exerting an anti-apoptotic effect in response to serum withdrawal in cardiac myocytes *via* an Erk 1/2-dependent pathway [103]. Urocortin, a peptide related to hypothalamic corticotrophin releasing factor, is released by myocytes in response to stressful stimuli such as ischemia [104]. Using neonatal rat myocytes, Brar *et al.* [105] demonstrated that after a prolonged episode of hypoxia, the presence of urocortin, at the time of reoxygenation, prevented cell death, by an anti-apoptotic action. Furthermore, activation of the PI3 kinase-Akt cascade has also been implicated in urocortin-mediated protection [98]. In this study, urocortin-mediated protection against hypoxia-reoxygenation injury was abrogated in rat myocytes treated with the specific PI3K inhibitors, wortmannin or LY294002. In addition, urocortin-induced protection in the same setting was abrogated in neonatal rat myocytes possessing a dominant negative mutation of PI3K-Akt [106].

Fibroblast growth factor-2 (also known as basic fibroblast growth factor, FGF) is a polypeptide growth factor, which has been shown to modulate cell proliferation, survival and apoptosis [107]. FGF has been demonstrated to induce cardio-protection, when administered during the reperfusion phase in a rat model of myocardial infarction in a nitric oxide dependent manner [108] and has been associated with attenuation of apoptotic cell death [109]. Studies have implicated PKC and the Erk 1/2 pathway in FGF-mediated cardio-protection [110].

Treatment with angiotensin-converting enzyme inhibitors (ACE-I) has been linked to cardio-protection in the setting of ischemia-reperfusion injury [111]. Studies have demonstrated that ACE-I-induced cardio-protection is mediated by bradykinin (acting at the B2 receptor) and is dependent on nitric oxide [112]. Interestingly, it has been shown that Gq-protein receptors, such as the bradykinin B2 receptor signal through the PI3K pathway in the guinea pig heart [113]. Recently, a study using cultured bovine aortic endothelial cells has shown that bradykinin can activate Erk 1/2 and eNOS activation, independent of the PI3-Akt pathway [114]. This suggests that the Erk 1/2 kinase pathway may also contribute to bradykinin-mediated cardio-protection at reperfusion. Xu *et al.* [115] demonstrated that AMP579 (an adenosine A1/A2a receptor agonist) given during the reperfusion phase limited infarct size using an *in vivo* rabbit heart model of ischemia-reperfusion injury.

PROTECTION AT REPERFUSION BY INHIBITION OF COMPLEMENT ACTIVATION

Carotenoids are a naturally occurring group of compounds that possess antioxidant properties and are known to be physical quenchers of singlet oxygen, as well as chain terminators of lipid peroxidation in cell membranes and intracellular membrane structures [116]. Most natural carotenoids display poor aqueous solubility and tend to form aggregates in solution. Disodium disuccinate astaxanthin (DDA; Cardax) is a water-dispersible synthetic carotenoid that rapidly and preferentially associates with serum albumin, thereby preventing the formation of supramolecular complexes and facilitating its efficacy after parenteral administration. DDA has been well characterized as a direct scavenger of biologically produced aqueous-phase super-oxide anion by electron paramagnetic resonance spectroscopy [117]. Coupled with the well established antioxidant ability of carotenoids, suggested that the mechanism(s) of action by which DDA reduces the tissue damage associated with reperfusion injury may include both antioxidant and anti-complement components [118].

Increasingly, there is interest in opportunities for protecting the myocardium in the ischemia/reperfusion setting, especially in the context of mechanical intervention where distal coronary embolization and resulting endothelial and myocytes dysfunction occur. It is well recognized that the inflammatory response accompanying myocardial ischemia and reperfusion plays a significant role in these phenomena and that activation of complement is a key component of this response [119]. Although the link between higher levels of inflammatory biomarkers and outcome in acute coronary syndromes is clear, whether and how modulation of inflammation might improve outcome is unknown.

Previously, two phase 2 interventions using humanized antibodies targeting leukocyte adhesion molecules in patients with myocardial infarction (MI) have failed to demonstrate clinical efficacy despite promising animal experimental data [120, 121]. Experimental data by Granger *et al.* that explored the role of pexelizumab, a monoclonal antibody against the C5 complement component as adjunctive therapy to primary PCI in 960 patients with ST elevation acute MI presenting within 6 hours of symptom onset in the Myocardial infarction treated with Angioplasty (COMMA) trial [27] indicated that although there was no reduction in the primary end point of MI size as assessed by CK-MB AUC, an unexpected dose-dependent reduction in 90-day mortality was observed. Whereas this mortality benefit was independent of a major impact on myocardial infarct size inhibiting complement activity might reduce mortality through attenuation of the inflammatory cascade that follows ischemic reperfusion or by reducing apoptosis [122]. This latter effect is an attractive hypothesis given that apoptosis has been identified as an important contributor to ultimate cell death in experimental MI; it is a significant determinant of remodeling and infarct healing in animal models, and complement has been shown to attenuate apoptosis in these models [123].

Protection by Soluble Complement Receptor Type-1

The complement system is an important mediator of the acute inflammatory response and an effective inhibitor of complement activation would suppress tissue damage in ischemia reperfusion injury. Such an inhibitor might be found among the endogenous regulatory proteins of complement that block the enzymes that activate C3 and C5. Of these proteins, complement receptor type 1 (CR1; CD35) has the most inhibitory potential, but its restriction to a few cell types limits its function *in vivo* [124]. This limitation was overcome by the recombinant soluble human CR1, sCRI, which lacks the transmembrane and cytoplasmic domains. The sCR1 bivalent bound dimeric forms of its ligand, C3b and methylamine-treated C4 (C4-ma) promoted their inactivation by sCRI factor-1 [124, 125]. It is reported that sCR1 had complement inhibitory and anti-inflammatory activities in a rat model of reperfusion injury of ischemic myocardium, reducing myocardial infarction size by 44% thus demonstrating that sCR1 as a potential agent for the suppression of complement dependent tissue injury in ischemia-reperfusion [124]. Similar to that TP10, another soluble complement receptor 1 had been shown to inhibit C3 and C5 convertase *in vitro* and *in vivo*, thus blocking activation of the 3 arms of the complement cascade at the level of C3 and C5 activation [125-127].

EMERGING POTENTIAL FOR PATENTS IN AVOIDING ISCHEMIA REPERFUSION INJURY

Ischemia-reperfusion injury is a multifactorial mechanism as explained earlier. Though many drugs have improved the treatment of cardiovascular disorders during the past decades, the quest for a novel treatment option has now shifted towards ischemia-reperfusion as the promising target, since this approach might provide the opportunity to prevent redox-inflammatory disorder and heart failure. In this context, patents with potential clinical use are still lacking and in this review we focus on the emerging potentials for new "drugable" targets for anti-ischemia-reperfusion therapies.

Polymers Incorporating Nitric Oxide Releasing/ Generating Substances

Diazeniumdiolates are compounds containing the X-[N(O)NO]$^-$ structural unit that as a class offer many advantages as tools for probing the roles of nitric oxide (NO) in biological redox injury (Fig. **3**) [128]. Available examples in which X is a secondary amine group spontaneously generate up to two molecules of NO per [N(O)NO]$^-$ unit when dissolved in aqueous media; their half-lives range from 2 s (for X = L-prolyl) to 20 h [for X =

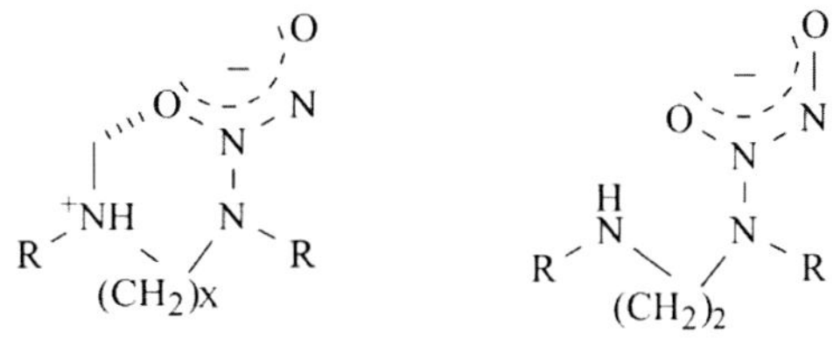

(A) **I.** **II.**

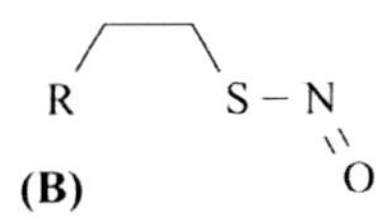

(B)

Fig. (3). Generic structures of two common NO donors: (**A**) zwitterionic (I) and a cation-stabilized (II) diazeniumdiolates and (**B**) an *S*-nitrosothiol [128].

$(H_2NCH_2CH_2)_2N]$ at pH 7.4 and 37°C, and are in general rarely influenced by medium effects or metabolism. When X = O^- (Angeli's salt), first-order dissociation produces NO^- rather than NO, but the ion becomes an NO source on 1-electron oxidation; diazeniumdiolate-derived NO can also be used to generate reactive nitrogen/oxygen species with higher nitrogen oxidation states (+3 and +4) in the presence of selected oxidizing agents. The advantages of diazeniumdiolates in biomedical research are briefly illustrated with examples from the recent literature probing NO's role in inhibiting oxidative drug metabolism, radical-induced lipid oxidation, the cytotoxicity of reactive oxygen species, and ischemia-induced vascular reoxygenation injury [129, 130].

The second class of NO-donor that has been utilized in developing NO-releasing polymers is S-nitrosothiols (RSNOs). *S*-Nitrosothiols are thought to serve as a reservoir and transporter of NO within biological systems [131]. S-Nitroso-serum albumin and S-nitrosoglutathione (GSNO) are the two most abundant naturally occurring S-nitrosothiols present in circulating blood, and GSNO is also found within cells [132]. The S-NO bond can be cleaved to release NO by three known mechanisms [133]. Copper mediated decomposition requires Cu^{+2} to be reduced to Cu^{+1}. Copper (I) then reacts with the nitrosothiols to release NO, forming a sulfhydryl anion product and regenerating Cu^{+2} [134]. Ascorbate and free thiolate ions are sufficient reducing agents to generate Cu^{1+} from Cu^{2+} under physiological conditions. A second reported decomposition pathway of S-nitrosothiols is the direct reaction of ascorbate, at concentrations greater than mM level, to release NO and produce a free thiol and dehydroascorbate [135]. The third mechanism of decomposition that has been reported is homolytic cleavage of the S-NO bond by light, using either 330-350 or 550-600 nm, releasing NO and producing disulfide bonds from the parent thiols [136]. It has been reported that smooth muscle cell proliferation was inhibited in solution phase cell cultures and platelet adhesion was inhibited on collagen-coated slides in the presence of these NO releasing hydro-gels. The proposed application of these materials is photopolymerization around arteries for site-specific delivery of NO with the eventual target application aimed at preventing restenosis after balloon angioplasty.

Shishido and co-workers blended the S-nitrosothiol GSNO and S-nitroso-*N*-acetylcysteine (SNAC) into poly(ethylene oxide) and poly(propylene oxide) copolymers or PEG [137, 138] for targeted delivery of NO in biomedical applications. A significant limitation of all of these materials is the potential loss of the NO-donors *via* leaching of the water-soluble RSNO donors and their reaction by-products from the polymer matrix under physiological conditions. This problem would be exacerbated under flow conditions experience by intravascular devices or extracorporeal circuits. The authors suggest that one potential application of these materials may be as transdermal NO-delivery device which may be more practical than using the materials for implanted devices although leaching of components from the polymer system would still be problematic.

Novel Inhibitor of p38 MAP Kinase as an Anti-TNF-α Drug (TAK-715)

The p38 mitogen-activated protein (MAP) kinase has been implicated in the proinflammatory cytokine signal pathway, and its inhibitors are potentially useful for the treatment of redox mediated inflammation. Miwatashi and co workers have recently synthesized a novel series of 4-phenyl-5-pyridyl-1,3-thiazoles and evaluated their inhibition of p38 MAP kinase, lipopolysaccharide (LPS)-stimulated release of tumor necrosis factor-α (TNF-α) from human monocytic THP-1 cells *in vitro*, and LPS-induced TNF-α production *in vivo* in mice (Fig. **4**) [139]. During the course of the study, the authors reported that these compounds risk the inhibition of cytochrome P450 (CYP) isoforms by coordination of the 4-pyridyl nitrogen with heme iron. As a result, *N*-[4-[2-ethyl-4-(3-methylphenyl)-1,3-thiazol-5-yl]-2-pyridyl]benzamide (TAK-715) exhibited potent inhibitory activity in these assays (inhibition of p38 α, IC_{50} = 7.1 nM; LPS-stimulated release of TNF-α from THP-1, IC_{50} = 48 nM; LPS-induced TNF-α production in mice, 87.6% inhibition at 10 mg/kg, and no inhibitory activity for major CYPs, including CYP3A4. This compound also showed good bioavailability in mice and rats and significant efficacy in a rat adjuvant-induced arthritis model. Compound TAK-715 was selected as a clinical candidate and is now under clinical investigation for the treatment of cardiovascular disorder.

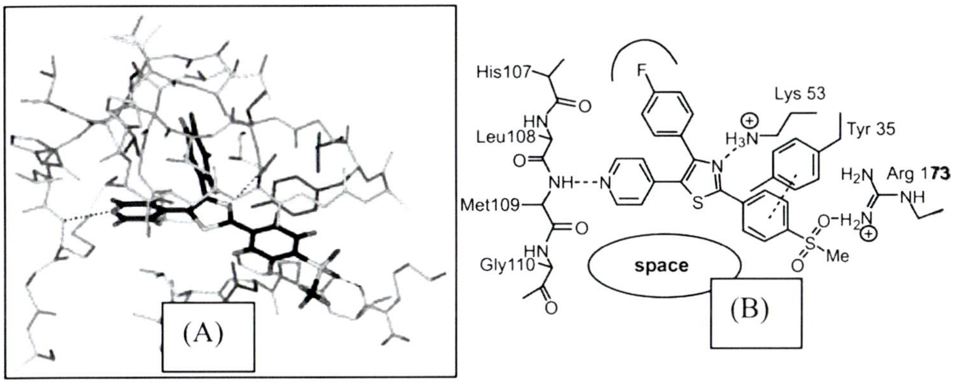

Fig. (4). Docking model of compound **1** (**A**) with p38 MAP kinase (**B**) [139].

Disodium Disuccinate Astaxanthin (Cardax™) on Multiple Independent Oxidative Stress Markers

Disodium disuccinate astaxanthin ('*rac*'-dAST; Cardax™) is a water-dispersible C40 carotenoid derivative [140] under development for oral and parenteral administration for cardioprotection of the at-risk ischemic cardiovascular patient (Fig. **5**). In experimental infarction models in animals (rats, rabbits, and dogs), significant myocardial salvage has been obtained, up to 100% at the appropriate dose in dogs. The documented mechanism of action *in vitro* includes direct scavenging of biologically produced superoxide anion *in vivo* in rabbits and the modulation of the serum complement activity has also been shown. A direct correlation between administration of the test compound in animals and reduction of multiple, independent markers of oxidative stress in serum was recently obtained in a rat experimental infarction model [141].

Extrapolation of the current mechanistic results to the human pathological situation may provide therapeutic efficacy in clinical indications including asthma, cardiovascular disease, and prostate cancer [142, 143]. Astaxanthin, the primary active antioxidant metabolite of Cardax™, may show improved efficacy over other chain-breaking antioxidants with activity against 5-LO (in particular vitamin E) [144] in the setting of cardiovascular disease, due to its excellent activity at low oxygen tension and low absolute physiologic concentration, and no demonstrated pro-oxidant activity at high oxygen tension to-date in model systems [145].

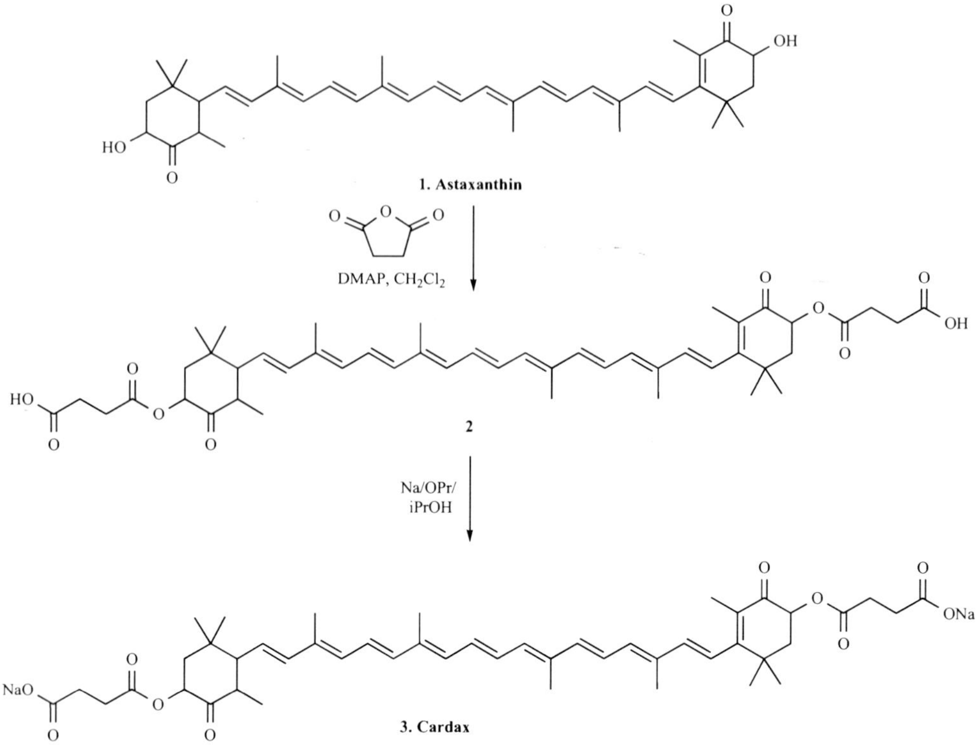

Fig. (5). Cardax™ ('racemic' disodium disuccinate astaxanthin; '*rac*'-dAST) was synthesized from crystalline astaxanthin [3*S*,3′*S*, 3*R*,3′*S*, 3*R*,3′*R* (1:2:1), a statistical mixture of stereoisomers obtained commercially [140].

Etanercept, a Soluble TNF Receptor (TNFR) Fusion Protein

Etanercept is a soluble TNF receptor (TNFR) fusion protein, initially developed and launched by Immunex for the treatment of early and moderate to severely active rheumatoid arthritis (RA) [Patents US375481; EU388846]. The drug was subsequently approved by the US FDA for use as a first-line therapy to treat patients with moderately to severely active RA [US375481]. However, recently the increasing understanding of the role of TNF in ischemia-reperfusion injury has led to its clinical assessment in this area. Following positive clinical results in phase II studies [US317562], [US315793], [US320666], [US359789], [US373980] in patients with chronic heart failure, etanercept entered phase III trials for this indication [US330068], and in 1997, US-patent 05605690 was issued to Immunex for methods of using etanercept to treat diseases mediated by TNF [146, 147].

CLINICAL IMPLICATIONS

Activation of the PI3K-Akt and Erk 1/2 kinase cascades appear to constitute a universal pro-survival kinase cascade mediating cardioprotection at reperfusion. However, it is interesting to note that the same kinase cascades have also been implicated in mediating the protection associated with the phenomenon of ischemic preconditioning (IPC) [163, 164]. In this scenario, activation of the kinase cascades occurs prior to the ischemic insult and acts as a preconditioning trigger and/or mediator for cardio-protection [165].

The evidence would tend to suggest that the pro-survival kinase cascades may therefore constitute a common path-way, mediating the cardioprotection induced by IPC on the one hand, as well as protecting the myocardium through their recruitment at the time of reperfusion on the other hand. However, the only direct evidence for this is largely with insulin-induced cardio-protection, and, therefore, more research is needed to elucidate whether the pro-survival kinase cascades actually constitute the common pathway for cardio-protection in these two settings.

We would therefore like to propose that therapeutic interventions which target and activate the pro-survival pathways during the reperfusion phase, can be used as an adjunct to current reperfusion therapy, and may provide an approach to salvaging viable myocardium and limiting infarct size in patients presenting with an acute myocardial infarction. Already, a large randomized control clinical study (named GIK II) is underway, examining the benefits of glucose insulin therapy (GIK) given at the time of reperfusion in patients presenting with an acute myocardial infarction [166].

An alternative strategy would be to investigate whether drugs that have been clearly demonstrated to be cardio-protective and are routinely used to treat chronic ischemic heart disease provide any benefit if given at the time of reperfusion. Clinical trials are required to investigate whether administration of these drugs, as an adjunct to current reperfusion therapy, offers protection against reperfusion injury following a myocardial infarction.

Recent studies have shown that fluoroscopic-guided intra-myocardial injection in the pig model is a feasible and safe procedure for targeting the delivery of therapeutic agents to the area of myocardium at risk from ischemia- reperfusion injury [167]. Therefore, the local delivery of growth factors themselves or the adenoviral vectors (carrying mutated genes which over-express growth factors) would provide a potential method for targeting and up-regulating these pathways in the clinical setting of reperfusion. Alternatively for patients undergoing an anticipated episode of ischemia-reperfusion injury, such as during CABG surgery or elective coronary angioplasty, gene transfer may be a possible method of delivering growth factors to myocardium at risk of lethal reperfusion-induced injury.

CURRENT & FUTURE DEVELOPMENTS

Recently, Tumor Necrosis Factor-alpha (TNF-α) and both of its cognate receptors have been identified in the myocardium and the ability of cardiomyocytes to produce TNF-α following ischemic injury has been demonstrated [168]. Although TNF-α signaling has been shown to modulate cardiac function and cardiomyocytes death [169] the role of this pleotropic cytokine in myocardial ischemia/ reperfusion injury remains controversial. Recent studies have revealed that TNF-α achieves this *via* the activation of nuclear factor-kappa-B (NF-κB) and the signal transducers and activators of transcription (STAT) family of transcription factors, leading to upregulation of the inducible iso-forms of nitric oxide synthase (iNOS) and NO itself [170, 171]. In general NO plays a protective function in the ischemia-reperfusion through multiple avenues but mostly *via* stimulation of sGC and production of cGMP-dependent protein kinase type-1 (PKG-I) as discussed earlier. In this regard, Pepys *et al.* [172] have shown that therapeutic inhibition of acute phase proteins that bind to ligands exposed in damaged tissue and those that activate complement may prove to be a promising new approach to cardioprotection.

More recently we have been able to demonstrate (unpublished work) the treatment of human blood with different concentrations of the NOS inhibitor revealed marked depletion of the inflammatory response (Fig. **6**). Further more, we demonstrated using a murine model of atherosclerosis that treatment with tea extract inhibited the production of both $ONOO^-$ and O_2^- and this led to elimination of oxidative stress-induced tissue damage (Fig. **7**).

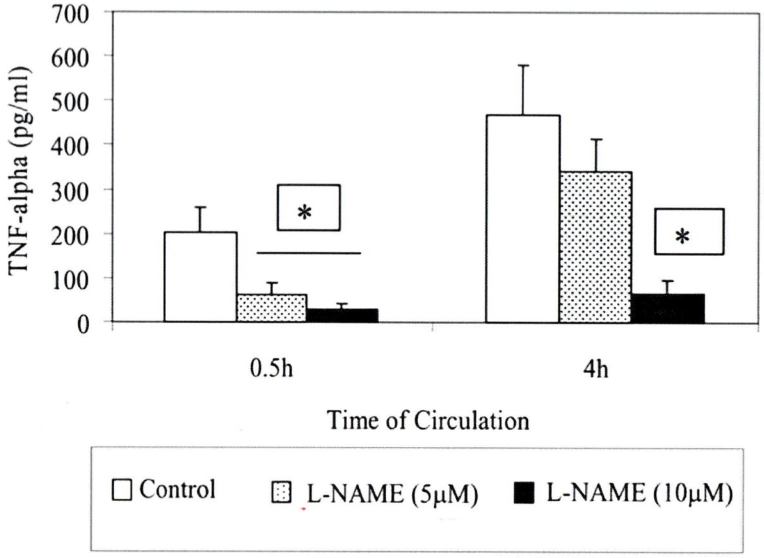

Fig. (6). Shows the levels of TNF-alpha in blood from healthy volunteers when treated with different concentrations of the NOS inhibitor L-NAME as compared with control at 0.5 and 4 h intervals. *P<0.05 compared with corresponding control values.

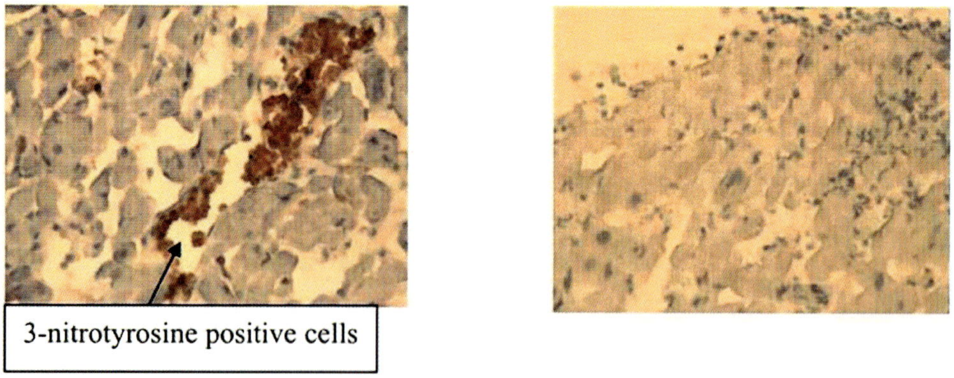

Fig. (7). (**A**) Shows immunohistological detection of ventricular myocardial cells staining positive (brown stain) for 3-nitrotyrosine, a known marker of oxidative stress-induced injury in a murine model of atherosclerosis. (**B**) Demonstrates the effectiveness of the tea plant extract (TE) in eliminating formation of 3-nitrotyrosine in the myocardium cells.

Hence, the inhibition of enzymes in blood that generate ROS may represent a novel approach for the effective reduction of systemic inflammatory reaction in patients undergoing cardiac surgery on cardiopulmonary bypass.

In conclusion, cardiovascular drug discovery remains a pivotal and rate-limiting step in the protracted process of clinical development and legislative review and regulation of novel therapeutics. A future direction of research is largely based on the discoveries highlighted in this review and that these should focus more on acceptable and safe replacements of physiological pathways during the early reperfusion phase. This affords an opportunity to attenuate reperfusion-induced injury, thereby salvaging viable myocardium and limiting infarct size.

ACKNOWLEDGEMENT

Special thanks to the Biomedical Research Department, Faculty of Medicine and Surgery, Lahore, Pakistan.

REFERENCES

[1] Park JL, Lucchesi BR. Mechanisms of myocardial reperfusion injury. Ann Thorac Surg 1999; 68: 1905-1912.

[2] Jolly SR, Kane WJ, Bailie MB, Abrams GD, Lucchesi BR. Canine myocardial reperfusion injury. Its reduction by the combined administration of superoxide dismutase and catalase. Circ Res 1984; 54: 277-285.

[3] Bolli R, Jeroudi MO, Patel BS, *et al.* Marked reduction of free radical generation and contractile dysfunction by antioxidant therapy begun at the time of reperfusion. Evidence that myocardial "stunning" is a manifestation of reperfusion injury. Circ Res 1989; 65: 607-612.

[4] Lauver DA, Lockwood SF, Lucchesi BR. Disodium Disuccinate Astaxanthin (Cardax) attenuates complement activation and reduces myocardial injury following ischemia/reperfusion. J Pharmacol Exp Ther 2005; 314: 686-692.

[5] Mehta JL, Nichols WW, Mehta P. Neutrophils as potential participants in acute myocardial ischaemia: relevance to reperfusion. J Am Coll Cardiol 1988; 11: 1309-1316.

[6] Mojcik CF, Levy JH. Aprotinin and the systemic inflammatory response after cardiopulmonary bypass. Ann Thorac Surg 2001; 71: 745-754.

[7] Kloner RA. Does reperfusion injury exist in humans? J Am Coll Cardiol 1993; 21: 537-545.

[8] Zhao ZQ, Nakamura M, Wang NP, *et al.* Dynamic progression of contractile and endothelial dysfunction and infarct extension in the late phase of reperfusion. J Surg Res 2000; 94: 133-134.

[9] Matsumura K, Jeremy RW, Schaper J, Becker LC. Progression of myocardial necrosis during reperfusion of ischemic myocardium. Circulation 1998; 97: 795-804.

[10] Hearse DJ. Reperfusion of the ischemic myocardium. J Mol Cell Cardiol 1977; 9: 605-606.

[11] Vanden Hoek TL, Shao Z, Li C, Zak R, Schumacker PT, Becker LB. Reperfusion injury on cardiac myocytes after simulated ischemia. Am J Physiol 1996; 270: 1334-1341.

[12] Elahi MM, Elahi M, Matata BM. Reactive oxidant species augment complement function in human blood independently of classical and MBL-pathways. Int J Mol Med Adv Sci 2005; 1: 382-391.

[13] Turner MW. The role of mannose-binding lectin in health and disease. Mol Immunol 2003; 40: 423-429.

[14] Weisman HF, Bartow T, Leppo MK, *et al.* Soluble human complement receptor type 1: *in vivo* inhibitor of complement suppressing post ischaemic myocardial inflammation and necrosis. Science 1990; 249: 146-151.

[15] Jordan JE, Montalto MC, Stahl GL. Inhibition of mannose-binding lectin reduces post-ischemic myocardial reperfusion injury. Circulation 2001; 104: 1413-1418.

[16] Collard CD, Vakeva A, Morrissey MA, *et al.* Complement activation after oxidative stress: role of the lectin complement pathway. Am J Pathol 2000; 156:1549-1556.

[17] Elahi MM, Matata BM. Blood-dependent redox activity during extracorporeal circulation in health and disease. Cardiology 2005; 1: 156-167.

[18] Elahi MM, Courtney JM, Matata BM. The interaction between reactive oxidant species and proinflammatory cytokines in human blood during extracorporeal circulation. Filtration 2005; 1: 89-94.

[19] Antoniades C, Tousoulis D, Tentolouris C, Toutouzas P, Stefanadis C. Herz Oxidative stress, antioxidant vitamins, and atherosclerosis. From basic research to clinical practice 2003; 28: 628-638.

[20] Clarke R, Armitage J. Antioxidant vitamins and risk of cardiovascular disease. Review of large-scale randomized trials. Cardiovasc Drugs Ther 2002; 16: 411-415.

[21] Fischer UM, Cox CS Jr, Allen SJ, Stewart RH, Mehlhorn U, Laine GA. The antioxidant N-acetylcysteine preserves myocardial function and diminishes oxidative stress after cardioplegic arrest. J Thorac Cardiovasc Surg 2003; 126: 1483-1488.

[22] Lassnigg A, Punz A, Barker R, *et al.* Influence of intravenous vitamin E supplementation in cardiac surgery on oxidative stress: a double-blinded, randomized, controlled study. Br J Anaesth 2003; 90: 148-154.

[23] Westhuyzen J, Cochrane AD, Tesar PJ, *et al.* Effect of preoperative supplementation with alpha-tocopherol and ascorbic acid on myocardial injury in patients undergoing cardiac operations. J Thorac Cardiovasc Surg 1997; 113: 942-948.

[24] Keith ME, Jeejeebhoy KN, Langer A, *et al.* A controlled clinical trial of vitamin E supplementation in patients with congestive heart failure. Am J Clin Nutr 2001; 73: 219-224.

[25] Maxwell SR, Lip GY. Free radicals and antioxidants in cardiovascular disease. Br J Clin Pharmacol 1997; 44: 307-317.

[26] Mahaffey KW, Granger CB, Nicolau JC, *et al.* and COMPLY Investigators. Effect of pexelizumab, an anti-C5 complement antibody, as adjunctive therapy to fibrinolysis in acute myocardial infarction: the COMPlement inhibition in myocardial infarction treated with thromboLYtics (COMPLY) trial. Circulation 2003; 108: 1176-1183.

[27] Granger CB, Mahaffey KW, Weaver WD, *et al.* and COMMA Investigators. Pexelizumab, an anti-C5 complement antibody, as adjunctive therapy to primary percutaneous coronary intervention in acute myocardial infarction: The Complement Inhibition in Myocardial Infarction Treated with Angioplasty (COMMA) Trial. Circulation 2003; 108: 1184-1190.

[28] Elahi MM, Naseem KM, Matata BM. Nitric oxide in blood. The nitrosative-oxidative disequilibrium hypothesis on the pathogenesis of cardiovascular disease. FEBS J 2007; 274: 906-923

[29] Elahi MM, Yii M, Matata BM. Significance of oxidants and inflammatory mediators in blood of patients undergoing cardiac surgery. J Cardiothorac Vasc Anesth 2008; 22: 455-467.

[30] Matata BM, Galinanes M. Cardiopulmonary bypass exacerbates oxidative stress but does not increase proinflammatory cytokine release in patients with diabetes compared with patients without diabetes: Regulatory effects of exogenous nitric oxide, J Thorac Cardiovasc Surg 2000; 120: 1-11.

[31] Elahi MM, Worner M, Khan JS, Matata BM Inspired Nitric Oxide and Modulation of Oxidative Stress during Cardiac Surgery. Curr Drug Saf. 2009, [Epub ahead of print].

[32] Cross TG, Scheel-Toellner D, Henriquez NV, Deacon E, Salmon M, Lord JM. Serine/threonine protein kinases and apoptosis. Exp Cell Res 2000; 256: 34-41.

[33] Mendelsohn ME. Viagra: now mending hearts. Nat Med 2005; 11: 115-116.

[34] Calderone A, Thaik CM, Takahashi N, Chang DL, Colucci WS. Nitric oxide, atrial natriuretic peptide, and cyclic GMP inhibit the growth-promoting effects of nor-epinephrine in cardiac myocytes and fibroblasts. J Clin Invest 1998; 101: 812-818.

[35] Wollert KC, Fiedler B, Gambaryan S, *et al.* Gene transfer of cGMP-dependent protein kinase I enhances the anti-hypertrophic effects of nitric oxide in cardiomyocytes. Hypertension 2002; 39: 87-92.

[36] Feil R, Lohmann SM, de Jonge H, Walter U, Hofmann F. Cyclic GMP-dependent protein kinases and the cardiovascular system: insights from genetically modified mice. Circ Res 2003; 93: 907-916.

[37] Fiedler B, Lohmann SM, Smolenski A, *et al.* Inhibition of calcineurin-NFAT hypertrophy signaling by cGMP-dependent protein kinase type I in cardiac myocytes. Proc Natl Acad Sci USA 2002; 99: 11363-11368.

[38] Cantley LC. The Phosphoinositide 3-kinase pathway. Science 2002; 296: 1655-1657.

[39] Cross TG, Scheel-Toellner D, Henriquez NV, Deacon E, Salmon M, Lord JM. Serine/threonine protein kinases and apoptosis. Exp Cell Res 2000; 256: 34-41.

[40] Latronico MV, Costinean S, Lavitrano ML, Peschle C, Condorelli G. Regulation of cell size and contractile function by AKT in cardiomyocytes. Ann N Y Acad Sci 2004; 101: 250-260.

[41] Matsui T, Rosenzweig A. Convergent signal transduction pathways controlling cardiomyocytes survival and function: the role of PI 3 kinase and Akt. J Mol Cell Cardiol 2005; 38: 63-71.

[42] Shioi T, McMullen JR, Kang PM, *et al.* Akt/protein kinase B promotes organ growth in transgenic mice. Mol Cell Biol 2002; 22: 2799-2809.

[43] Matsui T, Li L, Wu JC, *et al.* Phenotypic spectrum caused by transgenic over-expression of activated Akt in the heart. J Biol Chem 2002; 277: 22896-22901.

[44] McManus EJ, Alessi DR. TSC1-TSC2: a complex tale of PKB-mediated S6K regulation. Nat Cell Biol 2002; 4: 214-216.

[45] Tee AR, Fingar DC, Manning BD, Kwiatkowski DJ, Cantley LC, Blenis J. Tuberous sclerosis complex-1 and -2 gene products function together to inhibit mammalian target of rapamycin (mTOR)-mediated downstream signaling. Proc Natl Acad Sci USA 2002; 99:13571-13576.

[46] Proud CG. Ras, PI3-kinase and mTOR signaling in cardiac hypertrophy. Cardiovasc Res 2004; 63: 403-413.

[47] Morisco C, Zebrowski D, Condorelli G, Tsichlis P, Vatner SF, Sadoshima J. The Akt-glycogen synthase kinase 3beta pathway regulates transcription of atrial natriuretic factor induced by beta-adrenergic receptor stimulation in cardiac myocytes. J Biol Chem 2000; 275:14466-14475.

[48] Badorff C, Ruetten H, Mueller S, *et al.* Fas receptor signaling inhibits glycogen synthase kinase 3 beta and induces cardiac hypertrophy following pressure overload. J Clin Invest 2002; 109: 373-381.

[49] Morisco C, Seta K, Hardt SE, Lee Y, Vatner SF, Sadoshima J. Glycogen synthase kinase 3beta regulates GATA4 in cardiac myocytes. J Biol Chem 2001; 276: 28586-28587.

[50] Cohen P, Frame S. The renaissance of GSK3. Nat Rev Mol Cell Biol 2001; 2: 769-776.

[51] Michael A, Haq S, Chen X, *et al.* Glycogen synthase kinase-3beta regulates growth, calcium homeostasis, and diastolic function in the heart. J Biol Chem 2004; 279: 21383-21393.

[52] Li, Y.; Ruben, S.M.: US20056887683 (**2005**).

[53] Rockman HA, Koch WJ, Lefkowitz RJ. Seven-transmembrane-spanning receptors and heart function. Nature 2002; 415: 206-212.

[54] Mochly-Rosen D, Khaner H, Lopez J, Smith BL. Intracellular receptors for activated protein kinase C. Identification of a binding site for the enzyme. J Biol Chem 1991; 266:14866-14878.

[55] Hassouna A, Matata BM, Galinanes M. PKC-epsilon is upstream and PKC-alpha is downstream of mitoKATP channels in the signal transduction pathway of ischemic preconditioning of human myocardium. Am J Physiol Cell Physiol 2004; 287:1418-1425.

[56] Kedar V, McDonough H, Arya R, Li HH, Rockman HA, Patterson C. Muscle-specific RING finger 1 is a bona fide ubiquitin ligase that degrades cardiac troponin-I. Proc Natl Acad Sci USA 2004; 101:18135-18140.

[57] Heidkamp MC, Bayer AL, Scully BT, Eble DM, Samarel AM. Activation of focal adhesion kinase by protein kinase C epsilon in neonatal rat ventricular myocytes. Am J Physiol Heart Circ Physiol 2003; 285: 1684-1696.

[58] Iwata M, Maturana A, Hoshijima M, *et al.* PKCepsilon-PKD1 signaling complex at Z-discs plays a pivotal role in the cardiac hypertrophy induced by G-protein coupling receptor agonists. Biochem Biophys Res Commun 2005; 327: 1105-1113.

[59] Patrucco E, Notte A, Barberis L, *et al.* PI3K gamma modulates the cardiac response to chronic pressure overload by distinct kinase-dependent and -independent effects. Cell 2004; 118: 375-377.

[60] Datta SR, Dudek H, Tao X, *et al.* Akt phosphorylation of BAD couples survival signals to the cell-intrinsic death machinery. Cell 1997; 91: 231-241.

[61] Harada H, Andersen JS, Mann M, Terada N, Korsmeyer SJ. p70S6 kinase signals cell survival as well as growth, inactivating the pro-apoptotic molecule BAD. Proc Natl Acad Sci USA 2001; 98: 9666-9670.

[62] Tan Y, Ruan H, Demeter MR, Comb MJ. p90(RSK) blocks bad-mediated cell death *via* a protein kinase C-dependent pathway. J Biol Chem 1991; 274: 34859-34867.

[63] Zha J, Harada H, Yang E, Jockel J, Korsmeyer SJ. Serine phosphorylation of death agonist BAD in response to survival factor results in binding to 14-3-3 not BCL-X(L). Cell 1996; 87: 619-628.

[64] Yamaguchi H, Wang HG. The protein kinase PKB/Akt regulates cell survival and apoptosis by inhibiting Bax conformational change. Oncogene 2001; 20: 7779-7786.

[65] Tsuruta F, Masuyama N, Gotoh Y. The phosphatidylinositol 3-kinase (PI3K)-Akt pathway suppresses Bax translocation to mitochondria. J Biol Chem 2002; 277: 14040-14047.

[66] Marzo I, Brenner C, Zamzami N, *et al.* Bax and adenine nucleotide translocator cooperate in the mitochondrial control of apoptosis. Science 1998; 281: 2027-2031.

[67] Weston CR, Balmanno K, Chalmers C, *et al.* Activation of ERK1/2 by deltaRaf-1: ER* represses Bim expression independently of the JNK or PI3K pathways. Oncogene 2003; 22: 1281-1293.

[68] Mayo LD, Donner DB. A phosphatidylinositol 3-kinase/Akt pathway promotes translocation of Mdm2 from the cytoplasm to the nucleus. Proc Natl Acad Sci USA 2001; 98: 11598-11603.

[69] Kennedy SG, Kandel ES, Cross TK, Hay N. Akt/Protein kinase B inhibits cell death by preventing the release of cytochrome c from mitochondria. Mol Cell Biol 1999; 19: 5800-5890.

[70] Kroemer G, Dallaporta B, Resche-Rigon M. The mitochondrial death/life regulator in apoptosis and necrosis. Annu Rev Physiol 1998; 60: 619-622.

[71] Terada K, Kaziro Y, Satoh T. Analysis of Ras-dependent signals that prevent caspase-3 activation and apoptosis induced by cytokine deprivation in hematopoietic cells. Biochem Biophys Res Commun 2000; 267: 449-455.

[72] Cardone MH, Roy N, Stennicke HR, *et al.* Regulation of cell death protease caspase-9 by phosphorylation. Science 1998; 282: 1318-1321.

[73] Elahi MM, Matata BM, Galinanes M. Oxidant species are less effective in modulating proinflammatory cytokines turnover in ischaemic heart disease. J Mol Cell Cardiol 2004; 37: 245.

[74] Robertson AK, Hansson GK. T cells in atherogenesis: for better or for worse? Arterioscler Thromb Vasc Biol 2006; 26: 2421-2432.

[75] Valgimigli M, Agnoletti L, Curello S, Comini L, Francolini G, Mastrorilli F, Merli E, Pirani R, Guardigli G, Grigolato PG, Ferrari R. Serum from patients with acute coronary syndromes displays a proapoptotic effect on human endothelial cells. Circulation 2003; 107: 264-270.

[76] Daugherty A, Rateri DL. T lymphocytes in atherosclerosis: the yin-yang of Th1 and Th2 influence on lesion formation, Circ. Res 2002; 90: 1039-1040.

[77] Elahi MM, Matata BM. Functional adaptation to oxidative stress by memory T cells: an analysis of the role in the cardiovascular disease process. Biochem Biophys Res Commun. 2008; 376: 445-447.

[78] Romashkova JA, Makarov SS. NF-kappaB is a target of AKT in anti-apoptotic PDGF signalling. Nature 1999: 401: 86-90.

[79] Zingarelli B, Hake PW, Denenberg A, Wong HR. Sesquiterpene lactone parthenolide, an inhibitor of IkappaB kinase complex and nuclear factor-kappaB, exerts beneficial effects in myocardial reperfusion injury. Shock 2002: 17: 127-134.

[80] Zingarelli B, Hake PW, Yang Z, O'Connor M, Denenberg A, Wong HR. Absence of inducible nitric oxide synthase modulates early reperfusion-induced NF-kappaB and AP-1 activation and enhances myocardial damage. FASEB J 2002; 16: 327-332.

[81] Elahi MM, Matata BM, Galinanes M. Nitric Oxide modulates the inflammatory response to extracorporeal circulation of blood through activation of NF-Kappa B. Circulation 2004; 101: S1709.

[82] Walport MJ. Complement: first two parts. N Engl J Med 2001; 344: 1058-1066.

[83] Xu Y, Narayana SVL, Volanakis JE. Structural biology of the alternative pathway convertase. Immunol Rev 2001; 180: 123-125.

[84] Theil S, Vorup-Jensen T, Stover CM, *et al.* A second serine protease associated with mannan-binding lectin that activates complement. Nature 1997; 386: 506-510.

[85] Petersen SV, Thiel S, Jensenius JC. The Mannan-Binding Lectin Pathway of Complement Activation: Biology and Disease Association. Mol Immunol 2001; 38: 133-139.

[86] Turner MW. The Role of Mannose-Binding Lectin in Health and Disease. Mol Immunol 2003; 40: 423-429.

[87] Gadjeva M, Thiel S, Jensenius JC. The Mannan-Binding-Lectin Pathway of the Innate Immune Response. Curr Opin Immunol 2001; 13: 74-78.

[88] Schwaeble W, Dahl MR, Thiel S, Stover C, Jensenius JC. The mannan-binding lectin-associated serine proteases (MASPs) and Map19: four components of the lectin pathway activation complex encoded by two genes. Immunology 2002; 205: 455-456.

[89] Pangburn MK, Rawal N. Structure and function of complement C5 convertase enzymes. Biochem Soc Trans 2002; 30: 1006-1010.

[90] Weisman HF, Bartow T, Leppo MK, *et al.* Soluble human complement receptor type 1: *in vivo* inhibitor of complement suppressing post ischaemic myocardial inflammation and necrosis. Science 1990; 249: 146-151.

[91] Jordan JE, Montalto MC, Stahl GL. Inhibition of Mannose-Binding Lectin Reduces Post-ischemic Myocardial Reperfusion Injury. Circulation 2001; 104: 1413-1418.

[92] Yellon DM, Baxter GF. Reperfusion injury revisited: is there a role for growth factor signaling in limiting lethal reperfusion injury? Trends Cardiovasc Med 1999; 9: 245-249.

[93] Jonassen AK, Aasum E, Riemersma RA, Mjos OD, Larsen TS. Glucose-insulin-potassium reduces infarct size when administered during reperfusion. Cardiovasc Drugs Ther 2000; 14: 615-623.

[94] Jonassen AK, Brar BK, Mjos OD, Sack MN, Latchman DS, Yellon DM. Insulin administered at reoxygenation exerts a cardioprotective effect in myocytes by a possible anti-apoptotic mechanism. J Mol Cell Cardiol 2000; 32: 757-764.

[95] Jonassen AK, Sack MN, Mjos OD, Yellon DM. Myocardial protection by insulin at reperfusion requires early administration and is mediated *via* Akt and p70s6 kinase cell-survival signaling. Circ Res 2001; 89: 1191-1198.

[96] Gao F, Gao E, Yue TL, *et al.* Nitric oxide mediates the antiapop-totic effect of insulin in myocardial ischemia-reperfusion: the roles of PI3-kinase, Akt, and endothelial nitric oxide synthase phosphorylation. Circulation 2002; 105: 1497-1502.

[97] Otani H, Yamamura T, Nakao Y, *et al.* Insulin-like growth factor-I improves recovery of cardiac performance during reperfusion in isolated rat heart by a wortmannin-sensitive mechanism. J Cardiovasc Pharmacol 2000; 35: 275-281.

[98] Yamashita K, Kajstura J, Discher DJ, *et al.* Reperfusion-activated Akt kinase prevents apoptosis in transgenic mouse hearts overexpressing insulin-like growth factor-1. Circ Res 2001; 88: 609-614.

[99] Bai H, Pollman MJ, Inishi Y, Gibbons GH. Regulation of vascular smooth muscle cell apoptosis. Modulation of bad by a phosphatidylinositol 3-kinase-dependent pathway. Circ Res 1999; 85: 229-237.

[100] Wang L, Ma W, Markovich R, Chen JW, Wang PH. Regulation of cardiomyocytes apoptotic signaling by insulin-like growth factor I. Circ Res 1998; 83: 516-522.

[101] Lefer AM, Tsao P, Aoki N, Palladino, Jr. MA. Mediation of cardioprotection by transforming growth factor-beta. Science 1990; 249: 61-64.

[102] Baxter GF, Mocanu MM, Brar BK, Latchman DS, Yellon DM. Cardioprotective effects of transforming growth factor-beta1 during early reoxygenation or reperfusion are mediated by p42/p44 MAPK. J Cardiovasc Pharmacol 2001; 38: 930-939.

[103] Sheng Z, Knowlton K, Chen J, Hoshijima M, Brown JH, Chien KR. Cardiotrophin 1 (CT-1) inhibition of cardiac myocyte apoptosis via a mitogen-activated protein kinase-dependent pathway. Divergence from downstream CT-1 signals for myocardial cell hypertrophy. J Biol Chem 1997; 272: 5783-5791.

[104] Brar BK, Stephanou A, Okosi A, *et al.* CRH-like peptides protect cardiac myocytes from lethal ischaemic injury. Mol Cell Endocrinol 1999; 58: 55-63.

[105] Brar BK, Jonassen AK, Stephanou A, *et al.* Urocortin protects against ischemic and reperfusion injury via a MAPK-dependent pathway. J Biol Chem 2000; 275: 8508-8514.

[106] Brar BK, Stephanou A, Knight R, Latchman DS. Activation of protein kinase B/Akt by urocortin is essential for its ability to protect cardiac cells against hypoxia/reoxygenation-induced cell death. J Mol Cell Cardiol 2002; 34: 483-492.

[107] Szebenyi G, Fallon JF. Fibroblast growth factors as multifunc-tional signaling factors. Int Rev Cytol 1999; 185: 45-46.

[108] Cuevas P, Carceller F, Martinez-Coso V, *et al.* Cardioprotection from ischemia by fibroblast growth factor: role of inducible nitric oxide synthase. Eur J Med Res 1999; 4: 517-524.

[109] Cuevas P, Reimers D, Carceller F, *et al.* Fibroblast growth factor-1 prevents myocardial apoptosis triggered by ischemia reperfusion injury. Eur J Med Res 1997; 2: 465-468.

[110] Buehler A, Martire A, Strohm C, Wolfram S, Fernandez B, Palmen M, Wehrens XH, Doevendans PA, Franz WM, Schaper W, Zimmermann R. Angiogenesis-independent cardioprotection in FGF-1 transgenic mice. Cardiovasc Res 2002; 55: 768-777.

[111] Liu YH, Yang XP, Sharov VG, Sigmon DH, Sabbath HN, Carretero OA. Paracrine systems in the cardioprotective effect of angiotensin-converting enzyme inhibitors on myocardial ischemia/reperfusion injury in rats. Hypertension 1996; 27: 7-13.

[112] Hartman JC. The role of bradykinin and nitric oxide in the cardioprotective action of ACE inhibitors. Ann Thorac Surg 1995; 60: 789-792.

[113] Li Y, Sato T. Dual signaling via protein kinase C and phosphatidylinositol 3′-kinase/Akt contributes to bradykinin B2 receptor-induced cardioprotection in guinea pig hearts. J Mol Cell Cardiol 2001; 33: 2047-2053.

[114] Bernier SG, Haldar S, Michel T. Bradykinin-regulated interactions of the mitogen-activated protein kinase pathway with the endothelial nitric-oxide synthase. J Biol Chem 2000; 275: 30707-30715.

[115] Xu Z, Yang XM, Cohen MV, Neumann T, Heusch G, Downey JM. Limitation of infarct size in rabbit hearts by the novel adenosine receptor agonist AMP 579 administered at reperfusion. J Mol Cell Cardiol 2000; 32: 2339-2347.

[116] Cantrell A, McGarvey DJ, Truscott TG, Rancan F, Bohm F. Singlet oxygen quenching by dietary carotenoids in a model membrane environment. Arch Biochem Biophys 2003; 412: 47-54.

[117] Cardounel AJ, Dumitrescu C, Zweier JL, Lockwood SF. Direct superoxide anion scavenging by a disodium disuccinate astaxanthin derivative: relative efficacy of individual stereo-isomers versus the statistical mixture of stereoisomers by electron paramagnetic resonance imaging. Biochem Biophys Res Commun 2003; 307: 704-712.

[118] Lauver DA, Lockwood SF, Lucchesi BR. Disodium Disuccinate Astaxanthin (Cardax) attenuates complement activation and reduces myocardial injury following ischemia/reperfusion. J Pharmacol Exp Ther 2005; 314:686-692.

[119] Beranek JT. C-reactive protein and complement in myocardial infarction and postinfarction heart failure. Eur Heart J 1997; 18: 1834-1836.

[120] Faxon DP, Gibbons RJ, Chronos NA, Gurbel PA, Sheehan F. HALT-MI Investigators. The effect of blockade of the CD11/ CD18 integrin receptor on infarct size in patients with acute myocardial infarction treated with direct angioplasty: the results of the HALT-MI study. J Am Coll Cardiol 2002; 40: 1199-1204.

[121] Baran KW, Nguyen M, McKendall GR, *et al.* Limitation of Myocardial Infarction Following Thrombolysis in Acute Myocardial Infarction (LIMIT AMI) Study Group. Double blind, randomized trial of an anti-CD 18 antibody in conjunction with recombinant tissue plasminogen activator for acute myocardial infarction. Limitation of myocardial infarction following thrombolysis in acute myocardial infarction (LIMIT AMI) study. Circulation 2001; 104: 2778-2783.

[122] Frangogiannis NG, Smith CW, Entman ML. The inflammatory response in myocardial infarction. Cardiovasc Res 2002; 53: 31-37.

[123] Vakeva AP, Agah A, Rollins SA, Matis LA, Li L, Stahl GL. Myocardial infarction and apoptosis after myocardial ischemia and reperfusion, Circulation 1998; 97: 2259-2267.

[124] Weisman HF, Bartow T, Leppo MK, *et al.* Soluble human complement receptor type 1: *in vivo* inhibitor of complement suppressing post-ischemic myocardial inflammation and necrosis. Science 1990; 249: 146-151.

[125] Lazar HL, Hamasaki T, Bao Y, Rivers S, Bernard SA, Shemin RJ. Soluble complement receptor type 1 limits damage during revascularization of ischemic myocardium. Ann Thorac Surg 1998; 65: 973-977.

[126] Laser HL, Bokesch PM, van Lenta F, Fitzgerald C, Emmett C, Marsh HC, Ryan U. Soluble human complement receptor 1 limits ischemic damage in cardiac surgery patients at high risk requiring cardiopulmonary bypass. Circulation 2004; 110: 274-279.

[127] Li JS, Sanders SP, Perry AE, Stinnett SS, Jaggers J, Bokesch P, Reynolds L, Nassar R, Anderson PAW. Pharmacokinetics and safety of TP10, soluble complement receptor 1, in infants undergoing cardiopulmonary bypass. Am Heart J 2004; 147: 173-180.

[128] Reynolds MM, Zhou Z, Oh BK, Meyerhoff ME. Bis-diazeniumdiolates of dialkyldiamines: Enhanced nitric oxide loading of parent diamines. Org Lett 2005; 7: 2813-2816.

[129] Wu XA, Janczuk JJ, Cai T, Xian M, Wen Z, Wang PG. NO donors with anticancer activity. Exp Opin Ther Pat 2002; 12: 819-826.

[130] Fitzhugh AL, Keefer LK. Diazeniumdiolates: pro- and antioxidant applications of the "NONOates". Free Radic Biol Med 2000; 28: 1463-1469.

[131] Jourd'heuil D, Hallén K, Feelish M Grisham MB. Dynamic state of S-nitrosothiols in human plasma and whole blood. Free Rad Biol Med 2000; 28: 409-417.

[132] Tyurin VA, Tyurina YY, Liu SX, Bayir H, Hubel CA, Kagan VE, Quantitation of S-nitrosothiols in cells and biological fluids. Meth Enzymol 2002; 352: 347-349.

[133] Williams DLH, The chemistry of S-nitrosothiols. Acc Chem Res 1999; 32: 869-876.

[134] Dicks AP, Swift HR, Williams DLH, Butler AR, Al-Sadoni HH, Cox BGJ. Identification of Cu^{+} as the effective reagent in nitric oxide formation from S-nitrosothiols (RSNO). Chem Soc Perkin Trans-2 1996; 4: 481-487.

[135] Holmes AJ, Williams DLH. Reaction of ascorbic acid with S-nitrosothiols: clear evidence for two distinct reaction pathways. Chem Soc Perkin Trans-2 2000; 8: 1639-1644.

[136] Singh RJ, Hogg N, Joseph J, Kalyanaraman B. Mechanism of nitric oxide release from S-nitrosothiols. J Biol Chem 1996; 271: 18596-18603.

[137] Shishido SM, Seabra AB, Loh W, de Oliveira MG. Thermal and photochemical nitric oxide release from S-nitrosothiols incorporated into Pluronic F127 gel: potential uses for local and controlled nitric oxide release. Biomaterials 2003; 24: 3543-3553.

[138] Shishido SM, de Oliveira MG. Polyethylene glycol matrix reduces the rates of photochemical and thermal release of nitric oxide from S-nitroso-*N*-acetylcysteine. Photochem Photobiol 2000; 71: 273-280.

[139] Miwatashi S, Arikawa Y, Kotani E, Miyamoto M, Naruo K, Kimura H, Tanaka T, Asahi S, Ohkawa S. Novel inhibitor of p38 MAP kinase as an anti-TNF-alpha drug: discovery of *N*-[4-[2-ethyl-4-(3-methylphenyl)-1,3-thiazol-5-yl]-2-pyridyl]benzamide (TAK-715) as a potent and orally active anti-rheumatoid arthritis agent. J Med Chem 2005; 48: 5966-5969.

[140] Frey DA, Kataisto EW, Ekmanis JL, O'Malley S, Lockwood SF. The Efficient Synthesis of Disodium Disuccinate Astaxanthin (Cardax). Org Process Res Dev 2004; 8: 796-801.

[141] Lockwood SF, Penn MS, Hazen SL, Bikadi Z, Zsila F. The effects of oral Cardaxtrade mark (disodium disuccinate astaxanthin) on multiple independent oxidative stress markers in a mouse peritoneal inflammation model: influence on 5-lipoxygenase *in vitro* and *in vivo*. Life Sci 2006; 79: 162-164.

[142] Ghosh J, Myers CE. Inhibition of arachidonate 5-lipoxygenase triggers massive apoptosis in human prostate cancer cells. Proc Nat Acad Sci USA 1998: 95: 13182-13187.

[143] Myers CE, Ghosh J. Lipoxygenase inhibition in prostate cancer, Eur Urol 1999; 35: 395-398.

[144] Devaraj L, Jialal I. α-Tocopherol decreases tumor necrosis factor-α mRNA and protein from activated human monocytes by inhibition of 5-lipoxygenase. Free Radical Biol Med 2005; 38: 1212-1220.

[145] Beutner S, Bloedorn B, Frixel S, *et al.* Quantitative assessment of antioxidant properties of natural colorants and phytochemicals: carotenoids, flavonoids, phenols and indigoids. The role of β-carotene in antioxidant functions, J Sci Food Agric 2001; 81: 559-568.

[146] Weinblatt ME, Kremer JM, Bankhurst AD, *et al.* A trial of etanercept, a recombinant tumor necrosis factor receptor:Fc fusion protein, in patients with rheumatoid arthritis receiving methotrexate. N Engl J Med 1999; 340: 253-259.

[147] Yung RL. Etanercept Immunex. Curr Opin Investig Drugs 2001; 2: 216-221.

[148] Baker, J.E., Yang, S.: US20070173449 (**2007**).

[149] Oeltgen, P.R., Kindy, M.S.: US20056967192 (**2005**).

[150] Brooks, G.F., Donovan, S.: US20046767544 (**2004**).
[151] Liang, B.T., Jacobson, K.A.: US20036586413 (**2003**).
[152] Balu, P.: US6703480 (**2004**)
[153] Blackburn, B.K., Melville, C., Zablocki, J.A., Palle, V.P., Elzein, E.O., Wang, L.: US20036576619 (**2003**).
[154] Wink, D.A., Feelisch, M., Pagliaro, P., Kass, D.A., Paolocci, N., Miranda, K.M., Fukuto, J.M.: US20038947A1 (**2003**).
[155] Oeltgen, P.R., Kindy, M.S., Bishop, P.D.: US6294519B1 (**2001**).
[156] Kennedy, T.P.: US20006489311 (**2000**).
[157] Singh, I.: US5912019 (**1999**).
[158] Spada, A.P., Fink, C.A., Myers, M.R., Michael, R.: US5736554 (**1998**).
[159] Lau, J., Knutsen L.J.S., Sheardown, M., Hansen, A.J.: US5484774 (**1996**).
[160] Forman, M.B., Jackson, E.K.: US5206222 (**1993**).
[161] Shimamoto, N., Ogata, K.: US4948786 (**1990**).
[162] Nair, V.G., Joseph, J.P., Bernstein, S.: US4021545 (**1977**).
[163] Mocanu MM, Bell BM, Yellon DM. PI3 kinase and not p42/ p44 appears to be implicated in the protection conferred by ischemic preconditioning. J Mol Cell Cardiol 2002; 34: 661-668.
[164] Fryer RM, Pratt PF, Hsu AK, Gross GJ. Differential activation of extracellular signal regulated kinase isoforms in preconditioning and opioid-induced cardioprotection. J Pharmacol Exp 2001; 296: 642-649.
[165] Yellon DM, Downey JM. Preconditioning the myocardium: from cellular physiology to clinical cardiology. Physiol Rev 2003; 83: 1113-1121.
[166] Diaz R. Myocardial protection during acute myocardial infarction: the need for a simple large randomised trial with GIK. Cardiovasc Drugs The 2000; 14: 561-563.
[167] Gwon HC, Jeong JO, Kim HJ, *et al.* The feasibility and safety of fluoroscopy-guided percutaneous intra-myocardial gene injection in porcine heart. Int J Cardiol 2001; 79: 77-78.
[168] Irwin MW, Mak S, Mann DL, *et al.* Tissue expression and Immunolocalization of tumor necrosis factor-alpha in postinfarc-tion dysfunctional myocardium. Circulation 1999; 99: 1492-1498.
[169] Krown KA, Page MT, Nguyen C, *et al.* Tumor necrosis factor alpha-induced apoptosis in cardiac myocytes. Involvement of sphingolipid signalling cascade in cardiac cell death. J Clin Invest 1996; 98: 2854-2855.
[170] Xuan YT, Guo Y, Han H, Zhu Y, Bolli R. An essential role of the JAK-STAT pathway in ischemic preconditioning. Proc Natl Acad Sci USA 2001; 98: 9050-9055.
[171] Bolli R, Dawn B, Tang XL, *et al.* The nitric oxide hypothesis of late preconditioning. Basic Res Cardiol 1998; 93: 325-328.
[172] Pepys MB, Hirschfield GM, Tennebt GA, *et al.* Targeting C-reactive protein for the treatment of cardiovascular disease. Nature 2006; 440: 1217-1221.

The Role of Angiotensin Type 1 Receptor in Inflammation and Endothelial Dysfunction: Clinical Application

Dana Skultetyova*[,1], Adriena Sakalova[2], Pavol Chnupa[1] and Slavomira Filipova[2]

Dept. Cardiology,[1] National Institute of Cardiovascular Diseases and [2]Slovak Medical University, Bratislava, Slovak Republic

Abstract: Endothelial dysfunction plays an important role in all stages of atherosclerosis, and is characterized by an increased activity of vasoconstricting factors, proinflammatory and prothrombotic mediators. The aim of the review is to evaluate the role of angiotensin II (Ang II) and especially of angiotensin type 1 (AT_1) receptor in inflammation and endothelial dysfunction.

Ang II with AT_1 receptor are involved through several mechanisms in the progression of atherosclerosis. Stimulation of AT_1 receptor increases oxidative stress especially through activation of NADH/NADPH oxidase in the vascular cells. Oxidative stress is associated with activation of the inflammatory processes. Ang II via AT_1 receptor increases expression of adhesion molecules and stimulates the induction of monocyte chemoattractant protein-1 (MCP-1). AT_1 receptor enhances the activation of nuclear factor NF-κB, which stimulates the production of proinflammatory cytokines. Proinflammatory cytokines on the other side may induce acute-phase response in the liver. Activation of AT_1 receptor via inducible cyclooxygenase (COX)-2 promotes biosynthesis of matrix metalloproteinases (MMPs). Stimulation of proinflammatory cytokines activates profibrogenic transforming growth factor-beta 1 (TGF-β1). Ang II via NF-κB may regulate peroxisome proliferator activated receptors (PPARs) and the metabolism of glucose and lipids. Ang II is implicated in the process of angiogenesis. AT_1 receptor takes part in the regulation of vascular endothelial growth factor (VEGF), which is one of the most angiogenic factors and stimulates the activity of endothelial progenitor cells (EPC).

Recently some patents that were reported discussing the role of different compounds for the treatment of cardiovascular disease, renovascular disease nephropathy, peripheral vascular disease, portal hypertension and ophthalmic disorders, are cyclooxygenase-2 inhibitors. AT_1 receptor blockers are widely used in the treatment of cardiovascular, cerebral and renal diseases.

Keywords: Endothelial dysfunction, AT_1 receptor, oxidative stress, adhesive molecules, monocyte chemoattractant protein-1, cytokines, matrix metalloproteinases, vascular endothelial growth factor, peroxisome proliferator activated receptors.

---

*Corresponding author: Tel: + 421 2 59320281; Fax: + 421 2 59320282; E-mail: skultety@nusch.sk

Atta-ur-Rahman / M. Iqbal Choudhary (Eds.)

INTRODUCTION

Endothelial dysfunction is one of the earliest physiological hallmarks of atherosclerosis and plays an important role in the advanced stages of atherosclerosis. Endothelial dysfunction is characterized by an imbalance between vasodilating and vasoconstricting factors and contributes to an increased synthesis of vasoconstricting factors, vascular remodeling, increased synthesis of adhesive molecules, activation of apoptotic processes, and stimulation of coagulation cascade [1-3]. Common conditions predisposing to atherosclerosis, such as hypercholesterolemia, hypertension, diabetes, and smoking, are associated with endothelial dysfunction, lead to proinflammatory and prothrombotic phenotype of the endothelium [4]. Recent invention discusses the heterocyclic compounds for treating heart failure, hypertension, renovascular diseases, oxidative stress, endothelial dysfunction, peripheral vascular disease, portal hypertension etc [5-7].

Ang II regulates the electrolyte balance fluid volume, systemic blood pressure, aldosteron releases, sympathetic outflow via circulating endocrine system. The interstitial Ang II has a minimal acute effect on blood flow, but first of all it modulates lipid and carbohydrate metabolism in a tissue specific fashion [8]. Steele discussed the treatment of hypertension related disorders, congestive heart failure, coronary heart disease with the aldosterone synthase inhibitors, atherosclerosis, oxidative stress, hyperlipidemia alone or in combination with angiotensin I [9-11]. Recently Garvey has patented nitric oxide enhancing compounds as aldosterone antagonists for treating diseases i.e cardiovascular, diabetes, renovascular, oxidative stress, and endothelial dysfunction [12].

The aim of the article is to evaluate the mechanisms supporting the proatherogenic role of Ang II via AT_1 receptor, especially AT_1 receptor induced activation of inflammatory processes and endothelial dysfunction, and the application in clinical practice.

AT_1 RECEPTOR

The effects of Ang II are mediated by two plasma membrane receptors: AT_1 and AT_2 subtypes. AT_1 receptor is a member of 7 transmembrane-spanning G protein-coupled receptor family. This receptor binds to heterotrimeric G proteins, and lacks intrinsic tyrosine kinase activity [13]. There are at least four different aspects involved in AT_1 regulation. First, activation of AT_1 receptor with Ang II evokes internalization of the receptor protein and reduces receptor numbers on the cell surface. Second, prolonged Ang II stimulation reduces Ang II signaling via protein kinase C-protein translation. Third, alternative splicing of AT_1 receptor pre-mRNA can alter AT_1 receptor protein translation. Fourth, the most important mechanism is modulation of its gene expression. Human AT_1 receptor gene is mapped at the chromosome 3. AT_1 receptors are ubiquitously distributed in adult tissues. Ang II *via* AT_1 receptor can directly participate in the pathogenesis of cardiovascular diseases. Depending on the cell and organ type, Ang II can influence the cellular contraction, hypertrophy, proliferation or apoptosis [14,15]. Hypertension associated transcription factor-1 (HATF-1) and HATF-1 related protein-1 are discussed for the treatment of cardiovascular disorders, hypertension, heart failure or coronary artery disease [16].

AT_2 RECEPTOR

AT_2 receptors are highly expressed in the fetal organs that suggest their role in fetal development and organ morphogenesis. The expression of these receptors is dramatically decreased after birth. Then this activity is restricted to few organs, including the cardiovascular system. AT_2 receptor is a seven-transmembrane domain receptor. The gene is localized as a single copy on the X chromosome. In adult humans, low levels of AT_2 receptors are expressed in aorta and coronary arteries. The activation of AT_2 receptor occurs after cardiac or vascular injury and during wound healing, suggesting their role in tissue remodeling [17,18]. The effects of AT_1 and AT_2 receptors are antagonistic. Inhibition of AT_1 receptor leads to several-fold increase in plasma Ang II and to overstimulation of AT_2 receptor. AT_2 receptor promotes vasodilation in resistance microvessels and in large capacitance vessels. The vasodilating effect is mediated *via* AT_2 receptor – bradykinin - nitric oxid (NO) - cyclic quanosine-monophosphate (cGMP) pathway [19].

AT_1 RECEPTOR AND OXIDATIVE STRESS

There is an evidence that Ang II increases vascular oxidative stress. Stimulation of AT_1 receptor leads to activation of NADH/NADPH oxidase in vascular cells. This oxidative system, which is similar to the neutrophil oxidase, is the main source of reactive oxygen species (ROS) in endothelial cells, vascular smooth muscle, and adventitial fibroblasts. Nox proteins of the NADPH oxidase family are prominent sources of vascular ROS. The NOX-derived ROS have been implicated in a variety of vascular diseases, including hypertension, atherosclerosis, and vascular diabetic complications [14]. The increased vascular activity of NADH and NADPH oxidase enhances the production of ROS by several pathways, including the increased activation of xantine oxidase, the autooxidation of NADH, and the inactivation of superoxide dismutase. A variety of ROS are formed during the oxidative stress, such as superoxide (O_2^-), hydroxyl radical (HO^-), lipid radicals, and hydrogen peroxide (H_2O_2). Vascular O_2^- appears to function in two distinct ways: 1) extracellularly (paracrine), to modulate endothelium-dependent changes in vascular tone, and 2) intracellularly, as a second messenger to produce long-term phenotypic alterations of resident cells. Combination of O_2^- with NO leads to formation of peroxynitrite, which contributes to vasoconstriction and vascular injury. The peroxynitrite formation promotes lipid and protein oxidation in atherosclerotic lesions [20-22]. High levels of ROS induce apoptosis of endothelial cells. Ang II promotes apoptosis in endothelial cells *via* direct and indirect mechanisms. Ang II increases the activity of NADPH oxidase. On the other side Ang II and ROS can promote apoptosis of endothelial cells by inhibiting the function of antiapoptotic protein Bcl-2. Ang II may indirectly cause apoptosis via induction of Fas and Lectin-like oxLDL receptor-1 (LOX-1) [23]. Endothelial nitric oxide synthase (eNOS) can under certain pathophysiological conditions produce large amounts of O_2^-. This condition appears in the absence of tetrahydrobiopterin, which is the co-factor for eNOS function [24-26]. Ang II can directly increase release the production of endothelin (ET)-1. The vascular endothelium is the major source of ET-1 production, which is a potent vasoconstrictor and mitogen. ET-1 also increases the levels of O_2^- through activation of NADPH oxidase [27]. Oxidative stress is a key factor in the development of endothelial dysfunction and is associated with the activation of inflammatory processes. D-chiroinositol (DCI) acting as an antioxidant or glucose uptake promoter and metabolic normalizer used for treating oxidative stress [28].

AT_1 RECEPTOR AND INFLAMMATION

Vascular inflammation plays a major role in the atherosclerotic lesion formation, progression and rupture. Ang II increases the adhesiveness of endothelium *via* expression of adhesion molecules, such as vascular cell adhesion molecule-1 (VCAM-1), intercellular adhesion molecule-1 (ICAM-1), and E-selectin. These adhesion molecules are important in initiation and aggravation of atherosclerotic lesions, they induce adhesion and subsequent transendothelial migration of circulating leukocytes. The molecules bind very late antigen-4 on the surface of circulating leukocytes, initiating recruitment of leukocytes into the vessel wall. Focal expression of these adhesive molecules has been demonstrated in the human atherosclerotic plaques [29,30]. In smooth muscle cells, Ang II *via* AT_1 receptor stimulates the induction of MCP-1, which enhances the monocyte infiltration to the side of injury in the media of the vessel wall. MCP-1 is the key chemokine in mediating vascular monocyte-mediated inflammation. Ang II activates the interleukin-6 (IL-6) in smooth muscle cells, too. This cytokine has local (paracrine) actions to promote smooth muscle cell proliferation involving the local production of platelet-derived growth factor (PDGF), and it produces systemic effects by stimulating gene expression in distant organs [31,32].

Fatty streak contains an increased number of monocytes and T lymphocytes, and the formation is characterized by an increased oxidation of low density lipoproteins (LDL), uptake of oxLDL by macrophages, and foam cell formation [33]. Ang II has been reported to increase macrophage uptake of oxLDL and this effect may be mediated through the local actions of Ang II-induced IL-6 expression. AT_1 receptor enhances the expression LOX-1 receptor on endothelial cells, which stimulates the uptake of oxLDL in endothelial cells. Activation of this pathway leads to increased production of ROS and to stimulation of the proinflammatory NF-κB [34]. NF-κB plays a key signaling role in multiple proatherogenic insults. This factor induces the inflammatory vascular cytokine cascade, cellular recruitment, and is important in mediating atherosclerotic progression. Ang II has pleiotropic actions in multiple points in the NF-κB activation pathway in vascular smooth muscle cells.

There has been established a functional cross-regulation between the RAS and proinflammatory cytokine tumor necrosis factor-α (TNF-α), [35]. TNF-α is a pleiotropic cytokine, which through induction of imunomodulatory molecules may regulate the cell proliferation, differentiation and apoptosis [36-40]. Stimulated macrophages are the major source of TNF-α [41]. Activated endothelial cells also produce this cytokine but in a less amount as macrophages. TNF-α converting enzyme was found in activated endothelial cells, T-lymphocytes and smooth muscle cells [42]. TNF-α has detrimental effects on endothelial function. This cytokine reduces the expression of constitutive eNOS and activate the expression of inducible eNOS, which results in a large production of ROS [43].

Ang II together with TNF-α is capable of upregulating MMPs, which belong to a family of collagenolytic enzymes. Activation of MMPs facilitates progressive degradation of fibrillar collagen [44]. Expression of MMPs, especially 72-kDa (MMP-2) and 92-kDa (MMP-9) has been shown within the human atherosclerotic lesions. Enhanced expression of inducible cyclooxygenase (COX)-2, which is activated by AT_1 receptor, together with prostaglandin $(PG)E_2$-dependent synthase, stimulate the biosynthesis of these MMPs in macrophages. MMP-2 and MMP-9 are implicated in plaque rupture via weakening the fibrous cap of atherosclerotic plaque. Ang II, AT_1 receptor, and angiotensin converting enzyme (ACE) together with macrophages were found in human coronary arteries at the shoulder region of atherosclerotic plaques in patients with unstable angina [45]. Combined ACE and neutral endopeptidase (NEP) inhibitor, are used in the treatment of hypertension, diabetes, and cardiac and renal diseases [46]. Quinapril and new stabilized compositions of Quinapril and fosinoprilat with magnesium oxide are recently patented [47,48]. Renin-angiotensin inhibitors are useful for the prevention of conditions related with hypoxia or impaired metabolic function or efficiency [49]. P-thienylbenzylamides compounds act as agonists of angiotensin (1-7) receptor stimulants and patented for the cure of hypertension, cardiac insufficiency, angina pectoris or diabetes mellitus [50].

Proinflammatory cytokines may induce acute-phase response in the liver. This action involves a "transcriptional switch", by which proteins are synthesized de novo by the liver in response to circulating hormones elaborated at the site of injury. IL-6 *via* it's receptors plays the central role in the hepatic acute-phase reaction. Type I IL-6 signaling is mediated through a tyrosine kinase mechanism involving the janus kinase (JAK)/signal transducer and activator of transcription (STAT)-pathway, whereas type II IL-6 signaling is mediated through a Ras/mitogen-activated protein kinase/NF-IL-6 pathway. Type I (JAK/STAT) pathway is the major pathway responsible for acute-phase reactant synthesis [51]. The main acute-phase proteins such as C-reactive protein (CRP), serum amyloid A (SAA), fibrinogen and angiotensinogen may be the markers not only for the severity of vascular inflammation, but also have significant cardiovascular effects [52,53]. Novel organic nitric oxide compounds as anti-inflammatory agents act as therapeutic agent for the treatment of inflammation, pain and fever, inflammatory disease states or disorders, ophthalmic disorders, peripheral vascular diseases/diseases resulting from oxidative stress, and endothelial dysfunction [54].

Recent studies provide evidence for a functional link between Ang II and TGF-β1 in the cardiovascular system. RAS and TGF-β1 play the main role in the development of cardiac hypertrophy and heart failure. Ang II upregulates TGF-β expression *via* activation of AT_1 receptor in cardiac myocytes and fibroblasts. TGF-β1 induces the proliferation of fibroblasts, their conversion to myofibroblasts, and hypertrophic growth of cardiomyocytes [55]. TGF-β1 may be involved in vascular remodeling. This cytokine can accelerate vascular wall remodeling, arterial lesion growth, and vascular cell transdifferentiation. TGF-β1 as an immunomodulator and a fibrosis modulator may play a role in the maintenance of plaque stability [56]. In the study of healthy volunteers, correlations between TGF-β1 and ultrasound parameters (diameter and intima-media thickness of common carotid artery) were found. The authors suggest that these relationships may reflect artery remodeling [57].

There is an evidence of cross-talk between RAS and nuclear PPARs. Ang II, through activation of NF-κB, stimulates expression and downregulation of PPARα and PPARy [58]. PPAR-α plays a role in intracellular lipid metabolism. PPARy has an effect on glucose metabolism, stimulation of the receptor leads to improving insulin sensitivity and reducing triglyceride levels [59]. The other mechanism of insulin resistance regulation is the effect of Ang II on adiponectin production. Adiponectin is produced in adipose tissue and the levels are positively associated wth insulin sensitization, glucose use, β-oxidation and cardio-vascular protection. Dysregulation of adiponectin is associated with endothelial dysfunction and cardiovascular disease [60]. AT_1 receptor blockers (ARBs) are widely used in the treatment cardiovascular, cerebral and renal diseases. In addition to end-organ protection, they may improve glucose and lipid metabolism, resulting in an antiatherosclerotic affect.

AT_1 RECEPTOR AND ANGIOGENESIS

There is an evidence that Ang II via AT_1 receptor is implicated in the process of angiogenesis. Ang II is shown to upregulate VEGF. VEGF is an endogenous regulater of the endothelial integrity and is one of the most potent angiogenic factors, which enhances the number of EPCs. It is known that VEGF and NO have synergistic effects in the mobilization, migration, proliferation, and survival of endothelial cells [61]. VEGF is also responsible for Ang II induced vascular inflammation and structural changes on arterial wall in wall thickening. It is showed that VEGF induces migration and activation of monocytes through induction of adhesion molecules or chemokines such as MCP-1. Ang II induces VEGF production through stimulation of hypoxia-inducible factor-1α ($HIF\text{-}1_{\alpha}$), which plays the major in the control of VEGF expression. On the other side, blockade of VEGF by the soluble VEGF receptor 1 (sFlt-1) gene transfer attenuated the Ang II induced inflammation and remodeling [62,63]. sFlt-1 gene transfer reduced the early vascular inflammation and proliferation by inhibition of increased production of MCP-1, interleukin-1, PDGF. It is known as an interaction between VEGF and angiogenic growth factors as angiopoietin-1 and its antagonist angiopoietin-2. Angiopoietin-1 activates the recruitment of periendothelial cell support and reverses the enhanced permeability, induced by VEGF. Angiopoietin-2 stimulates the proinflammatory effects of VEGF [64].

Angiogenesis plays a pivotal role in tumor progression. Chronic inflammation has been identified as a risk for cancer. The local RAS appears to influence tumor growth and metastasis. Over-expression of AT_1 receptors has been reported in association with human cancers. Recent experimental studies provide strong evidence that drugs that inhibit RAS have the potential to reduce cancer risk or retard tumor growth and metastasis [65, 66].

AT_1 RECEPTOR AND STEM CELLS

There is an evidence that the vascular wall and the endothelium undergo a constant process of injury and repair in response to mechanical and chemical injuries. Bone marrow-derived endothelial stem cells and EPCs contribute to the repair of vascular injury and play a role in restoration of tissue repair. Endothelial dysfunction may be a relative deficiency of EPCs and the degree of dysfunction may correlate with the number of EPCs [67]. It is suggested that Ang II accelerates EPC senescence via AT_1 receptor and through induction of oxidative stress, and significantly diminished telomerase activity [68]. Treatment of heart failure by administration of a cortisol antagonist is reported [69].

AT_1 antagonists can act on hematopoietic stem-progenitor cells. Heringer-Walther *et al.* reported that Ang II metabolite, Ang-(1-7) positively stimulates the proliferation of CD34+ cord blood cells *in vitro*. The authors demostrated that continuous post-transplantation supplementation of Ang-(1-7) together with injection of cord blood mononuclear cells improved human hematopoietic progenitor engraftment. The results can reflect the important role of RAS in regulating hematopoietic progenitor differentiation and self-renewal. The use of Ang-(1-7), Ang II or manipulation of Ang II receptor binding may be important in bone marrow transplantation [70].

AT_1 RECEPTOR AND FIBRINOLYSIS

Ischemia and inflammation are associated with the activation of thrombosis. Fibrinolysis constitutes one of the endogenous defense mechanisms against intravascular thrombus formation. Experimental and clinical studies have shown a relationship between renin angiotensin system (RAS) and the fibrinolytic system. Plasminogen activator inhibitor type 1 (PAI-1) is the major physiologic inhibitor of tissue-type plasminogen activator (t-PA) and urokinase. Ang II binds to endothelial cells and stimulates PAI-1 production. The increased PAI-1 expression in atherosclerotic plague leads to a decreased formation of plasmin and reduces the activation of MMPs [71,72]. It is suggested that RAS influences vascular PAI-1 expression through the Ang II/AT_1 pathway [73].

CURRENT AND FUTURE DEVELOPMENTS

Ang II *via* AT_1 receptor increases oxidative stress, especially through the activation of NADH/NADPH oxidase in the vascular cells. AT_1 receptor enhances the adhesiveness of endothelial cells through the activation of ICAM-1, VCAM-1 and E-selectin. Induction of MCP-1 increases the monocyte infiltration in the vessel wall. Stimulation of NF-κB induces the expression of proinflammatory cytokines, such as TNF-α, IL-6, and the activation of MMPs. The activation of proinflammatory cytokines is associated with stimulation of TGF-β1. TGF-β1 is involved in remodeling process. There is also an evidence of cross-talk between RAS and PPARs, that plays an important role in glucose and lipid metabolism. Ang II *via* AT_1 receptor is implicated in the process of angiogenesis. ARBs are widely used in the treatment of cardiovascular, cerebral and renal diseases. Overexpression of AT_1 receptors has been reported in cancer. Inhibition of AT_1 receptors may be important in the treatment of the disease.

REFERENCES

[1] Pepine CJ. Clinical implications of endothelial dysfunction. Clin Cardiol 1998; 21: 795-799.

[2] Bachetti T. Endothelial dysfunction in chronic heart failure: some new basic mechanisms. Ital Heart J 2000; 1: 656-661.

[3] Ganz P, Vita JA. Testing endothelial vasomotor function. Nitric oxide, a multipotent molecule. Circulation 2003; 108: 2049-2053.

[4] Landmesser U, Hornig B, Drexler H. Endothelial function: a critical determinant in atherosclerosis ? Circulation 2004; 109 (suppl) II: II-27 – II-33.

[5] Worcel, M., Sabolinski, M., Tam, S.W., Mcnamara, D.M.: WO06110601A2 **(2006)**.

[6] Garvey, D. S.: WO06078995A1 **(2006)**.

[7] Garvey, D. S.: WO06102071A1 **(2006)**.

[8] Boschmann M, Jordan J, Adams F, *et al.* Tissue-specific response to interstitial angiotensin II in humans. Hypertension 2003; 41: 37-41.

[9] Steele, R.E.: NZ0521855A **(2004)**.

[10] Steele, R.E.: US20050059697A1 **(2005)**.

[11] Garvey, D.S., Cai, X., Lin, C.-E., Ranatunge, R.R., Stevenson, C. A., Wey, S-J.: WO06099058A2 **(2006)**.

[12] Garvey, D.S.: WO06093864A1 **(2006)**.

[13] Kim S, Iwao H. Molecular and cellular mechanisms of angiotensin II-mediated cardiovascular and renal diseases. Pharmacol Rev 2000; 52: 11-34.

[14] Bedard K, Krause KH. The NOX family of ROS-generating NADPH oxidases: physiology and pathophysiology. Physiol Rev 2007; 87: 245-253.

[15] Nickenig G, Harrison DG. The AT_1-type angiotensin receptor in oxidative stress and atherogenesis. Part II: AT_1 receptor regulation. Circulation 2002; 105: 530- 536.

[16] Herman, I.M., Siecwicz, G.J.: US20036521420 **(2003)**.

[17] Watanabe T, Barker TA, Berk BC. Angiotensin II and the endothelium. Diverse signals and effects. Hypertension 2005; 45: 163-169.

[18] Henrion D, Kubis N, Lévy BI. Physiological and pathophysiological functions of the AT_2 subtype receptor of angiotensin II. Hypertension 2001; 38: 1150-1157.

[19] Carey RM. Cardiovascular and renal regulation by the angiotensin type 2 receptor. Hypertension 2005; 45: 840-844.

[20] Műnzel T, Keaney JF, Jr. Are ACE inhibitors a "magic bullet" against oxidative stress? Circulation 2001; 104: 1571-1574.

[21] Sowers JR. Hypertension, angiotensin II, and oxidative stress. N Engl J Med 2002; 346: 1999-2001.

[22] Griendling KK, FitzGerald GA. Oxidative stress and cardiovascular injury. Part I: basic mechanisms and *in vivo* monitoring of ROS. Circulation 2003; 108: 1912- 1916.

[23] Li DY, Zhang YC, Philips MI, *et al.* Upregulation of endothelial receptor for oxidized low-density lipoprotein (LOX-1) in cultured human coronary artery endothelial cells by angiotensin II type 1 receptor activation. Circ Res 1999; 84: 1043-1049.

[24] Szmitko PE, Wang CH-H, Weisel RD, *et al.* Biomarkers of vascular disease linking inflammation to endothelial activation. Part II. Circulation 2003; 108: 2041-2048.

[25] Nickenig G, Harrison DG. The AT_1-type angiotensin receptor in oxidative stress and atherogenesis. Part I: oxidative stress and atherogenesis. Circulation 2002; 105: 393-396.
[26] Loscalzo J. Folate and nitrate-induced endothelial dysfunction. A simple treatment for a complex pathobiology. Circulation 2001; 104: 1086-1088.
[27] Pollock DM. Endothelin, angiotensin, and oxidative stress in hypertension. Hypertension 2005; 45: 477-480.
[28] Larner, J., Price, J., Brownlee, M., Fonteles, M.: US20060258754A1 **(2006)**.
[29] Blankenberg S, Rupprecht HJ, Bickel Ch, *et al.* Circulating cell adhesion molecules and death in patients with coronary artery disease. Circulation 2001; 104: 1336-1342.
[30] Wassmann S, Hilgers S, Laufs U, *et al.* Angiotensin II type 1 receptor antagonism improves hypercholesterolemia-associated endothelial dysfunction. Arterioscl Thromb Vasc Biol 2002; 22: 1208-1212.
[31] Brasier AR, Recinos III A, Eledrisi MS. Vascular inflammation and the renin- angiotensin system. Arterioscl Thromb Vasc Biol 2002; 22: 1257-1266.
[32] Gibbons GH. Endothelial function as a determinant of vascular function and structure: a new therapeutic target. Am J Cardiol 1997; 79(5A): 3-8.
[33] Pitt B. The potential use of angiotensin-converting enzyme inhibitors in patients with hyperlipidemia. Am J Cardiol 1997; 79(5A): 24-28.
[34] McFarlane SI, Kumar A, Sowers JR. Mechanisms by which angiotensin- converting enzyme inhibitors prevent diabetes and cardiovascular disease. Am J Cardiol 2003; 91(Suppl) : 30H-37H.
[35] Flesch M, Höper A, Dell'Italia L, *et al.* Activation and functional significance of the renin-angiotensin system in mice with cardiac restricted overexpression of tumor necrosis factor. Circulation 2003; 108: 598-604.
[36] Kishore R, Spyridopoulos I, Luedemann C, Losordo DW. Functionally novel tumor necrosis factor-α-modulated CHR-binding protein mediates cyclin A transcriptional repression in vascular endothelial cells. Circ Res 2002; 91: 307- 314.
[37] Krasinski K, Spyridopoulos I, Kearney M, *et al.* *In vivo* blockade of tumor necrosis factor-α accelerates functional endothelial recovery after balloon angioplasty. Circulation 2001; 104: 1754-1756.
[38] Francis GS. TNF-α and heart failure. The difference between proof of principle and hypothesis testing. Circulation 1999; 99: 3213-3224.
[39] Sakalova A, Skultetyova D, Bucova M, *et al.* Zapalove a protizapalove cytokiny pri zhubnych hematologickych ochoreniach. Klinicka Onkologie 2003; 16: 19-23.
[40] Skultety J, Labas P, Durdik S. Zytokinaktivität bei Patienten mit gastrointestinalen Karzinomen. In: Taschenbuch MMW. Systematische Enzymtherapy. Medizin Verlag: München 1996; pp. 251-253.
[41] Imaizumi T, Itaya H, Fujita K, *et al.* Expression of tumor necrosis factor-α in cultured human endothelial cells stimulated with lipopolysaccharide or interleukin-1α. Arterioscler Thromb Vasc Biol 2000; 20: 410-415.
[42] Blumm A, Miller H. Role of cytokines in heart failure. Am Heart J 1998; 135: 181-186.
[43] Libby P, Ridker PM, Maseri A. Inflammation and atherosclerosis. Circulation 2002; 105: 1135-1143.
[44] Cipollone F, Fazia M, Iezzi A, *et al.* Blockade of the angiotensin II type 1 receptor stabilizes atherosclerotic plaques in humans by inhibiting prostaglandin E_2-dependent matrix metalloproteinase activity. Circulation 2004; 109: 1482-1488.
[45] Kohlstedt K, Busse R, Fleming I. Signaling *via* the angiotensin-converting enzyme enhances the expression of cyclooxygenase-2 in endothelial cells. Hypertension 2005; 45: 126-132.
[46] Brown, N.J.: US20056887679 **(2005)**.
[47] Daniel, J.E., Harris, M.R., Hokanson, G.C., Weiss, J.: US20067015232 **(2006)**.
[48] Eyjolesson, R.: US20067045511 **(2006)**.
[49] Montgomery, H.E., Martin, J.F., Erusalimsky, J.D.: US20067071183 **(2006)**.
[50] Heitsch, H.: US20066984660 **(2006)**.
[51] Cesari M, Penninx BWJH, Newman AB, *et al.* Inflammatory markers and onset of cardiovascular events. Results from the Health ABC Study. Circulation 2003; 108: 2317-2322.
[52] Yeh ETH, Anderson V, Pasceri V, *et al.* C-reactive protein. Linking inflammation to cardiovascular complications. Circulation 2001; 104: 974-975.
[53] Verma S, Buchanan MR, Anderson TJ. Endothelial function testing as a biomarker of vascular disease. Circulation 2003; 108: 2054-2059.
[54] Garvey, D. S.: WO06127591A2 **(2006)**.
[55] Rosenkratz S. TGF-β_1 and angiotensin networking in cardiac remodeling. Cardiovasc Res 2004; 63: 423-432.
[56] Saura M, Zaragoza C, Herranz B, Griera M, Diez-Marqués L, Puyol DR, Puyol MR. Nitric oxide regulates transforming growth factor-β signaling in endothelial cells. Circ Res 2005; 97: 1115-1123.

[57] Skultetyova D, Filipova S, Riecansky I, *et al.* The relationship between the transforming growth factor-beta1, age and the ultrasound parameters of arterial wall. Vascular Disease Prevention 2008; 5: 140-144.

[58] Schupp M, Janke J, Clasen R, *et al.* Angiotensin type 1 receptor blockers induce peroxisome proliferator-activated receptor-activity. Circulation 2004; 109: 2054-2057.

[59] Inoue T, Node K. Telmisartan as a meabolic sartan for targeting vascular failure. Expert Opin Pharmacother 2008; 9: 1397-1406.

[60] Wang ZV, Scherer PE. Adiponectin, cardiovascular function, and hypertension. Hypertension 2008; 51: 8-14.

[61] Dzau VJ, Gnecchi M, Pachori AS. Therapeutic potential of endothelial progenitor cells in cardiovascular diseases. Hypertension 2005; 46: 7-18.

[62] Dzau Q, Ishibashi M, Hiasa K-I, *et al.* Essential role of vascular endothelial growth factor in angiotensin II-induced vascular inflammation and remodeling. Hypertension 2004; 44: 264-270.

[63] Morishita R. Is vascular endothelial growth factor a missing link between hypertension and inflammation? Hypertension 2004; 44: 253-257.

[64] Lim HS, Felmeden D, Lip GYH. Angiotensin II-mediated vascular inflammation: the balance between vascular endothelial growth factor and angiopoietins. Hypertension 2005; 45: e3.

[65] Smith GR, Missailidis S. Cancer, inflammation and the AT1 and AT2 receptors. J Inflamm 2004; 1: 3.

[66] Ager EI, Neo J, Christophi CH. The renin-angiotensin system and malignancy. Carcinogenesis 2008; 29: 1675-1684.

[67] Lerman A, Zeiher AM. Endothelial function. Cardiac events. Circulation 2005; 111: 363-368.

[68] Levy BI. Beneficial effects of circulating progenitor endothelial cells activated by angiotensin receptor antagonists. Hypertension 2005; 45: 491-502.

[69] Marin, P., Sorensen, S.: US20056881739 **(2005**).

[70] Heringer-Walther S, Eckert K, Schumacher S-M, *et al.* Angiotensin-(1-7) stimulates hematopoietic progenitor cells *in vitro* and *in vivo*. Haematologica 2009; 94: 857-860.

[71] Vaughan DE. The renin-angiotensin system and fibrinolysis. Am J Cardiol 1997; 79(5A): 12-16.

[72] Cody RJ. The integrated effects of angiotensin II. Am J Cardiol 1997; 79(5A): 9-11.

[73] Chen H-Ch, Bouchie JL, Perez AS, *et al.* Role of the angiotensin AT_1 receptor in rat aortic and cardiac PAI-1 gene expression. Arteriosc1 Thromb Vasc Biol 2000; 20: 2297- 2302.

B-Type Natriuretic Peptide for Diagnosis and Therapy

Marek Jankowski*

Laboratory of Cardiovascular Biochemistry, Centre de Recherche, Centre Hospitalier de l'Université de Montréal (RCCHUM) and Department of Medicine, University of Montreal, 3850 Saint Urbain Street, Montréal, Québec, H2W 1T7, Canada

Abstract: Brain natriuretic peptide (BNP) plays an important role in cardiovascular homeostasis. Plasma BNP increases markedly in left ventricular dysfunction from several causes, and its levels in heart failure (HF) correlate with symptoms severity. BNP has recently emerged as a potentially important clinical marker for the diagnosis of HF in patients with unexplained dyspnea. Other clinical applications of BNP, such as screening for asymptomatic ventricular dysfunction, establishing the prognosis or guiding the titration of drug therapy, are under investigation and have not yet been sufficiently validated for widespread clinical use. Laboratory-based and point-of-care analyses are available for BNP and N-terminal proBNP as fully-automated immunoassays. Several patented inventions and reagents for the diagnosis of various heart pathologies provide helpful information, particularly in conjunction with other clinical tests. They also have prognostic value for future cardiovascular events. Patents owned by Scios Inc. recommended recombinant BNP for managing acute decompensated HF. However, this treatment apparently has safety problems and no proven clinical advantage over existing treatments in terms of improved survival and prevention of subsequent hospitalizations.

Keywords: Human brain natriuretic peptide, atrial natriuretic peptide, BNP 32, NT-proBNP, heart failure, diagnosis, prognosis, treatment.

INTRODUCTION

Atrial natriuretic peptide (ANP) was discovered in 1981 by a team of researchers led by Adolfo J. de Bold in Ottawa after their seminal observation that injection of atrial (but not ventricular) tissue extracts into rats caused copious natriu-resis [1]. The substance responsible for these physiological effects was purified, then further characterized and named ANP. BNP (brain natriuretic peptide) is closely related to ANP and CNP (C-type natriuretic peptide), all of which share the same amino acid ring. The 4-amino acid (aa) N-terminal (NT) extended form of ANP (urodilatin) has been isolated from human urine [2]. BNP is produced in ventricular cardiomyocytes, [3-5] and CNP is synthesized predominantly in the brain, chondrocytes and endothelial cells [6]. In addition to the mammalian NPs (ANP, BNP, CNP), two other peptides with similar structure and properties have been isolated

*Corresponding author: Tel: 514-890-8000, Ext. 12925; Fax: 514-843-2719; E-mail: marek.jankowski@umontreal.ca

Atta-ur-Rahman / M. Iqbal Choudhary (Eds.)

from other species: salmon cardiac peptide [7] and dendroaspis natriuretic peptide (DNP) found in green mamba venom [8].

ANP and BNP are potent diuretics, natriuretics and vasodilators. They inhibit cell proliferation, cell hypertrophy, the sympathetic nervous system and hormones, such as renin/angiotensin/aldosterone, endothelins and vasopressin [2, 9]. Three natriuretic peptide receptors (NPR) have been cloned. Two of them are guanylate cyclases: receptor type A (NPR-A) is present in the large blood vessels, kidneys and adrenal glands and preferentially responds to ANP and BNP; the type B receptor (NPR-B) abundant in the brain, kidneys and adrenal tissue and binds CNP with the highest affinity. Their actions are mediated by cGMP. The third receptor has no hormonal effects and clears NPs from the plasma [10].

HUMAN BNP (hBNP)

BNP, produced by the heart ventricles, is not stored, but is under constant mRNA transcription and translation. Its levels rise in response to ventricular wall stretch and end-diastolic volume [11]. In human cardiac muscles, BNP is synthesized as a 134-aa preprohormone, which is processed into a 108-aa molecule Fig. (**1**). This precursor molecule of BNP, proBNP, is cleaved with the participation of various proteolytic enzymes, such as corin or furin, into 32 C-terminal aa (77-108) called BNP, NT 1-76 aa called NT-proBNP, and further breakdown products [12]. BNP and NT- pro-BNP are released in stochiometric amounts into the circulation.

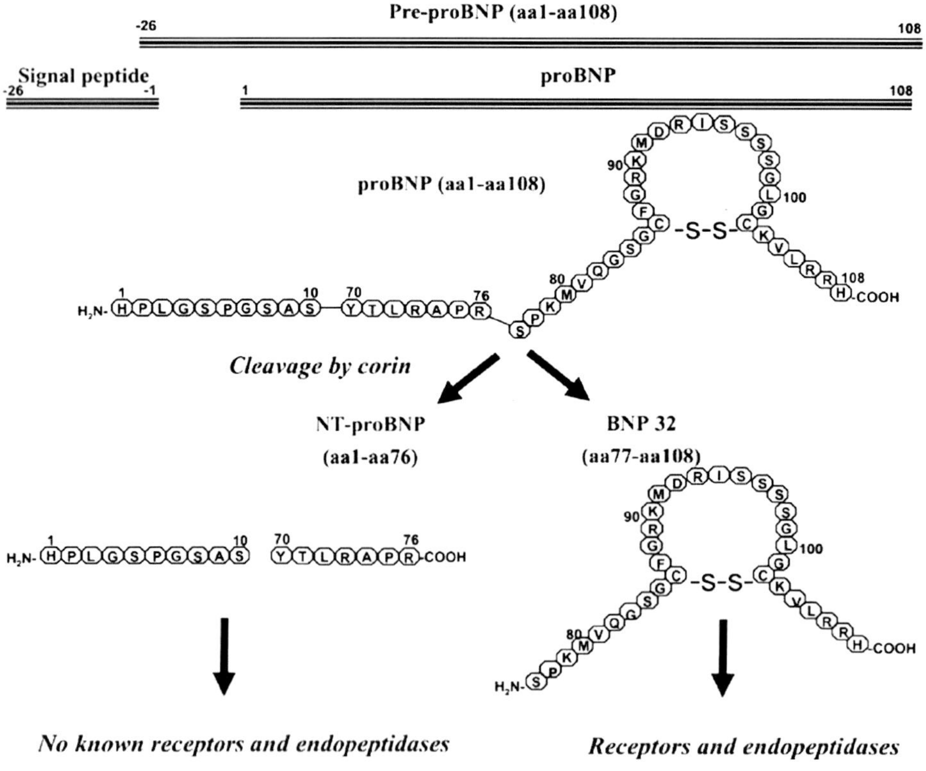

Fig. (1). Synthesis and secretion of B-type natriuretic peptide.

ANP and BNP are removed from the circulation by 2 pathways: receptor-mediated internalization and proteolytic degradation by neutral endopeptidase in the kidneys, vascular endothelium, lungs and heart. BNP has slower clearance by both pathways than ANP. Consequently, the circulating half-life of ANP is 3-5 minutes, whereas the half-life of BNP is about 20 minutes. The terminal fragment NT-proBNP has a longer half-life (60-120 minutes), which is relevant to its value in diagnostic tests [13]. BNP's shorter half-life may reflect changes in acute cardiac states to a greater extent than chronic cardiac states. In contrast, the long half-life of NT-proBNP results in much higher plasma levels, which are also more stable. Recent reports of intact plasma proBNP in heart failure (HF) suggest that increased cardiac BNP gene expression can surpass the biosynthetic capacity for proBNP maturation and lead to secretion of the unprocessed precursor peptide (proBNP 1-108), defective in cGMP activity [14]. A possible defect of corin in HF would inhibit pro-BNP processing, resulting in the release of uncleaved pro-BNP 1-108 [15].

Laboratory-based and point-of-care analyses are available for BNP and NT-proBNP as fully automated immunoassays. Although BNP assays are produced by numerous manufacturers, the original "patent" for BNP was owned by Scios Inc. Several other companies have obtained licenses to produce BNP assays (Biosite, Shinogi, Abbott, Beckman-Coulter and Bayer). The routine measurement of BNP is generally performed by non-competitive sandwich-type immunoassays that use non-radioactive labels for antigen/antibody reaction and two monoclonal antibodies or a combination of monoclonal and polyclonal antibodies for BNP binding. Usually one antibody binds to the ring structure, while the other either to the C- or N-terminal end of BNP, respectively. Roche Diagnostics owned patent for NT-proBNP assay (Roche Elecsys proBNP), includes two polyclonal antibodies directed against amino acid residues 1–21 and 39–50 of NT-proBNP. In addition, based on the same antibodies as the Roche NT-proBNP assay, the NT-proBNP assays are provided by Dade-Behring and Ortho Clinical Diagnostics.

MEASUREMENT OF hBNP

The role of proteolytic enzymes in the activation and degradation of natriuretic hormones raises issues concerning the stability of clinical samples. BNP has an intramolecular disulfide bridge and is not a very stable molecule. This is presumably due to its physiological function as a hormone that must be broken down quickly. Therefore, its use as a diagnostic marker requires careful and special attention in sample collection and processing [16]. On the other hand, NT-proBNP is relatively stable, even in separated serum without protease inhibitors for 24 h [17]. The collection of specimens for BNP assays requires the addition of EDTA, which will inhibit proteases and can be further assisted by protease inhibitors, such as aprotinin. To improve BNP stability in tested specimens, Belenky *et al.* [18] patented a method of stabilizing hBNP with at least 1 component from a group consisting of leupeptin, antipain, H-D-Phe-Phe-Arg-chloromethylketone, D-Phe-Pro-Arg-chloromethylketone, diisopropylfluorophosphate or their combination. Shimizu *et al.* [19, 20] invented glass containers coated with silicone to preserve BNP stability in collected specimens. Because natural and synthetic BNP is cleaved by proteases at the amino terminus between aa 78-79 and at the carboxy terminus between aa 106-108, Shih *et al.* [21, 22] developed antibodies that specifically bind to hBNP epitopes that are not cleaved by proteases. This strategy is continued in the recent patent [23]. Mischak *et al.* [24] patented reagents and methods for the rapid and direct quantification of BNP levels in biological fluids. The invention targeted 3 epitopes on the BNP 32 molecule which are recognized by monospecific antibodies. The antibody that is monospecific for a peptide epitope comprising aa 91-101 on the hBNP 32 molecule (M-D-R-I-S-S-S-S-G-L-G) is claimed to be a preferred reagent. The invention of Asada *et al.* [25] is an immunoradiometric assay kit with 2 different monoclonal antibodies which recognize the carboxyl terminal structure and the disulfide bond-mediated ring structure of hBNP. These authors have indicated that this method is specific for BNP 32 and does not detect the other molecular forms. To increase the test sensitivity of several clinical assays, including hBNP detection, Campbell *et al.* [26] proposed reaction with 3 monospecific antibodies that recognize different epitopes. On the other hand, Kono *et al.* [27] have produced a monoclonal antibody recognizing the C-terminus of hBNP with a minimum detection limit of 1 pg/ml. It can quantify hBNP levels directly in plasma without extraction. To improve diagnosis based on hBNP a new variants of BNP molecule are invented [28].

NT-PROBNP

NT-proBNP measurement specifically poses a problem because of its lack of biological activity. The production of NT-proBNP antibodies by means of peptide immunization is possible in principle, but affinity for the whole molecule is generally too low to reach the necessary sensitivity in diagnostic tests. Another difficulty derives from NT-proBNP heterogeneity in the circulation. Most immunoreactive NT-proBNP is significantly smaller in size than NT-proBNP1-76, with truncation at both termini. The smallest fragments can be detected by assays directed at the central part of NT-proBNP. The original patent [29] describes an immunological method of identifying NT-proBNP (aa 47-64). Correspondingly, the patent of Klemt *et al.* [30] refers to a small epitope on the NT-proBNP molecule (aa 41-46) and the methods for correlation of peptide level and HF. This research has resulted in several recent patents [31-33] claiming methodology for detecting proBNP with an antibody (or antibody combinations) specific for small epitope(s) inside NT-proBNP. The authors assert that this strategy detects "native proBNP", a marker more relevant clinically in the diagnosis of HF than total NT-proBNP measurements. Furthermore, de Bold [34] invented a monoclonal antibody with high affinity for NT-proBNP.

Therefore, important issues evolving around BNP assays include the choice of peptide to be measured and the measurement method. Failure to detect the active form of BNP and NT-proBNP could result in missed or incorrect diagnosis.

Combination of NPs

Hess and Horsch [35] patented a protocol combining tests for NT-proANP and NT-proBNP. Accordingly, NT-proANP in the presence of non- or weakly-increased NT-proBNP levels indicates an acute cardiac event, whereas augmented NT-proANP levels in the presence of highly-elevated NT-proBNP suggest chronic cardiac disease. They also presented invention facilitating to distinguish a diastolic dysfunction and systolic dysfunction [36]. Furthermore, Hess and Horsch [37] devised a 2-step procedure to diagnose the risk of cardiotoxic medications by quantitating ANP, NT-proANP, BNP, and NT-proBNP levels in body fluid or tissues. A similar method for the simultaneous detection of proANP and proBNP in samples tested for cardiac disease has been invented by Vuolteenaho *et al.* [38].

BNP Assays Combined with Other Clinical Tests

For the right diagnosis, BNP determination should be combined with other clinical tests. Ng [39] invented a method to screen patients for the likelihood of left ventricular systolic dysfunction on the basis of biomarker measurements (including BNP) and ECG analysis. Minamino *et al.* [40] hold that elevated plasma BNP correlates with loss of cardiomyocytes in the heart. Therefore, more accurate diagnosis of HF should include the study of apoptosis in heart biopsy combined with BNP assay in plasma. Recent reports indicate that the combined elevation of cardiac troponin and BNP in ambulatory patients with chronic HF contributes to the highest risk [41]. To provide a method for examining myocarditis or cardiomyopathy related to hepatitis C virus, BNP and NT-proBNP analysis in blood has been invented in addition to tests for viral antigens in cardiac biopsies and viral antibodies in the circulation [42]. Correspondingly, for diagnosis of some pulmonary or cardiovascular pathology is proposed combined assay of natriuretic peptides and interleukins [43].

hBNP in HF

Acute decompensated HF is a major public health problem throughout the world. HF, traditionally diagnosed by history and physical examination, is difficult to recognize clinically in its early stages. Supplementary diagnostic testing includes chest radiography, echocardiography, right-sided heart catherization, and the 6-minute walk test. Several studies have already demonstrated that HF diagnosis based on clinical history, physical signs and standard testing may be inadequate. NPs have been investigated as markers of HF diagnosis and management. Early studies in patients with HF showed that both ANP and BNP secretion from the ventricles increased in relation to the severity of ventricular dysfunction, as reflected by indices of left ventricular wall tension. These observations led to investigations of both ANP and BNP and their NT fragments as diagnostic tests for HF.

BNP increases more significantly than ANP in relation to the clinical severity of HF and, therefore, is a biomarker that detects risk, assesses the prognosis, and guides the management of HF.

BNP in Diagnosis

Studies have evaluated the diagnostic, prognostic and therapeutic monitoring value of BNP and NT-proBNP testing in HF patients. Plasma BNP and NT-proBNP concentrations correlate with elevated end-diastolic pressure, which closely parallels dyspnea in HF. This suggests that these biomarkers, increasing as HF progresses, are uniquely suited for accurate neurohormonal profiling. Elevated plasma BNP levels reflect the severity of myocardial ischemia, even before the appearance of necrosis, HF, acute atrial fibrillation and coronary heart disease. BNP levels are also elevated in patients with chronic obstructive pulmonary disease which forms the base for studies on the usefulness of BNP in distinguishing dyspnea due to HF from non-cardiac dyspnea [44, 45], pulmonary hypertension [46], and liver cirrhosis [47]. Patients with renal failure had markedly elevated plasma BNP levels [48]. Their BNP levels declined somewhat after dialysis sessions. It is unclear whether the elevations are due to volume overload (leading to increased BNP secretion), decreased metabolism and clearance of BNP, or decreased cardiac function.

These BNP tests to rule out HF may save patients from additional invasive and uncomfortable testing for HF, such as ECG and right heart catheterization, allowing care to focus on other reasons for shortness of breath. Based on diagnostic evidence, the Food and Drug Administration in the USA and other health authorities have approved BNP and NT-proBNP as blood tests to aid in the diagnosis of HF. Furthermore, the Task Force of the European Society of Cardiology for the diagnosis and treatment of chronic HF recently confirmed the recommendation that cardiac natriuretic hormone assay should be included in the first step of the algorithm for the diagnosis of both acute and chronic HF in adult patients [49]. In practice, in patients with dyspnea and BNP <100 pg/ml or NTproBNP <300 pg/ml, a diagnosis of HF is unlikely. BNP results in the 100-500 pg/ml range (NT-proBNP, 300-450 pg/ml) indicate an intermediate probability of HF, and values exceeding 500 pg/ml (NT-proBNP, 900 pg/ml) are consistent with a high likelihood of HF. Other diagnoses such as chronic left ventricular dysfunction, lung disease or pulmonary embolism, should also be taken into consideration. BNP levels may be affected by age, sex, weight, and renal function [50-53]. A recent invention, proposing the identification of an oxidized form of hBNP in samples as an indicator of HF [54], is based on the observation that the heart produces oxidized hBNP at methionine residues. In subjects experiencing cardiovascular disease, such as HF, oxidized BNP forms are released into the blood at higher than normal levels. As such, the detection of these oxidized BNP forms serves as an indication of cardiovascular disease. Amann-Zalan *et al.* [55] claimed to have invented an HF diagnosis test based on the amount of BNP in urine samples. It has been found in accordance with their invention that a urinary amount of BNP of at least 0.8 pg/ml is indicative for HF.

BNP as a Risk Predictor

Before cardiac pathologies become overt, and in the absence of HF, a modest increase in plasma BNP levels may serve as an important prognostic tool [56-58]. Plasma BNP and NT-proBNP concentrations correlate with elevated end-diastolic pressure, which closely parallels dyspnea in HF. BNP is heightened in patients with right ventricle HF, but the increase is not as great as the BNP increment from left ventricular dysfunction. Masson *et al.* [59], who directly compared BNP and NT-proBNP in patients with chronic and stable HF, concluded that both NPs showed subtle differences in their relationship to clinical characteristics and prognostic performance. It appears that NT-proBNP is better than BNP analysis for predicting death and the need of hospitalization in HF. BNP assay can help to predict the prognosis post-HF and post-infarction [60] as well as after HF with acute dyspnea [61]. Correspondingly, researchers associated with Roche Diagnostics [62, 63] claimed a procedure for the detection of NT-proBNP as well as a method for correlating NT-proBNP levels to HF severity. Despite the utility of NT-proBNP as a marker of HF, the influence of medical illnesses other than HF that raise NT-proBNP concentrations should be considered. In particular, chronic renal disease is associated with increased NT-proBNP levels due to reduced renal clearance. These potential problems are not trivial since a large number of HF patients also suffer renal failure.

BNP in Conditions Other than HF

BNP assays represent potential diagnostic tools for screening populations to identify asymptotic left ventricular dysfunction [64]. However, the prevalence of preclinical left ventricular systolic or diastolic dysfunction by screening with BNP for asymptomatic disease is considered suboptimal, requiring confirmatory echocardiography [65]. NT-proBNP is at least as effective as BNP in detecting left ventricular dysfunction in normal patients [66].

Increased plasma BNP in patients with coronary artery disease in the absence of ventricular dysfunction indicates that BNP production might also be enhanced by myocardial ischemia [67]. In this respect, for the early detection of coronary artery disease, the measurement of plasma BNP levels was invented to study patients before and after cardiac stress induced by either exercise or pharmacological agents [68]. Ample evidence supports the role of BNP and NT-proBNP in predicting mortality in patients with acute coronary syndrome [69] or stable coronary artery disease [70]. NT-proBNP is a strong predictor of adverse events in non-ST-segment elevation acute coronary syndrome and the NT-proBNP levels were particularly predictive for mortality, probably because they reflect larger infarct size, progressive remodeling, and thus a more pronounced degree of myocardial dysfunction [71]. The patent of Dahlen *et al.* [72] disclosed that BNP levels in patient samples, alone or in combination with other markers, provides prognostic information predicting near-term morbidity and/or mortality in acute coronary syndrome. The elevation of natriuretic peptides in the plasma samples can facilitate diagnosis of cardiac complications in patient subjected to coronary catherization [73] or for the stratification of therapy with erythropoietic stimulating agents [74].

There is reasonable evidence that therapies that reduce adverse clinical events in HF also lower BNP levels. BNP assay has been patented to assess the effectiveness of specific therapeutic interventions in other diseases, including the treatment of hypertension [75]. However, in hypertension, BNP levels are usually low, and high intra-individual assay variability precludes its use in this situation [76]. Further inventions view BNP as a marker of cardiovascular function in patients receiving Cox-2 inhibitors [68], cardiotoxic medications [38] and cardiac allograft rejection [77], to examine the risk of cardiovascular complications in osteoporosis patients [78]. On the other hand, inhibition of by blocking natriuretic peptide signaling *via* NPR-A is proposed for reducing inflammation [79].

hBNP as a Drug

The technology for producing nesiritide, hBNP designed for the treatment of cardiovascular pathologies, was invented by scientists associated with Scios Inc. [80, 81], which patented recombinant DNA encoding a BNP with potent natriuretic activity attributed to the aa sequence Cys-Phe-Gly-Arg-Lys-Met-Asp-Arg-Ile-Ser-Ser-Ser-Ser-Gly-Leu-Gly-Cys. Another patent presented by this company [82] provided an hBNP sequence with increased vasodilation and/or natriuresis potential. To improve the stability of the BNP molecule produced for the *in vivo* treatment of HF, new inventions proposed hBNP conjugates [83-86] which retain activity for stimulating cGMP production, binding to NPR-A, decreasing arterial blood pressure and have improved an half-life in the circulation. The proposed conjugates are constructed by various combinations, but the major peptide of the invention is a molecule containing a small aa sequence attached to Lys residues of hBNP. Another invention for improving hBNP stability in the body proposes the production of dipeptidyl peptidase-resistant molecules [87]. Dipeptidyl peptidases exist in various tissues and catalyze the sequential release of dipeptides from peptides, including hBNP. These inventions propose to replace the dipeptide moieties Xaa-Pro- or Xaa-Ala-, which are the targets of enzymes, with other aa sequences (Xaa = any aa). Another invention claims the pharmacological manipulation of δ-opioid receptors (e.g. by the administration of enkephalins) in intrinsic cardiac adrenergic cells to enhance BNP production and exert cardioprotection [88].

BNP Use in Therapy

Given the biological effects of NPs, their exploration in the treatment of HF patients is rational. Two synthetic NPs have been developed for use in HF: recombinant hBNP, nesiritide (commercial name Natrecor), distributed by Scios Inc. [81, 89], and ANP, carperitide, from the Daiichi Pharmaceutical Co. Ltd. Japan, [90]. These peptides mimic the action of endogenous NPs by binding to the same receptors in the heart, kidneys and vasculature, for the treatment of acute, decompensated, congestive HF in patients who have dyspnea at rest. Carperitide was approved for use in Japan in 1995 for the management of HF. ANP infusion reduces cardiac filling pressure, cardiac output, and stroke volume, an effect that has been attributed to ANP-induced venous vasodilatation in addition to fluid shifts or changes in diuresis and pulmonary or peripheral vascular resistance. Nesiritide was approved in the United States in 2001 for the treatment of HF patients. Nesiritide causes vasodilatation and may influence renal blood flow and natriuresis. Nesiritide produces dose-related reductions in pulmonary capillary wedge pressure (preload), right atrial pressure, and systemic vascular resistance (afterload) and indirectly leads to increases in stroke volume and cardiac output [90, 91]. However, clinical trials of nesiritide have not demonstrated any clinical advantage and revealed that, in comparison to non-inotrope-based control therapy, it is associated with an increased risk of renal dysfunction and greater mortality in patients with acutely-decompensated HF [92, 93]. In addition, several side-effects of nesiritide have been noted: asymptomatic hypotension (a decrease of 5 to 10 mmHg), nausea, headaches, insomnia and angina [94]. Some efforts are made to improve effects of nesiritide therapy. Intravenous nesiritide administration requires extended hospitalization of patients and, at current doses, ANP and BNP are rapidly degraded and removed by clearance receptors. To avoid this difficulty, the perioperative administration of low-dose nesiritide is proposed. Experiments in a dog model have demonstrated that such hBNP administration is biologically effective with increases of plasma cGMP and suppression of aldosterone [95]. In conclusion, nesiritide has not yet met the minimal criteria for safety and efficacy. Until a trial definitively proves that this drug reduces the risk of death or repeated hospitalization for HF, there will be questions about the appropriateness of the drug's use or even commercial availability.

New Technologies

The BNP is an example of polypeptides with high clearance from the body. This property of BNP poses problems when the peptide is applied as therapy. Alternatively, the BNP gene can be delivered by specific DNA vectors to achieve constitutive NP production in the body. Recently, Simari presented a method of administering of a DNA molecule encoding BNP, DNP, or chimeras of ANP, CNP, BNP or DNP, proposed for the inhibition or prevention of various cardiovascular diseases [96]. Both intracardiac and systemic administration of DNA is envisioned and may be accomplished by a recombinant adenovirus encoding NP sequences. Furthermore, Burnett and Lisy [97] patented peptides of Dendroaspis, including chimeric peptides of DNP and other NPs with potent natriuretic, diuretic, and/or vasodilator actions. A preferred peptide of the invention, a chimeric combining the core ring of the BNP molecule with the C-terminus of DNP, induces vasodilation with a focus on the pulmonary tree, natriuresis and the suppression of renin.

CURRENT AND FUTURE DEVELOPMENTS

The diagnostic measurement of plasma BNP and NT-proBNP is increasing the differentiation of HF from non-HF causes of dyspnea. These tests have been used effectively to assess the prognosis after myocardial infarction. BNP and NT-proBNP are better predictors of adverse events than predictors of death or HF.

Studies should not be limited to HF. New protocols are required with BNP as a marker of, for example, myocardial infarction, acute coronary syndrome, angina pectoris (stable and unstable), cardiomyopathy, myocarditis, and the diffe-rential diagnosis of heart-related conditions from lung-related conditions (such as pulmonary embolism). Because of the possibility of an increased risk of death, more controlled clinical investigations are necessary to understand the pathophysiological magnitude of BNP effects for the treatment of cardiac diseases to determine its clinical impact and relevance in comparison to traditional therapy.

REFERENCES

[1] De Bold AJ, Borenstein HB, Veress AT, *et al.* A rapid and potent natriuretic response to intravenous injection of atrial myocardial extract in rats. Life Sci 1981; 28: 89-94.

[2] Goetz K, Drummer C, Zhu JL, *et al.* Evidence that urodilatin, rather than ANP, regulates renal sodium excretion. J Am Soc Nephr 1990; 1: 867-874.

[3] Sudoh T, Kangawa K, Minamino M, *et al.* A new natriuretic peptide in porcine brain. Nature 1988; 332: 78-81.

[4] Cataliotti A, Chen HH, James KD, *et al.* Oral brain natriuretic peptide: A novel strategy for chronic protein therapy for cardiovascular disease. Trends Cardiovasc Med 2007; 17: 10-14.

[5] Mukoyama M, Nakao K, Hosoda K, *et al.* Brain natriuretic peptide as a novel cardiac hormone in humans - Evidence for an exquisite dual natriuretic peptide system, atrial natriuretic peptide and brain natriuretic peptide. J Clin Invest 1991; 87: 1402-1412.

[6] Sudoh T, Minamino N, Kangawa K, *et al.* C-type natriuretic peptide (CNP): a new member of natriuretic peptide family identified in porcine brain. Biochem Biophys Res Commun 1990; 168: 863-870.

[7] Tervonen V, Arjamaa O, Kokkonen K, *et al.* A novel cardiac hormone related to A-, B- and C-type natriuretic peptides. Endocrinology 1998; 139: 4021-4025.

[8] Singh G, Kuc RE, Maguire JJ, *et al.* Novel snake venom ligand dendroaspis natriuretic peptide is selective for natriuretic peptide receptor-A in human heart: downregulation of natriuretic peptide receptor-A in heart failure. Circ Res 2006; 99: 183-190.

[9] Lee CYW, Burnett JC Jr. Nariuretic peptides and therapeutic applications. Heart Fail Rev 2007; 12: 131-142.

[10] Koller KJ, Goeddel DV. Molecular biology of the natriuretic peptides and their receptors. Circulation 1992; 86: 1081 1088.

[11] De Bold AJ, Bruneau BG, de Bold KML. Mechanical and neuroendocrine regulation of the endocrine heart. Cardiovasc Res 1996; 31: 7-18.

[12] Hall C. Essential biochemistry and physiology of (NT-pro)BNP. Eur J Heart Fail 2004; 6: 257-260.

[13] Yandle TG, Richards AM, Gilbert A, *et al.* Assay of brain natriuretic peptide (BNP) in human plasma: evidence for high molecular weight BNP as a major plasma component in heart failure. J Clin Endocrinol Metab 1993; 76: 832-838.

[14] Heublein DM, Huntley BK, Boerrigter G, *et al.* Immunoreactivity and guanosine 3',5'-cyclic monophosphate activating actions of various molecular forms of human B-type natriuretic peptide. Hypertension 2007; 49:1114-1119.

[15] Giuliani I, Rieunier F, Larue C, *et al.* Assay for measurement of intact B-type natriuretic peptide prohormone in blood. Clin Chem 2006; 52:1054-1061.

[16] Shimizu H, Aono K, Masuta K, *et al.* Stability of brain natriuretic peptide (BNP) in human blood samples. Clin Chim Acta 1999; 285:169-172.

[17] van der Merwe DE, Henley R, Lane G, *et al.* Effect of different sample types and stability after blood collection of N-terminal pro-B-type natriuretic peptide as measured with Roche Elecsys system. Clin Chem 2004; 50: 779-780.

[18] Belenky, A., Livshin, L.A., Barbarakis, M.: WO2006102612 (**2006**).

[19] Shimizu, H., Asada, H., Endo, K.: WO99022235 (**1999**).

[20] Shimizu, H., Asada, H., Endo, K.: US20097534582 (**2009**).

[21] Shih, J. W., Pinkus, M. S., Tyner, J. D., Brophy, S. E., Tu, Bailin.: WO2007056507 (**2007**).

[22] Shih, J. W., Tyner, J. D., Matias M.S., Pinkus, M. S., Brophy, S. E., Daghfal D.J., Hawksworth, D.J.: WO2006088700 (**2006**).

[23] Buchler, K.F.: US20097524635 (**2009**).

[24] Mischak, R. P., Lim, G. A., Scardina, J. M.: WO97032900 (**1997**).

[25] Asada, H., Shimizu, H., Endou, K.: WO99013331 (**1999**).

[26] Campbell, J.E.L., Frank, P.A., Hawkes, M.E., Lobin, S.R., Miller, C.J.; Yang, Z.: WO2004011947 (**2004**).

[27] Kono, M., Tsuji, T., Inouye, K., Yamauchi, A., Igano, K.: US20046677124 (**2004**).

[28] Colocaru, G. S., Diber, A., Novik, A., Pollock, S., Levine, Z., Cohen, Y., Ayalon-Soffer, M.: US20080182299 (**2008**).

[29] Dzieglewska, H., Medinnova E, Hall, C.: WO93024531 (**1993**).

[30] Klemt, V., Borgya, A., Gallusser, A., Grol, M., Hallermayer, K., Seidel, C.: WO2004099253 (**2004**).
[31] Borgya, A., Gallusser, A., Grol, M., Hallermayer, K., Klemt, V., Seidel, C.: US20077264939 (**2007**).
[32] Borgya, A., Gallusser, A., Grol, M., Hallermayer, K., Klemt, V., Seidel, C.: US20077264938 (**2007**).
[33] Borgya, A., Gallusser, A., Grol, M., Hallermayer, K., Klemt, V., Seidel, C.: US20070117156 (**2007**).
[34] DeBold, A.: US20056960472 (**2005**).
[35] Hess, G., Horsch, A.: WO2006131529 (**2006**).
[36] Hess, G., Horsch, A.: US20080085862 (**2008**).
[37] Hess, G., Horsch, A.: WO2005124364 (**2005**).
[38] Vuolteenaho, O., Ala-Kopsala, M., Ruskoaho, H., Leppäluoto, J. Haapalahti.: WO2005003764 (**2005**).
[39] Ng, L.: WO2004034903 (**2004**).
[40] Minamino, T., Hori, M., Okada, K., Kitakaze, M.: US20070065850 (**2007**).
[41] Miller WL, Hartman KA, Burritt MF, *et al.* Serial biomarker measurements in ambulatory patients with chronic heart failure. Circulation 2007; 116: 249-257.
[42] Matsumori, A.: WO07023815 (**2007**).
[43] Snider, J.V., Jackobson, S.: WO131031 (**2007**).
[44] Maisel AS, Krishnaswamy P, Nowak RM, *et al.* Rapid measurement of B-type natriuretic peptide in the emergency diagnosis of heart failure. New Engl J Med 2002; 347:161-167.
[45] Mogelvang R, Goetze JP, Schnohr P, *et al.* Discriminating between cardiac and pulmonary dysfunction in the general population with dyspnea by plasma pro-b-type natriuretic peptide. J Am Coll Cardiol 2007; 50:1694-1701.
[46] Mueller C. B-type natriuretic peptides and the general practitioner. J Am Coll Cardiol 2007; 50:1702-1703.
[47] Wong F, Siu S, Liu P, Blendis LM. Brain natriuretic peptide: is it a predictor of cardiomyopathy in cirrhosis? Clin Sci 2001; 101:621-628.
[48] deFilippi CR, Seliger SL, Maynard S, *et al.* Impact of renal disease on natriuretic peptide testing for diagnosing decompensated heart failure and predicting mortality. Clin Chem 2007; 53:1511-1519.
[49] Swedberg K, Cleland J, Dargie H, *et al.* Guidelines for the diagnosis and treatment of chronic heart failure: executive summary (update 2005): the task force for the diagnosis and treatment of chronic heart failure of the European Society of Cardiology. Eur Heart J 2005; 26: 1115-1140.
[50] Winter WE, Elin RJ. The role and assessment of ventricular peptides in heart failure. Clin Lab Med 2004; 24: 235-274.
[51] Iwanaga Y, Kihara Y, Niizuma S, *et al.* BNP in overweight and obese patients with heart failure: an analysis based on the bnp-lv diastolic wall stress relationship. J Card Fail 2007; 13: 663-667.
[52] Krauser DG, Lloyd-Jones DM, Chae CU, *et al.* Effect of body mass index on natriuretic peptide levels in patients with acute congestive heart failure. A pro-BNP investigation of dyspnea in the emergency department (PRIDE) substudy. Am Heart J 2005; 149:744-750.
[53] Christ M, Laule-Kilian K, Hochholzer W, *et al.* Gender-specific risk stratification with B-type natriuretic peptide levels in patients with acute dyspnea: insights from the B-type natriuretic peptide for acute shortness of breath evaluation study. J Am Coll Cardiol 2006; 48:1808-1812.
[54] Protter, A.A.: WO2007041645 (**2007**).
[55] Amann-Zalan, I., Trauth, B., Rivera, O.J.M.: WO2006120152 (**2006**).
[56] Wang TJ, Larson MG, Levy D, *et al.* Plasma natriuretic peptide levels and the risk of cardiovascular events and death. N Engl J Med 2004; 350: 655-663.
[57] Struthers A, Lang C. The potential to improve primary prevention in the future by using BNP/N-BNP as an indicator of silent 'pancardiac' target organ damage: BNP/N-BNP could become for the heart what microalbuminuria is for the kidney. Eur Heart J 2007; 28: 1678-1682.
[58] McKie PM, Rodeheffer RJ, Cataliotti A, *et al.* Amino-terminal pro-B-type natriuretic peptide and B-type natriuretic peptide: biomarkers for mortality in a large community-based cohort free of heart failure. Hypertension 2006; 47: 874-880.
[59] Masson S, Latini R, Anad IS, *et al.* Direct comparison of B-type natriuretic peptide (BNP) and amino-terminal proBNP in a large population of patients with chronic and symptomatic heart failure: the valsartan heart failure (Val-HeFT) data. Clin Chem 2006; 106: 416-422.
[60] Uusimaa P, Ruskoaho H, Vuolteenaho O, *et al.* Plasma vasoactive peptides after acute myocardial infarction in relation to left ventricular dysfunction. Int J Cardiol 1999; 69: 5-14.
[61] McCullough PA, Nowak RM, McCord J, *et al.* B-type natriuretic peptide and clinical judgment in emergency diagnosis of heart failure: analysis from Breathing Not Properly (BNP) Multinational Study. Circulation 2002; 106: 416-422.
[62] Klemt, V., Borgya, A., Gallusser, A., Grol, M., Hallermayer, K., Seidel, C.: WO2004099253 (**2004**).
[63] Klemt, V., Borgya, A., Gallusser, A., Grol, M., Hallermayer, K., Seidel.: WO2004099252 (**2004**).
[64] McDonagh TA, Robb SD, Murdoch DR, *et al.* Biochemical detection of left-ventricular systolic dysfunction. Lancet 1998; 351: 9-13.

[65] Redfield MM, Rodeheffer RJ, Jacobsen SJ, *et al.* Plasma brain natriuretic peptide to detect preclinical ventricular systolic or diastolic dysfunction: a community-based study. Circulation 2004; 109: 3176-3181.

[66] Costello-Boerrigter LC, Boerrigter G, Redfield MM, *et al.* Amino-terminal pro-B-type natriuretic peptide and B-type natriuretic peptide in the general community: determinants and detection of left ventricular dysfunction. J Am Coll Cardiol 2006; 47: 345-353.

[67] Yeo K-T, Lee H-K, Wong K-C, *et al.* Can exercise-induced changes in B-type natriuretic peptides be used to detect cardiac ischemia? J Card Fail 2005; 11: S59-S64.

[68] Zoghbi, W.A., Win, H. K.: WO2004082639 (**2004**).

[69] Morrow DA, de Lemos JA, Blazing MA, *et al.* Prognostic value of serial B-type natriuretic peptide testing during follow-up of patients with unstable coronary artery disease. JAMA 2005; 294: 2866-2871.

[70] Ndrepepa G, Braun S, Schömig A, *et al.* Accuracy of N-terminal pro-brain natriuretic peptide to predict mortality in various subsets of patients with coronary artery disease. Am J Cardiol 2007; 100: 575-578.

[71] Eggers KM, Lagerqvist B, Venge P, *et al.* Prognostic value of biomarkers during and after non-ST-segment elevation acute coronary syndrome. J Am Coll Cardiol 2009; 54: 357-364.

[72] Dahlen, J.R.,Valkirs, G.E., Buechler, K. F.: WO02083913 (**2002**).

[73] Hess, G., Horsch, A., Zdunek, D.: WO08034750 (**2008**).

[74] Amann-Zalan, I., Moecks, J., Burger, H.U., Escrig, C., Scherhag, A., Dougherty, F.: US20080050749 (**2008**).

[75] Diamond. C., Man, A., Bremer, T.: US20050181386 (**2005**).

[76] Conen D, Pfisterer M, Martina B. Substantial intraindividual variability of BNP concentrations in patients with hypertension. J Humens Hypertens 2006; 20: 387-391.

[77] Spanuth, E.: WO2006077265 (**2006**).

[78] DeBold, A.: US20006117644 (**2000**).

[79] Mohapatra, S.S., Weidong, X., Kong, X., Wang, X.: US20070265204 (**2007**).

[80] Spanuth, E.: WO2007104682 (**2007**).

[81] Seilhamer, J.J., Lewicki J., Scarborough, R.M., Porter, J.G.: US5674710 (**1997**).

[82] Schreiner, G. F.: WO03081246 (**2003**).

[83] Seilhamer, J. J., Lewicki, J., Scarborough, R. M., Porter, G. J.: US20060030004 (**2006**).

[84] Kim, Y.M., Kim, D.J., Bae, S.M., Lim, C.K., Kwon, S.C., Lee, G.S., Song, D.H., Young H.: US20080085862 (**2008**).

[85] Bhaskar, V., Dubridge, R.B., Ramakrishnan, V., Jantzen, H.M., US20080181903 (**2008**).

[86] Whittaker, M.: US20080045444 (**2008**).

[87] James, K.: WO2006076471 (**2006**).

[88] Lambeir, A-M., Brandt, I., Scharpé, S., De Meester, I.: WO06108686 (**2006**).

[89] Huang, M., Uretsky, B.: WO2007033211 (**2007**).

[90] Pollitt, S. N., Buckley, D. I., Stathis, P. A., Hartman T. E., Zhong, Z.: US5114923 (**1992**).

[91] Masafumi K.: US20067026293 (**2006**).

[92] Sackner-Bernstein JD, Kowalski M, *et al.* Short-term risk of death after treatment with nesiritide for decompensated heart failure: a pooled analysis of randomized controlled trials. JAMA 2005; 293:1900-1905.

[93] Iglesias JI, Depalma L, Hom D, *et al.* Predictors of mortality in adult patients with congestive heart failure receiving nesiritide retrospective analysis showing a potential adverse interaction between neseritide and acute renal dysfunction. Nephrol Dial Transplant 2008; 23:144-153.

[94] Feldman DS, Sun B. Practical application of human B-type natriuretic peptide as a therapeutic intervention in the perioperative setting. Heart Fail Rev 2004; 9:203-208.

[95] Chen HH, Sundt DJ, Cook DJ, *et al.* Low dose nesiritide and the preservation of renal function in patients with renal dysfunction undergoing cardiopulmonary-bypass surgery: a double-blind placebo-controlled pilot study. Circulation 2007; 116: I-133- I-138.

[96] Simari, R.D.: US20060025367 (**2006**).

[97] Burnett, J.Jr., Lisy, O.: US2005059600 (**2005**).

Urokinase-An Important Anti-Thromboembolic Drug

Adinarayana Kunamneni*, Bhavani D. Ravuri, Vinjamuri Saisha, Poluri Ellaiah and Taadimalla Prabhakhar

Pharmaceutical Biotechnology Division, University College of Pharmaceutical Sciences, Andhra University, Visakhapatnam-530 003, India

Abstract: Urokinase (UK) [EC 3.4.99.26] is a serine protease that activates plasminogen to plasmin, which in turn degrades fibrin clots. Plasmin has diverse physiological roles apart from its fibrinolytic role in the regulation of blood clotting. It has been implicated in complement activation, cell migration, wound healing, and generation of localized extracellular proteolysis during tissue remodelling, pro-hormone conversion, carcinogenesis and neoplasia. Among the plasminogen activators, UK provides a superior alternative for the simple reasons of its being more potent as compared to tissue-plasminogen activator and non-antigenic by virtue of its human origin unlike streptokinase. Based on these observations, UK is an important anti-thromboembolic drug. Hence, UK, as one of the most potent plasminogen activators is attracting a great deal of attention. In this chapter, we will summarize recent patents related to the occurrence, mechanism of action, structure and function, physico-chemical properties, *in vitro* production, cloning and expression, purification and applications of UK.

Keywords: Urokinase (UK), plasminogen activators, fibrinolysis, cardiovascular agent, production, cloning and expression, purification, physico-chemical properties and applications.

INTRODUCTION

Plasminogen activators (PAs) are serine proteases that convert the zymogen plasminogen to the active protease plasmin by the cleavage of an Arg-Val peptide bond [1]. Urokinase (UK) [EC 3.4.99.26] is a strong plasminogen activator, which is involved, in many physiological processes. It activates plasminogen to plasmin by cleavage of Arg-Val bond. The active plasmin formed degrades the fibrin polymers of blood clots. It has been implicated in complement activation [2], cell migration [3], wound healing [4], and generation of localized extracellular proteolysis during tissue remodelling [5], pro-hormone conversion, carcinogenesis and neoplasia [6].

In recent years, thrombolytic therapy has revolutionized the treatment of these diverse circulatory disorders such as pulmonary embolism, myocardial infarction, deep vein thrombosis, thrombosis of the eye etc., [7].

* Corresponding author: E-mail: adikunamneni@rediffmail.com

Therapy in thrombosis has been directed towards interference with coagulation mechanism, activation of fibrinolytic system, interference with platelet aggregation or combination of these. In addition, surgical intervention to prevent embolization or to remove thrombi and restore blood flow is of critical importance.

Thrombolytic drugs play a crucial role in the management of patients with acute myocardial infarction, pulmonary embolism, deep vein thrombosis, arterial thrombosis, acute thrombosis of retinal vessels, extensive coronary emboli and peripheral vascular thromboembolism [8].

Thrombolytic agents have the unique ability to activate the components, intrinsic to the fibrinolytic system, resulting in degradation of blood clots which restores blood flow through occluded vessels. Recognition of the importance of fibrinolytic system in thrombus resolution has resulted in the development of different fibrinolytic agents [8,9].

The choice of a thrombolytic agent during therapy is dictated by a number of factors, which depends essentially upon the relative merits and demerits of individual PAs. These include the cost of the drug, side effects and their severity, *in vivo* stability and specificity towards the fibrin clots and immunological reactivity [10].

Among the PAs, UK provides a superior alternative for the simple reasons of its being more potent as compared to tissue plasminogen activator (t-PA) and non-antigenic by virtue of its human origin unlike streptokinase (SK). Based on these observations, UK is an important anti-thromboembolic drug. Hence, UK, as one of the most potent PAs is attracting a great deal of attention. Developments in cell lines and bioprocess technology have made it possible to produce UK from *in vitro* cell culture.

Most of the studies on UK are patented and only a few reports are available in literature on the production and purification of UK. This chapter will focus on reviewing recent patents related to the occurrence, mechanism of action, structure and function, physico-chemical properties, *in vitro* production, cloning and expression, purification and applications of UK.

SOURCES OF UK

UK was first discovered and isolated from human urine [11]. The UK activity in urine is elaborated from the cells lining the kidney tubules [12]. Isolation of UK from urine is a tedious, lengthy procedure and highly expensive also. Further, the yield obtained is very less i.e., 6 CTA (Committee on Thrombolytic Agents) units/L of urine. This value shows that a minimum of 1500 L of urine are required to produce one clinical dose of this enzyme (7500-8000 CTA units). In contrast, UK can be harvested at concentrations of order of 800 CTA units/ml from confluent cultures of human kidney cells.

Cells from different origin are known to produce UK, but generally in low concentration. Astedt *et al.* [13] measured fibrinolytic activity of liver, lung, bone marrow and kidney tissue explants of 16-20 weeks old human fetus and reported that the kidney tissues are the most active in the lysis of fibrin clots. However, human kidney cells are reported as the highest producers of UK [14,15].

Cultured cells have been reported to secrete larger quantities of UK (50-100 ng/ml) when compared to that present in urine (10-15 ng/ml) [12]. Human plasma also contains at least 10 μg/L of UK [16]. As such in recent years, human cell cultures are being used for

UK production and isolation. Different human cell lines which have been used for production of UK are listed in Table **1** [17-25].

Table 1. Production of UK Using Different Human and Recombinant Cell Lines and Their Activities

	UK activity	Reference
Human cell type		
Human kidney cell line (TCL-598)	76 PU/ml	Kohno *et al.* [17]
Human umbilical vein endothelial cells (HUVEC)	0.008 μg/ml	Booyse *et al.* [18]
Human kidney cell line (HT 1080)	140 PU/ml	Khaparde and Roychoudhury [19]
Human lung adenocarcinoma cell lines (CALU-3, HTB-55)	0.3 μg/ml	Khaparde and Roychoudhury [19]
Human kidney carcinoma (CAKI 1)	0.03 μg/ml	Khaparde and Roychoudhury [19]
Human kidney carcinoma (CAKI 2)	0.005 μg/ml	Khaparde and Roychoudhury [19]
Recombinant cell type		
Mouse cells LB6	0.8 mg/L/day	Nolli *et al.* [20]
Chinese hamster ovary cell line	1000 PU/ml	Avgerinors *et al.* [21]
Saccharomyces cerevisiae cells	1863 PU/ml	Turner *et al.* [22]
Namalwa KJM-1	3 μg/10^6 cells/day	Satoh *et al.* [23]
Escherichia coli cells	1500 PU/ml	Tang *et al.* [24]
Chinese hamster ovary cell line	860 PU/ml	Jo *et al.* [25]

Further investigations revealed that the UK is secreted by fibroblasts [26], epithelial cells [27], macrophages [28], cells of malignant tumors of different origin [29] and also by vascular endothelial smooth muscle cells (SMC) [6].

At present, UK is commercially produced by using primary cultures of human neonatal kidney cells [30]. However, these cells can be propagated for a limited period only (30-40 generations). Re-establishing of these primary cells requires extensive screening and testing of the kidney donors. Therefore, many of the continuous and recombinant cell lines are now being considered to be a useful alternative for the production of UK.

MECHANISM OF ACTION OF UK

It is a strong plasminogen activator which specifically cleaves the proenzyme, plasminogen to form the active enzyme plasmin (Fig. **1**). It is a trypsin like enzyme capable of hydrolysing L-lysine and L-arginine esters. It specifically catalyzes the cleavage of the Arg-Val bond in plasminogen by first order kinetics. The active plasmin is then able to break down the fibrin polymers of blood clots. Bell *et al.* [31] studied the mechanism of induction of fibrinolysis by UK and suggested that in systems containing UK, plasminogen and fibrinogen, UK may not activate plasminogen effectively until a plasminogen-fibrinogen complex has formed.

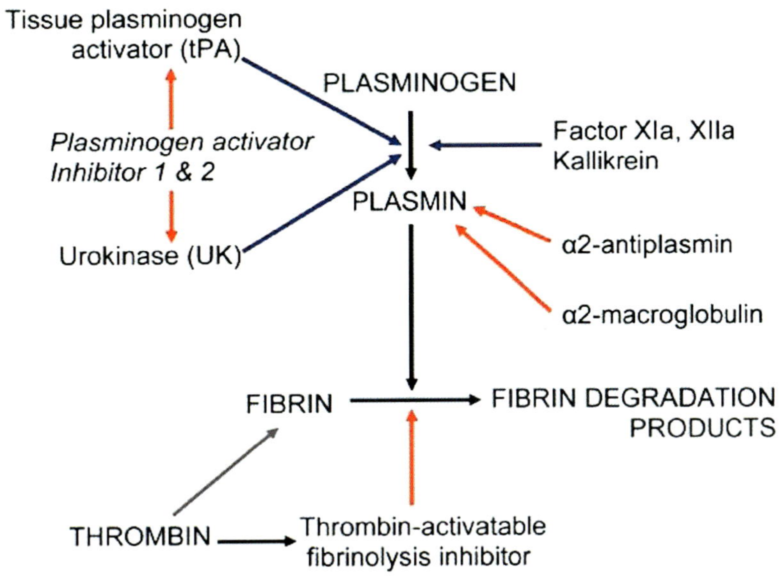

Fig. (1). Schematic representation of the fibrinolytic system with UK.

James and Francis [32] studied the mechanism of activation of rabbit plasminogen by UK. Their studies support a mechanism of activation of plasminogen by UK, which involves loss of peptide located at the NH_2- terminus of plasminogen. However, these same results showed that this NH_2- terminal peptide need not be released from rabbit plasminogen prior to the cleavage of the internal bond, which leads to the two-chain plasmin molecule.

Bernart and Francis [33], reported that human plasminogen (Glu-Pga) is activated by UK in the presence of pancreatic trypsin inhibitor. The plasmin produced (Glu-Pma) exclusively contains a heavy chain (Glu-Ha) derived intact from the original NH_2 terminus of Glu-Pga.

Picone *et al.* [34] identified a specific surface receptor for urokinase-type plasminogen activator (u-PA) which recognizes the amino-terminal growth factor-like sequence of u-PA, a region independent from and not required for the catalytic activity of this enzyme. The properties of the u-PA receptor and the localization and distribution of u-PA in tumor cell and tissues suggested that the u-PA /urokinasetype plasminogen activator receptor (u-PAR) interaction may be important in regulating extracellular proteolysis dependent processes.

STRUCTURE AND FUNCTION OF UK

Structure of UK

UK is synthesized by vascular endothelial and smooth muscle cells (SMC), by epithelial cells, fibroblasts, monocytes/macrophages, and also by cells of malignant tumors of different origin [35]. This protein is secreted by cells as a single-chain polypeptide with molecular weight of 55 kDa that consists of 411 amino acid residues [16,36]. The UK structure is subdivided into three domains: the N-terminal domain homologous to the epidermal growth factor, the kringle domain, and the C-terminal catalytic domain. The "growth factor-like domain" (GFD) is responsible for the interaction of UK with the u-PAR [37]. The protease domain of UK includes the active site of the enzyme represented by a specific for serine proteases amino acid triad His204, Asp255, and Ser356. The kringle domain of UK contains a sequence that interacts with the specific inhibitor PAI-1 (plasminogen activator inhibitor-1) [38]. Each domain of the protein has a rigid structure supported by internal disulfide bonds, three of which are located in the GFD, three in the kringle domain, and six bonds are located in the proteolytic domain. Site-specific mutagenic studies have shown that only the disulphide bridges in the catalytic domain are essential for maintaining amidolytic and fibrinolytic activities of the PA [39,40].

Structure of Pro-Urokinase (pro-UK)/Single-Chain Urokinase-Type Plasminogen Activator (sc-uPA)

Sc-uPA or pro-UK is the precursor of two-chain UK. Although the sc-uPA is a classic zymogen (pro-UK) and is inert in plasma at physiological concentrations, it has several unusual properties which distinguish it from other serine protease zymogens [41]. These include, its unique hypercatalytic transitional state which forms during the conversion of pro-UK to UK [42], its strong promotion by fibrin which gives the intrinsic activity of pro-UK, a catalytic activity against plasminogen equivalent to UK [36], its relatively high intrinsic catalytic activity [43] and its reversible inhibition by diisopropyl fluorophosphate (DFP) [44]. Although pro-UK does not bind to fibrin, it induces fibrin-specific clot lysis [45], but this property depends on its activation being confined to the fibrin clot surface. However, at therapeutic concentrations, pro-UK is subject to non-specific activation to UK in plasma [46], and recombinant pro-UK from *Escherichia coli* appears to be especially susceptible to this [47].

The sc-uPA has low intrinsic activity against synthetic substrates [48]. Therefore, this UK form was for a long time considered as the enzyme precursor, or pro-UK. However, pro-UK can convert plasminogen into plasmin. Plasmin, in its turn, activates UK and converts the sc-uPA into the two-chain form (tc-uPA) [49]. In addition to plasmin, activation of sc-uPA by kallikrein, trypsin, T-cell associated serine protease and the thiol proteinase cathepsin-B has also been reported [50-52]. A number of bonds in UK undergo proteolytic cleavage with formation of several variants of the protein on the cell surface.

Glycosylation of UK

UK is known to be a mosaic protein [53] by virtue of N-glycosylation of Asn302 in the proteolytic domain and O-glycosylation of Thr18 in the GFD. This glycosylation increases by 10-15% the molecular weight of the UK. The role of UK glycosylation has not been determined conclusively, but some data suggest that the Asn302-glycosylated UK is more susceptible to activation by plasmin and is more resistant to inhibitors [54]. The deglycosylation of the thr18 residue within the GFD of UK can cause the loss of the mitogenic properties, despite its unaltered affinity for u-PAR [55]. The neutral sugar content of high molecular weight (HMW) UK is 14.5% mole and that of low molecular weight (LMW) UK is 13.9% mole [56]. However, Li *et al.* [57] reported that the carbohydrate in sc-uPA is not important for its fibrinolytic activity in plasma.

There are conflicting reports in the literature regarding the importance of these glycosyl moieties in the catalytic role of UK. The recombinant non-glycosylated pro-UK from mammalian cells as well as from *E. coli* has been found to possess a higher catalytic efficiency against plasminogen than native pro-UK [54,58,59]. More recent report by Wang *et al.* [41] suggested that the glycosyl residue on pro-UK or UK is functionally important and modulates its activation and catalytic efficiency against its natural substrate.

UK Receptor (u-PAR): Localization of UK on the Cell Surface

Many cell types contain the specific receptor u-PAR, which binds UK with high affinity. The UK receptor was first identified on human monocytes and on U937 cell lines [60]. The mature receptor consists of 283 amino acids and has molecular weight 55-60 kDa [61,62]. The receptor molecule contains several N-glycosylation sites, and the weight of sugar residues comprises about half of the molecular weight of the mature protein [63]. The N-terminal GFD of UK is responsible for its binding to u-PAR. The UK receptor lacks a transmembrane sequence and is anchored in the plasma membrane by a glycosyl phosphatidylinositol (GPI) moiety [64,65]. The function of u-PAR is not limited by the locating of UK on the cell surface. The receptor-bound sc-uPA is activated by plasmin more efficiently than the free UK [66]. The u-PAR can also protect bound UK from further degradation by plasmin. Thus, u-PAR increases the half-life of the functionally active UK on the cell surface [67].

Physiological Role of UK

Studies on the roles of u-PAs in embryonic growth and differentiation, in neoplastic processes and on their involvement in invasion and metastasis have been extensively reviewed [68,69]. Quigley [70] reported that in addition to their action as thrombolytic agents, u-PA might play an important role in connective tissue degradation by activating plasmin and other proteinases.

Bode and Dziadek [71] observed that u-PA have different roles in different embryonic tissues and at different stages of development. Valinsky *et al.* [72] studied the association of controlled extracellular proteolysis mediated by u-PA with embryonic tissue remodeling and cell migration in the developing bursa fabricius of quail and chick embryos.

PHYSICO-CHEMICAL PROPERTIES OF UK

It is a colourless protein, with a high degree of stability over a wide range of pH and temperature. The amino terminal fragment (ATF) of UK is 130 amino acid residues long. It consists of 2-α-helics and two anti-parallel β-strands. The ATF contains 2 domains, a growth factor domain and a kringle domain. It binds to fucose (magenta) as a ligand. Fucose is a deoxy-sugar, a monosaccharide with one or more hydroxyl (-OH) groups replaced by a hydrogen (-H). The formula of fucose is $C_6H_{12}O_6$. The ATF also contains 6 disulphide bonds as follows, cys11-cys19, cys13-cys31, cys33-cys42, cys50-cys131, cys71-cys113 and cys102-cys126.

Harvey *et al.* [73] reported that the presence of PA activity related to u-PA in the conditioned medium of the human lung cancer cell line (HPL-SK-1) that was associated with a spectrum of MW's up to several million. These were fractionated into subspecies exhibiting size and charge differences. Also, these enzymes were found to be active towards the synthetic substrate, Spectozyme.

The enzyme is moderately stable, showing no appreciable loss in activity over years in lyophilized form or over months in sterile solutions at 1 mg/ml or more at refrigerator temperatures. Stability is decreased at salt concentrations below 0.03 M sodium chloride and precipitation with loss in activity occurs at very low salt concentrations. Vetterlein *et al.* [74] reported that, under certain conditions UK of approximately 60 kDa have been found in a variety of cell lines. Different forms of UK over a wide range of molecular weight have been reported from different sources (Table **2**) [75-80]. White *et al.* [81] established that two different sizes of UK are present in urine, a HMW form of 54 kDa and a LMW form of 31 kDa.

Several PAs, thrombolytic agents with different pharmacokinetic and pharmacodynamic properties have been developed to treat thrombolytic diseases [82]. No single agent has been approved by U.S.F.D.A. to be labelled for every indication and new agents, new dosage regimens are under constant investigation [8].

Five thrombolytics currently used in U.S.A. for myocardial infarction are SK, alteplase, antistreplase, reteplase and tenecteplase [8]. Two thrombolytic agents that are currently used in Canada are SK and t-PA. In India SK, UK and t-PA are being used [83].

Table 2. Different Sources of UK with Different Molecular Weights

Source	Molecular weight (kDa)	Reference
Urine	54	Sobel *et al.* [75]
Commercial UK preparation	100	Burges *et al.* [76]
Human cells	60	Vetterlein *et al.* [74]
Human kidney cells	53	Hiroyuki *et al.* [77]
Hep 3 cells	53	Wun *et al.* [16]
Urine	95-100	Hayashi *et al.* [78]
CALU-3, ATCC, HTB-55	53	Stump *et al.* [79]
HUVEC	95	Booyse *et al.* [18]
HT 1080 cells	64-55	Bansal and Roychoudhury [80]

Generation	Drug
1st Generation agents	SK*, UK*, t-PA
2nd Generation agents	alteplase*, activated anisoylated streptokinase-plasminogen activator complex (APSAC)*
3rd Generation agents	vampire bat-PA, reteplase*, tenecteplase*, lanoteplase, staphylokinase, recombinant glycosylated plasminogen activator.

* - indicates approved by F.D.A.

The Following are some of the Manufacturers of UK in India (CIMS [83]):

Manufacturer	Brand name
Dabur, Ghaziabad, U.P.	DABUNASE
VHB, Mumbai	KD-UNASE
Aristo (Otsira), Mumbai	SOLOKINASE
TTK, Chennai	UROKINASE
Unichem, Mumbai	UNI-KINASE
Chandra bhagat, Mumbai	UROKEN
Cadila, Ahmadabad	UROPASE

Contraindications of UK

Active internal bleeding, history of cerebrovascular accident, recent trauma of any kind including surgery, intracranial neoplasm, aneurysm, bleeding and severe uncontrolled hypertension are contraindicated for UK application [83].

Interactions of UK

Platelet inhibitors such as aspirin, indomethacin, can potentiate the action of UK and cause haemorrhage. Heparin and oral anticoagulants may increase risk of bleeding [83].

Adverse Reactions of UK

Superficial bleeding at the sites of venous cutdowns, vascular punctures, may occur. More serious internal bleeding could occur in any internal organ or site. Relatively mild allergic reactions such as bronchospasm or rash may occur occasionally. Other side effects include chills, blood pressure changes, dyspnoea, palpitation, cyanosis and hypoxia. Aspirin should not be given for fever [83].

Enzyme Units

In Great Britain, potency of UK is expressed in arbitrary units known as Plough units (PU). One PU is approximately equivalent to 1.5 IU (International units). In U.S.A., potency is expressed in CTA units (Committee on thrombolytic agents). One CTA unit is approximately equivalent to one IU. One FIP (Federation of International Pharmaceutique) unit is equivalent to 546 PU and approximately to 780 CTA units.

Advantages and Disadvantages of UK

Thrombolysis appears safer with UK than with alteplase with a lower incidence of haemorrhagic complication. It is preferable for local thrombolytic therapy due to increased efficacy of clot lysis and decreased rate of systemic fibrinolytic effect and bleeding complication [84]. It may provide an acceptable balance between thrombolytic efficacy and safety [8].

The increased efficacy and safety of UK makes it the preferred agent for intra-arterial infusion [85]. It is non-antigenic, non-pyrogenic and does not cause allergic reactions [85,86]. Hence, it can be administered repeatedly without antigenic problems [8]. It is the most appropriate agent for catheter-directed venous thromobolysis offering an advantageous compromise between fibrinolytic specificity and thromobolytic speed [87]. Its cost is more when compared to SK [8].

Inhibitors of UK

UK inhibitors belong to the superfamily of serpins (serine proteinase inhibitors). Primarily these include plasminogen activator inhibitors (PAI-1 and PAI-2), protease nexin-1 (PN-1) and protein C inhibitor [88-90]. PAI-1 is one of the main inhibitors of UK. The biological activity of UK is regulated post-translationally by a functional interplay between the proteinase, its receptor (u-PAR) and PAI-1. Amidine derivatives are competitive inhibitors of UK [91-96]. Amiloride is another inhibitor of UK, which reduces tumor growth and decreases the proliferation of tumor cells in hepatomas and intestinal carcinomas [97]. Benzothiophene, isocoumarine and guanidine derivatives are also inhibitors of UK [98-101].

Modulators of UK

The enhanced production of PA activity was shown to be a characteristic of many different cell types. The intracellular and extracelllular levels of PA were demonstrated to be substantially elevated in malignant cells [102], cells treated with a tumor promoter [103], activated macrophages [104], established cell lines [105,106], granulosa cells during ovulation [107], embryonic cells during differentiation [108] and hormone treated cells [109].

Lacroix and Fritz [110] reported that the rates of production and release of u-PA was greatly influenced by a variety of factors including cell density, presence of hormones, incubation temperature and duration of culture.

Modulation of uPA-mediated functions via the ATF of mannose-6-phosphate /insulin-like growth factor 2 receptor (CD222), reported by Stockinger *et al.* [111].

Deutheux *et al.* [112] examined the preparation of u-PA by culturing human diploid fibroblasts in a serum-free medium supplemented with peptones (eg. protease peptone) and K^+ ions for efficient expression of human gene in *E. coli.* In cultures of 3T3 fibroblasts, the PA activity increased by 20 fold when compared to control cells within 24 h when 100 uM of sulphur mustard (SM) was added. Also ryanodine (10 uM) amplified the u-PA up-regulation by 2-fold and dexamethasone (1 uM) added directly after SM treatment almost completely prevented the induction of u-PA at both the protein and mRNA levels [112].

IN VITRO PRODUCTION OF UK

Since 1885, urine has been known to show proteolytic activity, which was attributed due to proteolytic enzymes. The presence, in urine, of an activator substance capable of effecting transformation of plasminogen to plasmin was first described by Williams [11] and in the following year by Sobel *et al.* [76]. The latter groups have assigned the name Urokinase (UK) to this activator. Proof of the hypothesis that UK is elaborated in the kidneys was obtained, when renal cells in tissue culture produced a PA identical to urinary UK. The kidney activator was produced largely in the renal medulla, particularly by the Vasa-recta.

This localization of the activator suggested that it has a physiological role in maintaining the patency of the urinary tract by promoting the lysis of fibrous deposits [15].

In 1969, Bernik and Kwaan [14] demonstrated that fibrinolytic activity was present in cultures of human kidney cells. PA was found to be produced and released by cells emerging from small vessels in cultures of explants from human kidneys. By means of a histochemical fibrin slide technique, the fibrinolytic activity was accurately localized to the active cells. Immunological investigations showed that the PA was identical to UK.

Astedt *et al.* [13] measured fibrinolytic activity of liver, lung, bone marrow and kidney tissue explants of 16-20 weeks old human fetus. Their results showed, the kidney tissues to be the most active in the lysis of fibrin clots indicating the presence of PA. The PA secreted was found to be immunologically identical to the urinary activator.

Unkeless *et al.* [104] reported that activated macrophages, and cells from heart, lung and kidney were good sources of PA's. Nolan *et al.* [113] investigated the nature of the trypsin activatable PA produced by kidney cell cultures using human embryonic kidney (HEK) cell line in serum free medium. Comparison of immunological, physicochemical and enzymatic preparations indicated that the enzyme isolated from HEK cell conditioned culture media was similar to that from human urine, heart and blood vessels.

Kapina *et al.* [114] reported the RH-PA cell line as a source for obtaining the u-PA. This new cell line (RH-PA) was established on the basis of the HEK cell line (RH). This cell line produces u-PA with activities in the range of 150-200 IU/ml when estimated by fibrin plate method.

UK Production from Malignant Cells

Malignant cells have been reported to produce high levels of PA [115-118]. Rifkin *et al.* [118] reported the release of high levels of u-PA by avian and mammalian fibroblasts transformed *in vitro*, and by primary cultures of malignant tumors, such as chemically or virally induced carcinomas. Normal fibroblasts and cultures of normal control tissues released little or no activator. To determine whether similar fibrinolytic activity was associated with human neoplasia, the authors studied the properties of three tumor cell lines [osteosarcoma, melanoma and mesothelioma]. It was found that all of these cultures produced high levels of fibrinolytic activity.

Wilson *et al.* [119] conducted a survey of 56 normal and neoplastic tissues and showed that PA's were released by cultured human cells in several molecular forms distinguishable by their MW's and their susceptibility to inhibition by antibodies to the normal urinary enzyme UK.

Goldfart and Quigley [120] reported that rous sarcoma virus (RSV) transformed chick embryo fibroblasts produced a specific serine protease, u-PA at levels 25-100 fold greater than non-transformed cultures. A number of mammalian and avian cells in culture were shown to increase their production of u-PA after transformation by RNA or DNA viruses or chemical carcinogens.

Wun *et al.* [16] reported the production of PA by cell lines derived from a human tumor [Hep 3]. The activator was found to be indistinguishable from urinary urokinase and catalytically active when assayed by zymographic procedure. However, Freedman and Shui [121] stated that the existence of any casual relationship between transformation, cancer and the production of PA was not definitely proven. High levels of PAs were known to be produced by many normal cells, i.e., macrophages, polymorphonuclear leucocytes, lung and kidney. Transformants of lung, kidney and embryo cells were often less active in producing PA than their normal cells.

Cloning and Expression of UK

Since the advent of rDNA technology, attempts have been made to produce UK in bacteria [24,122-127], fungi [128], yeast [41,128,129], mammalian cells [130-133], insect cells [133] and in plants [134]. Different recombinant cell lines that have been used for production of UK are listed in Table **1**. Large-scale culture of bacteria or fungi is relatively easy but the main drawback of using prokaryotic system for UK production is the absence of post-translational modification machinery in these organisms. Therefore, the non-glycosylated UK so obtained does not have the same efficacy and pharmacodynamic properties as that of native UK. Mammalian cell lines are hence, preferred for production of UK. A considerable number of mammalian cell lines have been reported to date for UK production.

Kohno *et al.* [17] reported the establishment of a permanent cell line, TCL-598, which produces and secretes UK into the medium in smaller quantities.

Chinese hamster ovary (CHO) cells are considered ideal hosts for recombinant UK production [135]. These cells offer the advantages that they can be easily genetically manipulated, can be adapted for large-scale suspension culture and it can give rise to proteins with glycans which are similar, although not identical, to those found on human glycoproteins.

Interestingly, Kim and Swartz [136] have illustrated that UK could be efficiently synthesized in *E. coli* based cell-free systems using glutathione redox buffer coupled with the disulphide isomerase to facilitate formation of disulphide bonds. Recently, Roychoudhury *et al.* [9] reported that the CHO cell line is known for its unstable karyotype. Loss of recombinant gene copy number and appearance of non-producing populations of cells were predominant causes for instability of production.

Immobilization and Bioreactor Studies of UK

Senatore and Bernath [137] had immobilized UK to the inner surfaces of fibrocollagenous tubes in an attempt to develop a fibrinolytic biomaterial, which may be suitable for use as a small diameter vascular prosthesis. The enzyme was bound by adsorption followed by glutaraldehyde cross-linking.

Kang *et al.* [138] investigated kinetics of formation of UK from pro-UK in conditioned media and worked for a possibility of lowering the conversion to UK, by cultivating human cell lines under perfusion operations. A human kidney cell line, Caki-1, was cultivated in Dulbecco's modified Eagle's medium (DMEM) with fetal bovine serum (FBS), glutamine and gentamicin without Ca^{2+} to prevent clumping. Cells were then inoculated into a 2 L bioreactor with microcarriers. It was observed that better production of pro-UK was obtained with 5% serum containing media than 10% or serum free medium on cytodex II microcarrier under perfusion chemostat operations. Conversion of pro-UK was reduced in the serum containing media.

Wagner *et al.* [139] studied the production of pro-UK by a human kidney tumor cell line in long term cultures. Cells were grown on microcarriers, which were retained inside the reactor by sedimentation, or with a spin filter. Two modes of operation were compared: feed harvest at an average medium exchange rate of 0.3 ml/h and continuous perfusion at a higher dilution rate of 1.5 ml/h. In the two systems a stable production of pro-UK could be maintained for more than 400 h. Continuous perfusion yielded a higher cell density than feed harvest resulting in a 2-fold increase in the reactor productivity. But higher final enzyme activities were obtained with harvest recovered medium than in the perfusion medium. The cumulative medium consumption per mass of product was the same in the repeated batch and in the continuous operation mode.

Avgerinors *et al.* [21] used a 20 L stirred tank fermentor, for the continuous production of recombinant single chain urokinase-type plasminogen activator (rscu-PA) from CHO cells. The rscu-PA produced over the course of this continuous culture was purified and characterized both *in vitro* and *in vivo* and shown to be comparable to natural scu-PA produced from the transformed human kidney cell line, Tch-598.

Smidsrod *et al.* [140] stated that in recent years, entrapment of cells within spheres of Ca^{2+} alginate has become the most widely used technique for immobilizing living cells. This versatile method includes applications ranging from immobilization of living or dead cells in bioreactors, immobilization of plant protoplasts for micropropagation and immobilization of hybridoma cells for production of monoclonal antibodies, to entrapment of animal cells for implantation of artificial organs.

Tamponnet *et al.* [141] immobilized primary cultivated rabbit articular chondrocytes in calcium alginate beads. Both free and entrapped cells were allowed to grow under normal conditions. After long-term immobilization [38 days], the cells still exhibited metabolic activities, patterns of division, synthesis and secretion of extracellular matrix macromolecules such as type II collagen and proteoglycans. After bead lysis, harvested cells showed normal growth patterns when resuspended in culture medium. On the basis of these results, long-duration storage and large-scale production of extracellular matrix components were investigated.

Jen *et al.* [142] studied methods of immobilization of cells such as adhesion, matrix embedment and microencapsulation using hydrogels of u-PA producing human fetal (HF) cells from explants of neonatal fore skins.

Roychoudhury *et al.* [143] carried out studies in T-flasks and bioreactor to produce UK enzyme using HT 1080 human kidney cell line. While growing the cell line it has been observed that the lag phase is reduced considerably in the bioreactor as compared to T-flask culture. The HT 1080 cell adhesion rate and UK production were observed to be the function of serum concentration in the medium. The maximum UK activity of 3.1×10^{-4} CTA unit/ml was achieved in the bioreactor at around 65 h batch culture.

SEPARATION AND PURIFICATION OF UK

Cell culture products are under rigid quality regulations for therapeutic application. UK being an intravenously administered drug, it has to meet stringent quality standards with respect to quality, efficacy and purity.

UK generated a lot of curiosity in the scientific community immediately after its discovery in 1950's. The main source of UK was urine, it is the cheapest and most easily available. Several attempts were made to purify it (Table **3**) [144-149]. But purification of

Table 3. Purification of UK from Urine

Techniques employed	Number of steps	Recovery (%)	Reference
Ammonium sulphate precipitation, dialysis, Amberlite CG-50 gel permeation chromatography and Pyroglu-lys-leu-argal-Sepharose chromatography	4	90	Someno *et al.* [144]
Zn^{2+}-Sepharose chromatography, SP Sephadex C-50 chromatography, Sephadex G-100 chromatography, benzamidine-Sepharose chromatography and Immunoadsorption chromatography	5	70	Stump *et al.* [145,146]
Affinity ultrafiltration using a copolymer of *N*-acryloyl-*m*-aminobenzamidine and acrylamide	1	49	Male *et al.* [147]
D 160 resin adsorption and benzamidine-Sepharose 6B chromatography	2	12	Si *et al.* [148]
Metal ion precipitation and Benzidine-Sepharose affinity chromatography	2	90	Jan Kokai Tokkyo Koho [149]

UK from urine requires large amounts of urine, which makes it unsuitable for large scale use.

The crude commercial preparations of which are highly active but not homogenous, were used for designing purification strategies for UK (Table **4**) [150-161]. With the developments in cell culture technology, cell culture extract is fast replacing urine and other crude preparations as the source of UK (Table **5**) [162-172]. Developments in the area of UK separation from crude sources, over a period of last three decades, are discussed in the following section.

Many approaches for purification of UK have been utilized including ammonium sulphate precipitation [56, 144], gel permeation chromatography [56,144,165], ion exchange chromatography [156], immobilized metal ion chromatography [146,168] and affinity chromatography [145,146,155,156,164]. A complete overview on the purification of UK has been published recently [81]. Most of the isolation methods for UK use multi-step approaches, which lead to lower yields coupled with high capital and operating costs.

Preliminary concentration techniques such as salting out, dialysis, filtration and centrifugation have been unsuccessful in yielding any significant results in the purification of UK from crude preparations [173].

Koltsova *et al.* [174] developed an improved procedure for isolation of UK from human urine by means of ion exchange on carbonyl cationite SMT at pH 4.7, with subsequent stepwise elution by phosphate buffer, pH 7.0. Wun *et al.* [16] purifed u-PA from human epidermoid carcinoma HEp3. The enzyme was purified to apparent homogeneity from serum free conditioned medium by the combination of immunoaffinity chromatography and preparative gel electrophoresis. Skriver *et al.* [175] reported the purification of a PA with an approximate MW 48,000 from SV transformed murine cells.

UK was isolated from supernatants of bacterial cultures grown on sterilized soybeans or its powder suspension by repetitive centrifugation, precipitation with $(NH_4)_2SO_4$, dialyzing, and separating with Sephadex G100 and Sephacryl S-200 column [176]. UK from a culture supernatant of human kidney cells was purified by using a Streamline SP column and a phosphate buffer [171].

Table 4. Purification of UK from Crude Commercial Preparations

Techniques employed	Fold Purification	Recovery (%)	Reference
Sulpho-propyl cartridge and Zn(II)-IDA-cellulose chromatography	18	78	Hou and Zaniewski [150]
Amino-benzamidine dextran T-2000 chromatography	112	82	Cao *et al.* [151]
Separation process using benzamidine-polystyrene divinyl benzene copolymer	50	53	Pang *et al.* [152]
Benzidine-glycidyl methacrylate	21	89	Cao *et al.* [153]
Cefazoline-Sepharose 4B chromatography	99	78	Cao *et al.* [154]
Affinity chromatography (magnetic dextran microsphere (MDMS)/ *p*-aminobenzamide and L-arginine methyl ester or guanidine hexanoic acid)	15-33	40-61	Dong *et al.* [155]
Affinity chromatography (magnetic dextran microsphere, magnetic agarose microsphere, magnetic polyvinyl microsphere and magnetic polyhydroxyethyl methacrylate microsphere/*p*- aminobenzamide, L-arginine methyl ester, guanidine hexanoic acid or fibrinogen)	15–40	40–70	Dong *et al.* [156]
Size-exclusion chromatography, ion-exchange chromatography, heparin affinity chromatography or hydroxyapatite chromatography	-	-	Lin *et al.* [157]
Polysulfone ultrafiltration and Amberlite IRC-500 chromatography column	30	90	Morimoto *et al.* [158]
CNBr-activated agarose column	-	80-85	Morii *et al.* [159]
Bu agarose chromatography	8	95	Kondo *et al.* [160]
Ion-exchange column	1	-	Zhang *et al.* [161]

The refolded recombinant pro-UK was purified using size-exclusion chromatography, ion-exchange chromatography, heparin affinity chromatography, or hydroxyapatite chromatography [157]. Li *et al.* [177,178] reported that the affinity ligands can be used as inhibitors for preparation of high-purity pro-UK or UK.

Stump *et al.* [146] studied the purification of UK from the human lung adeno carcinoma line CALU-3 (ATCC, HTB-55), using a combination of chromatography on zinc chelate-Sepharose, SP- Sephadex C-50, and Sephadex G-100. Final yields of 65-100 µg/L of starting material were obtained with a 290-fold purification factor and a recovery of 30%. Edward *et al.* [179] studied the refolding and purification of a u-PA fragment by exclusion chromatography. Use of size-exclusion media with higher fractionation ranges resulted in an increase in the recovery of u-PA activity.

Table 5. Purification of UK from Cell Culture Extracts

Culture broth	Techniques employed	No. of steps	Fold purification	Recovery (%)	Reference
Mammalian cells	Dialysis and α-benzylsulfonyl-*p*-amino phenylalanine-Sepharose 4B chromatography	2	1500	50	Maciag *et al.* [162]
	Carboxylated polyethyleneimino-propyl trimethoxysilane chromatography	1	-	91	Edmunds *et al.* [163]
Mouse sarcoma 3T3 cells	Affinity chromatography, anion-exchange chromatography and gel filtration process	3	-	32	Dano *et al.* [164]
CALU-3 cells	Immobilized metal affinity chromatography, SP Sephadex C-50 chromatography and Sephadex G-100 chromatography	3	290	30	Stump *et al.* [145]
Escherichia coli BL21 mutant cells	SP-Sepharose chromatography, Sephacryl S-200 gel permeation and benzamidine-Sepharose chromatography	3	-	-	Xue *et al.* [165]
Recombinant CHO cells	Anti-sc-uPA-Sepharose 4B chromatography	1	50	90	Gao *et al.* [166]
Human umbilical vein endothelial cells	CM Sephadex C-50 anion exchange chromatography, anti-UK IgG-Seph-arose chromatography and benzamidine-agarose chromatography	3	-	41	Dong *et al.* [156]
HT 1080 cells	Sulpho-propyl-Sepharose chromatography	1	93	100	Khaparde *et al.* [167]
	Cu(II)-IDA-polyacrylamide cryogel chromatography	1	27	80	Kumar *et al.* [168]
Melanoma cells	Heparin-Sepharose column	1	-	90	Paques [169]
Tissue culture	Sulfopropyl cellulose catridge	1	9	87	Morimoto [170]
Human kidney cells	Stream SP column	1	-	-	Fujiwara *et al.* [171]
BHK cells	S-Sepharose chromatography and lysine- Sepharose chromatography	2	-	-	Johannessen *et al.* [172]

Takahashi *et al.* [180] developed an affinity chromatography for purification of two forms of UK from human urine. A new affinity chromatography (hydrophobic-mediated affinity chromatography) which was characterized by the matrix having affinity site to UK and hydrophobic site was established for the purification of UK from human urine. HMW and LMW forms of UK were obtained in high yield.

Integrated Production and Purification of UK from Bioreactor

One of the most successful approaches in improving the economy of bioprocesses is to reduce the number of steps involved, as each successive step amounts to considerable loss of the product.

Khaparde *et al.* [167] successfully developed a two-step integrated process for producing UK from HT 1080 cell line in a hollow fibre reactor to which a sterile 50 ml benzamidine-sepharose affinity column was coupled for on-line separation of UK. Approximately, 4.5×10^4 PU of UK was harvested per day from the integrated set-up continuously for more than 20 days.

An integrated system for UK production and simultaneous capture of UK was developed based on the application of continuous polyacrylamide sephacryl column [181].

Similarly, Kumar *et al.* [168] developed an integrated set-up of gelatin-pAAm cryogel bioreactor was further connected to a pAAm cryogel column carrying Cu(II)-iminodiacetic acid (Cu(II)-IDA-pAAm cryogel), which had been optimized for the capture of UK from the conditioned medium of the cell lines. Thus an automated system was built, which integrated the features of a hollow fibre reactor with a chromatographic protein separation system. The UK was continuously captured by the Cu (II)-IDA-pAAm cryogel column and periodically recovered through elution cycles. The UK activity increased from 280 PU/mg in the culture fluid to 1300 PU/mg after recovery from the capture column which gave about 4.5 fold purification of the enzyme. The integrated bioreactor system operated continuously for 32 days during which no backpressure was observed because of the porous structure of the cryogel matrix. The enzyme eluted from the Cu(II)-IDA-pAAm cryogel capture column was further purified on benzamidine-Sepharose affinity column which gave a preparation of different forms of UK with activity of 13550 PU/mg of protein. This is one of the very few successful UK production strategies using mammalian cell lines.

APPLICATIONS OF UK

UK is known as a thrombolytic agent and has been exploited for the treatment of pulmonary embolism, acute myocardial infarction, ophthalmic clot and haemorrhage and peripheral arterial occlusion [182-187]. UK is also a prognostic marker for human cancers and a target for anti-cancer therapy [188-199]. As a marker, high u-PA levels in primary tumor extracts correlate with high incidence of relapse and poor survival.

Recent data from X-ray crystallography and NMR screening have indicated a number of candidate molecules to block the uPA-mediated activation of plasminogen. Moreover, molecules designed on the uPAR-binding domain of u-PA are used either alone or fused to inhibiting activities to destroy the uPA–uPAR interaction or to prevent the proteolytic activity. Such molecules have also been recently used to selectively target the catalytic domain of toxins to uPAR-expressing cells [29,124,200-202].

CURRENT AND FUTURE DEVELOPMENTS

Thrombolytic therapy is widely available and can be promptly attended. However, the therapy causes haemorrhagic complications and cannot be administered to a sizable group due to contraindication. Current regimens are limited by the failure of initial reperfusion and reocclusion in 5-10% of patients and are associated with an increased risk of bleeding complications. The new protocol for administering t-PA, as a double bolus have not proven to be effective, further recombinant plasminogen activator (r-PA) [3rd generation agent] has failed to demonstrate superiority over t-PA [8]. Current available data fails to provide compelling evidence that newer plasminogen activators offer significantly greater efficacy and safety than well-established agents like UK when used to treat peripheral vascular thrombosis. Newer thrombolytic agents are expensive and still not available in India. SK and UK are widely used for the treatment of cardiovascular diseases in India due to their lower cost when compared to t-PA. SK is immunogenic because of its bacterial origin. Among these, UK is more potent, non-immunogenic and has lower cross reactivity. Hence, UK is a life saving, therapeutically important fibrinolytic enzyme used in treatment of many cardiac disorders including deep vein thrombosis, thrombosis of the eye, pulmonary embolism, myocardial infarction and many other disorders requiring dissolution of blood clots. To maximize the benefit of thrombolysis there is a great need for public education, reduced transport delays and improvise thrombolysis facilities in hospitals.

ABBREVIATIONS

UK	=	Urokinase
PA	=	Plasminogen activator
SK	=	Streptokinase
t-PA	=	Tissue plasminogen activator
CTA	=	Committee on thrombolytic agents
SMC	=	Smooth muscle cells
u-PA	=	Urokinase-type plasminogen activator
u-PAR	=	Urokinase-type plasminogen activator receptor
PAI-1	=	Plasminogen activator inhibitor-1
PAI-2	=	Plasminogen activator inhibitor-2
DFP	=	Diisopropyl fluorophosphate (DFP)
sc-uPA	=	Single-chain urokinase-type plasminogen activator
tc-uPA	=	Two-chain urokinase-type plasminogen activator
GFD	=	Growth factor-like domain
HMW	=	High molecular weight
LMW	=	Low molecular weight
GPI	=	Glycosyl phosphotidyl inositol
ATF	=	Amino terminal fragment

APSAC	=	Activated anisoylated streptokinase-plasminogen activator complex
PU	=	Plough unit
IU	=	International unit
FIP	=	Federation of international pharmaceutique
PN-1	=	Protease nexin-1
SM	=	Sulphur mustard
HEK	=	Human embryonic kidney
RSV	=	Rous sarcoma virus
rt-PA	=	Recombinant tissue-type plasminogen activator
CHO	=	Chinese hamster ovary
DMEM	=	Dulbecco´s modified Eagle´s medium
FBS	=	Fetal bovine serum
rscu-PA	=	Recombinant single-chain urokinase-type plasminogen activator
HF	=	Human fetal
r-PA	=	Recombinant plasminogen activator

ACKNOWLEDGEMENTS

Indian Council of Medical Research (ICMR) is thanked for the senior research fellowship of Dr. R. Bhavani Devi and for the Council of Scientific and Industrial Research (CSIR), India of Drs. V. Saisha and A. Kunamneni.

REFERENCES

[1] Irigoyen JP, Munoz-Canoves P, Montero L, Nagamine Y. The plasminogen activator system: biology and regulation. Cell Mol Life Sci 1999; 56: 104-132.

[2] Fust GY, Keresztes M. Plasminogen-plasmin system in complement activation induced by endotoxin. Ann Immunol Hung 1973; 17: 29-31.

[3] Quax PHA, Boxman ILA, Van Kesteren CAM, Verheijen JH, Ponec M. Plasminogen activators are involved in keratinocyte and fibroblast migration in wounded cultures *in vitro*. Fibrinolysis 1994; 8: 221-228.

[4] Zahm M, Kaplan H, Hérard AL, *et al*. Cell migration and proliferation during the *in vitro* wound repair of the respiratory epithelium. Cell Motil Cytoskeleton 1997; 37: 33-43.

[5] Collen D. Ham-Wasserman lecture: Role of the plasminogen system in fibrin-homeostasis and tissue remodelling. Haematology 2001; 1: 1-9.

[6] Helenius G, Heydarkhan HS, Siegbahn A, Risberg B. Tissue engineering expression of fibrinolytic and coagulation factors in cocultured human endothelial and smooth muscle cells. Tissue Eng 2004; 10: 353-360.

[7] Collen D, Stump JM, Gold HK. Thrombolytic therapy. Ann Rev Med 1988; 39: 405-423.

[8] Baruah DB, Rajendra ND, Chaudhari MR, Kadam SS. Plasminogen activators: A comparison. Vascul Pharmacol 2006; 44: 1-9.

[9] Roychoudhury PK, Kharparde SS, Mattiasson B, Kumar A. Synthesis, regulation and production of urokinase using mammalian cell culture: A comprehensive review. Biotechnol Adv 2006; 24: 514-528.

[10] Collen D. Coronary thrombolysis: streptokinase or recombinant tissue-type plasminogen activator? Ann Int Med 1990; 112: 529-538.

[11] Williams JRB. The fibrinolytic activity of urine. Br J Exp Pathol 1951; 32: 530-537.

[12] Vetterlein D, Calton GJ. Purification of urokinase from complex mixtures using immobilized monoclonal antibody against urokinase light chain. Thrombos Haemost 1983; 49: 24-27.

[13] Astedt B, Pandolfi J, Nilsson IM. Inhibitory effect of placenta on plasminogen activation in human organ culture. Proc Soc Biol Med 1972; 139: 1421-1424.

[14] Bernik MB, Kwaan HC. Plasminogen activator activity in cultures from human tissues. An immunological and histochemical study. J Clin Invest 1969; 48: 1740-1753.

[15] Lewis JL. Plasminogen activator (urokinase) from cultured cells. Thromb Haemost 1979; 42: 895-900.

[16] Wun TC, Schleuning WD, Reich E. Isolation and characterization of urokinase from human plasma. J Biol Chem 1982; 257: 3276-3283.

[17] Kohno T, Hopper P, Lillquist JS, Suddith RL, Greenlee R, Moir DT. Kidney plasminogen activator: A precursor form of human urokinase with high fibrin affinity. Biotechnol 1984; 2: 628-634.

[18] Booyse FM, Lin PH, Traylor M, Bruce R. Purification and properties of a single-chain urokinase-type plasminogen activator form produced by subcultured human umbilical vein endothelial cells. J Biol Chem 1988; 263: 15139-15145.

[19] Khaparde SS, Roychoudhury PK. Production of urokinase using hollow fiber bioreactor, in: Indian Chemical Engineering Conference, Technical Session Transcription 2004; 6: 11.

[20] Nolli ML, Sarubbi E, Corti A, *et al.* Production characterization of human recombinant single chain urokinase-type plasminogen activator from mouse cells. Fibrinolysis 1989; 3: 101-106.

[21] Avgerinos GC, Drapeau D, Socolow JS, Mao J, Hsiao K, Broeze RJ. Spin filter perfusion system for high density cell culture: production of recombinant urinary type plasminogen activator in CHO cells. Biotechnol 1990; 8: 54-58.

[22] Turner BG, Avgerinos GC, Melnick LM, Moir DT. Optimization of pro-urokinase secretion from recombinant *Saccharomyces cerevisiae*. Biotechnol Bioeng 1991; 37: 869-875.

[23] Satoh M, Hosoi S, Miyaji H, Itoh S, Satoh S. Stable production of recombinant pro-urokinase by human lymphoblastoid Namalwa KJM-1 cells: host-cell dependency of the expressed-protein stability. Cytotechnol 1993; 13: 79-88.

[24] Tang W, Sun Z, Pannell R, Gurewich V, Liu JN. An efficient system for production of recombinant urokinase-type plasminogen activator. Protein Exp Purif 1997; 11: 279-283.

[25] Jo EC, Yun JW, Jung KH, Chung SI, Kim JH. Performance study of perfusion cultures for the production of single-chain urokinase-type plasminogen activator (sc-uPA) in a 2.5 L spin-filter bioreactor. Bioprocess Eng 1998; 19: 363-372.

[26] Medcalf RL, Hamilton JA. Human synovial fibroblasts produce urokinase-type plasminogen activator. Arthritis Rheum 1986; 29: 1397-1401.

[27] Gibson PR, van de Pol E, Doe WF. Cell associated urokinase activity and colonic epithelial cells in health and disease. Gut 1991; 32: 191-195.

[28] Kusch A, Tkachuk S, Lutter S, *et al.* Monocyte-expressed urokinase regulates human vascular smooth muscle cell migration in a coculture model. Biol Chem 2002; 383: 217-221.

[29] Sidenius N, Blasi F. The urokinase plasminogen activator system in cancer: Recent advances and implication for prognosis and therapy. Canc Metastas Rev 2003; 22: 205-222.

[30] Hartnell GG, Gates J. The case of Abbokinase and the FDA: the events leading to the suspension of Abbokinase supplies in the United States. J Vasc Interv Radiol 2000; 11: 11841-11847.

[31] Bell PH, Dziobkowski CT, Englert ME. A sensitive fluorometric assay for plasminogen, plasmin, and streptokinase. Anal Biochem 1974; 61: 200-208.

[32] James MS, Francis JC. The mechanism of activation of rabbit plasminogen by urokinase. J Biol Chem 1975; 250: 3041-3049.

[33] Bernart NV, Francis JC. Mechanism of the urokinase-catalyzed activation of human plasminogen. J Biol Chem 1976; 251: 3906-3912.

[34] Picone R, Kajtaniak EL, Nielson LS, *et al.* Regulation of urokinase receptors in monocytelike U937 cells by phorbol ester phorbol myristate acetate. J Cell Biol 1989; 108: 693-702.

[35] Stepanova V, Tkachuk V. Urokinase as a multidomain protein and polyfunctional cell regulator. Biochem 2002; 67: 109-118.

[36] Holmes WE, Pennica D, Blaber M, *et al.* Cloning and expression of the gene for pro-urokinase in *Escherichia coli*. Biotechnol 1985; 3: 923-929.

[37] Appella E, Robinson EA, Ullrich SJ, *et al.* The receptor-binding sequence of urokinase. A biological function for the growth-factor module of proteases. J Biol Chem 1987; 262: 4437-4440.

[38] Mimuro J, Kaneko M, Murakami T, Matsuda M, Sakata Y. Reversal interactions between plasminogen activators and plasmi-nogen activator inhibitor-1. Biochem Biophys Acta 1992; 1160: 325-334.

[39] Hamelin J, Sarmientos P, Orsini G, Galibert F. Implication of cystiene residues in the activity of single-chain urokinase-plasminogen activator. Biochem Biophys Res Commun 1993; 194: 978-985.

[40] Kobayashi H, Gotoh J, Hirashima Y, Fujie M, Sugino D, Terao T. Inhibitory effect of a conjugate between human urokinase and urinary trypsin inhibitor on tumor cell invasion *in vitro*. J Biol Chem 1995; 270: 8361-8366.

[41] Wang P, Sun Z, Chen H, Liu JN. Glycosylation of pro-urokinase by *Pichia pastoris* impairs enzymatic activity but not secretion. Protein Exp Purif 2000; 20: 179-185.

[42] Liu J, Pannell R, Gurewich V. A transitional state of pro-urokinase that has a higher catalytic efficiency against Glu-plasminogen than urokinase. J Biol Chem 1992; 267: 15289-15292.

[43] Liu J, Tang W, Sun Z, *et al.* A site-directed mutagenesis of pro-urokinase which substantially reduces its intrinsic activity. Biochem 1996; 35: 14070-14076.

[44] Liu J, Gurewich V. Inactivation of the intrinsic activity of pro-urokinase by diisopropylfluorophosphate is reversible. J Biol Chem 1995; 270: 8408-8410.

[45] Gurewich V, Pannell R, Louie S, Kelley P, Suddith RL, Greenlee R. Effective and fibrin-specific clot lysis by a zymogen precursor form of urokinase (pro-urokinase). A study *in vitro* and in two animal species. J Clin Invest 1983; 73:1731-1739.

[46] Koster RW, Cohen AF, Hopkins GR, Beier H, Gunzler WA, van der Wouw PA. Pharmacokinetics and pharmacodynamics of saruplase, an unglycosylated single-chain urokinase-type plasminogen activator, in patients with acute myocardial infarction. Thromb Haemost 1994; 72: 740-745.

[47] Lenich C, Pannell R, Henkin J, Gurewich V. The influence of glycosylation on the catalytic and fibrinolytic properties of pro-urokinase. Thromb Haemost 1992; 68: 539-544.

[48] Lijnen HR, Van Hoef B, Nelles L, Collen D. Plasminogen activation with single-chain urokinase-type plasminogen activator (sc-uPA). Studies with active site mutagenized plasminogen (Ser-740-Ala) and plasmin-resistant sc-uPA (Lys 158-Glu). J Biol Chem 1990; 265: 5232-5236.

[49] Lijnen HR, Van Hoef B, Collen D. Activation with plasmin of two-chain urokinase-type plasminogen activator derived from single-chain urokinase-type plasminogen activator by treatment with thrombin. Eur J Biochem 1987; 169: 359-364.

[50] Ichinose A, Fujikawa K, Suyama T. The activation of pro-urokinase by plasma kallikrein and its inactivation by thrombin. J Biol Chem 1986; 261: 3486-3489.

[51] Brunner G, Simon MM, Kramer MD. Activation of pro-urokinase by the human T cell-associated serine proteinase HuTSP-1. FEBS Letts 1990; 260: 141-144.

[52] Kobayashi H, Schmitt M, Goretzki L, *et al.* Cathepsin B efficiently activates the soluble and the tumor cell receptor-bound form of the proenzyme urokinase-type plasminogen activator (Pro-uPA). J Biol Chem 1991; 266: 5147-5152.

[53] Toki N. Effect of pH on the platelet aggregating factor in porcine factor VIII concentrates. Thromb Haemost 1980; 43: 67.

[54] Lenich C, Pannell R, Henkin J, Gurewich V. The influence of glycosylation on the catalytic and fibrinolytic properties of pro-urokinase. Thromb Haemost 1992; 68: 539-544.

[55] Rabbani SA, Mazar AP, Bernier SM, *et al.* Structural requirements for the growth factor activity of the amino-terminal domain of urokinase. J Biol Chem 1992; 267; 14151-14156.

[56] Nobuhara M, Sakamaki M, Ohnishi H, Suzuki Y. A comparative study of high molecular weight urokinase and low molecular weight urokinase. J Biochem 1981; 90: 225-232.

[57] Li XK, Lijnen HR, Nelles L, Hu MH, Collen D. Biochemical properties of recombinant mutants of non-glycosylated single-chain urokinase-type plasminogen activator. Biochem Biophys Acta 1992; 1159: 37-43.

[58] Lijnen HR, Van Hoef B, Collen D. Comparative kinetic analysis of the activation of human plasminogen by natural and recombinant single-chain urokinase-type plasminogen activator. Biochem Biophys Acta 1986; 884: 402-408.

[59] Sasaki, K., Nishi, T., Yasumura, S., Sato, M., Itoh, S.: EP370205 A2 (**1990**).

[60] Vassali JD, Baccino D, Belin D. A cellular binding site for the Mr 55,000 form of the human plasminogen activator, urokinase. J Cell Biol 1985; 100: 86-92.

[61] Ploug M, Ronne E, Behrendt N, Jensen AL, Blasi F, Dano K. Cellular receptor for urokinase plasminogen activator. Carboxyl-terminal processing and membrane anchoring by glcosyl-phosphatidylinositol. J Biol Chem 1991; 266: 1926-1933.

[62] Mazar, A.P., Jones, T.R.: WO01025410 A2 (**2001**).

[63] Ploug M. Identification of specific sites involved in ligand binding by photoaffinity labeling of the receptor for the urokinase-type plasminogen activator. Residues located at equivalent positions in uPAR domains I and III participate in the assembly of a composite ligand-binding site. Biochem 1998; 37: 16494-16505.

[64] Moller LB, Pollanen J, Ronne E, Pedersen N, Blasi F. N-linked glycosylation of the ligand-binding domain of the human urokinase receptor contributes to the affinity for its ligand. J Biol Chem 1993; 268: 11152-11159.

[65] Danoe, K., Blasi, F., Roldan, A.L., Cubellis, M.V., Masucci, M.T., Appella, E., Schleuning, W.D., Behrendt, N., Roenne, E.: WO9012091 A1 (**1990**).

[66] Ellis V, Scully MF, Kakkar VV. Plasminogen activation initiated by single-chain urokinase-type plasminogen activator: potentiation by U937 monocytes. J Biol Chem 1989; 264: 2185-2188.

[67] Poliakov A, Tkachuk V, Ovchinnikova T, Potapenko N, Bagryantsev S, Stepanova V. Plasmin-dependent elimination of the growth-factor-like domain in urokinase causes its rapid cellular uptake and degradation. Biochem J 2001; 355: 639-645.

[68] Dano K, Anderson PA, Hansen GJ, Kristensen R, Niebar IS, Skriver L. Plasminogen activators, tissue degradation, and cancer. Adv Cancer Res 1985; 44: 139-266.

[69] Blasi F, Riccio A, Sebastio G. Human plasminogen activator. Genes and protein structure. In: Human genes and diseases. Blasi F, Ed. John Wiley and Sons, Ltd., London. 1986; 337-413.

[70] Quigley J. Phorbol ester-induced morphological changes in transformed chick fibroblasts: evidence for direct catalytic involvement of plasminogen activator. Cell 1979; 17: 131-141.

[71] Bode VC, Dziadek MA. Plasminogen activator secretion during mouse embryogenesis. Develop Biol 1979; 73: 272-289.

[72] Valinsky E, Reich E, Le Douarin NM. Plasminogen activator in the bursa of fabricius: correlations with morphogenetic remodeling and cell migrations. Cell 1981; 25: 471-476.

[73] Harvey SR, Minowade J, Takita H, Kover L, Markers G. Urokinase-like plasminogen activators of unusually high molecular weight secreted by a cell line derived from a human lung cancer case. J Biol Chem 1982; 257: 5645.

[74] Vetterlein D, Bell TE, Young PL, Roblin R. Immunological quantitation and imunoadsorption of urokinase-like plasminogen activators secreted by human cells. J Biol Chem 1980; 255: 3665-3672.

[75] Sobel GW, Mohler SR, Jones WW, Dawdy AB, Guest MM. Urokinase: an activator of plasma profibrinolysin extracted from urine. Am J Physiol 1952; 171: 768-769.

[76] Burges RA, Brammer KW, Coombes JD. Molecular weight of urokinase. Nature 1965; 208: 894.

[77] Hiroyuki S, Kosugi T, Matsuo O, Mihara H. Physicochemical properties of highly purified plasminogen activator (single chain urokinase) of kidney culture. Nippon Ketsueki Gakkai Zasshi 1982; 45: 119-128.

[78] Hayashi S, Yamada K, Ogikubo H. Urokinase with high fibrin affinity found in human urine. Ketsueki to Myakkan 1985; 16: 317-320.

[79] Stump DC, Stassen JM, Demarsin E, Collen D. Comparative thrombolytic properties of single-chain forms of urokinase-type plasminogen activator. Blood 1987; 69: 592-596.

[80] Bansal V, Roychoudhury PK. Production and purification of urokinase. Protein Exp Purif 2006; 45: 1-14.

[81] White WF, Barlow GH, Mozen MM. The isolation and characterization of plasminogen activators (urokinase) from human urine. Biochem 1966; 5: 2160-2169.

[82] Deitcher SR, Jaff MR. Pharmacologic and clinical characteristics of thrombolytic agents. Rev Cardiovasc Med 2002; 3: S25-S33.

[83] CIMS (Current Index of Medical Specialities), India 2006; 94: 173.

[84] Van Breda A, Katzen BT, Beutsch AS. Urokinase vs streptokinase in local thrombolysis. Radiology 1987; 165: 109-111.

[85] Belkin M, Belkin B, Bucknam CA, Straub JJ, Lowe R. Intra arterial fibrinolytic therapy, efficacy of streptokinase vs urokinase. Arch Surg 1986; 121: 769-773.

[86] Satoshkar RS, Bhandarkar SD, Ainapure SS. Pharmacology and Therapeutics. Revised 16th ed., Popular Prakashan, Mumbai, India. 1998; 460, 461, 1030,1031.

[87] Ouriel K, Welch EL, Shortell CK, Geary K, Fiore WM, Cimino C. Comparison of streptokinase, urokinase and recombinant tissue plasminogen activator in an *in vitro* model of venous thrombosis. J Vasc Surg 1995; 22: 593-597.

[88] Geiger M, Huber K, Wojta J, *et al.* Complex formation between urokinase and plasma protein C inhibitor *in vitro* and *in vivo*. Blood 1989; 74: 722-728.

[89] Manchanda N, Schwartz BS. Interaction of single chain urokinase and plasminogen activator inhibitor type 1. J Biol Chem 1995; 270: 20032-20035.

[90] Reinartz J, Schaefer B, Bechtel MJ, Kramer MD. Plasminogen activator inhibitor type-2 (PAI-2) in human keratinocytes regulates pericellular urokinase-type plasminogen activator. Exp Cell Res 1996; 223: 91-101.

[91] Billstrom A, Lecander I, Dagnaes-Hansen F, Dahllof B, Stenram U, Hartley-Asp B. Differential expression of uPA in an aggressive (DU 145) and a nonaggressive (1013L) human prostate cancer xenograft. Prostate 1995; 26: 94-104.

[92] Illig, C.R., Subasinghe, N.L., Hoffman, J.B., Wilson, K.J., Rudolph, M.J.: WO9940088 A1 (**1999**).

[93] Kuroiwa, K., Endo, K., Katayama, K., Nagasawa, T.: JP05279315 A (**1993**).

[94] Wosikowski-Buters, K., Schmalix, W.: DE10233632 A1 (**2004**).

[95] Sperl, S., Buergle, M., Schmalix, W., Wosikowski, K., Clement, B.: US2006142305A1 (**2006**).

[96] Bruncko M., McClellan, W.J.: US20036504031B1 (**2003**).

[97] Jankun JE, Skrzypczak-Jankun E. Binding site of amiloride to urokinase in different species. Int J Mol Med 2001; 8: 365-371.

[98] Dellaria, J.F.: US20016207701B1 (**2001**).

[99] Deck, L.M., Vander Jagt, D.L., Heynekamp, J.J.: US2006252823 A1 (**2006**).
[100] Sperl, S.: WO03103644 A2 (**2003**).
[101] Sturzebecher, J., Steinmetzer, T., Schweinitz, A.: WO03076391A2 (**2003**).
[102] Christman JK, Sulgi S, Newcomb EW, Silverstein SC. Correlated suppression by 5-bromodeoxyuridine of tumorigenicity and plasminogen activator in mouse melanoma cells. Proc Natl Acad Sci USA 1975; 72: 47-50.
[103] Wigler M, Weinstein IB. Tumor promoter induces plasminogen activator. Nature 1976; 259: 232-233.
[104] Unkeless J, Gardon S, Reich E. Secretion of plasminogen activator by stimulated macrophages. J Expt Med 1974; 139: 834-850.
[105] Mott DM, Tabisch PN, Sanc BP, Sorof S. Lack of correlation between fibrinolysis and the transformed state of cultured mammalian cells. Biochem Biophy Res Comm 1974; 61: 621-627.
[106] Rifkun DB, Pollack B. Production of plasminogen activator by established cell lines of mouse origin. J Cell Biol 1977; 73: 47-55.
[107] Strickland S, Beers WH. Studies on the role of plasminogen activator on ovulation: *in vitro* response of granulose cells to gonadotropins, cyclic nucleotides and prostaglandins. J Biol Chem 1976; 251: 5694-5702.
[108] Topp W, Hall JD, Massen N, *et al. In vitro* differentiation of teratomas and the distribution of creatine phosphokinase and plasminogen activator in teratocarcinoma-derived cells. Cancer Res 1976; 36: 4217-4223.
[109] Katz J, Troll W, Adler SW, Levitz M. Antipain and leupeptin restrict uterine DNA synthesis and function in mice. Proc Natl Acad Sci 1977; 74: 3754-3757.
[110] Lacroix M, Fritz IB. The control of the synthesis and secretion of plasminogen activator by rat Sertoli cells in culture. Mol Cell Endocrinol 1982; 26: 247-258.
[111] Stockinger, H., Binder, B., Leksa, V., Godar, S., Breuss, J.: WO04013177A1 (**2004**).
[112] Deutheux M, Jijaksi H, Lisson D. Effect of sulfur mustard on the expression of urokinase in cultured 3T3 fibroblasts. Arch Toxicol 1997; 71: 243-249.
[113] Nolan C, Hall LS, Barlow GH, Tribby IE. Plasminogen activator from human embryonic kidney cell cultures: evidence for a proactivator. Biochem Biophys Acta 1977; 496: 384-400.
[114] Kapina MA, Zelinin MG, Gluchova LA, Egorov BB. The RH-PA cell line-a source for obtaining the urokinase-type plasminogen activator. Antibiot Khimioter 1989; 34: 893-898.
[115] Unkeless JC, Tobia A, Ossowski L, Quigley JP, Riffin DB, Reich E. An enzymatic function associated with transformation of fibroblasts by oncogenic viruses. J Exp Med 1973; 137: 85-111.
[116] Goldberg AR. Increased protease levels in transformed cells: A casein overlay assay for the detection of plasminogen activator production. Cell 1974; 2: 95-102.
[117] Christman J, Acs G. Purification and characterization of a cellular fibronylic factor associated with oncogenic transformation. The plasmonogen activator from SV-40 transformed hamster cells. Biochem Biophys Acta 1974; 340: 339-347.
[118] Rifkin DB, Loet JN, Moore G, Reich E. Properties of plasminogen activators formed by neoplastic human cell cultures. J Expt Med 1974; 139: 1317-1328.
[119] Wilson EL, Michael LBB, Eileen GH, Eugene BD. Molecular species of plasminogen activators secreted by normal and neoplastic human cells. Cancer Res 1980; 40: 933-938.
[120] Goldfarb RH, Quigley JP. Purification of plasminogen activator from Rous sarcoma virus transformed chick embryo fibroblasts treated with the tumor promoter phorbol 12-myristate 13-acetate. Biochem 1980; 19: 5463-5471.
[121] Freedman VH, Shi SI. Cellular tumorigenicity in nude mice: correlation with cell growth in semi-solid medium. Cell 1974; 3: 355-359.
[122] Fahey EM, Chaudhuri PJB. Binding, refolding and purification of a urokinase plasminogen activator fragment by chromatography. J Chromatogr B 2000; 737: 225-235.
[123] Zhong, J., Liang, X., Huan, L.: CN1900289A (**2007**).
[124] Beaton, M., Mark, S., Pineda-Lucena, A.: WO05087917A2 (**2005**).
[125] Gurskii, Y.G., Belogurov, A.A., Bibilashvili, R.S., Grigoreva, N.V., Del'ver, E.P., Minashkin, M.M.: RU2247777C2 (**2005**).
[126] Sun, S., Yan, H., Chen, R.: CN1401662 A (**2003**).
[127] Kobayashi, H., Terao, T., Sugino, D., Okushima, M.: WO9725422A1 (**1997**).
[128] Hiramatsu R, Horinouchi S, Beppu T. Isolation and characterization of human pro-urokinase and its mutants accumulated within the yeast secretory pathway. Gene 1991; 99: 235-241.
[129] Hiramatsu, T., Kasai, S., Hirose, M., Tsukada, M., Tanabe, T., Kamimura, Y., Kawabe, H., Arimura, H.: JP 01252283 A (**1989**).
[130] Nelles L, Lijnen HR, Collen D, Holmes WE. Characterization of recombinant human single-chain urokinase-type plasminogen activator mutants produced by site-specific mutagenesis of lysine. J Biol Chem 1987; 262: 5682-5689.

[131] Hu, X., Gao, L., Chen, H., Pan, S., Yin, L., Yang, B., Zhang, Z.: CN1880449 A (**2006**).

[132] Okasinski, G.F., Schaefer, V.G., Suhar, T.S., Lesniewski, R.R.: WO96-US9345 (**1996**).

[133] Innis, M., Scott, E.: WO01032901 A1 (**2001**).

[134] Oishi, K.K., Zhou, D.: WO00000624 A1 (**2000**).

[135] Warner TG. Enhancing therapeutic glycoprotein production in Chinese hamster ovary cells by metabolic engineering endogenous gene control with antisense DNA and gene targeting. Glycobiology 1999; 9: 841-850.

[136] Kim DM, Swartz JR. Efficient production of a bioactive, multiple disulfide-bonded protein using modified extracts of *Escherichia coli*. Biotechnol Bioeng 2004; 85: 122-129.

[137] Senatore FF, Bernath FR. Urokinase bound to fibrocollagenous tubes: an *in vitro* kinetic study. Biotechnol Bioeng 1986; 28: 58-63.

[138] Kang JK, Choi SK, Lee HY. Kinetics of producing pro-urokinase in perfusion cultures. Biotechnol Lett 1990; 12: 173-178.

[139] Wagner A, Marc A, Engasser JM. Continuous production of pro-urokinase in feed harvest and perfusion cultures. Biotechnol Bioeng 1990; 36: 623-629.

[140] Smidsrod O, Skjak-Braek G. Alginate as immobilization matrix for cells. Trends Biotechnol 1990; 8: 71-78.

[141] Tamponnet C, Ramdi H, Guyot JB, Lievremont M. Rabbit articular chondrocytes in alginate gel: characterisation of immobilized preparations and potential applications. Appl Microbiol Biotechnol 1992; 37: 311-315.

[142] Jen AC, Wakes MC, Nikos AG. Hydrogels for cell immobilization. Biotechnol Bioeng 1996; 50: 357-364.

[143] Roychoudhury PK, Gomes J, Bhattacharyay SK, Abdullah N. Production of urokinase by HT1080 human kidney cell line. Artif Cells Blood Substit Immobil Biotechnol 1999; 27; 399-402.

[144] Someno T, Saino T, Katoh K, Miyazaki H, Ishii S. Affinity chromatography of urokinase on an agarose derivative coupled with pyroglutamyl-lysyl-leucyl-arginial. J Biochem 1985; 97: 1493-1500.

[145] Stump DC, Lijnen HR, Collen D. Purification and characterization of a novel low molecular weight form of single-chain urokinase-type plasminogen activator. J Biol Chem 1986; 261: 17120-17126.

[146] Stump DC, Thienpont M, Collen D. Urokinase related proteins in human urine. J Biol Chem 1986; 261: 1267-1273.

[147] Male KB, Nguyen AL, Luong JHT. Isolation of urokinase by affinity ultrafiltration. Biotechnol Bioeng 1990; 35: 87-93.

[148] Si S, Wang J, Li H, Song S. Purification of high molecular weight urokinase. Hebeisheng Kexueyuan Xuebao 1991; 4: 41-46.

[149] Japan Kokai Tokkyo Koho (Mokam Life Engineering Research Institute Foundation, S. Korea). JP104372 (**1990**).

[150] Hou KC, Zaniewski R. Purification of urokinase by combined cation exchanger and affinity chromatographic catridges. J Chromatogr 1990; 525: 297-306.

[151] Cao XJ, Zhu JW, Wang DW, Wus XY, Dai GC. Purification of urokinase by affinity cross-flow filtration using a water-soluble microligand. Ann NY Acad Sci 1996; 799: 454-459.

[152] Pang Z, Wu X, Cao X, Zhu J, Dai G. Affinity chromatographic purification of urokinase with a polystyrene-based medium. Huadong Ligong Daxue Xuebao 1996; 22: 417-421.

[153] Cao XJ, Tang M, Wu X, Dai GC. Purification of urokinase by affinity chromatography. Huadong Ligong Daxue Xue Bao 1998; 24: 515-520.

[154] Cao XJ, Tang M, Wu X, Dai GC. Affinity chromatography for purification of urokinase using cefazoline as ligand. Shengwu Huaxue Yu Shengwu Wuli Xuebao 1998; 30: 635-637.

[155] Dong YS, Liang F, Yu XY, Guo LA, Chang JH. Preparation of new magnetic dextran affinity adsorbents and their application to purify urokinase. Se Pu 2001; 19: 21-24.

[156] Dong YS, Liang F, Jin HX, Xi Q, Chang JH. Preparation of new magnetic affinity adsorbents and its application for purification of urokinase. Gaodeng Xuexiao Huaxue Xuebao 2002; 23: 1013-1017.

[157] Lin, X.: WO04094344A2 (**2004**).

[158] Morimoto, K., Kawahata, Y.: JP61146184A (**1986**).

[159] Morii, M., Ohoka, M., Kawashima, N., Morii, N., Suzuki, T.: EP210870A2 (**1987**).

[160] Kondo, M., Narita, S., Morimoto, K., Kawano, T.: JP60166621A (**1985**).

[161] Zhang, Y., Lu, J., Yang, S., Zhu, Z., Liu, C., Qu, X.: CN1613869A (**2005**).

[162] Maciag T, Weibel MK, Pye EK. In: Jakoby WB, Wilchek M, Eds. Affinity chromatography of urokinase. Methods Enzymology. Plenum, NewYork 1974; 451-459.

[163] Edmunds, T., Foley, S.: WO8912099A1 (**1989**).

[164] Dano K, Moller V, Ossowski L, Nielsen LS. Purification and characterization of a plasminogen activator from mouse cells transformed by an oncogenic virus. Biochem Biophys Acta 1980; 613: 542-555.

[165] Xue YM, Zhu H, Shi W, Liu W, Liu JN, Ma Z. Construction and characterization of a mutant of single-chain urokinase-type plasminogen activator (Ser (175)-His (187)-msc-uPA). Acta Biochem Biophys Sin 2000; 32: 26-30.
[166] Gao LH, Hu XW, Wu QF, Xiao CZ, Xu ZP, Zhang ZG. Single-chain urokinase-type plasminogen activator (sc-uPA) purification by immuno-affinity chromatography. Sheng Wu Gong Cheng Xue Bao 2002; 18: 356-359.
[167] Khaparde SS, Roychoudhury PK. Effect of temperature shift on urokinase production in hollow fiber bioreactor, Indian Chemical Engineering Conference, Technical Session Transcription 2005; 2: 255.
[168] Kumar A, Bansal V, Nandakumar KS, *et al.* Integrated bioprocess for the production and isolation of urokinase from animal cell culture using supermacroporous cryogels. Biotechnol Bioeng 2006; 93: 636-646.
[169] Paques, E.: DE3439980A1 (**1986**).
[170] Morimoto, K., Kawahata, Y.: JP61115492A (**1986**).
[171] Fujiwara, N., Saito, Y., Hattori, S., Ono, K., Amatsuji, Y., Miyake, S.: JP09187274 A (**1997**).
[172] Johannessen, M., Halkjaer, E., Petersen, L.C.: WO9400483A1 (**1994**).
[173] Bansal V, Roychoudhury PK, Mattiasson B, Kumar A. Integrated process for urokinase production from human kidney cell line HT1080 using supermacroporous monolithic scaffold, in: Indian Chemical Engineering Conference, Technical Session Transcription 2004; 6: 8.
[174] Koltsova SV, Shataeva LK, Sychareva TT. Isolation and purification of urokinase. Vopr Med Khim 1981; 27: 623-626.
[175] Skriver L, Nielsen LS, Stephens R, Dano SK. Plasminogen activator released as inactive proenzyme from murine cells transformed by sarcoma virus. Eur J Biochem 1982; 124: 409-414.
[176] Wu, Z., Qi, B., Peng, X.: CN1201070A (**1998**).
[177] Li, R., Zhou, X., Xiao, N.: CN1301694A (**2001**).
[178] Li, R., Zhou, X., Xiao, N., Liu, H., Wang, S.: CN1298869A (**2001**).
[179] Edward MF, Julian BC, Peter B. Refolding and purification of a urokinase plasminogen activator fragment by chromatography. J Chromatogr 2000; 737: 225-235.
[180] Takahashi R, Akiba K, Koika M, Noguchi T, Ezure Y. Affinity chromatography for purification of two urokinases from human urine. J Chromatogr B Biomed Sci Appl 2000; 742: 71-78.
[181] Zhang, Z., Chen, Z., Wu, S., Hu, X., Xu, Z., Xiao, C.: CN1778900A (**2006**).
[182] Sun, S., Yan, H., Chen, R., Chun, D.H.H.: WO03008594A1 (**2003**).
[183] Dadd, C., Stenland, C.J., Kent, J.D., Korneyeva, M.N., Baumbach, G.A., Cook, S.A., Bradley, R.T., Novokhatny, V., Villines, T.B.: WO01036611A1 (**2001**).
[184] Chen, Y., Liu, J.: CN1377969A (**2002**).
[185] Yi, J., Shen, H.: CN1311257A (**2001**).
[186] Amano, K., Sano, T., Nishitani, T.: JP103238 A (**2005**).
[187] Amano, K., Sano, T., Nishitani, K.: WO06094521 A1 (**2006**).
[188] Mazar, A.P., Ternansky, R.J., Parry, G., Gladstone, P.L., Gawlak, S.: WO05048822A2 (**2005**).
[189] Mennerich, D., Bruemmendorf, T., Heiden Castanos-Velez, E., Hermann, K., Kinnemann, H., Li, X., Roepcke, S., Staub, E., Hinzmann, B., Rosenthal, A., Pilarsky, C.: DE10316701A1 (**2004**).
[190] Eugen-olsen, J.: WO01038871A1 (**2001**).
[191] Harrison, R.G., Pento, T.J.: WO04112717A2 (**2004**).
[192] Verjat, T.: WO06131677A2 (**2006**).
[193] Hu, Q.: CN1288012A (**2001**).
[194] Resnati M., Blasi, F., Sidenius, N., Pallavicini, I.: WO06094828A2 (**2006**).
[195] Piironen, T., Hoyer-Hansen, G., Bruenner, N., Ploug, M., List, K., Laursen, B., Dano, K., Liljas, H., Haese, A., Hartwig, H., Tornblom, M., Gustafsson, O.: WO04099780A1 (**2004**).
[196] Killeen S, Hennessey A, El Hassan Y, Waldron B. The urokinase plasminogen activator system in cancer: a putative therapeutic target? Drugs News Perspect 2008; 21: 107-116.
[197] Ulisse S, Baldini E, Sorrenti S, D'Armiento M. The urokinase plasminogen activator system: a target for ant-cancer therapy. Curr Cancer Drug Targets 2009; 9: 32-71.
[198] Hildenbrand R, Schaaf A, Dorn-Beineke A, *et al.* Tumor stroma is the predominant uPA-, UPAR-, PAI-1-expressing tissue in human breast cancer: prognostic impact. Histol Histopathol 2009; 24: 869-877.
[199] Hildenbrand R, Schaaf A. The urokinase-system in tumor tissue stroma of the breast and breast cancer cell invasion. Int J Oncol 2009; 34: 15-23.
[200] Vallera, D.A., Hall, W. A.: US2003124147A1 (**2003**).
[201] Wilhelm, O., Buergle, M., Kessler, H., Schmiedeberg, N.: WO02016929A2 (**2002**).
[202] Perry, G.C.: WO05116077A2 (**2005**).

Anti-Inflammatory Effects of Endothelin Receptor Antagonists and their Importance for Treating Human Disease

Matthias Barton[*,1], Philipp C. Nett[2], Kerstin Amann[3], Mauro M. Teixeira[4]

[1]*Molecular Internal Medicine, University of Zürich, Switzerland*

[2]*Department of Visceral and Transplantation Surgery, University Hospital Bern, Switzerland*

[3]*Abteilung für Nephropathologie, Klinikum der Friedrich-Alexander Universität Erlangen-Nürnberg, Germany*

[4]*Departamento de Bioquimica e Imunologia, Instituto Ciencias Biologicas, Universidade Federal de Minas Gerais, Belo Horizonte, Brazil*

Abstract: Endothelin-1 (ET-1) is the main effector peptide of the endothelin family. Aside from being a potent endogenous vasoconstrictor and mitogen acting through its ET_A receptors, it contributes to the regulation of immune mechanisms, inflammatory cell activation, and release of cytokines. Thereby, endothelin promotes the developement of a number of chronic disease conditions characterized by inflammtory activation, including atherosclerosis and chronic renal failure. Studies using orally active endothelin receptor antogonists have shown that the ET_A receptor is mainly responsible for the immunomodulatory actions of endothelin. This review highlights recent findings in the field showing that the ET system, apart from being a marker and mediator of vascular injury, is directly involved in pathophysiology of these disease processes as an immunomodulatory factor. In this review, we summarize the current understanding of the mechanisms and signal transduction pathways triggered by ET-1 in inflammatory and immunomodulatory processes and discuss the findings of studies evaluating the use of selective and non-selective endothelin receptor antagonists in diseases associated with acute or chronic inflammatory activation, also discussing including the most recent clinical studies in the field using endothelin receptor antagonists.

Keywords: Disease, drug therapy, human, clinical, inflammation, interleukin, autoimmune, scleroderma, diabetes, kidney, atherosclerosis, infection, chronic, endothelin receptor antagonist.

1. THE ENDOTHELIN SYSTEM: COMPONENTS AND PHYSIOLOGICAL FUNCTIONS

Endothelin (ET-1), initially characterized as a potent vasoconstrictor [1-3], has a number of biological functions, including powerful mitogenic activity [4]. Endothelin has defined

*Corresponding author: E-mail: barton@access.uzh.ch

Atta-ur-Rahman / M. Iqbal Choudhary (Eds.)

activities during embryonic development and, after birth, within the cardiovascular, respiratory, renal, endocrine, gastrointestinal, and central nervous systems [4-7]. It is produced by several cell types, including endothelial cells, leukocytes, macrophages and monocytes [7-10]. ET-1 is the predominant of three endothelin isoforms [11] (Fig. **1**), being a product of

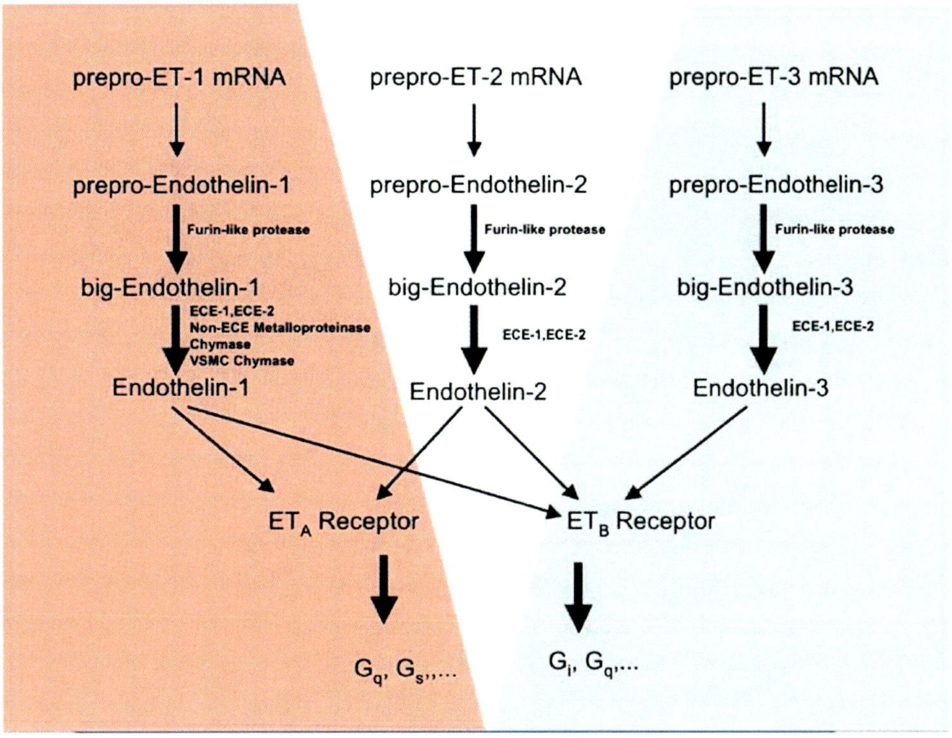

Fig. (1). Components of the endothelin pathway. Preproendothelins are formed following transcription and translation from prepro-endothelin mRNA and are subsequently processed by furin-like proteases to form big-ET intermediates that are further cleaved to three physiologically active endothelin peptides by endothelin-converting enzymes and other enzymes. Endothelin peptides interact with peptide-selective ET_B receptor or non-peptide selective ET_A receptors. These receptors couple to G proteins which result in the activation of different physiological responses. On the left, the components of the pre-pro ET-1 - ECE-1 - ET-1 - ET_A receptor axis is shown which is responsible for the development of embryonic cephalic and cardiac neural crest-derived craniofacial and cardiac outflow structures, vasoconstriction, cell growth, inflammation, among other actions. On the right, the components of the prepro ET-3 - ECE-1 - ET-3 - ET_B receptor axis is shown which is important for the development of neural crest-derived epidermal melanocytes and enteric neurons, natriuresis, melanocyte growth, and others. Also, ET_B receptor activation antagonizes many of the detrimental effects of mediated by ET_A receptors. Figure reproduced from Barton and Yanagisawa [4] with the permission of the publisher.

endopeptidasic cleavage of prepro-ET-1 to big ET-1 which is later transformed by ET-converting enzyme (ECE)-1 and/or ECE-2 into its active form (Fig. **1**) [6, 12]. Regulation of

ET production primarily occurs at the transcriptional level which is achieved by controlling the activity of the promoter and the stability of messenger RNA [13]. In a variety of cells, ET expression is controlled by autocrine and paracrine mechanisms [14] and induced by physiochemical factors such as blood flow, pulsatile stretch, sheer stress, hypoxia, pH or by cytokines, hormones and vasoactive agents [6, 12, 15-18] which also change the biological responsiveness to ET [12, 19].

In mammals, two ET receptors have been identified: ET receptor A (ET_A) and B (ET_B) which are members of the G protein-coupled superfamily [4-6, 12, 20]. ET_A receptors have selective affinity for ET-1 and ET-2, whereas ET_B receptors have similar affinity for all ET isoforms (Fig. **1**) [12, 21]. Both receptors stimulate phospholipase C which leads to increased formation of diaceylglycerol and inositol-1,4,5-triphosphate which activates the protein kinase C pathway and increases intracellular Ca^{2+}, respectively [22]. ET_A receptors are the predominant subtype mediating vasoconstriction and cell growth in humans whereas ET_B receptors are mainly expressed in vascular endothelial cells, mediating vasodilatation via release of nitric oxide (NO) and dilator prostanoids and thereby inhibiting cell proliferation [5, 6, 21]. Experimental studies using molecular and pharmacological inhibition of the ET system have demonstrated that ET-1 takes part in normal cardiovascular homeostasis [21, 23, 24]. Thus, ET-1 plays a major role in the functional and structural changes observed in arterial and pulmonary hypertension, glomerulosclerosis, atherosclerosis, largely via pressure-independent mechanisms [4, 12].

ET_A receptors are the predominant ET vasoconstrictor receptors in arteries. ET_A receptors on smooth muscle mediate contraction, cell proliferation, and hypertrophy [25]. Vasoconstrictor ET_B receptors are present in veins [26] and pulmonary vessels [27-29] in higher densities than in arteries, although ET_A receptors still predominate over ET_B receptors in these vessels. ET_B receptors are also localized on endothelial cells and act through the production of NO and prostacyclin to exert a vasodilator effect [24]. Whether vasoconstriction or vasodilatation is the predominant effect of ET-1 under normal conditions may depend on the vascular bed [30, 31]. It has been reported that in coronary arteries there are few endothelial vasodilator ET_B receptors [32]. As a result, ET-1 acts on coronary vessels mainly as a vasoconstrictor. In other vascular beds, however, ET-1 may function as a vasodilator under physiological conditions [33, 34].

2. GENERAL ASPECTS OF ENDOTHELIN AS AN IMMUNOMODULATOR

Endothelin is among the mediators released during inflammatory activation and together with different proinflammatory molecules, such as interleukin (IL)-1 and tumor necrosis factor (TNF)-α, may play a role in the cascade of events leading to tissue inflammation [35, 36]. In response to infectious and non-infectious stimuli, monocytes and macrophages release a number of mediators including cytokines which are involved in the inflammatory response [37]. These cytokines lead to further expression of mediators and co-stimulatory molecules which feed back into the inflammatory cascade [37, 38]. Increasing evidence supports a role for ET as a proinflammatory cytokine and fibrotic factor which is released in inflammatory and immune reactions [39, 40]. ET-1 acts as a proinflammatory peptide in vascular and non-vascular tisssues (Table **1**). ET-1 induces the release of proinflammatory cytokines [10, 39], provokes local ischemia [41] or alters the epithelial permeability allowing antigen translocation [42]. Thus, ET-1 has been implicated in many diseases characterized by inflammation and/or fibrotic remodeling, such as atherosclerosis [43], ischemia–reperfusion injury [44], alveolitis [45], dermatitis [46], Crohn's disease and ulcerative colitis

[41, 47,48], systemic sclerosis [49, 50], dermatomyositis/polymyositis [51], systemic lupus erythematodes [52], rheumatoid arthritis [53], liver cirrhosis [54], and glomeruloslerosis [55, 56]. In addition, ET-1 also contributes to diseases that are similarly characterized by chronic inflammatory processes such as pulmonary hypertension, systemic arterial hypertension, allograft rejection following solid organ transplantion, heart failure, cancer, and diabetes/obesity (Fig. **2**).

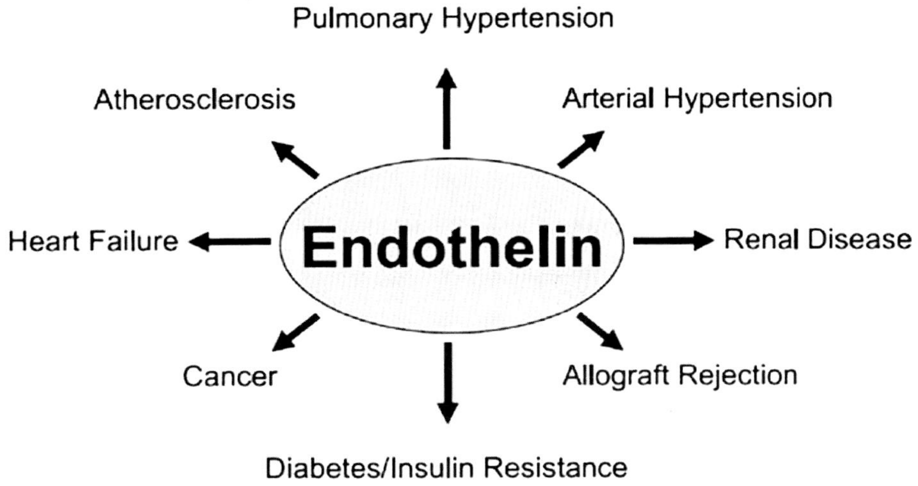

Fig. (2). A pathogenic role of endothelin-1 in several clinically important chronic disease processes with an acute or chronic inflammatory components. Figure reproduced from Barton and Yanagisawa [4] with the permission of the publisher.

Both ET_A and ET_B receptors appear to respond to these vascular and non-vascular related inflammatory disease processes [57-59]. In patients with Crohn's diesease and ulcerative colitis, plasma levels of ET-1 are significantly higher than in healthy controls and the density of ET positive cells as well as the expression of ET_A and ET_B receptors is increased [5, 41]. ET-1 is involved in many cell signaling pathways that include Ca^{2+} mobilization and activation of proinflammatory cytokines, extracellular signal-regulated kinases (ERK)1/2, and cyclin D1 [7, 60]. ET-1 also increases vascular permeability [61] as well as time- and dose-dependent entrapment of circulating platelets [62]. Recently, the downstream intracellular signal transduction pathways responsible for ET-1 have been in part identified. In this regard, a key role for mitogen-activated protein kinases (MAPK) has been suggested, which operate via phosphorylation cascades responsible for regulation of several substrates, mainly including transcription factors implicated in inflammation, development, cell proliferation and apoptosis [63, 64]. Three major MAPK subgroups are currently known, activated by dual phosphorylation on tyrosine and threonine residues and named c-Jun N-terminal kinases (JNK), p38, and ERK1/2, respectively [65]. In particular, ERK activation is crucially involved in mediating cell growth and differentiation induced by various stimuli, also including ET-1 [66, 67]. Important downstream targets of the MAPKs and ET-1 pathways are the cell cycle regulatory molecules such as cyclins, cyclin-dependent kinases and cyclin-dependent kinase inhibitors [68]. The cyclins are a target of both ET-1 and the MAPK pathway [69].

Table 1. Sites of Endothelin and Endothelin Receptor Expression During Inflammatory and Immunomodulatory Processes

Tissue	Cell Type
Brain	Neurons
	Astrocytes
	Microglia
Peripheral nerves	
Blood	Monocytes
	Leukocytes
Vascular system	Endothelial cells
	Vascular smooth muscle cells
	Macrophages
Heart	Cardiomyocytes
Liver	Kupfer cells
	Hepatocytes
Renal	Peritubular cells
	Mesangial cells
	Epithelial cells
	Podocytes (glomerular epithelial cells)
	Macrophages
Pancreas	Exocrine
	Endocrine
Gastro-intestinal	Epithelial cells
Lung	Epithelial cells
	Endothelial cells
	Vascular smooth muscle cells
	Macrophages
Prostate	

3. CELL-SPECIFIC ROLES OF ENDOTHELIN DURING INFLAMMATION

3.1. Effects on Leukocytes and Interleukins

ET-1 is known to stimulate neutrophils to release elastase [70, 71] and to stimulate monocytes to produce various cytokines, including IL-1 [39, 72], IL-6 [73, 74], IL-8 [75], IL-

10 [76], TNF-α [77], tumor growth factor (TGF)-β [45], granulocyte-macrophage colony-stimulating factor (GCSF) [78], monocyte chemoattractant protein (MCP)-1 [79, 80] and nuclear factor (NF)-κB [10, 81], promoting the inflammatory cascade (Table **2**). Overexpression of ET-1 stimulates expression of TNF-α, interferon (IFN)-γ, IL-1 and IL-6 [82]. Conversely, TNF-α and IL-1 modulate the expression of ET-1 in the inflammatory cascade [83, 84], which may further amplify its deleterious effects. Akin to ET-1, many of these mediators increase expression of cell adhesion molecules [85, 86], which promote the adhesion of circulating leucocytes to endothelial cells, an initial step in the events leading to cellular infiltrate in an inflamed tissue. Lopez-Farre *et al.* [87] demonstrated that ET-1 enhances neutrophil accumulation, suggesting a direct link between ET-1 and the inflammatory process. In addition to the neutrophil-activating properties of ET-1 it also acts as a chemoattractant for monocytes [88] and activator of mast cells [89-91] and inductor of significant eosinophil migration mediated by an increase in the local levels of eotaxin and IL-5 [92].

Table 2. Stimulatory Effects of Endothelin on Different Targets During Inflammatory and Immunomodulatory Processes

Cell Type	Activation of
Neutrophils, endothelia cells	Elastase
Pulmonary mast cells	Eotaxin
Monocytes	E-Selectin
Macrophages	GCSF
Monocytes	ICAM-1
Monocytes	IFN-γ
Monocytes, endothelial cells	IL-1
Pulmonary mast cells	IL-5
Monocytes, endothelial cells	IL-6
Endothelial cells	IL-8
Endothelial cells	IL-10
Fibroblasts	MCP-1
Macrophages, endothelial cells	NF-κB
-	TGF-β
Neutrophils, monocytes	TNF-α
Endothelial cells	Angiogenesis
Neutrophils, monocytes, macrophages	Cell adhesion
Monocytes	Chemotaxis

3.2. Effects on Monocytes and Macrophages

Macrophage, monocytes and polymorphonuclear leukocytes secrete ET-1 [9, 10, 93]. In addition to its ability to prime leukocytes for chemotaxis [94], ET-1 stimulates also the expression of adhesion molecules which are key players in the leukocyte-endothelial cell interaction [95]. Hayasaki *et al.* [96] documented that ET-1 induces intracellular adhesion molecule (ICAM)-1 expression on cultured cardiomyocytes and endothelial cells. Similarly, Zouki *et al.* [97] reported that ET-1 increased the expression of E-selectin and ICAM-1 on cultured human endothelial cells in a concentration-dependent fashion. The production of MCP-1, a potent chemoattractant for monocytes, can be also induced by ET-1 through ET_A receptor activation in endothelial cells. This effect is augmented by the proinflammatory cytokines TNF-α and IL-1β [98]. Although macrophages for more than a decade were believed to express only the ET_B receptor [99], very recent research has convincingly demonstrated that macrophages express also the ET_A receptor at the mRNA and protein level [100]. The fact that these cells express indeed the ET_A receptor may help to explain many the benefits of ET_A receptor blockade in numerous inflammatory or immune-mediated diseases [4] .

3.3. Effects on Vascular Endothelial Cells and Angiogenesis

In cultured endothelial cells, ET-1 promotes neutrophil aggregation [101] and stimulates surface expression of CD11b/CD1 on human neutrophils augmenting their adhesion to endothelial cells [87] and myocytes [96]. Activated endothelial cells are an important source of cytokines, adhesion molecules and growth factors enhancing inflammatory cells to migrate and accumulate in the extravascular tissue [102, 103]. Studies have demonstrated that ET-1 and ET-3, acting through the ET_B receptor, have dose-dependent stimulatory, proliferative and migratory effects on endothelial cells [104]. While ET-1 and ET-2 are reported to be equipotent in promoting DNA synthesis, ET-3 is less active [105]. During the formation of new blood vessels, endothelial cells migrate, proliferate and invade surrounding tissue to form capillaries [106]. ET-1, similar to VEGF, induces these angiogenic effects and, in concert with VEGF, displays a potent additive effect on the different stages of the angiogenic process. In this scenario, ET-1 signaling is mediated mainly by the ET_B receptor [107].

3.4. Effects on Vascular Smooth Muscle Cells and Fibroblasts

Fibroblasts and smooth muscle cells (or mesangial cells in the kidney) play a central role in disease processes such as glomerulosclerosis or atherosclerosis [108, 109]. ET-1 exerts mitogenic activity on smooth-muscle cells, myocytes, and fibroblasts [12, 110, 111]. In epithelial cells, ET-1 is known to induce gene expression and release of fibronectin [112] which is an important extracellular matrix component, as well as being chemoattractic factor for fibroblasts [113]. There is increasing evidence that ET-1 can function as a profibrotic cytokine by stimulating fibroblast chemotaxis and proliferation [114-116] and procollagen production [117, 118]. ET-1 may act in concert with several other profibrogenic molecules including TGF-β [119], platelet-derived growth factor (PDGF) [120], epidermal growth factor (EGF) [121], fibroblast growth factor (FGF) [122], insulin-like growth factor (IGF)-1 [123, 124], IL-11 [125] and insulin [67, 126, 127] to potentiate cellular transformation or replication. In particular, the synergistic interactions involving these mediators are crucial for implementing the tissue repair response leading to fibroblast proliferation, myofibroblast differentiation and collagen synthesis [123]. Within this context, MAPKs that participate in the cross-talk between ET-1 and the other fibrogenic factors at several levels play a pivotal role. Furthermore, cardiac fibroblasts have been shown to synthesize ET-1 [128], which induces collagen synthesis *via* both ET_A and ET_B receptors [129] as well as induces matrix metalloproteinase-2 expression [130].

3.5. Role of ET-1 in Bacterial and Parasite-induced Infection

The role of ET-1 in the pathogenesis of infectious diseases has only recently received attention. For example, ET-1 has been implicated in the etiology of vascular compromise and multi-organ dysfunction in the setting of septic shock [131, 132] and neuronal injury due to *Streptococcus pneumonia* meningitis [133]. Investigators have reported that circulating ET levels increase significantly in septic individuals which may be a beneficial effect in maintaining the blood pressure and organ perfusion during the early phase of septic shock [19, 102] and which correlates with mortality [134, 135]. Recent evidence also suggests that ET-1 plays a significant role in vascular dysfunction and organ failure associated with sepsis and septic shock [132]. It has been shown hat endotoxin administration results in upregulation of the ET system [136, 137] causing monocytes to produce proinflammatory cytokines such as TNF-α [39]. Endotoxin stimulates the production of TNF-α in monocytes and macrophages [10, 138]. Indeed, several reports have illustrated that antagonism of ET in septic animals improves metabolic acidosis as well as coronary, renal, splanchnic, pulmonary and intestinal perfusion [139-141]. In particular, release of ET-1 is stimulated by endotoxin [142]. Moreover, patients with *Rickettsia conorii*-induced vasculitis exhibit increased plasma levels of ET-1 [144]. *Rickettsia* share some important similarities with *Trypanosoma cruzi* (Chagas' disease) as both can reside within the endothelial cell cytoplasm and cause perturbations of the host cell [145]. ET is expressed during *Trypanosoma cruzi* infection in mice [68], and high plasma levels of immunoreactive ET were found in patients with severe chagasic cardiomyopathy [146]. Endogeneous ET-1 has protective effects during early chagas myocarditis [143, 155].

4. ENDOTHELIN RECEPTOR ANTAGONISTS AS ANTI-INFLAMMATORY DRUGS

4.1 Effects of Endothelin Receptor Antagonists on Leukocyte Activation

Activated leukocyte adhesion is the initial and rate-limiting step in the development of inflammatory cellular infiltrate. Both ET_A and ET_B receptors are involved in the ET-induced activation of leukocyte adhesion [96, 97, 147]. Based on these observations, selective and non-selective ET receptor antagonists might have the potential as immunomodulatory agents blocking the recruitment of leukocytes by reduction of leukocyte adhesion and preventing the ET-1-dependent progression of the inflammatory cascade. Indeed, Anthoni *et at.* [148] reported that bosentan, a non-selective ET_A/ET_B receptor antagonist, prevents the adhesion of leukocytes in colonic submucosal venules and reduces inflammation in a mouse model of inflammatory bowel disease. A comparable effect was also observed with the non-selective ET_A/ET_B receptor antagonist LU420627 [97]. Using a prevention study protocol, oral administration of bosentan reduced clinical inflammation and myeloperoxidase activity in colonic tissue in trinitrobenzene sulphonate-induced colitis in rats [149, 150]. The mechanisms of bosentan-induced reduction of leukocyte firm adherence remain speculative, but may depend on the blockade of ET-1-induced up-regulation of cell adhesion molecules on the endothelium and leukocytes [87, 96, 97, 151-153]. In particular, the finding that anti-inflammatory effects of ET-1 blockade are mediated by vascular cell adhesion molecule (VCAM)-1 in isolated endothelial cells suggests that this cell adhesions molecules may play a role in the attenuation of sticking and the elevation of rolling velocity in this study [152]. This is supported by the observation that treatment with an anti-VCAM-1 oligonucleotide exerts a more potent protective effect on leucocyte endothelial adhesion when compared to bosentan [154] which induces a reduction of the infection-associated increase in nitrate/nitrite (NOx) serum concentrations [155].

Previous in vitro studies using cardiac myocytes have shown that the selective ET_B receptor antagonist BQ-788 inhibits neutrophil-endothelial cell adhesion and ICAM-1 expression on endothelial cells [96], whereas the selective ET_B receptor antagonist S-0139 promotes neutrophil-cardiac myocytes adhesion and ICAM-1 production. This may be related to the differences in ET_A and ET_B receptor density on various cell types. For example, ET_A represents 90% of the receptors on the surface of cardiac myocytes, while the ET_B receptor is the dominant receptor on endothelial cells,. In contrast, macrophages express both the ET_A [100] and the ET_B receptor [156, 157]. However, different groups have reported varying results. Zouki *et al.* [97] reported that the ET_A-selective antagonist FR139317 markedly attenuated the ET-1 stimulated neutrophil adherence, suggesting a role of the ET_A receptor in neutrophil-endothelial attachment. It is possible that short- *versus* long-term exposure of endothelial cell to ET-1 may affect endothelial adhesiveness differently. The finding that the ET_A receptor-selective antagonist BQ610, but not the ET_B receptor-selective antagonist BQ788, decreased ET-1 induced MCP-1 expression suggests a role for the ET_A receptor in ET-1-mediated inflammation [98]. Recently, it has been shown that aryl-alkane-sulfonamides and their derivatives can also be used to reduce ET-1-mediated inflammation [158, 159] as well as a N-(5-isoxazolyl)benzene-sulfonamide ET receptor antagonist that can be modified in the 4-position with aryl and substituted aryl groups to generate a ET_A selective receptor antagonist [160, 161].

4.2. Endothelin Receptor Blockade and TNF-α Signaling

The mechanisms responsible for increased production of TNF-α by ET-1 and inhibition of TNF-α production by endothelin receptor antagonism remain unclear. ET-1 plays a proinflammatory role in different pathological conditions [162, 163]. Quehenberger *et al.* [164] for example demonstrated that the human ET-1 gene has NF-κB binding sites and reported that transcription of the ET-1 gene is controlled by NF-κB. These investigators demonstrated that binding of advanced glycation end products (AGEs) on the surface of erythrocytes, which occurs during oxidative stress, results in a NF-κB-dependent ET-1 induction *in vitro* [164]. It is likely that inhibition of TNF-α production by ET receptor antagonism is mediated by the NF-κB pathway. The effects of NF-κB in inflammation are well known, e.g., induction of synthesis of several proinflammatory cytokines including IL-1 and IL-6 [165]. Browatzki *et al.* [166] demonstrated that ET_A receptor activation induces IL-6 synthesis *via* NF-κB activation in human vascular smooth muscle cells, and extending these observations that ET-1 is also a potent stimulus for activation of NF-κB in human hepatic stellate cells [167]. These mechanisms may be responsible for the synthesis of most of these proinflammatory cytokines including the autocrine activation of ET-1 synthesis.

4.3. Endothelin Receptor Blockade and Allergic Inflammation

ET-1 stimulates eosinophil migration mediated by an increase in the local levels of eotaxin and IL-5 [92, 168] This observation explains previous reports showing the accumulation of eosinophils rather than neurophils, as well we an increase in immunoreactive ET in the broncho-alveolar fluid in experimental airway inflammation [169-171], and in a murine model of allergic pleurisy [172, 173]. Treatment of these animals with a selective ET receptor antagonist significantly decreased the production of proinflammatory mediators [45] and eosinophilia [168]. In this context recent patents mention the application of a novel class of indole-based ECE inhibitors to diminish the production of ET-1 to inhibit bronchoconstriction and pulmonary vasoconstriction in newborn mammals [174, 175].

4.4. Endothelin Receptor Blockade and Auto-immune Diseases

A number of studies emphasize a key inflammatory role of the endothelial cells, either by overexpression of inflammatory mediators or by stimulating formation of new blood vessels, in the disease processes of auto-immune diseases leading to the systemic organ involvement [176]. ET released after activation and/or damage of endothelial cells, might play an important role inflammatory processes and vasculopathy in autoimmune diseases [126, 127, 163, 177]. In particular, endothelin contributes to the inflammatory processes related to the onset of type 1 diabetes in well-characterized rodent models, as well as abnormal regulation of endothelin converting enzymes and endothelin receptors [163]. Increased plasma ET levels have been found in various autoimmune diseases such as systemic lupus erythematodes [52], systemic sclerosis [50] or rheumatoid arthritis [53]. Moreover, raised ET serum levels have been implicated in the pathophysiology of both fibrotic and vascular manifestations of systemic sclerosis [50]. Recently, increased urinary ET-1 excretion has been identified in patients with overt Lupus nephritis and the authors suggested that this could be used to monitor inflammatory activation related to the disease [178]. Indeed, a number of clinical studies have now shown that there is therapeutic potential for endothelin receptor antagonists in the treatment of complications related to connective tissue disorders [179-187].

4.5. Endothelin Receptor Blockade and Chronic Allograft Rejection

In the field of experimental and clinical organ transplantation, several studies have shown an involvement of ET-1 in ischemia-reperfusion injury in heart, lung, liver and kidney allografts [188-190]. Treatment with a selective ET_A receptor antagonist BSF208075 has also protective effects on microcirculation after ischemia/reperfusion. Uhlmann *et al.* [191, 192] were able to show that BSF208075 not only affects the expression of vasoactive genes, but also decrease gene expression of proinflammatory cytokines such as TNF-α, IL-1 and IL-6 *in vitro*. Ischemia/reperfusion injury promotes a microcirculation-associated inflammatory response, involving release of aggressive mediators, such as reactive oxygen species, TNF-α, IL-1, the upregulation of leucocytic and endothelial adhesion molecules such as selectins, integrins, intracellular adhesion molecule-1 and the interaction of platelets and leucocytes with the microvascular endothelium [191-193]. Based on these results selective antagonism of ET_A receptors may have anti-inflammatory potential through suppression of the mRNA of the genes of proinflammatory cytokines as TNF-α, IL-1β and IL-6. Several other studies support a role for ET-1 in ischemia/reperfusion injury of heart, lung, liver and kidney allografts [188, 194].

Elevated levels of ET-1 have been associated with inflammation and immune responses [12, 195, 196] as well as with transplant-associated diseases [189, 197]. High ET-1 expression in early post-transplant biopsy specimens was related to poor long-term allograft function following renal transplantation [198] and combined endothelial and myocardial protection could be achieved by ET antagonism enhancing transplant allograft preservation [199]. Multiple chemokines, cytokines and proinflammatory mediators are involved in the immune response following transplantation [200]. ET-1 accumulates during cold storage of allografts and can be detected in the effluent preservation solution [201]. In addition, ET-1 is appears to contribute to the development of chronic allograft dysfunction [202] which represents one of the major causes of late allograft loss [203]. Increased expression of components of the ET system has been reported in areas of neointimal proliferation, a hallmark of chronic allograft vasculopathy [197, 199, 201].

There is growing evidence that unwanted effects of calcineurin inhibitors (CNI) may be caused by an altered expression of ET-1 [40, 204]. These effects include enhanced vaso-constriction as well as induction of glomerulosclerosis. This is particularly complicating the therapeutic long-term success if the transplanted organ is the kidney. Enhanced levels of ET-1 lead to augmented constriction of smooth muscle cells and their advanced proliferation, as could be shown in cell culture experiments [205, 206]. Plasma levels of big ET-1 are dependent on cydosporin A plasma levels 1 year after successful cardiac transplantation in patients [207]. Previous studies using ET_A receptor antagonism have used concomitant immunosuppressive therapy [12]; thus, the potential immunomodulatory actions of ET-1 and the actual contribution of ET-1 to chronic rejection were masked because of the immunosuppressive agents. In a recent study - in the absence of any immunosuppression - we found that ET receptor antagonism markedly reduced or even normalized the increase in in circulating levels seen with IL-1 and TNF-α (Fig. **3**). These findings were independent of the development of graft atherosclerosis [202] and are compatible with a direct immunomodulatory role of ET_A receptors during allograft rejection [208]. Braun *et al.* [209] reported that ET_A receptor blockade with LU135252 prevented long-term deleterious changes on renal allograft function and morphology independently from systemic blood pressure and did not lower proteinuria strongly arguing against any effect on glomerular hemodynamics and upregulation of renal ET-1 synthesis in a rat model of chronic renal allograft rejection together with the implication of the ET_A receptor has been demonstrated [210]. On the other hand, Orth and collegues convincingly demonstrated that the ET_A receptor antagonist darusentan (LU 135252) is effective to reduce the development of graft disease after experimental kidney transplantation [190]. Importantly, these results were achieved without treating the animals with immunosuppressants after the acute rejection period [190]. Tripeptide derivative [211, 212], as well as pyrimidine sulfamides derivatives and benzo-fused heterocycles may be of benefit in the treatment of ischemia and proliferative disorders associated with increased tissue or circulating levels ET-1 [213, 214].

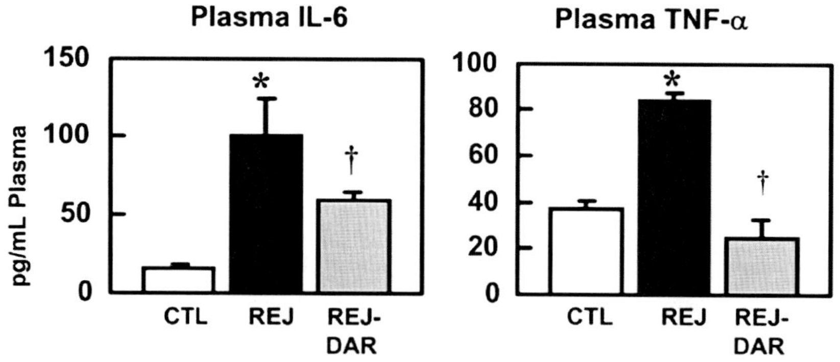

Fig. (3). Effect of chronic treatment with the ET_A receptor selective endothelin antagonist darusentan (DAR) on circulating cytokine levels in an experimental model of chronic allogeraft rejection (REJ) in the absence of immunosuppression. Treatment was associated with a marked reduction or even normalization of elevated cytokine levels. Data reproduced from Lattmann T, Hein M, Horber S, Ortmann J, *et al.* Activation of pro-inflammatory and anti-inflammatory cytokines in host organs during chronic allograft rejection: role of endothelin receptor signaling. Am J Transplant 2005; 5(5): 1042-1049. [202] with the permission of the publisher.

4.6. Endothelin Receptor Blockade and Infectious Diseases

Ono *et al.* [215] have reported that myocardial and plasma ET-1 levels increased in mice with encephalomyocarditis virus-induced myocarditis. The observation that ET-1 levels in the myocardium were higher than that in plasma suggested that the heart is a major source of endogenous ET-1 in myocarditis. The non-selective ET_A/ET_B receptor antagonist bosentan improved survival in these mice and reduced cellular infiltration and myocardial necrosis [215]. In addition, Pandey *et al.* [216] reported that another non-selective ET_A/ET_B receptor antagonist, SB217242, also improved impaired cardiac contractility and relaxation in these mice. ET-1 contributes to the pathogenesis of murine viral myocarditis and treatment with the non-selective ET_A/ET_B receptor antagonists bosentan or SB217242 significantly improved the pathological changes associated with the myocarditis [215, 216]. In another study, Albertini *et al.* [134] reported that ET_A receptor antagonist in rats completely prevented endotoxin-induced mortality and attenuated serum indices of myocardial, renal, liver and lung injury. Previous studies on experimental septic shock models evaluated the effects of ET_A receptor antagonists on injury and dysfunction of a single organ and showed that ET-1 has strong cardiodepressant effects in sepsis [141, 217].

We have recently reported that ET-1 contributes to the pathogenesis of chagasic cardiomyopathy *(Trypanosoma cruzi)* showing that interventions inhibiting endothelin synthesis or activation of endothelin receptors and/or endopeptidase may increase parasitemia and myocardial parasite infiltrates in chagasic cardiomyopathy [143, 155, 195, 218], indicating a protective function of endogenous ET-1 in this model. *Trypanosoma cruzi* infection induces ET-1 release from endothelial cells [219], and the released ET-1 contracts vascular smooth muscle via activation of ET_A receptors [220]. The mechanism by which ET-1 controls *Trypanosoma cruzi* infection are not investigated yet, however, ET-1 acting mainly on ET_A receptors can activate macrophages to release cytokines such as TNF-α [58]. As TNF-α-induced NO production by macrophages plays an important role in the acute phase of the infection [221], it is possible that the ability of ET-1 to release TNF-α may account for the effects observed. In this regard, we have shown that inflammatory mediators such as platelet-activating factors and chemokines, which like ET-1, act on G protein-coupled receptors, activate macrophages to produce NO and kill *Trypanosoma cruzi* [222].

4.7. Endothelin Receptor Blockade, Atherosclerosis, and Coronary Artery Disease

Inflammation of the vessel wall is a characteristic feature of atherosclerosis and seems to be responsible for the progression of the disease [109]. We have shown that ET-1 contributes to the pathogenesis of atherosclerosis and its acute complications [43, 58], and the anti-atherosclerotic effect of endothelin receptor antagonists has since been confirmed by several groups, utilizing either selective or non-selective drugs [58, 156, 223, 224]. Browatzki *et al.* [81] investigated the effect of ET-1 on the proinflammatory transcription factor NF-κB in human monocytes which are the major source of inflammatory mediators in atheroma and are located in rupture-prone plaque areas. In these monocytes, ET-1 caused NF-κB activation which could be blocked by inhibition of the I-κB-α-degrading proteasome complex as well as the ET_A receptor antagonist BQ123 but not by the ET_B receptor antagonist BQ788. ET-1 stimulated expression of the proinflammatory molecule CD40 but not of the cytokine IL-6 in a NF-κB-dependent manner. The data demonstrate the ability of ET-1 to differently activate inflammatory pathways in human monocytes [81]. Ammarguellat *et al.* [225, 226] reported that myocardial inflammation and fibrosis (which also occurs in patients with coronary artery disease) in hearts of deoxycorticosterone acetate hypertensive rats were, at least in part, mediated by ET-1. In this model, the selective ET_A

receptor antagonist A-127722 prevented cardiac fibrosis in hearts by normalizing the levels of procollagen I and III and FTGF. A-127722 also abrogates the activation of the inflammatory mediator NF-κB and the expression of platelet-endothelial cell adhesion molecule (PECAM)-1 and VCAM-1 [225, 226]. Hocher *et al.* [227] demonstrated that ET-1 plays an important role in the development of cardiac fibrosis in a two-kidney one-clip rat model of renovascular hypertension. In this model, the use of the ET_B-selective antagonist IRL1038, but not the ET_A-selective antagonist BQ-123, attenuated cardiac fibrosis. While benzo-1,3-dioxolyl- and benzofuranyl-substituted pyrrolidine derivatives as endothelin antagonists [228-231] might be useful for the treatment of congestive heart failure, one of the main consequences of coronary artery disease due to atherosclerosis, recent patents reveal that pyrrolidine and piperidine derivates act as selective ET_A and ET_B receptor antagonists and that novel alkanesulfonamides show beneficial effects in atherosclerosis [214, 232]. Possibly, wanted effects of ET_A endothelin receptor blockade may also include unexpected benefits, such as lowering of blood lipid levels [108, 233].

4.8. Endothelin Receptor Blockade, Glomerulosclerosis and Proteinuric Renal Disease

Endothelin is a key peptide promoting glomerular injury and subsequent proteinuria [108]. This process, which appears to be reversible if therapy is initiated in time [108] (Fig. 4), relates to inflammatory activation and changes in the protein filter of the kidney which is

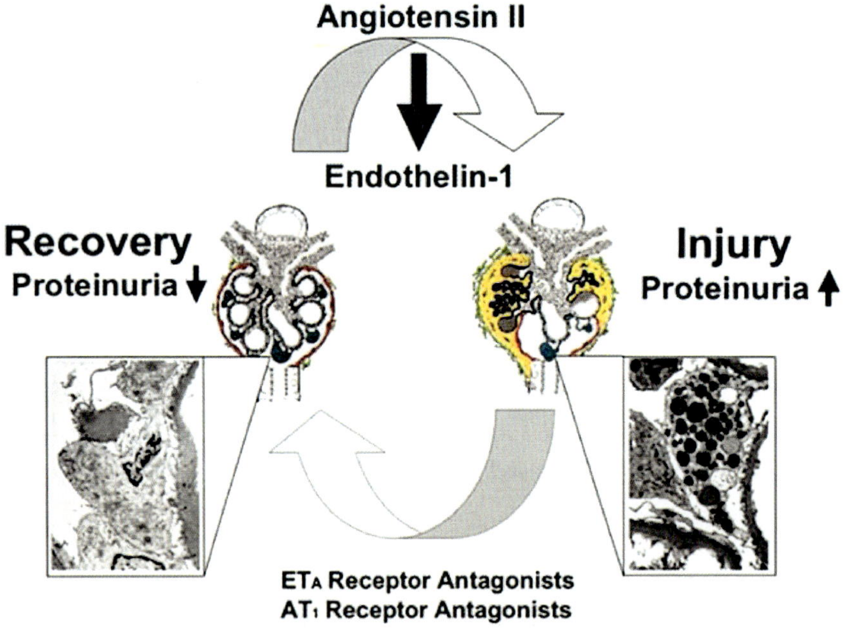

Fig. (4). Reversal of chronic inflammatory disease by ET_A antagonism as exemplified by glomerulosclerosis. Proteinuric renal disease as an example of chronic inflammatory processes that can be interfered with by blocking ET_A receptors. Treatment with endothelin receptor antagonists reverses functional injury due to glomerulosclerosis evident as proteinuria in rodents and humans and exerts these effects mainly *via* blood-pressure independent mechanisms. Figure reproduced from Barton M., Mullins J.J., Bailey M.A., Kretzler M., Role of endothelin receptors for renal protection and survival in hypertension: waiting for clinical trials. *Hypertension* 2006; 48(5): 834-7. [237] with the permission of the publisher.

formed by the glomerular epithelial cells, the pocodytes (reviewed in [108]). Aging, which is characterized by inflammatory activation as well, is associated with spontaneous development of focal-segmental glomerulosclerosis, which can be reversed by blockade of endothelin ET_A receptors [56], and similar effects can be seen in diabetic nephropathy [234]. Blockade of endothelin ET_A receptors can also attenuate the inflammatory responses associated with glomerulosclerosis development seen in diabetes [235]. First human trials have been completed ([236] and reviewed in [108]), and several studies with selective and non-selective antagonists are currently ongoing (reviewed in [108]).

5. CURRENT AND FUTURE DEVELOPMENTS FOR THERAPY OF HUMAN DISEASE

Endothelin (ET), a ubiquitously expressed polypeptide with a broad range of activities including vasoconstrictor, proinflammatory and profibrotic properties, has also been implicated in inflammatory and immunomodulatory processes that are characterized by vascular damage, inflammatory infiltrates and progressive fibrosis of the skin and internal organs. Plasma and local tissue concentrations of ET-1 are elevated in certain inflammatory reactions and may favor the inflammatory cascade by facilitating the recruitment of leukocytes, the expression of cell adhesion molecules and cytokines. ET-1 also induces fibrosis by activating fibrotic factors, increasing collagen synthesis, and stimulating fibroblast proliferation. ET-1 acts as a proinflammatory, profibrotic and mitogenic factor, thus ctivation of the ET system under these conditions is pathogenic and not simply adaptive. Mainly the ET_A receptor appear to be involved in these responses, as demonstrated by the results of studies using endothelin receptor blockers. Therefore, the ET axis represents a novel target for immunomodulation. Studies with selective ET_A or non-selective ET_A/ET_B receptor antagonists indicate that ET-receptor antagonism, indeed, holds the potential to markedly reduce consequences of local or systemic inflammatory processes with regard to improving symptoms and/or prognosis of the underlying disease. Several clinical [179, 233, 236] as well as randomized, placebo-controlled clinical trials [237, 238] have already been successfully completed and many more under way to further explore the therapeutic potential of this new type of immunomodulatory class of drugs in humans.

ACKNOWLEDGEMENTS

Supported by the Swiss National Science Foundation grants 3200-108258 and K-33KO122504/1, and the Interdiszipinäres Zentrum für Klinische Forschung, Universität Erlangen, Projekt A11. This work is based on and represents an extended and an updated version of our article previously published in Recent Pat Cardiovasc Drug Discov 2006; 1(3): 265-276.

REFERENCES

[1] Hickey KA, Rubanyi G, Paul RJ, Highsmith RF. Characterization of a coronary vasoconstrictor produced by cultured endothelial cells. Am J Physiol 1985; 248(5 Pt 1): C550-556.

[2] Gillespie MN, Owasoyo JO, McMurtry IF, O'Brien RF. Sustained coronary vasoconstriction provoked by a peptidergic substance released from endothelial cells in culture. J Pharmacol Exp Ther 1986; 236(2): 339-343.

[3] Yanagisawa M, Kurihara H, Kimura S, *et al.* A novel potent vasoconstrictor peptide produced by vascular endothelial cells. Nature 1988; 332(6163): 411-415.

[4] Barton M, Yanagisawa M, Endothelin: 20 years from discovery to therapy. Can J Physiol Pharmacol 2008; 86(8): 485-498.

[5] Rubanyi GM, Botelho LH, Endothelins. FASEB J 1991; 5(12): 2713-2720.

[6] Levin ER. Endothelins. N Engl J Med 1995; 333(6): 356-363.

[7] Kedzierski RM, Yanagisawa M. Endothelin system: the double-edged sword in health and disease. Annu Rev Pharmacol Toxicol 2001; 41: 851-876.

[8] Gray MO, Long CS, Kalinyak JE, Li HT, Karliner JS. Angiotensin II stimulates cardiac myocyte hypertrophy via paracrine release of TGF-beta 1 and endothelin-1 from fibroblasts. Cardiovasc Res 1998; 40(2): 352-363.

[9] Ehrenreich H, Anderson RW, Fox CH, *et al.* Endothelins, peptides with potent vasoactive properties, are produced by human macrophages. J Exp Med 1990; 172(6): 1741-1748.

[10] Cunningham ME, Huribal M, Bala RJ, McMillen MA. Endothelin-1 and endothelin-4 stimulate monocyte production of cytokines. Crit Care Med 1997; 25(6): 958-964.

[11] Inoue A, Yanagisawa M, Kimura S, *et al.* The human endothelin family: three structurally and pharmacologically distinct isopeptides predicted by three separate genes. Proc Natl Acad Sci USA 1989; 86(8): 2863-2867.

[12] Luscher TF, Barton M. Endothelins and endothelin receptor antagonists: therapeutic considerations for a novel class of cardiovascular drugs. Circulation 2000; 102(19): 2434-2440.

[13] Bloch KD, Friedrich SP, Lee ME, Eddy RL, Shows TB, Quertermous T. Structural organization and chromosomal assignment of the gene encoding endothelin. J Biol Chem 1989; 264(18): 10851-10857.

[14] Inoue A, Yanagisawa M, Takuwa Y, Mitsui Y, Kobayashi M, Masaki T. The human preproendothelin-1 gene. Complete nucleotide sequence and regulation of expression. J Biol Chem 1989; 264(25): 14954-14959.

[15] Rakugi H, Tabuchi Y, Nakamaru M, *et al.* Evidence for endothelin-1 release from resistance vessels of rats in response to hypoxia. Biochem Biophys Res Commun 1990; 169(3): 973-977.

[16] Malek A, Izumo S. Physiological fluid shear stress causes downregulation of endothelin-1 mRNA in bovine aortic endothelium. Am J Physiol 1992; 263(2 Pt 1): C389-396.

[17] Macarthur H, Warner TD, Wood EG, Corder R, Vane JR. Endothelin-1 release from endothelial cells in culture is elevated both acutely and chronically by short periods of mechanical stretch. Biochem Biophys Res Commun 1994; 200(1): 395-400.

[18] Wesson DE, Simoni J, Green DF. Reduced extracellular pH increases endothelin-1 secretion by human renal microvascular endothelial cells. J Clin Invest 1998; 101(3): 578-583.

[19] Battistini B, Forget MA, Laight D. Potential roles for endothelins in systemic inflammatory response syndrome with a particular relationship to cytokines. Shock 1996; 5(3): 167-183.

[20] Barton JR, Sibai BM, Whybrew WD, Mercer BM. Urinary endothelin-1: not a useful marker for preeclampsia. Am J Obstet Gynecol 1993; 168(2): 599-601.

[21] Barton M, Luscher TF. Endothelin antagonists for hypertension and renal disease. Curr Opin Nephrol Hypertens 1999; 8(5): 549-556.

[22] Simonson MS, Dunn MJ. Cellular signaling by peptides of the endothelin gene family. FASEB J 1990; 4(12): 2989-3000.

[23] Benigni A, Remuzzi G. Endothelin antagonists. Lancet 1999; 353(9147): 133-138.

[24] Schiffrin EL. Endothelin: role in hypertension. Biol Res 1998; 31(3): 199-208.

[25] de Nucci G, Thomas R, D'Orleans-Juste P, *et al.* Pressor effects of circulating endothelin are limited by its removal in the pulmonary circulation and by the release of prostacyclin and endothelium-derived relaxing factor. Proc Natl Acad Sci USA 1988; 85(24): 9797-800.

[26] Moreland S, McMullen DM, Delaney CL, Lee VG, Hunt JT. Venous smooth muscle contains vasoconstrictor ET_B-like receptors. Biochem Biophys Res Commun 1992; 184(1): 100-106.

[27] Russell FD, Davenport AP. Characterization of endothelin receptors in the human pulmonary vasculature using bosentan, SB209670, and 97-139. J Cardiovasc Pharmacol 1995; 26 (Suppl 3): S346-347.

[28] Sato K, Oka M, Hasunuma K, Ohnishi M, Kira S. Effects of separate and combined ET_A and ET_B blockade on ET-1-induced constriction in perfused rat lungs. Am J Physiol 1995; 269(5 Pt 1): L668-672.

[29] Davie N, Haleen SJ, Upton PD, *et al.* ET(A) and ET(B) receptors modulate the proliferation of human pulmonary artery smooth muscle cells. Am J Respir Crit Care Med 2002; 165(3): 398-405.

[30] Russell FD, Skepper JN, Davenport AP. Detection of endothelin receptors in human coronary artery vascular smooth muscle cells but not endothelial cells by using electron microscope autoradiography. J Cardiovasc Pharmacol 1997; 29(6): 820-826.

[31] Widmer CC, Mundy AL, Kretz M, Barton M. Marked heterogeneity of endothelin-mediated contractility and contraction dynamics in mouse renal and femoral arteries. Exp Biol Med (Maywood) 2006; 231(6): 777-781.

[32] Bacon CR, Davenport AP. Endothelin receptors in human coronary artery and aorta. Br J Pharmacol 1996; 117(5): 986-992.

[33] Verhaar MC, Strachan FE, Newby DE, *et al.* Endothelin-A receptor antagonist-mediated vasodilatation is attenuated by inhibition of nitric oxide synthesis and by endothelin-B receptor blockade. Circulation 1998; 97(8): 752-756.

[34] Goddard J, Johnston NR, Hand MF, *et al.* Endothelin-A receptor antagonism reduces blood pressure and increases renal blood flow in hypertensive patients with chronic renal failure: a comparison of selective and combined endothelin receptor blockade. Circulation 2004; 109(9): 1186-1193.

[35] Saleh D, Furukawa K, Tsao MS, *et al.* Elevated expression of endothelin-1 and endothelin-converting enzyme-1 in idiopathic pulmonary fibrosis: possible involvement of proinflammatory cytokines. Am J Respir Cell Mol Biol 1997; 16(2): 187-193.

[36] Graido-Gonzalez E, Doherty JC, Bergreen EW, Organ G, Telfer M, McMillen MA. Plasma endothelin-1, cytokine, and prostaglandin E2 levels in sickle cell disease and acute vaso-occlusive sickle crisis. Blood 1998; 92(7): 2551-2555.

[37] Luster AD. Chemokines--chemotactic cytokines that mediate inflammation. N Engl J Med 1998; 338(7): 436-445.

[38] Keane MP, Strieter RM. Chemokine signaling in inflammation. Crit Care Med 2000; 28(4 Suppl): N13-26.

[39] McMillen MA, Sumpio BE. Endothelins: polyfunctional cytokines. J Am Coll Surg 1995; 180(5): 621-637.

[40] Solini A, Santini E, Ferrannini E. Enhanced angiotensin II-mediated effects in fibroblasts of patients with familial hypercholesterolemia. J Hypertens 2005; 23(2): 367-374.

[41] Murch SH, Braegger CP, Sessa WC, MacDonald TT. High endothelin-1 immunoreactivity in Crohn's disease and ulcerative colitis. Lancet 1992; 339(8790): 381-385.

[42] Oktar BK, Coskun T, Bozkurt A, *et al.* Endothelin-1-induced PMN infiltration and mucosal dysfunction in the rat small intestine. Am J Physiol Gastrointest Liver Physiol 2000; 279(3): G483-491.

[43] Barton M, Haudenschild CC, d'Uscio LV, Shaw S, Munter K, Luscher TF. Endothelin ET_A receptor blockade restores NO-mediated endothelial function and inhibits atherosclerosis in apolipoprotein E-deficient mice. Proc Natl Acad Sci USA 1998; 95(24): 14367-14372.

[44] Bajory Z, Hutter J, Krombach F, Messmer K. The role of endothelin-1 in ischemia-reperfusion induced acute inflammation of the bladder in rats. J Urol 2002; 168(3): 1222-1225.

[45] Finsnes F, Lyberg T, Christensen G, Skjonsberg OH. Effect of endothelin antagonism on the production of cytokines in eosinophilic airway inflammation. Am J Physiol Lung Cell Mol Physiol 2001; 280(4): L659-665.

[46] Griswold DE, Douglas SA, Martin LD, *et al.* Endothelin B receptor modulates inflammatory pain and cutaneous inflammation. Mol Pharmacol 1999; 56(4): 807-812.

[47] Letizia C, Boirivant M, De Toma G, *et al.* Plasma levels of endothelin-1 in patients with Crohn's disease and ulcerative colitis. Ital J Gastroenterol Hepatol 1998; 30(3): 266-269.

[48] MacCarthy PA, Grocott-Mason R, Prendergast BD, Shah AM. Contrasting inotropic effects of endogenous endothelin in the normal and failing human heart: studies with an intracoronary ET(A) receptor antagonist. Circulation 2000; 101(2): 142-147.

[49] Becvar R, Stork J, Pesakova V, *et al.* Clinical correlations of potential activity markers in systemic sclerosis. Ann N Y Acad Sci 2005; 1051: 404-412.

[50] Vancheeswaran R, Magoulas T, Efrat G, *et al.* Circulating endothelin-1 levels in systemic sclerosis subsets--a marker of fibrosis or vascular dysfunction? J Rheumatol 1994; 21(10): 1838-1844.

[51] Mayes MD. Endothelin and endothelin receptor antagonists in systemic rheumatic disease. Arthritis Rheum 2003; 48(5): 1190-1199.

[52] Yoshio T, Masuyama J, Mimori A, Takeda A, Minota S, Kano S. Endothelin-1 release from cultured endothelial cells induced by sera from patients with systemic lupus erythematosus. Ann Rheum Dis 1995; 54(5): 361-365.

[53] Haq A, El-Ramahi K, Al-Dalaan A, Al-Sedairy ST. Serum and synovial fluid concentrations of endothelin-1 in patients with rheumatoid arthritis. J Med 1999; 30(1-2): 51-60.

[54] Rockey DC, Chung JJ. Endothelin antagonism in experimental hepatic fibrosis. Implications for endothelin in the pathogenesis of wound healing. J Clin Invest 1996; 98(6): 1381-1388.

[55] Barton M, Vos I, Shaw S, *et al.* Dysfunctional renal nitric oxide synthase as a determinant of salt-sensitive hypertension: mechanisms of renal artery endothelial dysfunction and role of endothelin for vascular hypertrophy and glomerulosclerosis. J Am Soc Nephrol 2000; 11(5): 835-845.

[56] Ortmann J, Amann K, Brandes RP, *et al.* Role of podocytes for reversal of glomerulosclerosis and proteinuria in the aging kidney after endothelin inhibition. Hypertension 2004; 44(6): 974-981.

[57] Teder P, Noble PW. A cytokine reborn? Endothelin-1 in pulmonary inflammation and fibrosis. Am J Respir Cell Mol Biol 2000; 23(1): 7-10.

[58] Barton M. Endothelial dysfunction and atherosclerosis: endothelin receptor antagonists as novel therapeutics. Curr Hypertens Rep 2000; 2(1): 84-91.

[59] Traupe T, Ortmann J, Munter K, Barton M. Endothelial therapy of atherosclerosis and its risk factors. Curr Vasc Pharmacol 2003; 1(2): 111-121.

[60] Suzuki E, Nagata D, Kakoki M, Hayakawa H, Goto A, Omata M, Hirata Y. Molecular mechanisms of endothelin-1-induced cell-cycle progression: involvement of extracellular signal-regulated kinase, protein kinase C, and phosphatidylinositol 3-kinase at distinct points. Circ Res 1999; 84(5): 611-619.

[61] Helset E, Kjaeve J, Hauge A. Endothelin-1-induced increases in microvascular permeability in isolated, perfused rat lungs requires leukocytes and plasma. Circ Shock 1993; 39(1): 15-20.

[62] Helset E, Lindal S, Olsen R, Myklebust R, Jorgensen L. Endothelin-1 causes sequential trapping of platelets and neutrophils in pulmonary microcirculation in rats. Am J Physiol 1996; 271(4 Pt 1): L538-546.

[63] Widmann C, Gibson S, Jarpe MB, Johnson GL. Mitogen-activated protein kinase: conservation of a three-kinase module from yeast to human. Physiol Rev 1999; 79(1): 143-180.

[64] Chang L, Karin M. Mammalian MAP kinase signalling cascades. Nature 2001; 410(6824): 37-40.

[65] MacCorkle RA, Tan TH. Mitogen-activated protein kinases in cell-cycle control. Cell Biochem Biophys 2005; 43(3): 451-461.

[66] Whelchel A, Evans J, Posada J. Inhibition of ERK activation attenuates endothelin-stimulated airway smooth muscle cell proliferation. Am J Respir Cell Mol Biol 1997; 16(5): 589-596.

[67] Nett PC, Ortmann J, Celeiro J, *et al.* Transcriptional regulation of vascular bone morphogenetic protein by endothelin receptors in early autoimmune diabetes mellitus. Life Sci 2006; 78(19): 2213-2218.

[68] Petkova SB, Tanowitz HB, Magazine HI, *et al.* Myocardial expression of endothelin-1 in murine Trypanosoma cruzi infection. Cardiovasc Pathol 2000; 9(5): 257-265.

[69] Petkova SB, Ashton A, Bouzahzah B, Huang H, Pestell RG, Tanowitz HB. Cell cycle molecules and diseases of the cardiovascular system. Front Biosci 2000; 5: D452-460.

[70] Hafstrom I, Ringertz B, Lundeberg T, Palmblad J. The effect of endothelin, neuropeptide Y, calcitonin gene-related peptide and substance P on neutrophil functions. Acta Physiol Scand 1993; 148(3): 341-346.

[71] Halim A, Kanayama N, el Maradny E, Maehara K, Terao T. Activated neutrophil by endothelin-1 caused tissue damage in human umbilical cord. Thromb Res 1995; 77(4): 321-327.

[72] Fabricio AS, Rae GA, Zampronio AR, D'Orleans-Juste P, Souza GE. Central endothelin ET(B) receptors mediate IL-1-dependent fever induced by preformed pyrogenic factor and corticotropin-releasing factor in the rat. Am J Physiol Regul Integr Comp Physiol 2006; 290(1): R164-171.

[73] Saito Y, Nakao K, Mukoyama M, Imura H. Increased plasma endothelin level in patients with essential hypertension. N Engl J Med 1990; 322(3): 205.

[74] Stankova J, D'Orleans-Juste P, Rola-Pleszczynski M. ET-1 induces IL-6 gene expression in human umbilical vein endothelial cells: synergistic effect of IL-1. Am J Physiol 1996; 271(4 Pt 1): C1073-1078.

[75] Zidovetzki R, Chen P, Chen M, Hofman FM, Endothelin-1-induced interleukin-8 production in human brain-derived endothelial cells is mediated by the protein kinase C and protein tyrosine kinase pathways. Blood 1999; 94(4): 1291-1299.

[76] Huribal M, Kumar R, Cunningham ME, Sumpio BE, McMillen MA. Endothelin-stimulated monocyte supernatants enhance neutrophil superoxide production. Shock 1994; 1(3): 184-187.

[77] Ruetten H, Thiemermann C. Endothelin-1 stimulates the biosynthesis of tumour necrosis factor in macrophages: ET-receptors, signal transduction and inhibition by dexamethasone. J Physiol Pharmacol 1997; 48(4): 675-688.

[78] Waters CE, Shi-Wen X, Denton CP, Abraham DJ, Pearson JD. Signaling pathways regulating intercellular adhesion molecule 1 expression by endothelin 1: comparison with interleukin-1beta in normal and scleroderma dermal fibroblasts. Arthritis Rheum 2006; 54(2): 649-660.

[79] Luft FC. Proinflammatory effects of angiotensin II and endothelin: targets for progression of cardiovascular and renal diseases. Curr Opin Nephrol Hypertens 2002; 11(1): 59-66.

[80] Duerrschmidt N, Wippich N, Goettsch W, Broemme HJ, Morawietz H. Endothelin-1 induces NAD(P)H oxidase in human endothelial cells. Biochem Biophys Res Commun 2000; 269(3): 713-717.

[81] Browatzki M, Pfeiffer CA, Schmidt J, Kranzhofer R. Endothelin-1 induces CD40 but not IL-6 in human monocytes via the proinflammatory transcription factor NF-kappaB. Eur J Med Res 2005; 10(5): 197-201.

[82] Yang LL, Gros R, Kabir MG, *et al.* Conditional cardiac overexpression of endothelin-1 induces inflammation and dilated cardiomyopathy in mice. Circulation 2004; 109(2): 255-261.

[83] Maemura K, Kurihara H, Morita T, Oh-hashi Y, Yazaki Y. Production of endothelin-1 in vascular endothelial cells is regulated by factors associated with vascular injury. Gerontology 1992; 38(Suppl 1): 29-35.

[84] Klemm P, Warner TD, Hohlfeld T, Corder R, Vane JR. Endothelin 1 mediates *ex vivo* coronary vasoconstriction caused by exogenous and endogenous cytokines. Proc Natl Acad Sci USA 1995; 92(7): 2691-2695.

[85] Arndt H, Bolanowski MA, Granger DN. Role of interleukin 8 on leucocyte-endothelial cell adhesion in intestinal inflammation. Gut 1996; 38(6): 911-915.

[86] Panes J, Granger DN. Leukocyte-endothelial cell interactions: molecular mechanisms and implications in gastrointestinal disease. Gastroenterology 1998; 114(5): 1066-1090.

[87] Lopez Farre A, Riesco A, Espinosa G, *et al.* Effect of endothelin-1 on neutrophil adhesion to endothelial cells and perfused heart. Circulation 1993; 88(3): 1166-1171.

[88] Achmad TH, Rao GS. Chemotaxis of human blood monocytes toward endothelin-1 and the influence of calcium channel blockers. Biochem Biophys Res Commun 1992; 189(2): 994-1000.

[89] Sessa WC, Kaw S, Hecker M, Vane JR. The biosynthesis of endothelin-1 by human polymorphonuclear leukocytes. Biochem Biophys Res Commun 1991; 174(2): 613-618.

[90] Uchida Y, Ninomiya H, Sakamoto T, *et al.* ET-1 released histamine from guinea pig pulmonary but not peritoneal mast cells. Biochem Biophys Res Commun 1992; 189(2): 1196-1201.

[91] Maurer M, Wedemeyer J, Metz M, *et al.* Yanagisawa M.M., Tsai M., Galli S.J., Mast cells promote homeostasis by limiting endothelin-1-induced toxicity. Nature 2004; 432(7016): 512-516.

[92] Cui P, Sharmin S, Okumura Y, *et al.* Endothelin-1 peptides and IL-5 synergistically increase the expression of IL-13 in eosinophils. Biochem Biophys Res Commun 2004; 315(4): 782-787.

[93] Sessa WC, Kaw S, Zembowicz A, Anggard E, Hecker M, Vane JR. Human polymorphonuclear leukocytes generate and degrade endothelin-1 by two distinct neutral proteases. J Cardiovasc Pharmacol 1991; 17 (Suppl 7): S34-38.

[94] Langenfeld MR, Nakhla S, Death AK, Jessup W, Celermajer DS. Endothelin-1 plus oxidized low-density lipoprotein, but neither alone, increase human monocyte adhesion to endothelial cells. Clin Sci (Lond) 2001; 101(6): 731-738.

[95] Springer TA. Traffic signals for lymphocyte recirculation and leukocyte emigration: the multistep paradigm. Cell 1994; 76(2): 301-314.

[96] Hayasaki Y, Nakajima M, Kitano Y, Iwasaki T, Shimamura T, Iwaki K. ICAM-1 expression on cardiac myocytes and aortic endothelial cells via their specific endothelin receptor subtype. Biochem Biophys Res Commun 1996; 229(3): 817-824.

[97] Zouki C, Baron C, Fournier A, Filep JG. Endothelin-1 enhances neutrophil adhesion to human coronary artery endothelial cells: role of ET(A) receptors and platelet-activating factor. Br J Pharmacol 1999; 127(4): 969-979.

[98] Chen P, Shibata M, Zidovetzki R, Fisher M, Zlokovic BV, Hofman FM. Endothelin-1 and monocyte chemoattractant protein-1 modulation in ischemia and human brain-derived endothelial cell cultures. J Neuroimmunol 2001; 116(1): 62-73.

[99] Bacon CR, Cary NR, Davenport AP. Endothelin peptide and receptors in human atherosclerotic coronary artery and aorta. Circ Res 1996; 79(4): 794-801.

[100] Mencarelli M, Pecorelli A, Carbotti P, Valacchi G, Grasso G, Muscettola M. Endothelin receptor A expression in human inflammatory cells. Regul Pept 2009; 158(1-3): 1-5.

[101] Gomez-Garre D, Guerra M, Gonzalez E, *et al.* Aggregation of human polymorphonuclear leukocytes by endothelin: role of platelet-activating factor. Eur J Pharmacol 1992; 224(2-3): 167-172.

[102] Krishnaswamy G, Kelley J, Yerra L, Smith JK, Chi DS. Human endothelium as a source of multifunctional cytokines: molecular regulation and possible role in human disease. J Interferon Cytokine Res 1999; 19(2): 91-104.

[103] Majka M, Janowska-Wieczorek A, Ratajczak J, *et al.* Numerous growth factors, cytokines, and chemokines are secreted by human CD34(+) cells, myeloblasts, erythroblasts, and megakaryoblasts and regulate normal hematopoiesis in an autocrine/paracrine manner. Blood 2001; 97(10): 3075-85.

[104] Noiri E, Hu Y, Bahou WF, Keese CR, Giaever I, Goligorsky MS. Permissive role of nitric oxide in endothelin-induced migration of endothelial cells. J Biol Chem 1997; 272(3): 1747-1752.

[105] Battistini B, Chailler P, D'Orleans-Juste P, Briere N, Sirois P. Growth regulatory properties of endothelins. Peptides 1993; 14(2): 385-399.

[106] Distler O, Neidhart M, Gay RE, Gay S. The molecular control of angiogenesis. Int Rev Immunol 2002; 21(1): 33-49.

[107] Salani D, Taraboletti G, Rosano L, *et al.* Endothelin-1 induces an angiogenic phenotype in cultured endothelial cells and stimulates neovascularization in vivo. Am J Pathol 2000; 157(5): 1703-1711.

[108] Barton M. Reversal of proteinuric renal disease and the emerging role of endothelin. Nat Clin Pract Nephrol 2008; 4(9): 490-501.

[109] Barton M, Minotti R, Haas E. Inflammation and atherosclerosis. Circ Res 2007; 101(8): 750-751.

[110] Matsuya M, Sasaki H, Aoto H, *et al.* Cell adhesion kinase beta forms a complex with a new member, Hic-5, of proteins localized at focal adhesions. J Biol Chem 1998; 273(2): 1003-1014.

[111] Gallelli L, Pelaia G, D'Agostino B, *et al.* Endothelin-1 induces proliferation of human lung fibroblasts and IL-11 secretion through an ET(A) receptor-dependent activation of MAP kinases. J Cell Biochem 2005; 96(4): 858-868.

[112] Marini M, Carpi S, Bellini A, Patalano F, Mattoli S. Endothelin-1 induces increased fibronectin expression in human bronchial epithelial cells. Biochem Biophys Res Commun 1996; 220(3): 896-899.

[113] Malemud CJ. Matrix metalloproteinases (MMPs) in health and disease: an overview. Front Biosci 2006; 11: 1696-1701.

[114] Shahar I, Fireman E, Topilsky M, *et al.* Effect of endothelin-1 on alpha-smooth muscle actin expression and on alveolar fibroblasts proliferation in interstitial lung diseases. Int J Immunopharmacol 1999; 21(11): 759-775.

[115] Gray MJ, Zadoks RN, Fortes ED, *et al. Listeria monocytogenes* isolates from foods and humans form distinct but overlapping populations. Appl Environ Microbiol 2004; 70(10): 5833-5841.

[116] Hafizi S, Wharton J, Chester AH, Yacoub MH. Profibrotic effects of endothelin-1 via the ET_A receptor in cultured human cardiac fibroblasts. Cell Physiol Biochem 2004; 14(4-6): 285-292.

[117] Kahaleh MB. Endothelin, an endothelial-dependent vasoconstrictor in scleroderma. Enhanced production and profibrotic action. Arthritis Rheum 1991; 34(8): 978-983.

[118] Dawes KE, Cambrey AD, Campa JS, *et al.* Changes in collagen metabolism in response to endothelin-1: evidence for fibroblast heterogeneity. Int J Biochem Cell Biol 1996; 28(2): 229-238.

[119] Shimojo N, Jesmin S, Zaedi S, *et al.* Eicosapentaenoic acid prevents endothelin-1-induced cardiomyocyte hypertrophy in vitro through the suppression of TGF-{beta}1 and phosphorylated JNK. Am J Physiol Heart Circ Physiol 2006; 291(2): H835-H845.

[120] Yahiaoui L, Villeneuve A, Valderrama-Carvajal H, Burke F, Fixman ED. Endothelin-1 regulates proliferative responses, both alone and synergistically with PDGF, in rat tracheal smooth muscle cells. Cell Physiol Biochem 2006; 17(1-2): 37-46.

[121] Beaucage P, Moreau P. EGF Receptor transactivation in angiotensin II and endothelin control of vascular protein synthesis *in vivo*. J Cardiovasc Pharmacol 2004; 44 (Suppl 1): S20-23.

[122] Li P, Oparil S, Sun JZ, Thompson JA, Chen YF. Fibroblast growth factor mediates hypoxia-induced endothelin-- a receptor expression in lung artery smooth muscle cells. J Appl Physiol 2003; 95(2): 643-651; discussion 863.

[123] Zhang S, Smartt H, Holgate ST, Roche WR. Growth factors secreted by bronchial epithelial cells control myofibroblast proliferation: an *in vitro* co-culture model of airway remodeling in asthma. Lab Invest 1999; 79(4): 395-405.

[124] Holgate ST, Davies DE, Lackie PM, Wilson SJ, Puddicombe SM, Lordan JL. Epithelial-mesenchymal interactions in the pathogenesis of asthma. J Allergy Clin Immunol 2000; 105(2 Pt 1): 193-204.

[125] Vignola AM, Mirabella F, Costanzo G, *et al.* Airway remodeling in asthma. Chest 2003; 123(3 Suppl): 417S-422S.

[126] Ortmann J, Traupe T, Nett P, *et al.* Upregulation of Vascular ET_B Receptor Gene Expression after Chronic ET_A Receptor Blockade in Prediabetic NOD Mice. J Cardiovasc Pharmacol 2004; 44: S105-S108.

[127] Ortmann J, Nett PC, Celeiro J, *et al.* Endothelin inhibition delays onset of hyperglycemia and associated vascular injury in type I diabetes: evidence for endothelin release by pancreatic islet beta-cells. Biochem Biophys Res Commun 2005; 334(2): 689-695.

[128] King KL, Winer J, Phillips DM, Quach J, Williams PM, Mather JP. Phenylephrine, endothelin, prostaglandin F2alpha and leukemia inhibitory factor induce different cardiac hypertrophy phenotypes *in vitro*. Endocrine 1998; 9(1): 45-55.

[129] Guarda E, Katwa LC, Myers PR, Tyagi SC, Weber KT. Effects of endothelins on collagen turnover in cardiac fibroblasts. Cardiovasc Res 1993; 27(12): 2130-2134.

[130] Bergman MR, Cheng S, Honbo N, Piacentini L, Karliner JS, Lovett DH. A functional activating protein 1 (AP-1) site regulates matrix metalloproteinase 2 (MMP-2) transcription by cardiac cells through interactions with JunB-Fra1 and JunB-FosB heterodimers. Biochem J 2003; 369(Pt 3): 485-496.

[131] Iskit AB, Senel I, Sokmensuer C, Guc MO. Endothelin receptor antagonist bosentan improves survival in a murine caecal ligation and puncture model of septic shock. Eur J Pharmacol 2004; 506(1): 83-88.

[132] Mitaka C. [Septic shock and endothelin]. Nippon Rinsho 2004; 62 (Suppl 9): 661-664.

[133] Pfister LA, Tureen JH, Shaw S, *et al.* Endothelin inhibition improves cerebral blood flow and is neuroprotective in pneumococcal meningitis. Ann Neurol 2000; 47(3): 329-335.

[134] Albertini M, Clement MG, Hussain SN. Role of endothelin ETA receptors in sepsis-induced mortality, vascular leakage, and tissue injury in rats. Eur J Pharmacol 2003; 474(1): 129-135.

[135] Forni M, Mazzola S, Ribeiro LA, *et al.* Expression of endothelin-1 system in a pig model of endotoxic shock. Regul Pept 2005; 131(1-3): 89-96.

[136] Pittet JF, Morel DR, Hemsen A, *et al.* Elevated plasma endothelin-1 concentrations are associated with the severity of illness in patients with sepsis. Ann Surg 1991; 213(3): 261-264.

[137] Gandhi CR, Stephenson K, Olson MS. A comparative study of endothelin- and platelet-activating-factor-mediated signal transduction and prostaglandin synthesis in rat Kupffer cells. Biochem J 1992; 281 (Pt 2): 485-492.

[138] McMillen MA, Huribal M, Kumar R, Sumpio BE. Endothelin-stimulated human monocytes produce prostaglandin E2 but not leukotriene B4. J Surg Res 1993; 54(4): 331-335.

[139] Weitzberg E, Lundberg JM, Rudehill A. Elevated plasma levels of endothelin in patients with sepsis syndrome. Circ Shock 1991; 33(4): 222-227.

[140] Wanecek M, Oldner A, Rudehill A, Sollevi A, Alving K, Weitzberg E. Cardiopulmonary dysfunction during porcine endotoxin shock is effectively counteracted by the endothelin receptor antagonist bosentan. Shock 1997; 7(5): 364-370.

[141] Wanecek M, Weitzberg E, Alving K, Rudehill A, Oldner A. Effects of the endothelin receptor antagonist bosentan on cardiac performance during porcine endotoxin shock. Acta Anaesthesiol Scand 2001; 45(10): 1262-1270.

[142] Sugiura M, Inagami T, Kon V. Endotoxin stimulates endothelin-release in vivo and in vitro as determined by radioimmunoassay. Biochem Biophys Res Commun 1989; 161(3): 1220-1227.

[143] Camargos ER, Machado CR, Teixeira Jr AL, *et al.* Role of endothelin during experimental *Trypanosoma cruzi* infection in rats. Clin Sci (Lond) 2002; 103 (Suppl 48): 64S-67S.

[144] Davi G, Giammarresi C, Vigneri S, *et al.* Demonstration of *Rickettsia Conorii*-induced coagulative and platelet activation in vivo in patients with Mediterranean spotted fever. Thromb Haemost 1995; 74(2): 631-634.

[145] Shi RJ, Simpson-Haidaris PJ, Lerner NB, Marder VJ, Silverman DJ, Sporn LA. Transcriptional regulation of endothelial cell tissue factor expression during *Rickettsia rickettsii* infection: involvement of the transcription factor NF-kappaB. Infect Immun 1998; 66(3): 1070-1075.

[146] Salomone OA, Caeiro TF, Madoery RJ, *et al.* High plasma immunoreactive endothelin levels in patients with Chagas' cardiomyopathy. Am J Cardiol 2001; 87(10): 1217-1220; A7.

[147] Boros M, Massberg S, Baranyi L, Okada H, Messmer K. Endothelin 1 induces leukocyte adhesion in submucosal venules of the rat small intestine. Gastroenterology 1998; 114(1): 103-114.

[148] Anthoni C, Mennigen RB, Rijcken EJ, *et al.* Bosentan, an endothelin receptor antagonist, reduces leucocyte adhesion and inflammation in a murine model of inflammatory bowel disease. Int J Colorectal Dis 2005: 1-10.

[149] Hogaboam CM, Muller MJ, Collins SM, Hunt RH. An orally active non-selective endothelin receptor antagonist, bosentan, markedly reduces injury in a rat model of colitis. Eur J Pharmacol 1996; 309(3): 261-269.

[150] Gulluoglu BM, Kurtel H, Gulluoglu MG, *et al.* Role of endothelins in trinitrobenzene sulfonic acid-induced colitis in rats. Digestion 1999; 60(5): 484-492.

[151] Sanz MJ, Johnston B, Issekutz A, Kubes P. Endothelin-1 causes P-selectin-dependent leukocyte rolling and adhesion within rat mesenteric microvessels. Am J Physiol 1999; 277(5 Pt 2): H1823-1830.

[152] Ishizuka T, Takamizawa-Matsumoto M, Suzuki K, Kurita A, Endothelin-1 enhances vascular cell adhesion molecule-1 expression in tumor necrosis factor alpha-stimulated vascular endothelial cells. Eur J Pharmacol 1999; 369(2): 237-245.

[153] McCarron RM, Wang L, Stanimirovic DB, Spatz M. Endothelin induction of adhesion molecule expression on human brain microvascular endothelial cells. Neurosci Lett 1993; 156(1-2): 31-34.

[154] Rijcken E, Krieglstein CF, Anthoni C, *et al.* ICAM-1 and VCAM-1 antisense oligonucleotides attenuate in vivo leucocyte adherence and inflammation in rat inflammatory bowel disease. Gut 2002; 51(4): 529-535.

[155] Camargos ER, Rocha LL, Rachid MA, *et al.* Protective role of ET_A endothelin receptors during the acute phase of *Trypanosoma cruzi* infection in rats. Microbes Infect 2009; 6(7): 650-656.

[156] Babaei S, Picard P, Ravandi A, *et al.* Blockade of endothelin receptors markedly reduces atherosclerosis in LDL receptor deficient mice: role of endothelin in macrophage foam cell formation. Cardiovasc Res 2000; 48(1): 158-167.

[157] Sakurai-Yamashita Y, Yamashita K, Yoshida A, *et al.* Rat peritoneal macrophages express endothelin ET(B) but not endothelin ET(A) receptors. Eur J Pharmacol 1997; 338(2): 199-203.

[158] Boss C, Bolli MH, Weller T, Fischli W, Clozel M. Bis-sulfonamides as endothelin receptor antagonists. Bioorg Med Chem Lett 2003; 13(5): 951-954.

[159] Weller, T.; Bolli, M.; Boss, C.; Clozel, M.; Fischli, W.: 2006: US7091201.

[160] Chan MF, Kois A, Verner EJ, *et al.* The discovery and structure-activity relationships of nonpeptide, low molecular weight antagonists selective for the endothelin ET(B) receptor. Bioorg Med Chem 1998; 6(12): 2301-2316.

[161] Chan, M.F.; Raju, B.G.; Kois, A.; Verner, E.J.; Wu, C.; Castillo, R.S.; Yalamoori, V.; Balaji, V.N.; Ramnarayan, K.: 2003: US2000000749716.

[162] Parissis JT, Korovesis S, Giazitzoglou E, Kalivas P, Katritsis D. Plasma profiles of peripheral monocyte-related inflammatory markers in patients with arterial hypertension. Correlations with plasma endothelin-1. Int J Cardiol 2002; 83(1): 13-21.

[163] Nett PC, Teixeira MM, Candinas D, Barton M. Recent developments on endothelin antagonists as immunomodulatory drugs--from infection to transplantation medicine. Recent Pat Cardiovasc Drug Discov 2006; 1(3): 265-276.

[164] Quehenberger P, Bierhaus A, Fasching P, *et al.* Endothelin 1 transcription is controlled by nuclear factor-kappaB in AGE-stimulated cultured endothelial cells. Diabetes 2000; 49(9): 1561-1570.

[165] Gaddipati JP, Sundar SV, Calemine J, Seth P, Sidhu GS, Maheshwari RK. Differential regulation of cytokines and transcription factors in liver by curcumin following hemorrhage/resuscitation. Shock 2003; 19(2): 150-156.

[166] Browatzki M, Schmidt J, Kubler W, Kranzhofer R. Endothelin-1 induces interleukin-6 release via activation of the transcription factor NF-kappaB in human vascular smooth muscle cells. Basic Res Cardiol 2000; 95(2): 98-105.

[167] Gallois C, Habib A, Tao J, *et al.*Role of NF-kappaB in the antiproliferative effect of endothelin-1 and tumor necrosis factor-alpha in human hepatic stellate cells. Involvement of cyclooxygenase-2. J Biol Chem 1998; 273(36): 23183-23190.

[168] Sharmin S, Shiota M, Murata E, *et al.* A novel bioactive 31-amino acid ET-1 peptide stimulates eosinophil recruitment and increases the levels of eotaxin and IL-5. Inflamm Res 2002; 51(4): 195-200.

[169] Finsnes F, Skjonsberg OH, Tonnessen T, Naess O, Lyberg T, Christensen G. Endothelin production and effects of endothelin antagonism during experimental airway inflammation. Am J Respir Crit Care Med 1997; 155(4): 1404-1412.

[170] Finsnes F, Christensen G, Lyberg T, Sejersted OM, Skjonsberg OH. Increased synthesis and release of endothelin-1 during the initial phase of airway inflammation. Am J Respir Crit Care Med 1998; 158(5 Pt 1): 1600-1606.

[171] Finsnes F, Skjonsberg OH, Lyberg T, Christensen G. Endothelin-1 production is associated with eosinophilic rather than neutrophilic airway inflammation. Eur Respir J 2000; 15(4): 743-750.

[172] Sampaio AL, Rae GA, Henriques MG. Participation of endogenous endothelins in delayed eosinophil and neutrophil recruitment in mouse pleurisy. Inflamm Res 2000; 49(4): 170-176.

[173] Sampaio AL, Rae GA, Henriques MM. Role of endothelins on lymphocyte accumulation in allergic pleurisy. J Leukoc Biol 2000; 67(2): 189-195.

[174] Brands M, Erguden JK, Hashimoto K, *et al.* Novel, selective indole-based ECE inhibitors: lead optimization via solid-phase and classical synthesis. Bioorg Med Chem Lett 2005; 15(19): 4201-4205.

[175] Weigand, S., Frey, R., Stasch, J.P., 2006: WO06037491A1.

[176] Libby P, Sukhova G, Lee RT, Galis ZS. Cytokines regulate vascular functions related to stability of the atherosclerotic plaque. J Cardiovasc Pharmacol 1995; 25 (Suppl 2): S9-12.

[177] Ortmann J, Nett PC, Celeiro J, Hofmann-Lehmann R, Tornillo L, Terracciano LM, Barton M. Downregulation of renal endothelin-converting enzyme 2 expression in early autoimmune diabetes. Exp Biol Med (Maywood) 2006; 231(6): 1030-1033.

[178] Dhaun N, Lilitkarntakul P, Macintyre IM, *et al.* Urinary endothelin-1 in chronic kidney disease and as a marker of disease activity in lupus nephritis. Am J Physiol Renal Physiol 2009; 296(6): F1477-1483.

[179] Denton CP, Humbert M, Rubin L, Black CM. Bosentan treatment for pulmonary arterial hypertension related to connective tissue disease: a subgroup analysis of the pivotal clinical trials and their open-label extensions. Ann Rheum Dis 2006; 65(10): 1336-1340.

[180] Ryan MJ. The pathophysiology of hypertension in systemic lupus erythematosus. Am J Physiol Regul Integr Comp Physiol 2009; 296(4): R1258-1267.

[181] Ferraccioli G, Romano G. Renal interstitial cells, proteinuria and progression of lupus nephritis: new frontiers for old factors. Lupus 2008; 17(6): 533-540.

[182] Denton CP, Black CM, Abraham DJ. Mechanisms and consequences of fibrosis in systemic sclerosis. Nat Clin Pract Rheumatol 2006; 2(3): 134-144.

[183] Kowal-Bielecka O. Targeting vascular disease in systemic sclerosis. Endocr Metab Immune Disord Drug Targets 2006; 6(4): 401-407.

[184] Sticherling M. The role of endothelin in connective tissue diseases. Rheumatology (Oxford) 2006; 45 (Suppl 3): iii8-10.

[185] Hinchcliff M, Varga J. Systemic sclerosis/scleroderma: a treatable multisystem disease. Am Fam Physician 2008; 78(8): 961-968.

[186] van Laar JM, Stolk J, Tyndall A. Scleroderma lung: pathogenesis, evaluation and current therapy. Drugs 2007; 67(7): 985-996.

[187] Riemekasten G, Sunderkotter C. Vasoactive therapies in systemic sclerosis. Rheumatology (Oxford) 2006; 45 (Suppl 3): iii49-51.

[188] Behrend M. The endothelin receptor antagonist TAK-044 in the treatment of reperfusion injury in organ transplantation. Expert Opin Investig Drugs 1999; 8(7): 1079-1091.

[189] Guttmann RD, Forbes RD, Zheng SX. The pathophysiology of chronic rejection. Am J Med Sci 1997; 313(5): 302-304.

[190] Orth SR, Odoni G, Amann K, Strzelczyk P, Raschack M, Ritz E. The ET(A) receptor blocker LU 135252 prevents chronic transplant nephropathy in the "Fisher to Lewis" model. J am Soc Nephrol 1999; 10(2): 387-391.

[191] Uhlmann D, Gabel G, Ludwig S, *et al.* Effects of ET(A) receptor antagonism on proinflammatory gene expression and microcirculation following hepatic ischemia/reperfusion. Microcirculation 2005; 12(5): 405-419.

[192] Uhlmann D, Gaebel G, Armann B, *et al.* Attenuation of proinflammatory gene expression and microcirculatory disturbances by endothelin A receptor blockade after orthotopic liver transplantation in pigs. Surgery 2006; 139(1): 61-72.

[193] Witzigmann H, Ludwig S, Armann B, *et al.* Endothelin(A) receptor blockade reduces ischemia/reperfusion injury in pig pancreas transplantation. Ann Surg 2003; 238(2): 264-274.

[194] Hansen A, Bekeredjian R, Filusch A, *et al.* Cardioprotective Effects of the Novel Selective Endothelin-A Receptor Antagonist BSF 461314 in Ischemia-Reperfusion Injury. J Am Soc Echocardiogr 2005; 18(11): 1213-1220.

[195] Rachid MA, Camargos ER, Rocha LL, *et al.* Blockade of endothelin ET(A)/ET(B) receptors favors a role for endothelin during acute *Trypanosoma cruzi* infection in rats. Microbes Infect 2006; 8(8): 2113-2119.

[196] Sampaio AL, Rae GA, Henriques MG. Effects of endothelin ETA receptor antagonism on granulocyte and lymphocyte accumulation in LPS-induced inflammation. J Leukoc Biol 2004; 76(1): 210-216.

[197] Ravalli S, Szaboles M, Albala A, Michler RE, Cannon PJ. Increased immunoreactive endothelin-1 in human transplant coronary artery disease. Circulation 1996; 94: 2096-2102.

[198] Takeda M, Ishida T, Ishimura T, Fujisawa M. Correlation between endothelin expression in early post-transplant biopsy specimens and long-term allograft function in living-related renal transplantation. Clin Transplant 2006; 20(1): 26-29.

[199] Fedak PW, Rao V, Verma S, *et al.* Combined endothelial and myocardial protection by endothelin antagonism enhances transplant allograft preservation. J Thorac Cardiovasc Surg 2005; 129(2): 407-415.

[200] Mueller TF, Ma C, Lederer JA, Perkins DL. Differentiation of stress, metabolism, communication, and defense responses following transplantation. J Leukoc Biol 2003; 73(3): 379-390.

[201] Gottmann U, van der Woude FJ, Braun C. Endothelin receptor antagonists: a new therapeutic option for improving the outcome after solid organ transplantation? Curr Vasc Pharmacol 2003; 1(3): 281-299.

[202] Lattmann T, Hein M, Horber S, Ortmann J, *et al.* Activation of pro-inflammatory and anti-inflammatory cytokines in host organs during chronic allograft rejection: role of endothelin receptor signaling. Am J Transplant 2005; 5(5): 1042-1049.

[203] Nett PC, Heisey DM, Fernandez LA, Sollinger HW, Pirsch JD. Association of cytomegalovirus disease and acute rejection with graft loss in kidney transplantation. Transplantation 2004; 78(7): 1036-1041.

[204] Busauschina A, Schnuelle P, van der Woude FJ. Cyclosporine nephrotoxicity. Transplant Proc 2004; 36(2 Suppl): 229S-233S.

[205] Bunchman TE, Brookshire CA. Cyclosporine-induced synthesis of endothelin by cultured human endothelial cells. J Clin Invest 1991; 88(1): 310-314.

[206] Komuro I, Kurihara H, Sugiyama T, Yoshizumi M, Takaku F, Yazaki Y. Endothelin stimulates c-fos and c-myc expression and proliferation of vascular smooth muscle cells. FEBS Lett 1988; 238(2): 249-252.

[207] Kocik M, Malek I, Glagolicova A, Pirk J. The effect of cyclosporin A on the level of big endothelin in patients one year after orthotopic heart transplantation. Transpl Int 2004; 17(2): 65-70.

[208] Adams DH, Russell ME, Hancock WW, *et al.* Chronic rejection in experimental cardiac transplantation: studies in the Lewis-F344 model. Immunol Rev 1993; 134: 5-19.

[209] Braun C, Conzelmann T, Vetter S, *et al.* Treatment with a combined endothelin A/B-receptor antagonist does not prevent chronic renal allograft rejection in rats. J Cardiovasc Pharmacol 2000; 36(4): 428-437.

[210] Knoll T, Oltersdorf J, Gottmann U, *et al.* Influence of acute selective endothelin-receptor-A blockade on renal hemodynamics in a rat model of chronic allograft rejection. Transpl Int 2003; 16(6): 425-429.

[211] Liu, K., Yu, W., Liang, Y., Wang, H., Zhao, Y., Ding, Z.: 2005: US6953780.

[212] Yu W, Liang Y, Liu K, Zhao Y, Fei G, Wang H. The chemical syntheses and bioactivities of novel peptide-based endothelin antagonists. J Pept Res 2002; 59(3): 134-138.

[213] Bolli MH, Boss C, Clozel M, Fischli W, Hess P, Weller T. The use of sulfonylamido pyrimidines incorporating an unsaturated side chain as endothelin receptor antagonists. Bioorg Med Chem Lett 2003; 13(5): 955-959.

[214] Bolli MH, Marfurt J, Grisostomi C, *et al.* Novel benzo[1,4]diazepin-2-one derivatives as endothelin receptor antagonists. J Med Chem 2004; 47(11): 2776-2795.

[215] Ono K, Matsumori A, Shioi T, Furukawa Y, Sasayama S. Contribution of endothelin-1 to myocardial injury in a murine model of myocarditis: acute effects of bosentan, an endothelin receptor antagonist. Circulation 1999; 100(17): 1823-1829.

[216] Pandey AS, Stewart DJ, Cernacek P, Dawood F, Wen WH, Liu P. Chronic endothelin-1 blockade preserves myocardial contractility in dilated cardiomyopathy. J Cardiovasc Pharmacol 1998; 31 (Suppl 1): S306-308.

[217] Wanecek M, Oldner A, Sundin P, Alving K, Weitzberg E, Rudehill A. Effects on haemodynamics by selective endothelin ET(B) receptor and combined endothelin ET(A)/ET(B) receptor antagonism during endotoxin shock. Eur J Pharmacol 1999; 386(2-3): 235-245.

[218] Jelicks LA, Chandra M, Shirani J, *et al.* Cardioprotective effects of phosphoramidon on myocardial structure and function in murine Chagas' disease. Int J Parasitol 2002; 32(12): 1497-1506.

[219] Wittner M, Christ GJ, Huang H, *et al. Trypanosoma cruzi* induces endothelin release from endothelial cells. J Infect Dis 1995; 171(2): 493-497.

[220] Tanowitz HB, Wittner M, Morris SA, *et al.* The putative mechanistic basis for the modulatory role of endothelin-1 in the altered vascular tone induced by Trypanosoma cruzi. Endothelium 1999; 6(3): 217-230.

[221] Brener Z, Gazzinelli RT. Immunological control of Trypanosoma cruzi infection and pathogenesis of Chagas' disease. Int Arch Allergy Immunol 1997; 114(2): 103-110.

[222] Aliberti JC, Machado FS, Souto JT, *et al.* beta-Chemokines enhance parasite uptake and promote nitric oxide-dependent microbiostatic activity in murine inflammatory macrophages infected with Trypanosoma cruzi. Infect Immun 1999; 67(9): 4819-4826.

[223] Iwasa S, Fan J, Miyauchi T, Watanabe T. Blockade of endothelin receptors reduces diet-induced hypercholesterolemia and atherosclerosis in apolipoprotein E-deficient mice. Pathobiology 2001; 69(1): 1-10.

[224] Watson AM, Li J, Schumacher C, de Gasparo M, *et al.* The endothelin receptor antagonist avosentan ameliorates nephropathy and atherosclerosis in diabetic apolipoprotein E knockout mice. Diabetologia 2009.

[225] Ammarguellat F, Larouche I, Schiffrin EL. Myocardial fibrosis in DOCA-salt hypertensive rats: effect of endothelin ET(A) receptor antagonism. Circulation 2001; 103(2): 319-324.

[226] Ammarguellat FZ, Gannon PO, Amiri F, Schiffrin EL. Fibrosis, matrix metalloproteinases, and inflammation in the heart of DOCA-salt hypertensive rats: role of ET(A) receptors. Hypertension 2002; 39(2 Pt 2): 679-684.

[227] Hocher B, George I, Rebstock J, *et al.* Endothelin system-dependent cardiac remodeling in renovascular hypertension. Hypertension 1999; 33(3): 816-822.

[228] Liu G, Kozmina NS, Winn M, von Geldern TW, *et al.* Design, synthesis, and activity of a series of pyrrolidine-3-carboxylic acid-based, highly specific, orally active ET(B) antagonists containing a diphenylmethylamine acetamide side chain. J Med Chem 1999; 42(18): 3679-3689.

[229] Jae HS, Winn M, von Geldern TW, *et al.* Pyrrolidine-3-carboxylic acids as endothelin antagonists. 5. Highly selective, potent, and orally active ET(A) antagonists. J Med Chem 2001; 44(23): 3978-3984.

[230] Winn, M., Boyd, S.A., Hutchins, C.W., Jae, H.S., Tasker, A.S., Vongeldern, T.W., Kester, J.A., Sorensen, B.K., 2005: CA2195677C.

[231] Winn, M., Boyd, S.A., Hutchins, C.W., Jae, H.S., Tasker, A.S., Vongeldern, T.W. V., Kester, J.A., Sorensen, B.K., Szczepankiewicz, B.G., Henry, K.J.J., Liu, G., Wittenberger, S.J., King, S.A., 2006: EP0885215B1.

[232] Actelion Pharmaceuticals Ltd. A.P., 2005: IL0162534A0.

[233] Raichlin E, Prasad A, Mathew V, *et al.* Efficacy and safety of atrasentan in patients with cardiovascular risk and early atherosclerosis. Hypertension 2008; 52(3): 522-528.

[234] Gagliardini E, Corna D, Zoja C, *et al.* Unlike each drug alone, lisinopril if combined with avosentan promotes regression of renal lesions in experimental diabetes. Am J Physiol Renal Physiol 2009; 297(5): F1448-F1456.

[235] Sasser JM, Sullivan JC, Hobbs JL, *et al.* Endothelin A receptor blockade reduces diabetic renal injury via an anti-inflammatory mechanism. J Am Soc Nephrol 2007; 18(1): 143-154.

[236] Wenzel RR, Littke T, Kuranoff S, *et al.* Avosentan reduces albumin excretion in diabetics with macroalbuminuria. J Am Soc Nephrol 2009; 20(3): 655-664.

[237] Barton M, Mullins JJ, Bailey MA, Kretzler M. Role of endothelin receptors for renal protection and survival in hypertension: waiting for clinical trials. Hypertension 2006; 48(5): 834-837.

[238] Weber MA, Black H, Bakris G, *et al.* A selective endothelin-receptor antagonist to reduce blood pressure in patients with treatment-resistant hypertension: a randomised, double-blind, placebo-controlled trial. Lancet 2009; 374(9699): 1423-1431.

Levosimendan in Heart Failure

Charalambos Antoniades*, Michael Demosthenous,
Dimitris Tousoulis, Costantinos Bakogiannis, Nikolaos Koumallos
and Christodoulos Stefanadis

1st Cardiology Department, Athens University Medical School, Athens Greece

Abstract: Heart failure is characterised by decreased cardiac output, which results in the development of both peripheral hypoperfusion and pulmonary congestion and can lead to the development of acute pulmonary edema. The primary objective in treating a patient with decompensated heart failure is hemodynamic stabilization, which is usually achieved by inotropic support. Classic inotropic agents provide short-term hemodynamic improvement, but their use has been correlated with poor prognosis. Levosimendan, a new calcium sensitizer, offers hemodynamic and symptomatic improvement without increasing cAMP and intracellular calcium concentrations. This agent improves contractility without increasing the risk of cardiac events such as arrhythmias. By combining a positive inotropic action mediated via calcium sensitization and a vasodilatory effect via ATP-dependent potassium channels, it appears to be superior than classic positive inotropic agents. Furthermore, it seems to have prolonged benefit in heart failure patients, and it also has anti-inflammatory and antiapoptotic properties. In conclusion, levosimendan seems to be a particularly promising agent for the treatment of decompensated heart failure, as in addition to improving cardiac output, it has a more favorable side-effect profile than classic inotropic agents, and it affects multiple pathways with key role in the pathophysiology of heart failure.

Keywords: Levosimendan, heart failure, inotropes, calcium sensitizers, apoptosis.

INTRODUCTION

Heart failure has become an increasingly common clinical condition over recent decades due to the escalating growth of the ageing population. Despite the use of "triple" therapy (beta-blockers, angiotensin converting enzyme (ACE) inhibitors and aldosterone antagonist) and high-dose loop diuretics combined with thiazides, severe heart failure resistant to therapy is still common. Unfortunately inotropic agents are of little symptomatic benefit , and have often increased mortality [1,2]. Thus far all inotropic agents investigated in major clinical trials have operated through the adrenergic nervous signaling pathway or the sodium potassium pump. This leads to an increase in intracellular calcium, which may have deleterious effects on cardiac myocyte relaxation, cell survival, and arrhythmia induction. Levosimendan is a new calcium-sensitizing drug that opens adenosine triphosphate–dependent potassium (KATP) channels, which increases myocardial contraction and

*Corresponding author: Tel: +30-210-6616466; E-mail: antoniad@well.ox.ac.uk

Atta-ur-Rahman / M. Iqbal Choudhary (Eds.)

vasodilation. Importantly, this improvement of myocardial contractility occurs without increasing oxygen requirements, thereby reducing ventricular preload, [3]. This pharmacologic profile of levosimendan offers new therapeutic possibilities in patients with heart failure.

THERAPEUTIC STRATEGIES

The fundamental problem in heart failure is a blunting of the heart's pumping activity, resulting either in excessive filling pressures, insufficient "forward" output or both. Cardiac dysfunction sets in motion a chain reaction of neuroendocrine activation, vasoconstriction, end-organ dysfunction and a further decline in cardiac function, and these events are believed to be responsible for generating the symptoms of heart failure. Most pharmacological agents used for the treatment of heart failure exert their benefit by either directly interfering with the hemodynamic alterations or through inhibition of the neurohormonal activation underlying these alterations. These medications fall into several categories: diuretics, beta-blockers, ACE inhibitors and inotropic agents.

Diuretics have long played an important role in the symptomatic treatment of heart failure [4]. The induced diuresis and natriuresis reduce extracellular volume and ventricular filling pressures, thereby ameliorating congestive symptoms. This effect occurs without a significant decrease in cardiac output or systemic blood pressure unless excessive diuresis and intravascular volume depletion occur. It should be noted that while diuretics are beneficial in controlling symptoms and improving exercise capacity in patients with heart failure, diuretic use has not resulted in a decrease in mortality [5]. Furthermore patients treated with diuretics require close monitoring of their renal function and serum electrolytes.

Beta-blockade is another drug category offering great help to patients with heart failure. These agents can inhibit the adverse affects of norepinephrine on the myocardium, leading to up-regulation of cardiac beta adrenergic receptors. The long term administration of these agents is associated with a reversal of left ventricular (LV) remodelling, resulting in decreased LV volume and increased ejection fraction with concomitant improvement in hemodynamics [6]. Large clinical trials [7-9] have demonstrated a 35% reduction in mortality and 40% reduction in hospitalization due to heart failure in patients treated with beta-blocking agents. Additionally, treatment with beta-blockers reduces symptoms of heart failure and improves exercise capacity, although these affects may not be evident for several weeks or months after initiation of treatment.

ACE inhibitors have a variety of beneficial effects on the pathophysiology of heart failure [10,11]. As potent potent vasodilators, they reduce both pre-load and after-load. The subsequent fall in intracardiac pressures and reduction in wall stress lead to reduced myocardial oxygen demand, potentially reducing ischemia, and a decrease in sympathetic nervous system activity, thereby reducing electrical instability. Additionally, the ACE inhibitor-induced reduction in angiotensin II, as well as the subsequent reduction in adrenal aldosterone release, may have direct effects on the extent of fibrosis and collagen deposition that characterize myocardial remodelling and heart failure. The effects of ACE inhibitors are primarily mediated by inhibition of the enzyme responsible for the conversion of angiotensin I to angiotensin II thereby decreasing production of the latter. However, some of the benefit of the ACE inhibitors may result in part from their effects on the kinin system. ACE inhibitors decrease the degradation of kinins and thereby enhance their vasodilatory effects and potentiate kinin-mediated synthesis of vasodilatory prostaglandins. However use of ACE inhibitors may be limited by the development of side effects such as hypotension, worsening of renal function, electrolyte imbalance and a dry cough.

Traditional inotropic agents affect myocardial contractility. Several drugs belong to this category and act via different pathways. Digoxin is a selective inhibitor of the membrane bound Na-K-ATPase with a relatively small effect on left ventricular systolic function. Its use is largely being replaced by newer drugs [12]. Dopamine is an endogenous catecholamine that functions through stimulation of alpha and beta-adrenergic receptors [13]. A unique feature of this agent is that it has distinctly different hemodynamic affects in different doses: vasodilation in low doses, increase in myocardial contractility at moderate doses and vasoconstriction and tachycardia at high doses. Dobutamine is a synthetic catecholamine that acts by direct stimulation of adrenergic receptors. In contrast to dopamine, the inotropic affect of dobutamine is associated with relatively little increase in heart rate and with a modest reduction in left ventricular filling pressure and peripheral resistance [14]. On the other hand milrinone and amrinone are phosphodiesterase inhibitors that increase cardiac contractility and vasodilation. They are useful in the management of patients with decompensated heart failure that is characterized by elevated peripheral resistance and elevated filling pressures [15]. However, there is evidence that prolonged use of both beta-adrenergic agonists and phosphodiesterase inhibitors may have adverse effects on mortality in the longer term [16] suggesting a clear need for novel therapeutic options in treatment of heart failure.

INOTROPIC AND VASODILATORY EFFECTS

Levosimendan is a new inotropic and vasodilator agent. It has been proposed as a novel therapeutic approach by which cardiac performance may be enhanced without predisposition to calcium-induced arrhythmias or an increase in myocardial oxygen demand [17]. Via its interaction with cardiac contractile proteins, levosimendan increases the contractile force generated for a given amount of cytoplasmic free calcium compared with agents that do not possess this activity. Additionally, by increasing the sensitivity of the contractile proteins to calcium without enhancing calcium influx into myocytes, this agent precludes the intracellular calcium overload and increased calcium turnover associated with positive inotropic treatment, thus reducing the risk of arrhythmias [18]. The mechanisms of action, the pharmacokenitics, and the most recent clinical studies concerning levosimendan will be outlined below.

PHARMACOKINETICS

Levosimendan has a complex pharmacokinetic profile. Although it has high oral bioavailability, thus far it has only been developed for intravenous administration [18-21]. Steady state is achieved within 5 hours of a constant dose infusion. Levosimendan has an elimination half-life of approximately 1 hour. Only a small proportion (about 4%) of the drug is free in plasma, the majority being bound to albumin. Approximately 5% of levosimendan is acetylated to form two active metabolites, OR-1896 and OR-1855. Their elimination half-lives are approximately 80 hours [19] and their pharmacologic effects may persist for approximately 1 week. OR-1855 is formed by the action of intestinal bacteria on levosimendan excreted by the biliary route. It is an intermediate metabolite that forms OR-1896. However both metabolites are active. Approximately 40% of these metabolites are bound to plasma proteins. Rapid acetylators may further prolong the duration of effect but does not seem to influence the short-term pharmacodynamic response to levosimendan.. Finally, no tolerance to the effects of levosimendan [19] and no rebound decline in hemodynamic variables after withdrawal of the drug have been observed.

Acetylator status does not influence the pharmacokinetics of levosimendan, but rapid acetylators appear to form more of the active metabolite OR-1896. This formation does not appear to influence the short-term pharmacodynamic response to levosimendan but may further prolong the duration of effect. The cytochrome-P450 enzyme system does not play a role in the metabolism of levosimendan or its active metabolite.

No tolerance to the effects of levosimendan has been observed, despite infusions lasting as long as 7 days [19]. Furthermore, no rebound decline in hemodynamic variables has been observed after withdrawal of levosimendan.

Renal dysfunction has little effect on the plasma concentration of levosimendan, although it does prolong the elimination half-life of OR-1896. Liver cirrhosis prolongs the elimination half-life of levosimendan slightly, but the effects on production or metabolism of OR-1896 are unknown.

PHARMACODYNAMICS

Levosimendan is a "calcium sensitizer" with multiple mechanisms of action (Fig. **1**). It exerts its inotropic effect by increasing the affinity of troponin-C for calcium, directly stabilising the calcium-induced conformation of troponin-C, or acting distal to the troponin-C molecule [17]. Levosimendan binds in a calcium-dependent manner to the N-terminal domain of troponin-C, thus magnifying the extent of the contraction produced by troponin-C when it is calcium-activated [18]. It binds only to the calcium-bound conformation of

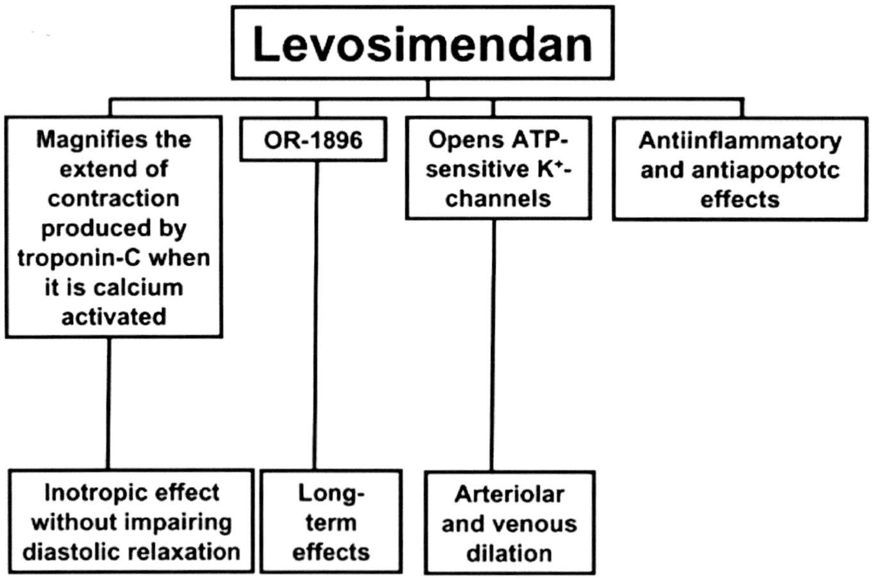

Fig. (1). Levosimendan is a "calcium sensitizer" with multiple mechanisms of action. It exerts its inotropic effect by increasing the affinity of troponin-C for calcium and induces arteriolar and venous dilatation because of its ability to open ATP-sensitive potassium channels on vascular smooth muscle. Recent studies have also shown an anti-inflammatory and antiapoptotic effect of levosimendan. OR-1896 is an active, potent, acetylated metabolite which is responsible for most of the longer-term effects of levosimendan (Figure adopted from reference [51]).

troponin-C and this leads to a maximum effect when intracellular calcium levels are high with minimal effects observed during cardiac relaxation. This leads to a positive inotropic effect without impairing diastolic relaxation [22-24] or causing cytosolic calcium ion overload, which might provoke cardiac myocyte dysfunction, arrhythmogenesis, and cell death. Levosimendan may also increase calcium dependent inotropic effects by enhancing release and reuptake of calcium into the sarcoplasmic reticulum [25]. Finally, levosimendan has an active, metabolite, OR-1896, that has a long half-life and is a calcium concentration-dependent calcium sensitizer; this may be responsible for most of the longer-term effects of levosimendan [19].

Levosimendan not only increases cardiac performance, but has also been shown to induce arteriolar and venous dilatation because of its ability to open ATP-sensitive potassium channels in vascular smooth muscle [26-28]. It is also a selective phosphodiesterase III inhibitor *in vitro*, although this effect probably occurs only at concentrations outside the therapeutic dose range [29,30]. Improved contractile performance and vasodilatation leads to a reduction in both preload and afterload in the failing heart with reduced myocardial oxygen consumption [31]. Combined with coronary vasodilatation [32], also has antiischemic effects via the opening of ATP-sensitive potassium channels in vascular smooth-muscle cells [33].

Hemodynamic Effects

It is now well documented that levosimendan has beneficial hemodynamic effects in heart failure [19,34-37]. Cardiac output is increased by 0.4 to 0.8 l/min (increases both stroke volume and heart rate), pulmonary capillary wedge pressure (PCWP) is reduced by 4 to 6 mmHg and systemic vascular resistance is reduced while transpulmonary gradient remains unchanged (Table **1**).

The LIDO (Levosimendan Infusion Versus Dobutamine in Severe Low Output Heart Failure) study [36], a randomized double-blinded clinical trial, compared infusions of levosimendan or dobutamine over a period of 24 hours in 203 patients with severe chronic heart failure. After 30 hours treatment, levosimendan increased cardiac output and reduced PCWP to a greater extent than dobutamine. Levosimendan also reduced systolic blood pressure more and tended to cause more vasodilatation. The haemodynamic effects of levosimendan, unlike those of dobutamine, were not attenuated by the concomitant use of β-blockers. This finding is important, in view of the increasing evidence for and the usefulness of β-blockers for the management of severe heart failure.

The Dose-Ranging Study [35] compared five different doses of levosimendan with placebo and dobutamine when infused over a period of 24 hours. The study included 151 patients with New York Heart Association (NYHA) class II to IV heart failure. All doses of levosimendan caused a greater reduction in PCWP than placebo or dobutamine. Both levosimendan and dobutamine had similar effects on stroke volume, but higher doses of levosimendan had a greater effect on cardiac output because of a greater increase in heart rate. Systemic vascular resistance fell equally with both treatments at recommended doses, although further vasodilatation occurred with higher doses of levosimendan. A fall in mean systemic arterial pressure of 5 to 10 mm Hg was noted with higher doses of levosimendan. Pulmonary vascular resistance declined with higher doses of levosimendan while the transpulmonary gradient remained unchanged.

The Dose Escalation Study [34] included 146 patients with NYHA class III to IV heart failure. Infusion of levosimendan was increased hourly up to a maximum of 0.4μg/kg/min,

Table 1. Hemodynamic Effects of Levosimendan

	Population	Methods	Conclusion
LIDO study [36]	203 patients with severe chronic heart failure	Infusion of levosimendan or dobutamine over a period of 24 hours. Measurements after 30 hours.	Levosimendan increased cardiac output and reduced PCWP to a greater extent than dobutamine. Levosimendan reduced systolic blood pressure more and tended to cause more vasodilatation. Six hours after stopping the infusion, the effects of dobutamine had disappeared, but those of levosimendan persisted.
Dose-ranging study [35]	151 patients with NYHA class II to IV heart failure	Compared 5 different doses of levosimendan with a placebo and with dobutamine when infused over a period of 24 hours.	All doses of levosimendan exerted a greater reduction in PCWP than placebo or dobutamine. Both exerted similar effects on stroke volume. Systemic vascular resistance fell equally with levosimendan and dobutamine. Further vasodilatation occurred with higher doses of levosimendan. A fall in mean systemic arterial pressure of 5 to 10 mm Hg was noted with higher doses of levosimendan. Pulmonary vascular resistance declined with higher doses of levosimendan while the transpulmonary gradient remained unchanged.
Dose Escalation study [34]	146 patients with NYHA class III to IV heart failure	Infusion of levosimendan followed by hourly increments up to a maximum of 0.4μg/kg/min. Patients randomized to levosimendan then received open-label drug for the remainder of the 24 hours. Subsequently, patients were randomized to continue levosimendan for 24 hours or to have it withdrawn. Further hemodynamic measurements were made at 48 hours.	Only 70% of patients were titrated to the maximum dose of levosimendan. Levosimendan increased stroke volume and cardiac index with significant effects even at the lowest dose. Heart rate increased by an average of 6 bpm at higher doses while systemic and pulmonary vascular resistance declined, and mean systemic arterial pressure dropped by 4 mm Hg. Transpulmonary gradient was not affected. Hemodynamic effects persisted or increased over the subsequent 48 hours for those who remained on the infusion.
Seven-day study [19]	24 patients with NYHA class III to IV heart failure	Randomized to an infusion of 0,05 or 0,1 μg/kg/min for seven days, during which time heart rate, blood pressure and ECG were monitored.	Heart rate rose to a peak 18 bpm and 26 bpm respectively while blood pressure fell by 6 mmHg and 11 mmHg. Blood pressure returned to baseline within 3 days of cessation of therapy in contrast to the heart rate which remained increased even 14 days after cessation of infusion. Metabolite concentrations peaked about 24 hours after cessation of therapy and were still detectable at therapeutic concentrations 2 weeks after.
Bolus study [37]	24 patients with severe chronic heart failure	5 min bolus infusions of levosimendan ranging from 0.25 to 4 mg.	The heart rate and cardiac output increased while the filling pressures reduced. The peak was reached after 10 min and the results were dose related.

with 70% of patients reaching the maximum dose. Reduction in PCWP to less than 10 mm Hg and increase in heart rate above baseline of more than 15 bpm (beats per minute) was the most common reason for not attaining the top dose. Patients randomized to levosimendan then received open-label drug for the remainder of the 24 hours, with patients then randomized to continue levosimendan for 24 hours or to have it withdrawn. Levosimendan increased stroke volume and cardiac index with significant effects even at the lowest dose. Heart rate increased by an average of 6bpm at higher doses while systemic and pulmonary vascular resistance declined, and mean systemic arterial pressure dropped by 4mmHg. Transpulmonary gradient was not affected.

In the Seven-Day Study [19] 24 patients were randomized to infusions of 0.05 or 0.1 µg/kg/min for seven days. Heart rate rose to a peak 18 bpm and 26 bpm respectively while blood pressure fell by 6 mmHg and 11 mmHg. Blood pressure returned to baseline within 3 days of cessation of therapy in contrast to the heart rate, which remained elevated 14 days after treatment cessation. Metabolite concentrations peaked 24 hours after cessation of therapy and were still detectable at therapeutic concentrations after2 weeks.

The Bolus study [37] randomized 24 patients to 5 min bolus infusions of levosimendan ranging from 0.25 to 4 mg. The heart rate and cardiac output increased while the filling pressures reduced. The peak was reached after 10 min and the results were dose-dependent.

Anti-Inflammatory and Anti-Apoptotic Effects

The failing myocardium is a major source of proinflammatory cytokines [38,39], which contribute to the pathophysiology of heart failure [39-41]. Cytokines promote the transition from asymptomatic to symptomatic heart failure [42] since they depress myocardial contractility [43], while also promoting cardiomyocyte apoptosis subsequent cardiac remodeling [44].

Two randomized placebo-controlled trials [45,46] have shown that levosimendan administration causes a significant reduction of the circulating proinflammatory cytokine interleukin-6 (even one month after infusion), and soluble apoptosis mediators such as the apoptotic marker soluble FAS (sFAS) and Fas ligand in patients with decompensated heart failure. The improved hemodynamics may partly explain the decreased expression of cytokines from the failing myocardium, while levosimendan also seems to inhibit the stimuli for myocardial cytokine production and spillover into circulation [23]. Additionally, levosimendan-induced improvement of systolic function and peripheral vasorelaxation may also attenuate peripheral tissue hypo-perfusion, leading to down-regulation of cytokine extra-cardiac production by transcriptional factors such us NF-kB [39,47]. These immunomodulatory effects may lead to improvement of symptoms and echocardiographic markers of cardiac contractile performance.

Effects of Levosimendan on Heart Failure Symptoms

Symptoms have been assessed in three studies: the Randomized Study on Safety and Effectiveness of Levosimendan in Patients with Left Ventricular Failure After an Acute Myocardial Infarct (RUSSLAN) [38], LIDO study [36] and Dose Escalation Study [34].

The RUSSLAN study randomized 504 patients with acute pulmonary edema after myocardial infarction to four different 6-hour dosing regimens of levosimendan or placebo in addition to conventional background therapy with the exception of other intravenous inotropic agents. The objective of the study was to examine the safety of levosimendan in this high-risk population, targeting the risk of ischemia and hypotension. Levosimendan use did not exacerbate these problems except at the highest dose. Overall, levosimendan did not affect symptoms. However, worsening heart failure was less likely with levosimendan than with placebo at 6 hours (P = 0.033) and at 24 hours (P = 0.044). Also, patients treated with levosimendan experienced less dyspnea (P = 0.042) and fatigue (P = 0.047).

In the Dose Escalation Study [34], patients were more often improved on levosimendan than on placebo at the end of the 6-hour, double-blind phase. Similar trends were observed for fatigue.

In the LIDO study [36], nonsignificant trends towards greater improvement in breathlessness and fatigue were noted among patients receiving levosimendan compared with dobutamine.

Effects of Levosimendan on Morbidity and Mortality

In the RUSSLAN study [38], the composite outcome of death or worsening heart failure at 24 hours was reduced from 8.8% to 4.0% (P = 0.04). All-cause mortality at 14 days was reduced from 19.6% to 11.7% (P = 0.03). At 180 days, mortality on levosimendan was 22.6% compared with 31.4% on placebo. The reduction in mortality was similar independently of the dose of levosimendan used in the study.

In the LIDO study [36], three deaths occurred during infusion of dobutamine, but none occurred with placebo. After one month, there was a significantly lower mortality with levosimendan than with dobutamine and a reduction in the composite of death or worsening heart failure reported as an adverse event.

In addition to improving haemodynamic performance, lower mortality was seen in the levosimendan group than in the dobutamine group for up to 180 days (26% versus 38%, 0·57 [0·34–0·95]; p=0·029). A reduction in the composite outcome of death or hospitalization with heart failure and of an increase in days alive and out of hospital during six months of follow-up was also observed. The LIDO study is the largest randomized trial of dobutamine for heart failure ever conducted. The results of the study have led to much speculation. Dobutamine may have had an adverse effect on survival. Acute exposure to powerful adrenergic stimulants may not only provoke arrhythmias but also accelerate programmed cell death of cardiac myocytes, worsening both short-term and long-term outcome. On the other hand levosimendan might exert a sustained beneficial effect on hemodynamics, with possible secondary neuroendocrine benefits without the hazards of arrhythmogenesis, cellular calcium overload, and induction of cell death. This combination of effects may lead to an improvement in medium-term and long-term survival, and especially when combined with beta blockers. Mebazaa *et al.* [48] with a study involving 692 patients with chronic heart failure (CHF) who were on beta-blocker therapy before receiving a single intravenous infusion of levosimendan or dobutamine revealed all-cause mortality benefits of levosimendan treatment over dobutamine when all-cause mortality was lower in the CHF/levosimendan group than in the CHF/dobutamine group (3.4 *vs.* 5.8%; HR, 0.58, CI 0.33-1.01, P = 0.05 at day 5 and 7.0 *vs.* 10.3%; HR, 0.67, CI 0.45-0.99, P = 0.045 at day 14).

LEVOSIMENDAN IN THE CLINICAL PRACTICE: CURRENT AND FUTURE DEVELOPMENTS

Levosimendan is the most popular calcium sensitizer that has been introduced into clinical practice. First launched in Sweden in 2000, it has subsequently received final marketing authorization in a number of other countries through the Mutual Recognition Process. In several countries, the drug is already used routinely in patients with heart failure, in particular those with decompensated heart failure with low cardiac output and high filling pressures that require inotropic support. Preliminary results using levosimendan in patients with ventricular dysfunction after coronary bypass surgery or after angioplasty are encouraging, although randomized controlled trials of sufficient size are still lacking for these applications [49,50]. In industrialised countries, the incidence of heart failure will continue to increase due to the escalating growth of the ageing population. Under these circumstances levosimendan has the potential to play a critical role in the management of the disease in the following years.

CONCLUSIONS

Levosimendan is a calcium sensitizer and KATP channel opener that has multiple mechanisms of action. It offers new therapeutic possibilities in the treatment of heart failure, providing symptomatic and hemodynamic improvement within a few hours of treatment initiation. These benefits are achieved without increasing arrhythmogenicity, oxygen requirements and without impairing diastolic relaxation, thus offering clinical advantages over traditional inotropic agents. In several countries, the drug is already routinely used in patients with heart failure requiring inotropic support. If further studies confirm that, uniquely among inotropic agents, it reduces mortality, it is likely to become the inotropic agent of first choice in severe heart failure.

DISCLOSURE

This is an invited submission of an updated version of our previous publication: Koumallos N, Antoniades C, Tousoulis D, Shirodaria C, Stefanadis C. Levosimendan: a novel agent in heart failure. Recent Pat Cardiovasc Drug Discov. 2006;1(2):185-91.

REFERENCES

[1] Thackray S, Coletta A, Jones P, Dunn A, Clark AL, Cleland JG. Clinical trials update: Highlights of the Scientific Sessions of Heart Failure 2001, a meeting of the Working Group on Heart Failure of the European Society of Cardiology. CONTAK-CD, CHRISTMAS, OPTIME-CHF. Eur J Heart Fail 2001; 3: 491-494.

[2] Rossinen J, Harjola VP, Siirila-Waris K, *et al.* The use of more than one inotrope in acute heart failure is associated with increased mortality: a multi-centre observational study. Acute Card Care 2008; 10: 209-213.

[3] Ukkonen H, Saraste M, Akkila J, *et al.* Myocardial efficiency during levosimendan infusion in congestive heart failure. Clin Pharmacol Ther 2000; 68: 522-531.

[4] Brater DC. Diuretic therapy. N Engl J Med 1998; 339: 387-395.

[5] Pitt B, Zannad F, Remme WJ, *et al.* The effect of spironolactone on morbidity and mortality in patients with severe heart failure. Randomized Aldactone Evaluation Study Investigators. N Engl J Med 1999; 341: 709-717.

[6] Bristow MR. beta-adrenergic receptor blockade in chronic heart failure. Circulation 2000; 101: 558-569.

[7] The Cardiac Insufficiency Bisoprolol Study II (CIBIS-II): a randomised trial. Lancet 1999; 353: 9-13.

[8] Colucci WS, Packer M, Bristow MR, *et al.* Carvedilol inhibits clinical progression in patients with mild symptoms of heart failure. US Carvedilol Heart Failure Study Group. Circulation 1996; 94: 2800-2806.

[9] Hjalmarson A, Goldstein S, Fagerberg B, *et al.* Effects of controlled-release metoprolol on total mortality, hospitalizations, and well-being in patients with heart failure: the Metoprolol CR/XL Randomized Intervention Trial in congestive heart failure (MERIT-HF). MERIT-HF Study Group. JAMA 2000; 283: 1295-1302.

[10] Demers C, Mody A, Teo KK, McKelvie RS. ACE inhibitors in heart failure: what more do we need to know? Am J Cardiovasc Drugs 2005; 5: 351-359.

[11] Cruden NL, Newby DE. Angiotensin antagonism in patients with heart failure: ACE inhibitors, angiotensin receptor antagonists or both? Am J Cardiovasc Drugs 2004; 4: 345-353.

[12] Hauptman PJ, Kelly RA. Digitalis. Circulation 1999; 99: 1265-1270.

[13] Maskin CS, Ocken S, Chadwick B, LeJemtel TH. Comparative systemic and renal effects of dopamine and angiotensin-converting enzyme inhibition with enalaprilat in patients with heart failure. Circulation 1985; 72: 846-852.

[14] Ruffolo RR, Jr. The pharmacology of dobutamine. Am J Med Sci 1987; 294: 244-248.

[15] Colucci WS, Wright RF, Jaski BE, Fifer MA, Braunwald E. Milrinone and dobutamine in severe heart failure: differing hemodynamic effects and individual patient responsiveness. Circulation 1986; 73: III175-183.

[16] Levine BS. Intermittent positive inotrope infusion in the management of end-stage, low-output heart failure. J Cardiovasc Nurs 2000; 14: 76-93.

[17] Haikala H, Pollesello P. Calcium sensitivity enhancers. IDrugs 2000; 3: 1199-1205.

[18] Haikala H, Linden IB. Mechanisms of action of calcium-sensitizing drugs. J Cardiovasc Pharmacol 1995; 26 (Suppl 1): S10-19.

[19] Kivikko M, Antila S, Eha J, Lehtonen L, Pentikainen PJ. Pharmacodynamics and safety of a new calcium sensitizer, levosimendan, and its metabolites during an extended infusion in patients with severe heart failure. J Clin Pharmacol 2002; 42: 43-51.

[20] Sandell EP, Hayha M, Antila S, *et al.* Pharmacokinetics of levosimendan in healthy volunteers and patients with congestive heart failure. J Cardiovasc Pharmacol 1995; 26 (Suppl 1): S57-S62.

[21] Antila S, Huuskonen H, Nevalainen T, Kanerva H, Vanninen P, Lehtonen L. Site dependent bioavailability and metabolism of levosimendan in dogs. Eur J Pharm Sci 1999; 9: 85-91.

[22] Haikala H, Nissinen E, Etemadzadeh E, Levijoki J, Linden IB. Troponin C-mediated calcium sensitization induced by levosimendan does not impair relaxation. J Cardiovasc Pharmacol 1995; 25: 794-801.

[23] Hasenfuss G, Pieske B, Castell M, Kretschmann B, Maier LS, Just H. Influence of the novel inotropic agent levosimendan on isometric tension and calcium cycling in failing human myocardium. Circulation 1998; 98: 2141-2147.

[24] Pagel PS, Harkin CP, Hettrick DA, Warltier DC. Levosimendan (OR-1259), a myofilament calcium sensitizer, enhances myocardial contractility but does not alter isovolumic relaxation in conscious and anesthetized dogs. Anesthesiology 1994; 81: 974-987.

[25] Edes I, Kiss E, Kitada Y, *et al.* Effects of Levosimendan, a cardiotonic agent targeted to troponin C, on cardiac function and on phosphorylation and Ca2+ sensitivity of cardiac myofibrils and sarcoplasmic reticulum in guinea pig heart. Circ Res 1995; 77: 107-113.

[26] Bowman P, Haikala H, Paul RJ. Levosimendan, a calcium sensitizer in cardiac muscle, induces relaxation in coronary smooth muscle through calcium desensitization. J Pharmacol Exp Ther 1999; 288: 316-325.

[27] Kaheinen P, Pollesello P, Levijoki J, Haikala H. Levosimendan increases diastolic coronary flow in isolated guinea-pig heart by opening ATP-sensitive potassium channels. J Cardiovasc Pharmacol 2001; 37: 367-374.

[28] Pataricza J, Hohn J, Petri A, Balogh A, Papp JG. Comparison of the vasorelaxing effect of cromakalim and the new inodilator, levosimendan, in human isolated portal vein. J Pharm Pharmacol 2000; 52: 213-217.

[29] Hasenfuss G, Pieske B, Kretschmann B, Holubarsch C, Alpert NR, Just H. Effects of calcium sensitizers on intracellular calcium handling and myocardial energetics. J Cardiovasc Pharmacol 1995; 26 (Suppl) 1: S45-51.

[30] Haikala H, Kaheinen P, Levijoki J, Linden IB. The role of cAMP- and cGMP-dependent protein kinases in the cardiac actions of the new calcium sensitizer, levosimendan. Cardiovasc Res 1997; 34: 536-546.

[31] Todaka K, Wang J, Yi GH, *et al.* Effects of levosimendan on myocardial contractility and oxygen consumption. J Pharmacol Exp Ther 1996; 279: 120-127.

[32] Lilleberg J, Nieminen MS, Akkila J, *et al.* Effects of a new calcium sensitizer, levosimendan, on haemodynamics, coronary blood flow and myocardial substrate utilization early after coronary artery bypass grafting. Eur Heart J 1998; 19: 660-668.

[33] Pollesello P, Papp Z. The cardioprotective effects of levosimendan: preclinical and clinical evidence. J Cardiovasc Pharmacol 2007; 50: 257-263.

[34] Slawsky MT, Colucci WS, Gottlieb SS, *et al.* Acute hemodynamic and clinical effects of levosimendan in patients with severe heart failure. Study Investigators. Circulation 2000; 102: 2222-2227.

[35] Nieminen MS, Akkila J, Hasenfuss G, *et al.* Hemodynamic and neurohumoral effects of continuous infusion of levosimendan in patients with congestive heart failure. J Am Coll Cardiol 2000; 36: 1903-1912.

[36] Follath F, Cleland JG, Just H, *et al.* Efficacy and safety of intravenous levosimendan compared with dobutamine in severe low-output heart failure (the LIDO study): a randomised double-blind trial. Lancet 2002; 360: 196-202.

[37] Lilleberg J, Sundberg S, Nieminen MS. Dose-range study of a new calcium sensitizer, levosimendan, in patients with left ventricular dysfunction. J Cardiovasc Pharmacol 1995; 26 (Suppl 1): S63-S69.

[38] Moiseyev VS, Poder P, Andrejevs N, *et al.* Safety and efficacy of a novel calcium sensitizer, levosimendan, in patients with left ventricular failure due to an acute myocardial infarction. A randomized, placebo-controlled, double-blind study (RUSSLAN). Eur Heart J 2002; 23: 1422-1432.

[39] Adamopoulos S, Parissis JT, Kremastinos DT. A glossary of circulating cytokines in chronic heart failure. Eur J Heart Fail 2001; 3: 517-526.

[40] Hasper D, Hummel M, Kleber FX, Reindl I, Volk HD. Systemic inflammation in patients with heart failure. Eur Heart J 1998; 19: 761-765.

[41] Anker SD, Egerer KR, Volk HD, Kox WJ, Poole-Wilson PA, Coats AJ. Elevated soluble CD14 receptors and altered cytokines in chronic heart failure. Am J Cardiol 1997; 79: 1426-1430.

[42] Ceconi C, Curello S, Bachetti T, Corti A, Ferrari R. Tumor necrosis factor in congestive heart failure: a mechanism of disease for the new millennium? Prog Cardiovasc Dis 1998; 41: 25-30.

[43] Yokoyama T, Vaca L, Rossen RD, Durante W, Hazarika P, Mann DL. Cellular basis for the negative inotropic effects of tumor necrosis factor-alpha in the adult mammalian heart. J Clin Invest 1993; 92: 2303-2312.

[44] Krown KA, Page MT, Nguyen C, *et al.* Tumor necrosis factor alpha-induced apoptosis in cardiac myocytes. Involvement of the sphingolipid signaling cascade in cardiac cell death. J Clin Invest 1996; 98: 2854-2865.

[45] Parissis JT, Adamopoulos S, Antoniades C, *et al.* Effects of levosimendan on circulating pro-inflammatory cytokines and soluble apoptosis mediators in patients with decompensated advanced heart failure. Am J Cardiol 2004; 93: 1309-1312.

[46] Trikas A, Antoniades C, Latsios G, *et al.* Long-term effects of levosimendan infusion on inflammatory processes and sFas in patients with severe heart failure. Eur J Heart Fail 2006; 8: 804-809.

[47] Yokoshiki H, Katsube Y, Sunagawa M, Sperelakis N. Levosimendan, a novel Ca2+ sensitizer, activates the glibenclamide-sensitive K+ channel in rat arterial myocytes. Eur J Pharmacol 1997; 333: 249-259.

[48] Mebazaa A, Nieminen MS, Filippatos GS, *et al.* Levosimendan vs. dobutamine: outcomes for acute heart failure patients on beta-blockers in SURVIVE. Eur J Heart Fail 2009; 11: 304-311.

[49] Sonntag S, Sundberg S, Lehtonen LA, Kleber FX. The calcium sensitizer levosimendan improves the function of stunned myocardium after percutaneous transluminal coronary angioplasty in acute myocardial ischemia. J Am Coll Cardiol 2004; 43: 2177-2182.

[50] Follath F, Franco F, Cardoso JS. European experience on the practical use of levosimendan in patients with acute heart failure syndromes. Am J Cardiol 2005; 96: 80G-85G.

[51] Koumallos N, Antoniades C, Tousoulis D, Shirodaria C, Stefanadis C. Levosimendan: a novel agent in heart failure. Recent Pat Cardiovasc Drug Discov 2006; 1: 185-191.

Thyroid Hormone in Heart Failure: Potential Therapeutic Implications

Alessandro Pingitore* and Giorgio Iervasi

Institute of Clinical Physiology, C.N.R., Pisa, Italy

Abstract: Interest in the role of thyroid hormones (TH) in heart failure is steadily increasing due to evidence for a physiological, homeostatic role of TH and the effects of altered TH metabolism on the cardiovascular system, particularly in presence of heart failure.

Experimental studies have shown that altered TH metabolism modifies cardiovascular homeostasis by inducing alterations of cardiac histology, cardiomyocyte morphology and gene expression and consequently, of diastolic and systolic myocardial function. Clinical studies have shown that mild forms of thyroid dysfunction, both primary (subclinical hypothyroidism and subclinical hyperthyroidism) and secondary (low T_3 syndrome) have negative prognostic impacts on patients with heart failure. In these patients, the administration of synthetic triiodothyronine (T_3) was well tolerated and induced significant improvement in cardiac function without increased heart rate and metabolic demand. Large multicenter, placebo-controlled prospective studies are necessary to evaluate the safety and prognostic effects of chronic treatment with TH replacement therapy in patients with heart failure. The article also discusses recent patents in this field.

Keywords: Thyroid hormone, triiodothyronine, heart failure.

THYROID AND HOMEOSTASIS IN THE CONTEXT OF HEART FAILURE

Heart failure (HF) is a relentless progressive syndrome, the final common passage of different anatomic, functional and biological alterations interacting in a complex manner and involving all body systems over a sustained period of time. HF begins as a single-organ disease, characterized by heart dysfunction alone, but it becomes a systemic disease during its evolution and progression. Neuroendocrine activation has a pivotal role as a compensatory mechanism for reduced cardiac output, increased atrial pressure, arterial underfilling and/or inadequate systemic arterial volume [1, 2] and is a suitable explanation of the systemic involvement in HF. When referring to pathophysiology of chronic stress stimuli [3], HF should be viewed in a unique scenario of altered systemic homeostasis in which heart dysfunction, peripheral organ dysfunction and neuroendocrine and immuno-mediatory system derangement represent a chronic stress stimuli with a continuous activation of the stress response that predisposes to allostatic load, defined by McEwan as "*the cumulative strain on the body produced by repeated ups and downs of physiologic response, as well as by the elevated activity of physiologic system under challenge and the changes in metabolism and the impact of wear and tear on a number of organs and tissues,*

*Corresponding author: Tel: +39-050-3152605; Fax: +39-050-3152166; E-mail: alessandro.pingitore@ifc.cnr.it

Atta-ur-Rahman / M. Iqbal Choudhary (Eds.)

can predispose the organism to disease" [3]. In other words, allostatic load refers to the price the body pay for being continuously forced to adapt to adverse physical and pathophysiological situations [4]. In the case of HF the continuous up-regulation when neuroendocrine and immunoreactive systems shift their effects from compensatory to unfavorable and finally to toxic ones as documented by induction of calcium overload and apoptosis, and stimulation of myocardial fibrosis, promote the left ventricular remodeling process and also systemic impairment.

In this scenario, it is suggestive the hypothesis that whether left ventricular dysfunction is more important prognostic variable at early phases of HF when this is still an organ disease, in the continuing evolution HF can progress into two mainly different arms, i.e. the cardiac and the systemic ones in which clinical status and patients outcome are mainly dominated by the progressive left ventricular dysfunction and the systemic derangement respectively.

Thyroid hormone (TH) system is profoundly involved in the cardiovascular and systemic homeostasis [5,6]. TH influences diastolic and systolic functions both directly and indirectly. Increased left ventricular (LV) relaxation is mediated through the activation of the sarcoplasmic reticulum Ca^{2+}-ATPase (SERCA), which reduces cytosolic calcium from the high systolic to the low resting levels in diastole, and the concomitant inhibition of phospholamban, which inhibits SERCA through a decrease in the enzyme's affinity for Ca^{2+} [7-10]. The direct TH effects on contractility are mediated by increasing the α-myosin heavy chain (MHC) content, which have a high contractility state, and decreasing β-myosin expression, which is associated with a better energetic efficiency and economy of force maintenance. The indirect TH effects on diastolic and systolic functions are mediated by favorable changes in cardiac loading conditions. In particular, experimental and clinical evidence clearly documents that one of the earliest responses to TH administration is decreased total peripheral vascular resistance [10]. Thus the final result of all these effects is a positive TH-mediated ventricle-arterial coupling, which leads to a more favorable balance for the work of the heart [10].

The importance of TH in maintaining cardiovascular homeostasis can also be deduced from data showing that mild forms of TH abnormalities, i.e. subclinical hypothyroidism and subclinical hyperthyroidism significantly alter cardiovascular function [11,12]. A mild hypothyroidism is associated with impaired LV diastolic function characterized by slowed myocardial relaxation and impaired ventricular filling. Also, impaired systolic function has been documented both at rest and on effort and has been related to the altered working load condition of the heart. The negative effect induced by a mild hypothyroidism, on the cardiovascular system can be reversed by restoring euthyroidism with levothyroxine replacement therapy [11,12].

The role of TH system in maintaining systemic homeostasis is determined by the effects on the function of different organs and systems, i.e. the same organs and systems that are found to be altered in HF, and the interaction with several hormonal pathways. Altered thyroid metabolism determines renal insufficiency and mood alterations with symptoms of depression and anxiety. In hypothyroid patients serum creatinine is higher than in controls and the severity of thyroid dysfunction correlates with renal function [13]. The main psychological symptoms in hypothyroidism are working memory decrement, somatic complaints, anxiety and depressive features [14]. Patients with coronary artery disease and depressive symptoms had higher incidence of HF and lower triiodothyronine (T3) circulating levels, suggesting the association between altered thyroid profile, depression and cardiac dysfunction [15]. The relationship between thyroid system and other hormone pathways is particularly crucial in the HF context in which neuroendocrine activation plays a pivotal pathophysiological role. The thyroid-adrenergic synergy is bidirectional [16], with TH potentiating beta-1 adrenergic receptor signals both increasing the number of receptors and cAMP production through the stimulation of adenylyl cyclase activity [17,18] whereas adrenergic system promotes T4 to T3 peripheral conversion [18]. The gene expression of angiotensin type I and II receptors significantly increases in rats with thyroidectomy-induced hypothyroidism [19]. Cytokines, in particular tumor necrosis factor, interleukin 1 and 6, have been implicated in the pathogenesis of low T3 syndrome in several group of patients and in particular in patients with HF [20]. The cytokine-induction of low T3 syndrome is similar to that documented in HF, i.e. the reduction in peripheral T4 to T3 conversion through inhibiting deiodination activity [21]. TH increases serum brain natriuretic peptide (BNP) probably through a direct stimulatory effect on the secretion of BNP both at the level of the atrial and ventricular myocytes [22]. BNP secretion, BNP mRNA levels, and BNP promoter activity increased 3-6 fold following T3 treatment [23]. In patients with both subclinical and overt hyperthyroidism BNP levels were significantly higher than in controls [24].

The more frequent alteration of TH metabolism in HF is the low T3, that mimics hypothyroid syndrome, sharing both similar cardiovascular and systemic alterations (Fig. **1**). The new hypothesis is that low T3 syndrome may participate directly in HF progression. This is supported by the findings of the direct detrimental effect induced by hypothyroidism on cardiac morpho-structure, histology and systolic and diastolic function of left ventricle, as shown in experimental setting, and of the reversibility of alterations after TH profile normalization [25]. Further clinical findings showed the negative prognostic impact of low T3 syndrome in HF patients having a significantly higher incidence of cardiac and cumulative death when compared to those without low T3 syndrome [26-29].

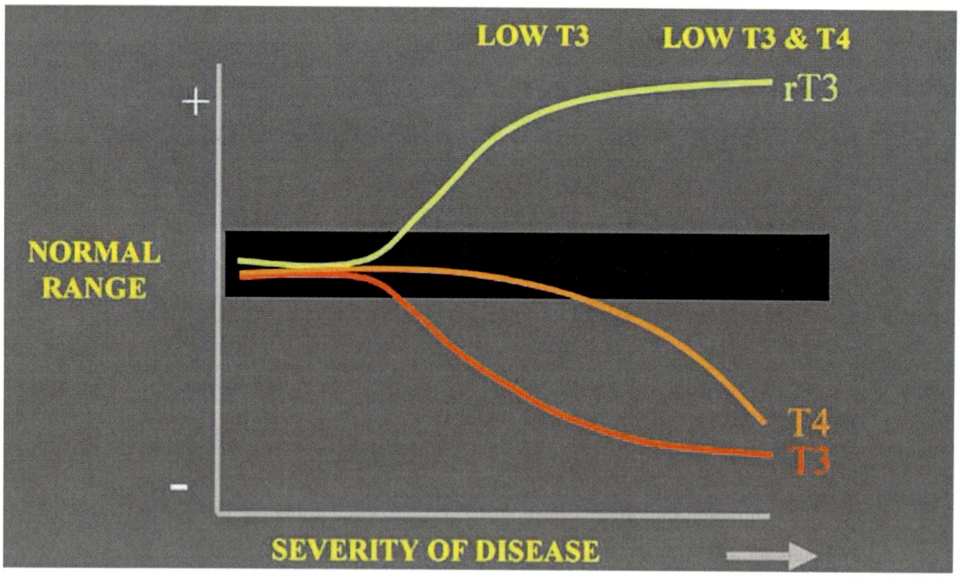

Fig. (1). Thyroid hormone profile evolution in heart failure.

Thus it is plausible that a normal thyroid status is essential for maintaining systemic and cardiovascular homeostasis; when persistently lost, increased whole-body and cardiovascular vulnerability is observed. The restoration of normal TH metabolism appears to be useful in order to interrupt the vicious circle of HF, that involves heart dysfunction, systemic impairment and neuroendocrine and immuno-inflammatory systems activation, altogether impairing systemic and cardiovascular homeostasis. In this context, TH replacement therapy may be considered a new therapeutical frontier in HF patients, in addition to the current neuroendocrine treatment portfolio.

THYROID HORMONES AND HEART FAILURE IN EXPERIMENTAL MODELS

Pathophysiological Effects of Altered TH Metabolism on the Cardiovascular System

Several experimental studies have clearly shown that an altered TH metabolism modifies cardiovascular homeostasis by inducing alterations of cardiac histology, cardiomyocyte morphology and gene expression, and consequently, of diastolic and systolic myocardial function. All these alterations may be at least partly responsible for the progression of HF (Fig. **2**). In a rat model of starvation-induced low-T_3 syndrome the mRNA content of α-MHC gene decreased by 46% when compared with controls; importantly, the decline was linearly related to the decrease in serum T_3 [30]. A similar result was observed regarding SERCA2 mRNA content. Systolic and diastolic LV function was impaired significantly, with +DP/dt (a measure of LV contractility) reduced by 13%, and the mean LV relaxation time (a measure of diastolic (dys)function) increased by 21%. Importantly, supplementation with synthetic T_3 normalized the α-MHC isoform and SERCA2 contents despite persistence of food restriction, as well as improved systolic and diastolic heart performance. Moreover, in the Bio-T0-2 hamster model of primitive dilated cardiomyopathy, which develops spontaneous subclinical hypothyroidism [31], thyroid dysfunction was associated with a decreased number of myocytes and increased myocardial fibro-necrosis. Also, resting myocardial blood flow and maximal coronary vasodilatation after adenosine administration were significantly decreased [31]. All these alterations normalized after supplementation with synthetic thyroxine (T4). These findings fit well with previous evidences showing a coronary microcirculatory dysfunction secondary to rarefaction of myocardial arterioles [32]. A potential mechanism of arteriolar rarefaction is the reduced availability of nitric oxide synthesis that has been shown to be reduced in hypothyroidism [33,34]. The functional and anatomical alteration of coronary microcirculation is also in line with the evidence that progression of HF may also depend on the process of oncosis, a pathologic mechanism of myocyte death due to ischemic reasons, aside from apoptosis [35]. This experimental evidence has an important clinical impact since abnormal coronary microcirculatory flow, potentially causing impairment of myocardial perfusion and regional metabolic changes compatible with myocardial ischemia, has been shown in patients with dilated cardiomyopathy [36]. Moreover, severely depressed myocardial blood flow has been found to be a predictor of poor prognosis in patients with idiopathic LV dysfunction independently of the degree of LV functional impairment, and of the presence of overt HF [37]. Alteration of the cardiomyocyte cyto-skeleton induced by thyroid dysfunction may favor the progression of HF as documented by myocyte lengthening and subsequent LV chamber dilatation and dysfunction [25] in a rat model of 6-week propylthiouracil-induced hypothyroidism. Alteration in the myocyte cyto-skeleton has also been documented in a human model of prolonged (10-day) T_3-deprived atrial myocardial cultured tissue [38]. In this study cellular remodeling consisted of enlargement of myocyte surface area and transversal diameter, leading to cellular degeneration including atrophy, cell death and fibrosis. These morpho-structural alterations were associated with a significantly reduced expression of alpha sarcomeric actin, an essential protein for preserving the cytoskeleton, that has been related to LV remodeling in human HF [39]. Another potential link between thyroid dysfunction and HF progression is the activation of the fetal gene program, indicated as "recapitulation of the fetal phenotype" [40,41]. This process consists of reversal of genotype/phenotype to a more fetal-like cardiac state and is characterized by: 1) decreased fast-contracting α-MHC; 2) increased slow-contracting β-MHC; 3) decreased SERCA2.

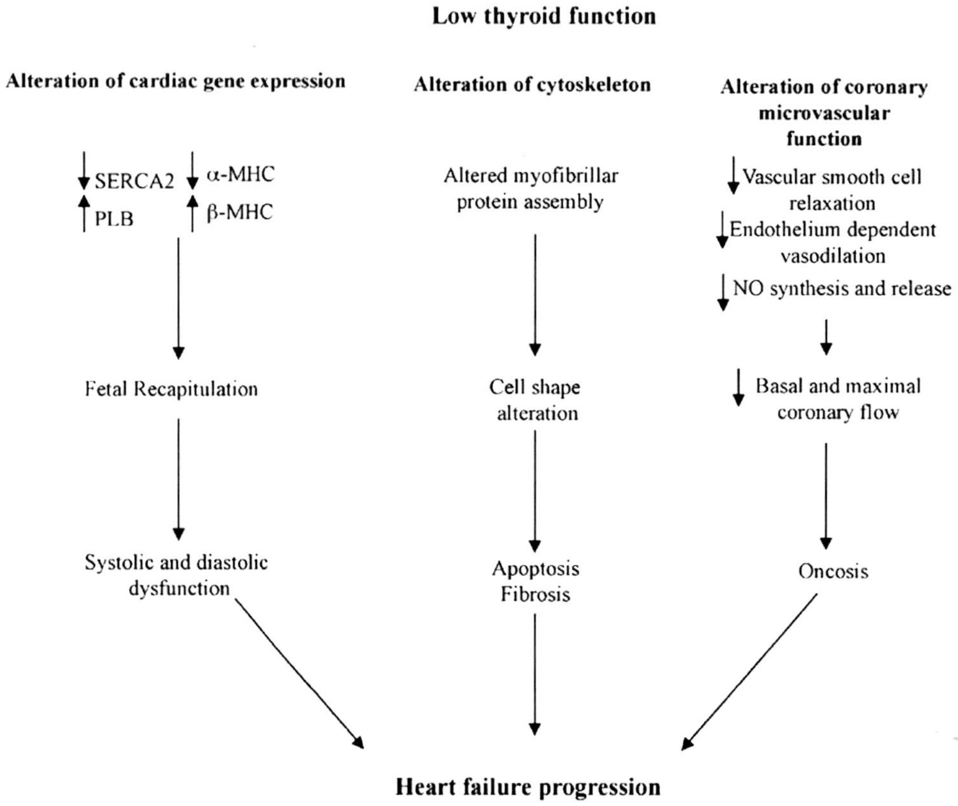

Fig. (2). Potential mechanisms of thyroid and heart relationship during the progression of heart failure.

Effects of Thyroid Hormone Administration in Experimental Settings

Different experimental models of normal and failing hearts were used to assess the effects and the potential molecular mechanisms of T_3 administration. The observed T_3-induced improvement of cardiac performance has been related to several mechanisms including: 1) a cardioprotective action in both ischemia and post-ischemic LV remodeling. 2) peripheral and coronary vasodilation; 3) cardiomyocyte preservation and hypertrophy. In isolated dog's heart, administration of T_3 infused before and after global hypothermic ischemia had positive cardiac inotropism, which was not accomplished with oxygen wasting effects [42]. Improved cardiac efficiency and function after ischemia-reperfusion was partially explained by T_3-induced modulation of glucose metabolism. In fact T_3 administration during reperfusion soon improved coupling of glycolysis to glucose oxidation by increasing the activity of pyruvate dehydrogenase. This metabolic effect was associated with a reduced cellular concentration of protons (H^+) produced from glycolysis, which negatively influences cardiac efficiency. In fact H^+ are exchanged with extra-cellular Na^+ via the Na^+ /H^+ exchanger, thus reducing Ca^{2+} efflux and resulting in Ca^{2+} overload and cell death [43].

Post-ischemic LV remodeling is characterized by recapitulation of the fetal phenotype consisting in the overexpression of β-MHC isoform and decreased α-MHC in the non-infarcted myocardium [44]. TH administration soon after infarction reversed this process by increasing α-MHC expression, reducing beta-MHC expression, and increasing SERCA/PLB ratio [44]. Further cardioprotection following T_3 administration is also provided by modulating the protein kinase C (PKC) pathway, that directly (and negatively) affects cardiac function through myofilament phosphorylation [45]; the PKC route also has a pivotal role in the development of cardioprotective effects of ischemic preconditioning [46].

In the model of ischemia-reperfusion, decreased coronary resistance and increased coronary flow were documented after T3 administration [42]. This finding fits well with the evidence of a relaxant effect of TH in different vascular districts, including coronary arteries, that is independent from cAMP and nitric oxide formation [47]. Both T_3 and T_4 have direct vasodilatory effects, with the former more prominent than the latter. The T_3 vasodilatory effect has both an endothelium-independent (which is more evident in physiological concentrations of T_3) and an endothelium-dependent component, more evident in supraphysiological concentrations of T_3 [48]. In a hamster cheek pouch, microcirculation T_3 treatment consistently induced dose-dependent dilation of arterioles more rapidly than that induced by T_4 administration (2 vs 16 minutes) [49]. In the same study, local conversion of T_4 to T_3 was documented to be a crucial step for the dilation of the microcirculatory system by considering that: 1) iopanoic acid, a strong inhibitor of both 5′ type 1 and type 2 deiodinase, abolished the dilation elicited by T_4 but not that of T_3; 2) 6-propyl-2-thiouracil, which inhibits 5′-type 1 deiodinase but does not alter T_3 production from T_4 by 5′-type 2 deiodinase, did not affect the dilation induced by T_4. Further, a neo-angiogenic response has been documented after TH treatment. This response, consisting in capillary proliferation, is rapid in onset and occurs after a single injection of synthetic L-T_4, primarily in the venous capillaries, and is linked to the overexpression of Beta FGF, as well as to mechanical factors, i.e. wall tension, shear stress, increased capillary flow [50].

Interestingly, many cardiac effects induced by TH can be partially explained by the activation of the Akt signal that has both hypertrophic [51], and anti-apoptotic effects [52], also enhancing cardiac contractility without affecting beta adrenergic receptor activity [53]. In neonatal isolated rat ventricular cardiomyocytes T_3 treatment induced phosphorylation of Akt after 24 h and protected against starvation-induced cell death [54]. A more rapid T_3-mediated activation of Akt signal has been documented in cultured cardiomyocytes. Continuous 24-h T_3 administration induced physiological cell growth by increasing P13K activity which resulted in increased phosphorylation of Akt. The evidence that the T_3-induced P13K-Akt signaling pathway was mediated through cytosolic-localized alpha-1 thyroid receptors support cytosolic non-genomic actions of TH that are rapid in onset and able to maintain long-term effects [55].

Another potential T_3-induced mechanism of cardiac hypertrophy is the stimulation of cardiomyocyte proliferation through activation of the cyclin and cyclin-dependent kinase system [56]. Cyclic D1 mRNA cytosolic levels were enhanced in the hearts of T_3-treated rats, and, most importantly, also in the nuclear fraction indicating that T_3 has the ability to induce translocation of the cyclin from the cytoplasm to the nucleus. Moreover, nuclear translocation of cyclin D1 was associated with increased cardiomyocyte DNA synthesis, as demonstrated by increased levels of cyclin A, a specific marker of the S-phase of the cell-cycle, and the incorporation of bromodeoxyuridine into DNA.

Modulation of calcium handling through the sarcoplasmic reticulum is strongly influenced by TH which up-regulates protein levels of sarcoplasmic reticulum calcium-ATPase (SERCA2) and down-regulates those of phospholamban (PLB). Another potential T_3-activated pathway is the overexpression of ryanodine receptors, an important protein in the junctional sarcoplasmic reticulum, which mediates calcium release to trigger muscle contraction [57]. Unloaded heart is characterized by reduced cardiac performance and impaired LV relaxation, and at the cellular level by increased phospholamban activity with a reduced SERCA2/PLB protein ratio [58]. Treatment with physiological doses of T_3 induced normalization of the SERCA2/ PLB ratio, and improved ventricular relaxation and contractility. Interestingly, neither MHC isoform shift nor induction of LV hypertrophy was observed, thus suggesting that the observed beneficial effect of T_3 is partially due to the restoration of calcium handling [59]. These results could have important clinical implications if we consider that unloading heart is induced in patients with the implantation of the LV assisted device and that myocardial dysfunction is frequently documented after weaning and removal of the device [60].

All the above mentioned experimental findings offer a mechanistic bases for a TH-system based therapy in patients with left ventricular dysfunction and low/borderline levels of T3. The restoration of a normal TH profile might counteract progression of heart disease by 1) a positive remodeling through the modulation of myocardial gene expression and cell protection and proliferation; 2) improving cardiac systo-diastolic function and reducing vascular resistance with a consequent improvement in hemodynamic; 3) improving myocardial perfusion, known to be impaired in the early stage of dilated cardiomyopathy and leading to progression towards HF and death.

THYROID HORMONE AND HEART FAILURE IN PATIENTS

Clinical and Prognostic Relevance of TH Abnormalities in Patients with Heart Failure

Experimental findings on the pathophysiological effects of an altered thyroid profile on the cardiovascular system have relevant clinical and prognostic confirmation in patients with cardiac disease, and in particular in those with HF [26-29,61-63]. Low T_3 syndrome is the first and most common alteration of TH metabolism in patients with cardiac disease, with an incidence of almost 30% in patients with HF [26,28]. This syndrome is characterized by a reduction in serum total and free-T_3 concentrations in presence of normal levels of T_4 and thyrotropin (TSH) [64]. Several factors are documented to contribute to thyroid abnormalities: 1) inhibition of the activity of type I 5′-deiodinase, the enzyme catalyzing the deiodination of T_4 and reverse-T_3 to T_3 and 3, 3′-diiodothyronine, 2) decreased transport of T_4 into tissues and probably 3) reduced activity of type II deiodinase which is believed to be responsible for local cellular demand of T_3 [64]. In patients with HF the incidence of low T_3 syndrome correlates with clinical status, with significantly higher incidence in patients with NYHA functional class III-IV than in those with NYHA I-II; also alterations in cardiac index, ventricular filling pressures, and LV functional impairment are more significant in patients than in those without low T_3 syndrome [27].

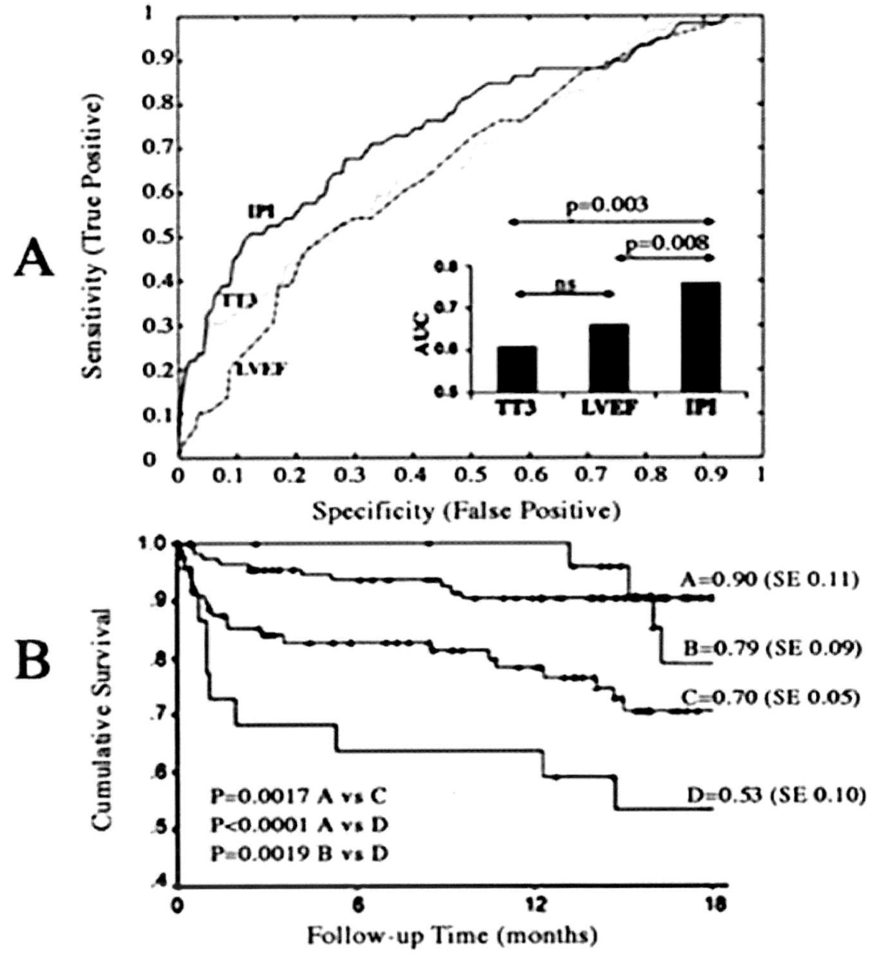

Fig. (3). Panel A: Receiver operating characteristics (ROC) curves for left ventricular ejection fraction (LVEF), total T_3 (TT_3) and integrated prognostic index (IPI). Histograms show the area under the curve AUC for the 3 variables. Panel B: Kaplan-Meier 18-month survival curves of the subgroups A (ejection fraction > 20 % and total T_3 > 1.2 nmol/L), B (ejection fraction ≤ 20 % and total T_3 > 1.2 nmol/L), C (Ejection fraction > 20 % and total T_3 ≤ 1.2 nmol/L), D (Ejection fraction ≤ 20 % and total T_3 ≤ 1.2 nmol/L). Data from Pingitore *et al.* (2005), modified.

Additional clinical studies have shown the important negative prognostic impact of low T_3 syndrome in patients with HF [26-29]. In the study by Hamilton and Opasich [26,27] an altered thyroid profile, i.e. low free T_3 index/reverse T_3 ratio and reduced circulating levels of T_3, was associated with a poor outcome, with moderate-to-severe HF. The study by Kozdag [29], which enrolled inpatients (n = 111) with ischemic and non-ischemic dilated cardiomyopathy, confirmed the relatively higher probability of cardiac death in patients with a low free-T_3/free-T_4 ratio when the cut-off value ≤1.7 was used. In 281 in-patients with non-ischemic and ischemic HF total T_3 and LV ejection fraction were found to be the only independent predictive variables at multivariate analysis of both cardiac and cumulative death. When evaluating the prognostic power of these two predictors by receiver operating characteristics (ROC) curve, the area under ROC curves (AUC: Area Under the Curve) showed a slightly higher prognostic accuracy for LV ejection fraction (AUC = 0.659, $p<0.0001$) as compared to total T_3 (AUC = 0.610, $p<0.0001$), although the difference between the two areas was not statistically significant ($p=0.733$) (Fig. **3**) [27]. When a new prognostic index was obtained by integrating both LV ejection fraction and total T_3, the AUC curve of this integrated index was significantly higher than that of the total T_3 and LV ejection fraction alone. The reason for the increased prognostic power of the integrated prognostic index arises from the analysis of the ROC curves showing that the sensitivity of total T_3 was higher than that of LV ejection fraction in the higher specificity region of the ROC, indicating that the prognostic incremental value of total T_3 was particularly evident in patients with severely reduced LV ejection fraction, i.e. < 0.20. Kaplan-Meyer survival curves of patients with reduced LV ejection fraction as well as T_3 showed the highest mortality when compared to that of patients with similar LV ejection fraction but normal T_3, thereby indicating the power of T_3 concentration in distinguishing patients at very high risk for death (Fig. **3**). These findings fit well with the common observation in clinical practice of different outcomes in patients with similar and severely impaired LV ejection fraction. Similarly, the negative prognostic power of low T3 syn-drome was particularly enhanced in patients with higher BNP concentration. In particular, the combination of high BNP and low fT3 identified the group of patients with HF having the higher mortality rate (Fig. **4**) [65].

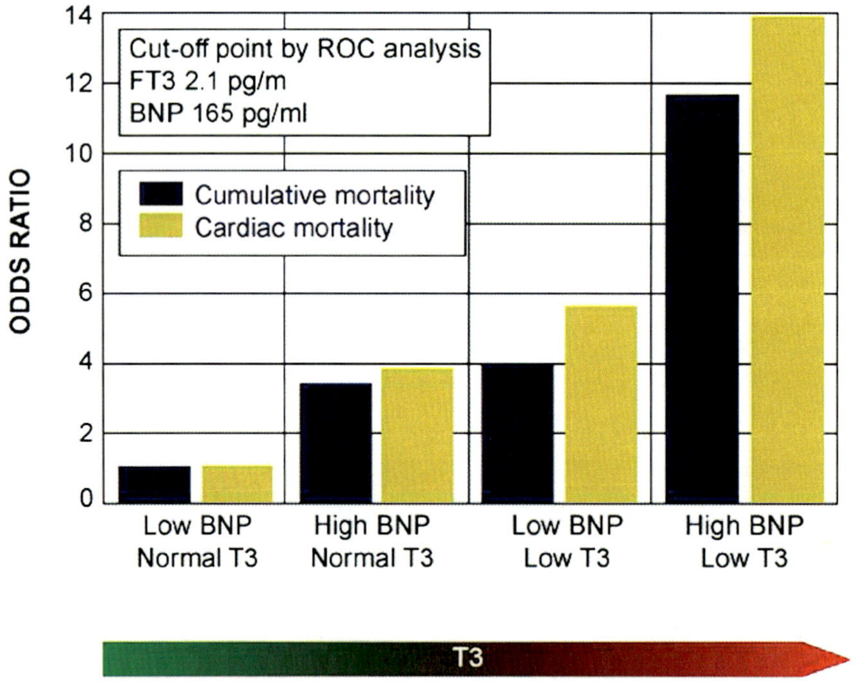

Fig. (4). Probability of cardiac and cumulative death by combining T3 and BNP results.

Also, subclinical mild hyperthyroidism and subclinical mild hypothyroidism, characterized respectively by increased and decreased thyrotropin levels in the presence of normal values of free THs have been also linked to an increased mortality rate in patients with diagnosed ischemic or non-ischemic cardiac disease [61]. Differently from the low T_3 syndrome, which can be considered a disorder of peripheral TH metabolism that progressively develops during the evolution of several systemic diseases, subclinical hyperthyroidism and subclinical hypothyroidism are primary disorders of the thyroid gland. In the above-cited large prospective observational study, survival time was significantly lower in both subclinical hypothyroidism and subclinical hyperthyroidism than in euthyroid patients when cardiac and cumulative deaths were considered.

TREATMENT OF HEART FAILURE WITH SYNTHETIC THYROID HORMONE

The potential therapeutical strategies that can be employed to optimize TH signaling in presence of HF and non thyroidal illness syndrome can be summarized in the following points: 1) administration of synthetic L-T4; by this approach the main physiological pathway of secretion and peripheral metabolism of TH system is guaranteed; 2) administration of L-T3 that is, the biological active form of THs; 3) administration of a TH analog, that is, of a synthetic and, as possible, cardiotropic compound showing similar positive but lower adverse effects than the natural TH; 4) genetic manipulation of the TH cardiac signaling

T3 Administration

Nowadays, there are three reports in which T_3 was used intravenously in patients with HF and low T_3 syndrome [66-68]. These studies are difficult to compare with each other due to the different T_3 dose regimen applied. The study by Hamilton *et al.* adopted a protocol based on administration of intravenous bolus dose followed or not by a few-hour infusion of T_3, whereas, in the two studies of our group T_3 was continuously administered for 3 days at an initial dose of 20 mcg/m2/b.s./day diluted in 100 ml of saline; the dose was adjusted, when necessary, in order to maintain T_3 circulating levels within the physiological range (Fig. **5**) [68]. Independently of the adopted T_3 administered regimen, all cited studies documented an improvement in cardiac performance, associated with a reduction in systemic vascular resistance [66]. Importantly, heart rate did not change nor did metabolic demand, as assessed by indirect calorimetry [66]. These results were confirmed in an invasive hemodynamic study, and in a non-invasive study that assessed LV performance with cardiac magnetic resonance. In the invasive study T_3 constant infusion induced a progressive reduction in systemic vascular resistance and an increase in ejection fraction and cardiac output, the latter invasively monitored by Swan-Ganz catheter; urinary output was also improved, whereas no changes in heart rate and systemic arterial blood pressure were observed [67]. An improvement in overall cardiac performance characterized by increased stroke volume and LV end-diastolic diameter was also non-invasively documented in 20 patients with chronic and clinically stable dilated cardiomyopathy and low T_3 syndrome (Fig. **6**) [68]. The observed enlargement of the endiastolic LV volume can be interpreted as the expression of the recruitment of residual ventricular filling reserve, a fundamental compensatory mechanism for maintaining cardiac output in patients with HF [69]. This finding may result from the positive effects of biologically active T3 on diastolic relaxation secondary to the increase in calcium ATPase of SERCA pump [70] and to the inhibition of its counter-regulatory phospholamban [70]. The improvement in cardiac performance induced by T3 did not correspond to increased myocardial oxygen consumption, as indirectly estimated by calculation of the rate pressure product as well as total cardiac work. The benefit of T3 infusion on cardiac function parallels with a deactivation of neuroendocrine profile, as a result from the significant reduction in vasoconstrictor/sodium retaining noradrenaline, aldosterone, and in the counterpart NT-proBNP plasma levels (Fig. **6**). It is uncertain whether the neuroendocrine rearrangement is indirect, due to improved cardiac performance, rather than direct T3-mediated action. In fact, as previously mentioned, THs "per se" are able to increase rather than decrease catecolamines, BNP and aldosterone release. However, the potential clinical relevance of T3-induced neuroendocrine deactivation in patients with LV dysfunction is clearly deducible from analysis of reported data in the literature showing highly beneficial effects of aldosterone and β-adrenergic antagonists in terms of survival, rate of hospitalization, symptoms and cardiac performance.

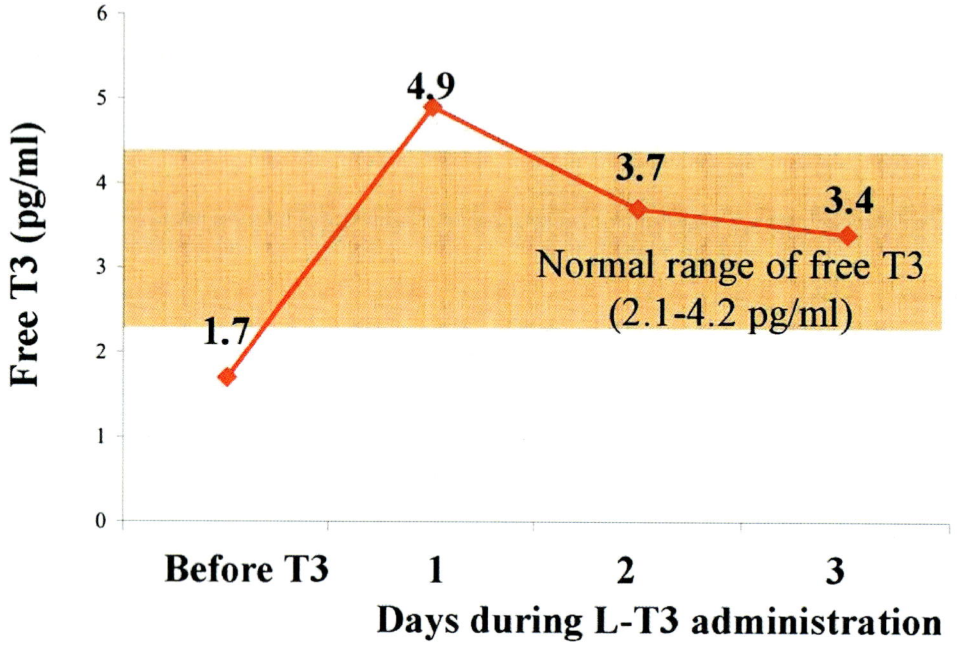

Fig. (5). An example of L-T3 circulating levels during 3-day continuous infusion of L-T3. The initial infusion dose of L-T3 was 20 µg/m2; during the 3-day infusion T3 dose was changed in order to maintain circulating T3 levels within normal range.

The rationale for treating patients with T_3 instead of T_4 is based on the evidence that the physiological pattern of peripheral conversion from T_4 into T_3 is impaired in presence of a non-thyroidal illness syndrome, and thus the administration of T_3 by-passes this critical point through direct application of the biologically active TH. Moreover, the chosen protocol of infusion, that is continuous 3-day administration of T_3 and with the dose only adjusted in order to maintain circulating levels of T_3 within normal range, was based on the evidence that this modality of T_3 infusion promotes more effective nuclear action of T_3 and T_3-mediated transcription in the myocardium compared to multiple bolus injection or oral regimen [71]: and that the restoration of serum bioactive T_3 by constant infusion of T_4 was unable to normalize tissue levels of T_3, including the myocardium [72]. This may be even more evident in presence of an impaired peripheral conversion of T_4 into T_3 as in presence of a low T_3 syndrome.

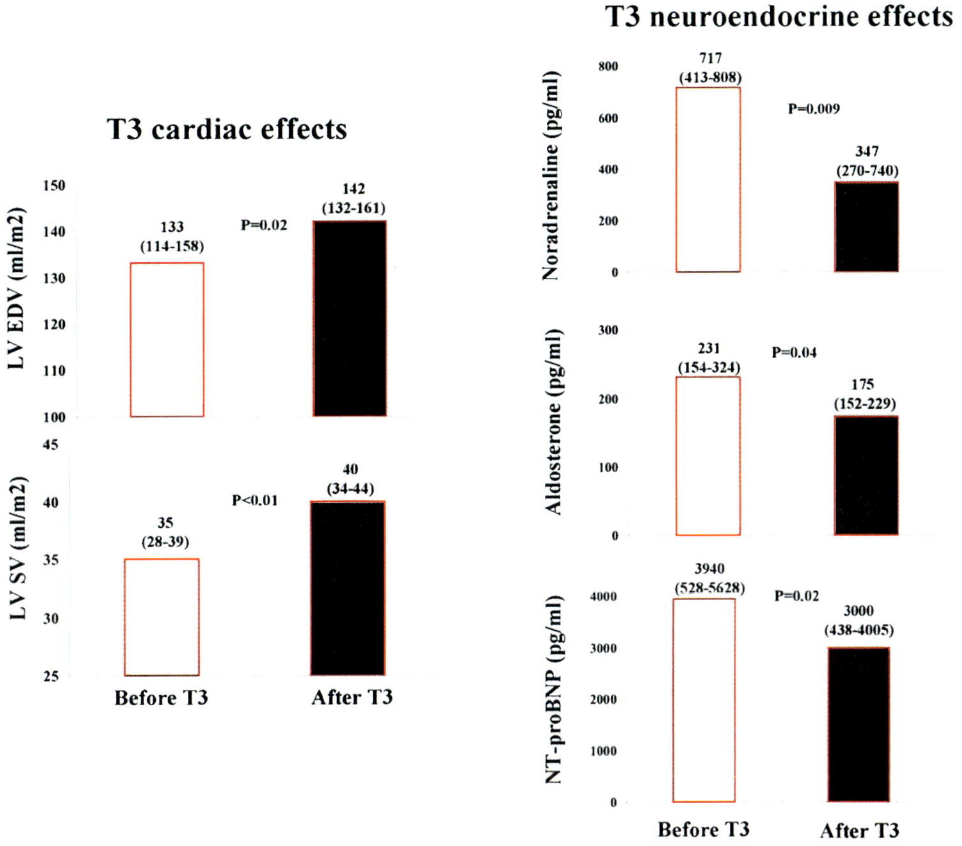

Fig. (6). T3 effect on cardiac function and neuroendocrine system in patients with HF.

LVSV = Left ventricular stroke volume

LVEDV = Left ventricular end-diestolic volume

T4 Administration

Moruzzi *et al.* published two studies in which synthetic T_4 was given orally at the "physiological" dose of 0.1 mg per day with assessment of cardiovascular effects after short-term (1 week) and after continuous 3-month treatment [73, 74]. In both studies T_4 was well tolerated and induced a significant improvement in cardiac pump function consisting in enhanced resting LV ejection fraction, resting cardiac output, and exercise capacity. Furthermore, the response to dobutamine increased in treated patients, with significant improvement in cardiac output and heart rate. The latter finding may be linked to enhanced adrenergic sensitivity in accordance with experimental data showing the beta 1 upregulating effect of TH [75]. The beneficial hemodynamic effects of intravenous thyroxine administration (20 microgr/h) have been also documented in 10 patients with cardiogenic shock unresponsive to conventional pharmacological inotropic therapy and intra-aortic balloon counterpulsation. In this study, T3 was sampled at baseline in three patients only and all of them had low T3 syndrome. The cardiovascular effects of continuous infusion of L-T4 were maintained for a long enough time to accomplish a definite surgical treatment consisting of heart transplantation or LV assist device [76].

3,5-Diiodothyropropionic Acid (DITPA)

The 3,5-diiodothyropropionic acid (DITPA), a TH analog, has cardiac inotropic selectivity compared with TH itself, accompanied by minimal effects on heart rate and metabolic activity [77]. DITPA binds to T_3 nuclear receptors, and induces a T_3-like transcription response [78]. Long-term administration of DITPA also stimulates coronary arteriolar growth without inducing cardiac hypertrophy, by upregulating key angiogenic growth factors [79]. In recent randomized placebo controlled clinical study, DITPA was administered in patients with NYHA functional class II-III for 2 to 4 weeks [80]. DITPA increased cardiac index, and decreased systemic vascular resistance, and low-density lipoprotein cholesterol. Although the positive hemodynamic results, DITPA was poorly tolerated with increasing fatigue and discontinued in more than 50% of patients. No evident outcome benefits were manifest, and complex arrhythmias were recorded in the DITPA group. An explanation of the absence of scarce tolerance to DITPA and the occurrence of side effects, may be the induction of iatrogenic induced thyrotoxicosis, that is, weight loss, increased heart rate, fatigue, and suppressed TSH, all well-known signs and symptoms of this syndrome [81].

Which dose Regimen Choice for the Thyroid Hormone Treatment in Heart Failure

The dose regimen of substitutive TH treatment, both with synthetic TH and TH analog, in patients with HF is mandatory in order to avoid the appearance of side effects. Experimental and clinical data strongly suggest the opportunity to maintain T_3 circulating levels within physiological ranges. In fact, experimental data clearly documented that myocardial hypertrophy, induced by high doses of T_3 was only initially associated with improved cardiac performance, and it was followed by a decline after 1-month treatment [82]. This finding was also associated with an increased expression of uncoupling proteins (UCP2 and 3) that may be responsible for the decrease in mitochondrial efficiency during thyroid hyperfunction [83]. Beyond the above-cited study with DITPA, previous studies already documented the incidence of side effects using high dose regimen of TH inducing iatrogenic hyperthyroid state. In 1961, Jones *et al.* administered 4-8 mg of sodium D-thyroxine daily (corresponding, in terms of biological effect, to a dose of 300-350 mcg of L-thyroxine that is, 3-5 times the daily production of L-thyroxine by thyroid gland) in euthyroid patients with the aim of reducing serum cholesterol [84]. Although this objective was reached, weight loss, increased oxygen consumption, tongue tremor, all typical signs and symptoms of overt hyperthyroidism, occurred. Further cardiac symptoms, consisting of episodes of typical chest pain and congestive HF, imposed the discontinuation of sodium D-thyroxine. The authors concluded that this treatment is not recommended in patients with cardiac diseases. Similar results have been also confirmed in the cardiac drug project study [85]. Therefore, taken as a whole, these experimental and clinical data strongly suggest that substitutive TH treatment in cardiac patients has to drive at restoring normal circulating levels of THs and thus avoiding dysthyroidism. Accordingly, we recently started a phase II, randomized, double blind, placebo-controlled study with long-term substitutive L-T3 treatment targeting restoration and maintenance of normal circulating levels of T3, T4, and TSH in patients with acute myocardial infarction and low T3 syndrome. The principal aim of the study will be to evaluate safety and feasibility of TH treatment and its effects on cardiac performance and remodeling [81].

Other TH Therapeutic Approaches

Genic manipulation of thyroid genes has enormous potential in order to augment the intramyocardial TH signaling. The strategies are multiple and still limited to experimental settings. The increase in deiodinase 2 activity expression enhances the local production and bioavailability of T3, favoring T4 to T3 conversion [86,87]. This prevents the expression of markers of pathological hypertrophy or alterations in calcium handling. Similarly, the overexpression of thyroid receptors (TRalfa1 or TRbeta1), using adeno-associated viruses, enhances the hormonal signaling in presence of normal or even low bio-available T3. Alternatively, the reduction in D3 deiodinases, that inactivate the biological active form of T3 into reverse T3, and the inactivation of micro-RNA that inhibit myosin heavy chain gene regulated by TH can be alternative pathways increasing intramyocardial TH signaling. The adoption of a new target-organ strategy based on genetic manipulation, makes it possible to overcome all the limitations related to a systemic administration of synthetic native hormone or TH analogs.

According to the above mentioned approaches two strategies of TH substitutive therapy in HF patients are suggested: 1) the cardiosystemic one pursued with synthetic T4 or T3 administration; 2) the cardio-selective one provided with TH analogs, or specific intramyocardial TH targets through gene therapy. The rationale of these two approaches is based on the pathophysiology of HF progression that is linked to the progressive impairment of systo-diastolic cardiac function and also to the systemic disturbance, which frequently progresses independently from cardiac function worsening. At early stages of HF, when it is still an organ disease, specifically cardiac, the cardiac-selective strategy may be preferable in order to avoid worsening of cardiac function. On the contrary, when HF becomes a systemic disease, in which cardiac dysfunction parallels the systemic impairment, or this last dominates clinical status, the cardio-systemic strategy of TH treatment probably is preferable.

Whether the systemic effects of TH therapy in HF have been assessed, the fact is that hypothyroidism mimics HF in terms of systemic dyshomeostasis, and the positive effects of TH substitutive therapy in other clinical settings suggests that hypothyroidism may generate a vicious circle potentially impairing cardiovascular and systemic homeostasis in HF, and also that the same vicious circle may be interrupted with the normalization of TH profile.

In conclusion, TH therapy in HF setting is still a full-opened chapter. Several questions remain still without answers: type, dosage and schedule of TH treatment, the effects of TH therapy on systemic homeostasis. Large multicenter, placebo controlled prospective studies are thus necessary to provide safety and prognostic information of the chronic treatment with TH replacement therapy.

ACKNOWLEDGEMENT

We would like to thank Laura Mazza for her secretarial assistance.

REFERENCES

[1] Kjaer A, Hesse B. Heart failure and neuroendocrine activation: diagnostic, prognostic and therapeutic perspectives. Clin Physiol 2001; 21: 661-672.

[2] Swedberg K. Is more better? About dose levels of ACE inhibitors in chronic heart failure. Eur Heart J 2000; 2: 229-233.

[3] McEwen BS, Stellar E. Stress and the individual. Mechanisms leading to disease. Arch Intern Med 1993; 153: 2093-20101.

[4] McEwan BS. The neurobiology of stress: from serendipity to clinical relevance. Brain Res 2000; 886: 172-189.

[5] Kahaly GJ, Dillmann DH. Thyroid hormone action in the heart. Endocr Rev 2005; 26: 704-728.

[6] Davis PJ, Davis FB. Nongenomic actions of thyroid hormone on the heart. Thyroid 2002; 12: 459-466.

[7] Koss KL, Kranias EG. Phospholamban: a prominent regulator of myocardial contractility. Circ Res 1996; 79: 1059-1063.

[8] Ojamaa K, Petrie JF, Balkman C, Hong C, Klein I. Posttranscriptional modification of myosin heavy-chain gene expression in the hypertrophied rat myocardium. Proc Natl Acad Sci USA 1994; 91: 3468-3472.

[9] Klein I, Ojamaa K. Mechanism of disease. Thyroid hormone and the cardiovascular system. N Engl J Med 2001; 344: 501-509.

[10] Klein I. Thyroid hormone and the cardiovascular system. Am J Med 1990; 88: 631-637.

[11] Biondi B. Cardiovascular effects of mild hypothyroidism. Thyroid 2007; 17: 625-630.

[12] Ripoli A, Pingitore A, Favilli B, *et al.* Does subclinical hypothyroidism affect cardiac pump performance? Evidence from a mag-netic resonance imaging study. J Am Coll Cardiol 2005; 45: 439-445.

[13] Den Hollander JG, Wulkan RW, Mantel MJ, *et al.* Correlation between severity of thyroid dysfunction and renal function. Clin Endocrinol 2005; 62: 423-427.

[14] Samuels MH. Cognitive function in untreated hypothyroidism and hyperthyroidism. Curr Opin Endocrinol Diabetes Obes 2008; 15: 429-433.

[15] Bunevicius R, Varoneckas G, Prange AJ Jr, *et al.* Depression and thyroid axis function in coronary artery disease: impact of cardiac impairment and gender. Clin Cardiol 2006; 29: 170-174.

[16] Silva JE, Bianco SD. Thyroid-adrenergic interactions: physiological and clinical implications. Thyroid 2008; 18: 157-165.

[17] Bumgarner JR, Ramkumar V, Stiles GL. Altered thyroid status regulates the adipocyte A1 adenosine receptor-adenylate cyclase system. Life Sci 1989; 44: 1705-1712.

[18] Silva JE, Larsen PR. Adrenergic activation of triiodothyronine production in brown adipose tissue. Nature 1983; 305: 712-713.

[19] Carneiro-Ramos MS, Diniz GP, Almeida J, *et al.* Cardiac angiotensin II type I and type II receptors are increased in rats submitted to experimental hypothyroidism. J Physiol 2007; 583: 213-223.

[20] Papanas N, Papatheodorou K, Papazoglou D, *et al.* Post-thyroidectomy thyroxine replacement dose in patients with or without compensated heart failure: the role of cytokines. Cytokine 2008; 41: 121-126.

[21] Bartalena L, Bogazzi F, Brogioni S, Grasso L, Martino E. Role of cytokines in the pathogenesis of the euthyroid sick syndrome. Eur J Endocrinol 1998; 138: 603-614.

[22] Kohno M, Horio T, Yasunari K, *et al.* (1993) Stimulation of brain natriuretic peptide release from the heart by thyroid hormone. Metabolism 1998; 42: 1059-1064.

[23] Liang F, Webb P, Marimuthu A, *et al.* Triiodothyronine increases brain natriuretic peptide (BNP) gene transcription and amplifies endothelin-dependent BNP gene transcription and hypertrophy in neonatal rat ventricular myocytes. J Biol Chem 2003; 278: 15073-15083.

[24] Ertugrul DT, Gursoy A, Sahin M, *et al.* Evaluation of brain natriuretic peptide levels in hyperthyroidism and hypothyroidism. J Natl Med Assoc 2008; 100: 401-405.

[25] Tang YD, Kuzman JA, Said S, *et al.* Low thyroid function leads to cardiac atrophy with chamber dilatation, impaired myocardial blood flow, loss of arterioles, and severe systolic dysfunction. Circulation 2005; 112: 3122-3130.

[26] Hamilton MA, Stevenson LW, Luu M, Walden JA. Altered thyroid hormone metabolism in advanced heart failure. J Am Coll Cardiol 1990; 16: 91-95.

[27] Opasich C, Pacini F, Ambrosino N, *et al.* Sick euthyroid syndrome in patients with moderate-to-severe chronic heart failure. Eur Heart J 1996; 17: 1860-1866.

[28] Pingitore A, Landi P, Taddei MC, Ripoli A, L'Abbate A, Iervasi G. Triiodothyronine levels for risk stratification of patients with chronic heart failure. Am J Med 2005; 118: 132-136.

[29] Kozdag G, Ural D, Vural A, *et al.* Relation between free triiodothyronine/free thyroxine ratio, echocardiographic parameters and mortality in dilated cardiomyopathy. Eur J Heart Fail 2005; 7: 113-118.

[30] Katzeff HL, Powell SR, Ojamaa K. Alterations in cardiac contractility and gene expression during low-T3 syndrome: prevention with T3. Am J Physiol 1997; 273: E951-E956.

[31] Kopechy J, Sigurdson L, Park IR, Himms-Hagen J. Thyroxine 5'-deiodinase in brown adipose tissue of myopathic hamsters. J Am Physiol Endocrinol Metab 1986; 251: E8-E13.

[32] Heron MI, Rakusan K. Short- and long-term effects of neonatal hypo- and hyperthyroidism on coronary arterioles in rat. Am J Heart Circ Physiol 1996; 271: H1746-H1754.

[33] McAllister RM, Albarracin I, Price EM, Smith TK, Turk JR, Wyatt KD. Thyroid status and nitrix oxide in rat arterial vesseils. J Endocrinol 2005; 185: 111-119.

[34] Taddei S, Caraccio N, Virdis A, *et al.* Impaired endothelium-dependent vasodilatation in subclinical hypothyroidism: beneficial effect of levothyroxine therapy. J Clin Endocrinol Metab 2003; 88: 3731-3737.

[35] Ryoke T, Gu Y, Ikeda Y, *et al.* Apoptosis and oncosis in the early progression of left ventricular dysfunction in the cardiomyopathic hamster. Basic Res Cardiol 2002; 97: 65-75.

[36] van den Heuvel AF, van Veldhuisen DJ, van der Wall EE, *et al.* Regional myocardial blood flow reserve impairment and metabolic changes suggesting myocardial ischemia in patients with idiopathic dilated cardiomyopathy. J Am Coll Cardiol 2000; 35: 19-28.

[37] Neglia D, Michelassi C, Trivieri MG, *et al.* Prognostic role of myocardial blood flow impairment in idiopathic left ventricular dysfunction. Circulation 2002; 105: 186-193.

[38] Forini F, Paolicchi A, Pizzorusso T, *et al.* 3,5,3'-Triiodothyronine deprivation affects phenotype and intracellular [Ca^{2+}] of human cardiomyocytes in culture. Cardiovasc Res 2001; 51: 322-330.

[39] Hein S, Kostin S, Heling A, Maeno Y, Schaper J. The role of the cytoskeleton in heart failure. Cardiovasc Res 2000; 45: 273-278.

[40] Colucci WS. Molecular and cellular mechanisms of myocardial failure. Am J Cardiol 1997; 80: 15L-25L.

[41] Pantos C, Malliopoulou V, Varanos DD, Cokkinos DV. Thyroid hormone and phenotypes of cardioprotection. Bas Res Cardiol 2004; 99: 101-120.

[42] Klemperer JD, Klein I, Gomez M, *et al.* Thyroid hormone treatment after coronary artery bypass surgery. N Engl J Med 1995; 333: 1522-1527.

[43] Liu G, Clanachan AS, Lopaschuk GD. Acute effects of triiodothyronine on glucose and fatty acid metabolism during reperfusion of ischemic rat heart. Am J Physiol 1998; 275: E392-E399.

[44] Pantos C, Mourouzis I, Markakis K, *et al.* Thyroid hormone attenuates cardiac remodeling and imporves hemodynamics early after acute myocardial infarction in rats. Eur J Cardiothorac Surg 2007; 32: 333-339.

[45] Hambleton M, Hahn H, Pleger ST, *et al.* Pharmacological- and gene therapy-based inhibition of protein kinase C alpha/beta enhances cardiac contractility and attenuates heart failure. Circulation 2006; 114: 574-582.

[46] Ytrehus K, Liu Y, Downey J. Preconditioning protects ischemic rabbit heart by protein kinase C activation. Am J Physiol 1994; 266: H1145-H1152.

[47] Ojamaa K, Klemperer JD, Klein I. Acute effects of thyroid hormone on vascular smooth muscle. Thyroid 1996; 6: 505-512.

[48] Park KW, Dai HB, Ojamaa K, Lowenstein E, Klein I, Sellke FW. The direct vasomotor effect of thyroid hormones on rat skeletal muscle resistance arteries. Anest Analg 1997; 85: 734-738.

[49] Colantuoni A, Marchiafava PL, Lapi D, Forini FS, Iervasi G. Effects of tetraiodothyronine and triiodothyronine on hamster cheek pouch microcirculation. Am J Physiol Heart Circ Physiol 2005; 288(4): H1931-1936.

[50] Tomanek RJ, Doty MK, Sandra A. Early coronary angiogenesis in response to thyroxine: growth characteristics and upregulation of basis fibroblast growth factor. Circ Res 1998; 82: 587-593.

[51] Oh H, Fujio Y, Kunisada K, *et al.* Activation of phosphatidylinositol 3-kinase through glycoprotein 130 induces protein kinase B and p70 S6 kinase phosphorylation in cardiac myocytes. J Biol Chem 1998; 273: 9703-9710.

[52] Fujio Y, Nguyen T, Wencker D, Kitsis RN, Walsh K. Akt promotes survival of cardiomyocytes *in vitro* and protects against ischemia-reperfusion injury in mouse heart. Circulation 2000; 101: 660-667.

[53] Condorelli G, Drusco A, Stassi G, *et al.* AKT induces enhanced myocardial contractility and cell size *in vivo* in transgenic mice. Proc Natl Acad Sci USA 2002; 99: 12333-12338.

[54] Kuzman JA, Gerdes AM, Kobayashi S, Liang Q. Thyroid hormone activates AKT and prevents serum starvation-induced cell death in neonatal rat cardiomyocytes. J Mol Cell Cardiol 2005; 39: 841-844.

[55] Kenessey A, Ojamaa K. Thyroid hormone stimulates protein synthesis in the cardiomyocyte by activating the AKT-mTOR and p70S6K pathways. Biol Chem 2006; 281: 20666-20672.

[56] Ledda-Columbano GM, Molotzu F, Pibiri M, Cossu C, Perra A, Columbano A. Thyroid hormone induces cyclin D1 nuclear translocation and DNA synthesis in adult rat cardiomyocytes. FASEB J 2006; 20: 87-94.

[57] Jiang M, Xu A, Tokmakejian S, Narayanan N. Thyroid hormone-induced overexpression of functional ryanodine receptors in the rabbit heart. Am J Physiol Heart Circ Physiol 2000; 278: H1429-H1438.

[58] Ito K, Nakayama M, Hasan F, Yan X, Schneider MD, Lorell BH. Contractile Reserve and calcium regulation are depressed in myocytes from chronically unloaded hearts. Circulation 2003; 107: 1176-1182.

[59] Minatoya Y, Ito K, Kagaya Y, *et al.* Depressed contractile reserve and impaired calcium handling of cardiac myocytes from chronically unloaded hearts are ameliorated with the administration of physiological treatment dose of T3 in rats. Acta Physiol 2007; 189; 221-231.

[60] Wohlschlaeger J, Schmitz KJ, Schmid C, *et al.* Reverse remodeling following insertion of left ventricular assist devices (LVAD): a review of the morphological and molecular changes. Cardiovasc Res 2005; 68: 376-386.

[61] Iervasi G, Molinaro S, Landi P, *et al.* Association between increased mortality and mild thyroid dysfunction in cardiac patients. Arch Intern Med 2007; 167: 1526-1532.

[62] Murzi B, Iervasi G, Masini S, Moschetti R, Vanini V, Zucchelli GB. A Thyroid hormones homeostasis in pediatric patients during and after cardiopulmonary by-pass Ann Thorac Surg 1995; 59: 481-485.
[63] Utiger RD. Altered thyroid function in nonthyroidal illness and surgery. To treat or not to treat? N Engl J Med 1995; 333: 1562-1563.
[64] Kohrle J. Local activation and inactivation of thyroid hormones: the deiodinase family. Mol Cell Endocrinol 1999; 151: 103-119.
[65] Passino C, Pingitore A, Landi P, *et al.* Prognostic valure of combined measurement of brain natriuretic peptide and triidothyronine in heart failure. J Cardiac Fail 2009; 15: 35-40.
[66] Hamilton MA, Stevenson LW, Fonarow GC. Safety and hemodynamic effects of intravenous triiodothyronine in advanced congestive heart failure. Am J Cardiol 1998; 81: 443-447.
[67] Iervasi G, Emdin M, Colzani RMP, *et al.* Beneficial effects of long-term triiodothyronine (T3) infusion in patients with advanced heart failure and low T3 syndrome. Kimchi A, Ed. Medimond Medical Publications, 2001; pp. 549-553.
[68] Pingitore A, Galli E, Barison A, *et al.* Acute effects of triiodothyronine replacement therapy in patients with chronic heart failure and low-t3 syndrome: a randomized, placebo-controlled study. J Clin Endocrinol Metab 2008; 93: 1351-1358.
[69] Colucci WS, Braunwald E. Pathophysiology of heart failure. In: Braunwald's Heart Disease, 7th edition. A Textbook of Cardiovascular Medicine. Zipes DP, Libby P, Bonow RO, Braunwald E, Eds. Elsevier Saunders 2005; 509-538.
[70] Park CW, Shin YS, Ahn SJ, *et al.* Thyroxine treatment induces upregulation of rennin-angiotensin-aldosterone system due to decreasing effective plasma volume in patients with primay myxoedema. Nephrol Dial Transplant 2001; 16: 1799-1806.
[71] Danzi S, Dubon P, Klein I. Effect of serum triiodothyronine on regulation of cardiac gene expression: role of histone acetylation. Am J Physiol Heart Circ Physiol 2005; 289: H1506-1511.
[72] Escobar-Morreale HF, del Rey FE, Obregon MJ, de Escobar GM. Only the combined treatment with thyroxine and triiodothyronine ensures euthyroidism in all tissues of the thyroidectomized rat. Endocrinology 1996; 137: 2490-2502.
[73] Moruzzi P, Doria E, Agostoni PG, Capacchione V, Sganzerla P. Usefulness of L-thyroxine to improve cardiac and exercise performance in idiopathic dilated cardiomyopathy. Am J Cardiol 1994; 73: 374-378.
[74] Moruzzi P, Doria E, Agostoni PG. Medium-term effectiveness of L-thyroxine treatment in idiopathic dilated cardiomyopathy. Am J Med 1996; 101: 461-467.
[75] Hammond HK, White FC, Buxton IL, Saltzstein P, Brunton LL, Longhurst JC. Increased myocardial beta-receptors and adrenergic responses in hyperthyroid pigs. Am J Physiol 1987; 252: H283-H290.
[76] Malik FS, Mehra MR, Uber PA, *et al.* Intravenous thyroid hormone supplementation in heart failure with cardiogenic shock. J Card Fail 1999; 5: 31-37.
[77] Pennock GD, Raya TE, Bahl JJ, Goldman S, Morkin E. Cardiac effects of 3,5 diiodothyropropionic acid, a thyroid hormone analog with inotropic selectivity. J Pharmacol Exp Ther 1992; 263: 163-169.
[78] Morkin E, Pennock G, Spooner PH, Bahl JJ, Underhill FK, Goldman S. Pilot studies on the use of 3,5-diiodothyropropionic acid, a thyroid hormone analog, in the treatment of congestive heart failure. Cardiology 2002; 97: 218-225.
[79] Wang X, Zheng W, Christensen LP, Tomanek RJ. DITPA stimulates bFGF, VEGF, angiopoietin, and Tie-2 and facilitates coronary arteriolar growth. Am J Physiol Heart Circ Physiol 2003; 284: H613-H618.
[80] Goldman S, McCarren M, Morkin E, *et al.* DITPA (3,5-diiodothyropropionic acid) a thyroid hormone analog to treat heart failure: phase II trial veterans affairs cooperative study. Circulation 2009; 119: 3093-3100.
[81] Pingitore A, Gerdes MA, Iervasi G. DITPA, a thyroid hormone analog to treat heart failure: a phase II trial Veterans Affair Cooperative Study. Letter to the Editor. Circulation 2009; (In press).
[82] Degens H, Gilde AJ, Lindhout M, Willemsen PHM, Van Der Vusse GJ, Van Bilsen M. Functional and metabolic adaptation of the heart to prolonged thyroid hormone treatment. Am J Physiol Heart Circ Physiol 2003; 284: H108-H115.
[83] Boehm EA, Jones BE, Radda GK, Veech RL, Clarke K. Increased uncoupling proteins and decreased efficiency in palmitate-perfused hyperthyroid rat heart. Am J Physiol Heart Circ Physiol 2001; 280: H977-H983.
[84] Jones RJ, Cohen L. Sodium dextro-thyroxine in coronary disease and hypercholesteremia. Circulation 1961; 24: 164-170.
[85] The coronary drug project. Findings leading to further modifications of its protocol with respect to dextrothyroxine. The coronary drug project research group. JAMA 1972; 15: 220: 996-1008.
[86] Trivieri MG, Oudit GY, Sah R, *et al.* Cardiac-specific elevations in thyroid hormone enhance contractility and prevent pressure overload-induced cardiac dysfunction. Proc Natl Acad Sci 2006; 103: 6043-6048.

[87] Belke DD, Gloss B, Swanson EA, Dillmann WH. Adeno-associated virus-mediated expression of thyroid hormone receptor isoforms-alpha1 and -beta1 improves contractile function in pressure overload-induced cardiac hypertrophy. Endocrinology 2007; 148: 2870-2877.

Skeletal Muscle Derived Stem Cells for Myocardial Repair

Husnain K. Haider[*,1], Lei Ye[2] and Muhammad Ashraf[1]

[1]*Department of Pathology and Laboratory of Medicine, 231-Albert Sabin Way, University of Cincinnati Ohio-45267-0529, USA*

[2]*National University Medical Institutes, National University of Singapore-117597, Singapore*

Abstract: Treatment of patients with heart failure secondary to myocardial infarction remains a therapeutic challenge. Extensive myocyte death in the heart and post-ischemic remodeling accentuate progressive expansion of the scar area and compromise left ventricular contractile function. The scarcity of resident stem cells in the heart and limited proliferative capacity of adult cardiomyocytes warrant novel strategies of outside intervention to supplement the inept intrinsic repair mechanism. Heart cell therapy using patient's own skeletal muscle derived myoblasts (SkMs) provides a relatively simple and inexpensive therapeutic option. Phase-I and II clinical trials supported by plethora of pre-clinical studies have shown the safety and effectiveness of SkM engraftment in the treatment of infarcted heart. However, before widespread application of this approach in the clinical settings, there remain some fundamental issues including extensive donor cell death during acute phase after SkMs engraftment, failure of SkMs to adopt cardiac phenotype and transient ventricular arrhythmias subsequent to SkMs transplantation which require serious considerations. This review will provide profound analysis of merits and limitations of SkMs as the choice cells for heart cell therapy and will summarize the potential of genetic and pharmacological manipulation SkMs to enhance their therapeutic efficacy for myocardial repair.

Keywords: Cells, cardiac, heart, myocardium, skeletal myoblasts.

BACKGROUND

Despite the recent progress in the pharmacological and surgical interventions to salvage the functional and hibernating myocardium, morbidity and mortality following heart failure remain significantly high [1]. Extensive loss of cardiomyocytes through apoptosis and left ventricular dysfunction are the common features of heart failure. Subsequent to infarction, myocytes in the peri-infarct region undergo compensatory hypertrophy in order to support the compromised left ventricular contractile function. Even though rewarding in the beginning, this soon becomes maladaptive and results in apoptotic loss of hypertrophied myocytes and progressive infarct size expansion. Moreover, the neurohormonal changes

*Corresponding author: E-mail: haiderkh@ucmail.uc.edu

Atta-ur-Rahman / M. Iqbal Choudhary (Eds.)

which occur as part of the intrinsic repair mechanism accentuate the left ventricular remodeling process which is characterized by changes in extracellular matrix and expanded area of fibrosis [2].

The long standing dogma about the heart as being terminally differentiated organ has been challenged recently. There is mounting evidence that cardiomyocytes are capable of re-entering into cell cycle and become mitotically active in response to myocardial ischemia [3,4]. The existence of resident cardiac stem and progenitor cells and their possible superior efficacy to repair infarcted hearts has been reported [5,6]. Nonetheless, their number is too little to fully compensate for the functional cardiomyocytes loss which occurs especially in the large infarcts. Myocardial ischemia mobilizes stem cells from bone marrow niches which show tropism for the ischemic myocardium and home into the damaged myocardium where they undergo milieu dependent differentiation to adopt cardiac phenotype [7]. Their cumulative contribution in the intrinsic repair process is however, too small to fully replenish the lost myocytes unless supplemented by an outside intervention for effective therapeutic outcome [8].

MOLECULAR AND CELLULAR APPROACHES FOR HEART FAILURE TREATMENT

Various molecular and cellular approaches have been devised for treatment of the failing heart. Initiation of mitosis in cardiomyocyte through oncogene induction or cyclin A2 delivery [9] and genetic modulation of fibroblasts in scar tissue to form contractile cells by forced expression of genes that mediate its myogenic differentiation have been attempted [10,11]. A less complex but innovative approach however, is heart cell therapy which invovles introduction of stem cells into scar tissue with angiogenic as well as myogenic potential. This compensates for the cardiomyocytes loss and positively influences the remodeling process [7,8,12,13]. In some case stem cell therapy has been combined with cytokine administration or with simultaneous therapeutic gene delivery to promote their effectiveness in the cardiac repair process [14]. The objective of stem cell therapy is to repopulate post-infarction scar tissue with contractile cells that can supply sufficient cell number and be functionally integrated into the host tissue. Furthermore, this strategy is based on assumption that grafted cells demonstrate a normal response to physiological stimuli. The cells employed for cardiac repair can be grossly classified as non-myogenic and myogenic (Table **1**).

Non-Myogenic Cells

Non-myogenic cells including fibroblast, endothelial and endothelial progenitor cells have been implanted into the heart to assess their feasibility and effectiveness for cardiac repair. Nevertheless, their use has been restricted to pre-clinical experimental studies only. Myogenic differentiation of fibroblasts was achieved by forced expression of MyoD gene [15,16]. The primary cardiac fibroblasts overexpressing MyoD showed overly expressed myogenic markers such as myosin heavy chain and myocyte enhancer factor-2 [15]. These observations suggested that cardiac fibroblasts can be converted into potentially functioning myocytes. The risk in the use of fibroblasts as donor cells is that even few of the non-transduced fibroblasts in the cell preparation will produce undesired fibrosis in the infarcted heart after engraftment. A safer approach would be the transduction of MyoD gene into myocardial granulation tissue in the scar area and replace the fibrous tissue with myocytes.

Table 1. Cell Types for Cellular Cardiomyoplasty

Cell Type	Reference
Non-myogenic cell	
Fibroblast	[15,16]
Endothelial cell	[17, 114]
Myogenic cell	
Smooth muscle cell	[24,25]
ES cell	[32,33]
Cardiomyocyte	
Fetal	[70,115]
Neonatal	[116,117]
HL-1	[19]
AT-1	[20]
BMDSC	[118-120]
Skeletal myoblast	
C2C12	[73,105]
L6	[95]
Primary culture	[43,62,95]

BMDSC: Bone marrow derived stem cells; **ES:** Embryonic stem cells.

Aortic endothelial cells and endothelial progenitor cells derived from bone marrow are vasculogenic and angiogenic [17]. Endothelial progenitor cells can also adopt cardiac phenotype with similar electrical activity upon co-culture with cardiomyocytes [18]. Nevertheless, these results have not been reported by other research groups. Considering the fact that endothelial cells may be recruited from peripheral circulation by angiogenic factors, transplantation of endothelial progenitor cells may not be an ideal strategy to strengthen the injured heart at least in terms of myogenesis.

Stem Cells with Myogenic Potential

The cells with inherent ability to form muscle fibers have been extensively investigated for their possible use in heart cell therapy. The underlying principle for their application is to replace scar tissue with new muscle to enhance contractile function of the injured myocardium. Cardiomyocytes may be the most ideal cells for replacement of scar tissue and were the first ones used for cellular cardiomyoplasty. The transplanted cardiomyocytes formed stable grafts in the recipient heart [19]. Their main advantage was the ability to develop functional links with the host cardiomyocytes [20,21]. Indeed, their use during cell transplantation studies provided the much needed proof-of-concept evidence regarding safety and effectiveness of the approach in experimental myocardial infarction models. Despite having near ideal characteristics, ethical concerns and availability issues remained major hurdles in their clinical application. Currently, cardiomyocytes derived from embryonic stem cells and induced pluripotent stem cells (iPS cells) are gaining popularity as an alternative source of cardiomyocytes for engraftment [22,23]. On the other hand, smooth muscle cells are better substitute of cardiomyocytes as donor cells and may form contractile tissue in the myocardial scar and improve the pump function in infarcted heart [24,25]. In comparison with these cells, bone marrow stem cells have a consenting nature and are capable to differentiate into various cell lineages [26,27]. The multifactorial mechanism of their reparative action is related to neomyogenesis, angiogenesis and the release of paracrine factors [28,29]. Encouraged by the results from pre-clinical studies, bone marrow stem cell engraftment has also been carried out in patients as an adjunct procedure with routine interventional procedure or as a sole therapy [30,31]. Notwithstanding the encouraging results about their safety and effectiveness, intriguing questions have been raised viv-a-vis their multilineage potential, age related altered activity in elderly patients and long-term safety and efficacy when used as a sole therapy. These issues warrant intensive investigation. Additionally, pluripotent embryonic stem cells can differentiate into cardiomyocytes and endothelial cells [32,33] albeit the ethical issues, religious considerations, immunological complexities and teratoma formation significantly reduce enthusiasm for their clinical use [32]. Cardiomyocytes derived from embryonic stem cells may thus provide a safer source of cells for transplantation to avoid untoward effects associated with the use of embryonic stem cells [34,35]. More recently, regenerative potential of cardiac stem cells is being explored to for possible use in heart cell therapy [14].

SkMs ENGRAFTMENT FOR CARDIAC REPAIR

SkMs are muscle-building cells, which are endogenous to the human body and maintain the regenerative potential of skeletal muscle. Upon activation by appropriate stimulus, SkMs re-enter into cell cycle, differentiate into myotubes and eventually form new muscle fibers capable of contraction. Their use in the heart cell therapy avoids ethical issues, tumorigenesis, immunological considerations and availability problems [36]. Ease of in vitro propagation and that too without pre-mature differentiation helps to achieve the required number of cells before transplantation. SkMs have been isolated from various species such as mice, rat, rabbit, sheep, pigs and humans. They have been characterized and investigated for their potential to repair infarcted heart in experimental animal models (Table **2**) and clinical studies (Table **3**).

SkMs TRANSPLANTATION FOR CARDIAC REPAIR IN EXPERIMENTAL ANIMALS

Since the pioneering work of Marelli and colleagues, SkMs have been extensively studied in regenerative medicine for cardiac repair in various small as well as large experimental animal heart models [37] . Although, the mechanism by which implanted SkMs improve heart function remain undetermined, this is considered to be multifactorial: (1) Inhibiting scar formation within the infarct area by providing a body of viable cells (2) they have the potential to actively contribute to myocardial contractility (3) by providing a scaffold [38] to support the weakened infarcted wall and attenuate remodeling process by preservation of remote matrix architecture [39] and (4) *via* release of multiple growth factors which may act in paracrine fashion to protect host myocytes [40]. (5) A newer concept in this regard is that SkMs transplantation brings about increased in situ oxygenation in cells in the infarcted heart [41]. The myocardial pO2 changes were detected with oxygen-sensing paramagnetic spin probes (OxySpin) and measured by electron paramagnetic resonance (EPR) spectroscopy [42].

Table 2. **Animal Studies of SkMs Transplantation for Cardiac Repair**

Model	Animal	Cell Source	RAO	Pre-treatment	References
Normal	mice	C2C12	I/A	No	[121]
	syngenic	IMI	No		[70]
	rat	L6	IMI	Heat Shock	[95]
	syngenic	IMI	No		[51]
	rabbit	autologous	ICI/IMI	No	[43]
	pig	autologous	EV	No	[122]
Cryoinjury	rat	xenogenic	IMI	VEGF expression	[74]
	syngenic	IMI	No		[116]
	neonatal	IMI	No		[50]
	rabbit	autologous	IMI	No	[38,43]
	dog	autologous	IMI	No	[37]
Ligation	rat	syngenic	IMI	Connexin 43	[110]
	neonatal	IMI	No		[45,104]
	autologous	IMI	No		[85]
	pig	xenogenic	IMI	VEGF	[62]
	sheep	autologous	IMI	No	[49]
Toxin	rat	syngenic	ICI	No	[123]
	sheep	autologous	IMI	No	[124]
Ischemia	pig	xenogenic	IMI	No	[61]
Hypertrophy	rat	syngenic	IMI	cardiotrophin-1	[112]

E/V: endoventricular; I/A: Intra-arterial administration; ICI: Intra-coronary infusion; IMI: Intra-myocardial injection; ROA: Route of administration; VEGF: Vascular endothelial growth factor.

A landmark study by Taylor and colleagues demonstrated the effectiveness of SkM transplantation for improvement of cardiac function in rabbit heart model of croy-injury [43]. Islands of elongated, striated cells which retained characteristics of skeletal and cardiac muscle cells were found in the infarct region with subsequent improvement in regional contractility. Functional studies also showed an improvement and compliance in cryoinfarcted myocardium after SkMs implantation. Interestingly, improved diastolic compliance was observed prior to systolic performance *via* neomyogenesis in the cryo-

Table 3. Clinical Trials Using SkMs as Donor Cells for Cardiac Repair

Research gp.	AP	Patients	Cell Number	Marker/Purity	Results
[57]	CABG	10	Average $871x10^6$	CD56+/86%	Improved NYHA (2.7 to 1.6), LVEF from 23.8% to 32.1% with systolic thickening. Four patients had VT and implanted with an automatic internal cardioverter-defibrillator (AICD).
[106]	CABG or LVAD	12+CABG 6+LVAD	$10\sim300\ x10^6$	CD56/43-98%	LVEF increased from 21% to 29%. One patient had non-sustained ventricular tachycardia.
[86]	CABG. Autologous serum for cell culture	12	Average 221×10^6	CD56/65.6%	LVEF from 35.5% to 53.5% with improved regional contractility. Amiodarone for 3 months to prevent cardiac arrhythmia.
[60]	Transcatheter	5	$196\pm105x10^6$	Desmin /55±30%	LVEF increased from 36% to 41% (3 months) and 45% (6 months). Increased wall thickening. No serious adverse events. One patient had non-sustained VT.
[107]	Percutaneous catheter	2	Average $1.2x10^6$	Unavailable	Uneventful recovery of both patients. No ventricular arrhythmia.
[125]	CABG	3	Unavailable	Unavailable	Decreased LV diastolic diameter, improved LVEF by 1~11%, improved wall thickness and perfusion.
[64]	CABG	1	$374x10^6$	desmin/98%	LVEF from 30% to 37% Reduced perfusion defect.
[63]	CABG Allograft	3	110 and $120x10^6$	Desmin />98%	LVEF increased 14.6% and 10.5%. Reduced perfusion defect.
[126]	CABG Autologous serum for cell culture	20	$300\pm20x10^6$	CD56+desmin/ 78±5%	LVEF increased from 28% to 52%. Regional wall motion score index decreased from 3.1 to 1.4 in cell-treated segments. Improved NYHA from 2.5 to 1.2. No malignant cardiac arrhythmias.
[127]	CABG Autologous	10	4×10^5 to 5×10^7	Desmin / 65.4± 5.5%	LVEF increased from 35.2% to 42.0%. Sustained VT in 2 patients in the early postoperative period and in the other 2 patients after 2 weeks of follow-up. Prophylactic amiodarone used for remaining 8 patients to prevent sustained VT episodes.

AP: Adjunct procedure; **CABG:** coronary artery bypass grafting; **LV:** Left ventricle; **LVAD:** Left ventricular assist device; **LVEF:** Left ventricular ejection fraction; **NYHA:** New York Heart Association.

injured myocardium [38]. Later studies have duplicated these results and predominantly showed that morphologically, SkMs differentiated into multinucleated skeletal myotubes, formed viable myoblast implants to repopulate the infarcted heart to the extent of replacing large portion of the scar tissue [44,45]. The engraftment capacity SkMs in the scar tissue can be further enhanced by a special delivery device with the option of electrical stimulation post engraftment [46]. In the latest development, a three-dimensional hydrogel microenvironments consisting of naturally derived proteins, proteoglycans and/or polysaccharides has been proposed to embed stem cells for their delivery. The well defined 3-dimensional microenvironment improved their engraftment capacity and provided a guide for the differentiating stem cells [47]. Using a rat model of a pressure-overloaded right ventricle, transplantation SkMs sheet improved the diastolic dysfunction and suppressed ventricular fibrosis with increased capillary density [48].

Long term studies inferred that the engrafted SkMs successfully colonized the scarred myocardium and replaced fibrosis by skeletal muscle cells with the expression of myosin heavy chain for up to one year [49]. Despite encouraging results, fate of SkMs engrafted into normal or injured myocardium remained a matter of debate because they were initially reported to acquire some characteristics of cardiomyocytes [43] or retain skeletal muscle properties [50]. Furthermore, their ability to electrically couple and integrate with the host cardiomyocytes is controversial. There are reports which showed that the newly formed fibers survived as independent islands of muscle fibers in the infarcted heart without showing synchronous contractility with the host myocardium [51]. Besides myogenic differentiation, SkM also release multiple growth factors which act in paracrine fashion for recruitment of resident cardiac stem cells and stem and progenitor cells from peripheral circulation with contributory effects in myocardial regeneration and angiogenesis at the site of the cell graft. Thus, there was significantly improved regional as well as global heart function [44,45,49,52]. A causal relationship has been observed between cell number and degree of improvement; larger number of SkMs favor better prognosis in terms of improvement in cardiac function. However, this relationship may not hold well with the immortalized cell lines of SkMs which possess ability of extensive proliferation. Dose-escalation studies are therefore required to better characterize the relationship between the number of grafted cells and the functional outcome. This also brings into consideration the importance of massive donor cell death which occurs during acute phase after cell transplantation (discussed in the later part of review). Besides extensive cell death, faulty and inefficient delivery strategy significantly influences the rate of SkMs engraftment [53]. The problem can be overcome by multi-site injection strategy.

Efficacy of SkM has been compared with other types of donor cells in experimental animal heart models [54,55]. SkM or bone marrow cell transplantation resulted in a similar degree of improvement in a derivative of stroke work. Indeed, the multilineage potential of bone marrow derived stem cells remains unmatched by unipotent SkMs. Taken together; these studies provide good evidence that SkMs engraftment is safe and results in improved global contractile function.

CLINICAL STUDIES

In the light of encouraging results of pre-clinical studies, SkMs transplantation has been performed clinically on patients by various research groups, mostly for safety and feasibility assessment of the approach. Capitalizing on their first-in-human pioneering study results [56], Menasche and colleagues in France reported 10 patients who received autologous SkM engraftment as an adjunct procedure to the routine coronary artery bypass grafting (CABG) [57]. Following combined procedure of CABG and cell therapy, the patient's left ventricle ejection fraction increased from 23.8% to 32.1% with concomitant systolic wall thickening and improved New York Heart Association (NYHA) class from 2.7 to 1.6 on average. One of the 10 patients died acutely from complications unrelated to myoblast injection. There were no cell transplantation related complications except for unwanted ventricular tachycardia in 4 patients which was pharmacologically treatable. The first patient who underwent SkM engraftment died from a stroke caused by acute occlusion of the left subclavian artery at 17.5 months after SkM therapy. Immunohistological studies on the heart of this patient showed successful engraftment and survival of SkMs which formed myotubes within the infarcted myocardium [58]. These results were confirmed in a later study when autologous SkMs were injected into the hearts of the patients receiving left ventricle assist device (LVAD) implantation as a bridge to the heart replacement therapy [59]. This novel approach allowed experimental use of human heart to study the fate of donor cells post engraftment. Immunohistological studies confirmed the formation of islands of skeletal myotubes in the recipient hearts. Most of these clinical studies involved intramyocardial injection of cells.

While the intramyocardial injection of stem cells is the most straightforward strategy, intravascular delivery approach should have numerous advantages by way of greater practicality in clinical routine as it would be less invasive and obviate the need for cardiac surgery. The feasibility of trans-catheter delivery approach was adopted in 5 patients [60]. SkM transplantation was performed endocardially under NOGA-guided catheter system (Biosense-Webster, Waterloo, Belgium) in the infarcted myocardium without any adverse effects. Only one patient received an implantable cardioverter-defibrillator after transplant-tation because of asymptomatic runs of non-sustained ventricular tachycardia.

Extrapolating the results of our animal studies showing long term survival of xenomyoblasts using transient immunosuppression in porcine heart model of myocardial infarction [61,62], the first allomyoblast transplantation was performed in Russia [63]. Three patients received successful allomyoblasts transplantation supported by transient immunosuppression for two months without any untoward events. The use of SkMs from allogenic source is significant to overcome the economic and logistic concerns associated with the use of autologous SkMs. This will also provide flexibility of time frame for cell transplantation post infarction in patients which otherwise is restricted by the purification and ex-vivo expansion of the cells for each patient in the case of autologous SkMs transplantation.

The first-in-man SkMs transplantation on beating heart was carried out in Singapore [64]. Under direct vision and stabilization with the Octopus III tissue stabilizer, 3.70 x 108 autologous SkMs in 3 ml of the patient's own serum were injected into the myocardium in 20 sites on the anterior wall and near the apex on the posterior wall, in and around the infarcted myocardium.

Long-term follow-up report of the first worldwide cohort of grafted patients (n = 9) at a median 52 (18 to 58) months after cell transplantation in conjunction with CABG showed stable beneficial effects in terms of left ventricle ejection fraction and improvement in NYHA class [65]. Despite stability in clinical status as indicated by a strikingly low incidence of hospitalizations for heart failure (0.13/patient-years), the events of arrhythmia were reported in 5 patients which were controlled by medical therapy and/or on-request ACD implantation. Although these results appear supportive for a possible role of SkMs in the clinical perspective, it should not go without mention that most of the published clinical trials have been carried out as an adjunct procedure and that too without a control group of patients which poses difficulty in the assessment of true beneficial effects of SkM transplantation.

DIFFERENTIATION OF SkMs IN THE HEART: CARDIOMYOCYTES OR HETEROKARYONS?

Transdifferentiation of stem cells to adopt cardiac phenotype has been projected as the primary mechanism by which heart cell therapy contributes to improved cardiac function. There are reports in which differentiation of cells has not been observed post engraftment [51,66]. The general perception about the fate of engrafted SkMs is their development into skeletal myofibers [58,59]. The earlier observations of their milieu-dependent differentiation into cardiac muscle have failed to gather support from researchers. Later studies however proposed that SkMs became fatigue-resistant, slow twitch cardiac-like cells (not cardiac cells) in the heart, that were more suitable for a cardiac work [50]. An alternative proposed mechanism is that they fuse with host myocardium to form mosaic muscle fibers. SkMs are " fusigenic cells" and fusion between the donor and the host skeletal muscle cells to form heterokaryon is a commonly reported phenomenon observed when SkMs were transplanted for skeletal muscle repair. The ability of SkMs to fuse with cardiomyocytes to achieve similar fate is still under scrutiny. Expectedly, cell fusion may result in the rescue of damaged myocytes which otherwise undergo apoptosis and results in the formation of hybrid [67]. The hybrid cells carry genetic material from the parent fusing cells and may resemble in characteristics with them. The newly formed fusion cells may be capable of releasing biologically and therapeutically active factors into the cardiac milieu. Cell fusion has been demonstrated in vitro as well as in vivo. Despite the fact that incidence and rate of fusion between cells can be facilitated and increased by providing favorable conditions and the presence of fusogens, the electrophysiological, contractile and coupling properties of the hybrid cells remain undetermined.

In a co-culture system of neonatal cardiomyocytes and SkMs, the latter expressed cardiac troponin-T, atrial natriuretic peptide (ANP) and gap junction proteins [68]. However, these observations do not correlate well with the in vivo data. Reinecke *et al.* rebuffed the idea of transdifferentiation of SkMs into cardiomyocytes [51]. Immunofluorescent study on the human cardiac tissue receiving SkM transplantation further confirmed the absence of cardiac differentiation of the engrafted SkMs at 17.5 months after transplantation findings [56]. Quantitative analysis showed that more than 35% of these myotubes expressed myosin heavy chain (MHC) (fast isoform), while another 32% expressed MHC (slow isoform), and remaining 33% co-expressed both the MHC isoforms, with no expression of connexin-43, desmosomes and pan-cadherin. Similar results have been reported by Pagani *et al.* who showed that only skeletal myotubes were formed by the transplanted SkM [59]. Using Cre/lox reporter system to activate Lac-z only upon cell fusion, Reineke *et al.* has shown that SkMs grafting gives rise to a subpopulation of SkM-cardiomyocyte hybrid cells [69]. Similar observations have also been reported between transplanted SkMs and host myocytes in a mice model [70]. Despite some evidence in support of transdifferentiation to form cardiomyocytes and fusion to form hybrid cells; the debate continues and the fact remains that the outcome will have significant bearing on defining the underlying mechanism as to how SkMs bring about improvement in cardiac function.

SkMs AS CARRIERS OF THERAPEUTIC GENES

A novel strategy to improve effectiveness of heart cell therapy is to combine cell transplantation with therapeutic gene delivery to promote angiogenesis [71]. Myogenesis without restoration of blood flow to the infarcted myocardium may be less effective in restitution of the infarcted heart. The combined cell and gene therapy approach will achieve concurrent angiogenesis and myogenesis which is will facilitate alleviation of myocardial ischemia and improved pump function of the left ventricle. Additionally, cell based gene delivery using genetically engineered cells has more advantages including localized, steady and regulatable gene expression, and reduced inflammation [72]. SkMs are excellent carriers of therapeutic genes and have been extensively used for the delivery of genes encoding for growth factors with angiogenic potential. In a previous study, genetically modified SkMs were used for long-term delivery of recombinant transforming growth factor- β (rTGF-β) to the murine heart [73]. Immunohistological studies on the mice heart revealed the presence of grafted SkMs stably expressing TGF-β at the site of the cell graft. However, many aspects in this regard need to be explored. We have studied the potential of human SkMs carrying human VEGF165 for myogenesis and angiogenesis porcine heart model of chronic infarction [62]. Immunostaining for vWF-VIII expression showed significantly higher capillary density at low power field (x100) which was 57.13± 4.20 in VEGF-myoblast transplanted animal groups which was significantly higher than the other groups. Regional blood flow was significantly improved 6 and 12 weeks after VEGF-myoblast transplantation which was 2.41±0.11 and 3.39±0.11 ml/ min/g respectively. Furthermore, the systolic and diastolic functions were best preserved in the VEGF group after myocardial infarction. Similar results were obtained in a rat heart model of cryoinjury [74]. Keeping in view that the angiogenic cascade involves multiple growth factors and cells, therefore a single growth factor delivery may be too little to achieve the desired results. In order to overcome this deficiency, multiple gene delivery approach has been adopted [75]. Our group reported the first bicistronic adenoviral vector encoding for VEGF and angiopoietin-1; two of the main players in angiogenic cascade involved in angiogenic response and maturation of the newly formed blood vessels. SkMs were transduced with bicistronic vectors which continued to simultaneously overexpress VEGF and angiopoietin-1 post engraftment in a pig heart [76]. Double fluorescent immunostaining of the tissue sections for vWFactor-III and smooth muscle actin showed significantly higher vascular density of mature blood vessels per low power microscopic field in bicistronic vector delivered pig heart at 6- and 12-weeks. Most of these studies involve recombinant replication deficient viral vector transduction of SkMs which may have some drawbacks related with the use of viral vectors. To alleviate the safety concerns with the use of viral vectors, non-vrial vectors have been designed for genetic modulation of SkMs. However, low transfection efficiency with the use of non-viral vectors remains a big hurdle in their clinical application.

We have reported the efficiency of cationic polymer polyethylenimine (PEI) nanoparticle for genetic modulation of SkMs to over express VEGF (^{VEGF}SkMs) [77,78]. PEI is considered to be a gold standard compared to other polymers, as it facilitates effective DNA binding and protection, combined with a high endosomolytic competence, which all contribute to the superior transfection efficacy of the corresponding non-viral vectors [79,80]. ^{VEGF}SkMs continued to over express VEGF for 18 days of observation under optimized condition. Transplantation of ^{VEGF}SkMs in a rat model of acute myocardial infarction resulted in reduced cardiomyocyte apoptosis, improved wall thickness, increased neovascularization and regional blood flow in the infarcted myocardium with globally improved heart function.

Using optimized conditions for transfection of stromal cell derived factor (SDF-1α) gene into syngenic SkMs, we have shown that FuGene6 efficiently transferred human SDF-1α transgene (3:2v/w Fugene6/ human SDF, 4 h transfection) in the presence of 125 μM $ZnCl_2$ [81]. The genetically modified cells continued to over express human SDF-1α in the rat heart of acute myocardial infarction. Our results showed significant mobilization of CD31, CD34 and ckit positive cells which homed into the infarcted heart in response to the positive SDF-1α gradient developed due to overexpression of SDF-1α transgene. Heart function studies at showed improved contractile function of left ventricle and attenuation of remodeling. These results warrant for large animal studies to study the feasibility of the approach.

Taking into account that myocardial ischemia is a recurring and often progressive disease and long-term uncontrolled over-expression of VEGF results in angioma formation [82, 83], a more controlled and regulated expression of VEGF is expected to give better prognosis and abrogation of undesired effects [84]. We designed and manufactured one hypoxia-regulated VEGF plasmid (pHRE-VEGF) expression system, and investigated the efficacy of PEI nanoparticle mediated pHRE-VEGF gene transfer into rabbit SkMs for repair of acute myocardial infarction [Our unpublished data]. We found that this approach improved donor cell survival in early stage of acute myocardial infarction, increased angiogenesis and regional perfusion, and recovered left ventricular function of the infarcted heart.

CHALLENGES AND UNRESOLVED ISSUES IN SkMs TRANSPLANTATION

Ex-Vivo SkMs Purification and Culture

Purity of SkM culture is crucial for success of the procedure. Any contaminating cell population (e.g. fibroblast) in SkM preparation may jeopardize the success of the procedure and hence generate undesired results. Our study involving xenomyoblast transplantation in a porcine heart model revealed no left ventricle ventricular arrhythmia [62]. The purity of human SkMs used in our study was >95% for desmin and >93% for CD56 expression as revealed by flow cytometry. The secondary contributory factors in this regard might be related to *in vitro* processing of SkM culture [85]. Use of non-human serum in the cell culture medium might be responsible for this complication. Theoretically, the animal serum proteins get deposited on SkM' surface and serve as an antigenic trigger for immunological adverse effects that intrigue the incidence of arrhythmia. Although missing a clear link between the use of animal proteins for *in vitro* culture of SkMs and their arrhythmogenic behavior, expansion of SkMs *in vitro* using autologous human serum clearly showed uneventful transplantation of cells and recovery of the patients [86,87]. Moreover, the culture conditions need to be optimized for undifferentiated propagation of SkMs *in vitro* while still retaining their differentiation competence post transplantation [88].

Donor Cell Death and Pro-Survival Strategies

Substantial donor cell death during the early phase after engraftment is one of the prime challenges confronting heart cell therapy [89]. A significantly high percentage of SkMs undergoes necrosis within hours after transplantation, thus compromising the optimal outcome of the procedure. In some of the reported studies, more than 70–80% of the cultured SkMs were lost within 48-72 hours after transplantation [90-92]. Pagani *et al.* showed a meager 1% survival of the transplanted SkM in patient hearts [59]. Although the underlying cause of the unusually high and accelerated cell mortality after cell transplantation generally remains undefined, it is considered as multifactorial [58]. Potential contributing factors include mechanical injury associated with the transplantation procedure, maladaptation in the ischemic environment at the site of the scar tissue and host inflamematory response. Skuk *et al.* have determined the role of immune cells on the early death of donor cells following SkMs transplantation using outbreed mice as host for transplantation of primary cultured muscle cells and T-antigen-immortalized SkM [93]. No net loss of the donor cells was observed from 1 hour to 7 days. However, there was a brief neutrophil invasion within 48 hours followed by macrophage infiltration from day 1 to day 7.

Considering that cell survival may greatly enhance the effectiveness of transplantation therapy, several remedial approaches have been suggested. Physiologically relevant hyperthermia has been shown to selectively overexpress heat shock protein-70 in cardiac myoblasts and thus confers protection against oxidant stress [94,95]. Transplantation of genetically modulated SkMs to over-express interleukin-1 receptor antagonist showed better survival [90]. Similarly, exhaustion of host C3 complement significantly increased the initial endurance of donor SkMs [92,96]. Use of cyclosporine or FK506 gives improved survival of SkMs [97]. Transient immunosuppression may give long-term retention of allogenic SkMs [62]. Using transient immunosuppression starting 5 days prior to and until 6 weeks after human SkMs transplantation, we observed that xenomyoblasts successfully survived in porcine heart for up to 7 months of observation. This lends credence to the interesting concept that human SkMs under certain well defined engraftment conditions enjoy a conditionally immunoprivileged status. Down regulation of major histocompatibility complex class- I and II markers on SkMs during the process of differentiation also contribute to the survival of cells by escaping the host immune response [98]. Administration of growth factors promoting angiogenesis would improve blood perfusion in the scar thus leading to the longer term survival of the cell graft. Treatment of donor cells with survival enhancing factors prior to transplantation has been proposed to protect the cells against apoptosis in the host tissue [99]. Ischemic preconditioning has been shown to improve tolerance in various body tissues including the heart [100]. These effects can be mimicked by the use of pharmacological mimetics of ischemic preconditioning. Our group has adopted this novel approach having powerful cytoprotective effects with heart cell therapy to overcome the problem of extensive SkMs death post transplantation [101]. Our study demonstrated that preconditioning was extremely effective to promote SkMs survival under oxidative stress *in vitro* as well as *in vivo* in experimental rat model of acute myocardial infarction. Besides cytoprotection *via* upregulation of survival signaling, preconditioning induced the cells to release paracrine factors which promoted angiomyogenesis in the heart resulting in an overall improvement in the indices of LV heart function.

Electromechanical Coupling and Arrythmogenicity

Cardiac cells are electrically coupled with each other via specialized junctions which are composed of hexamers of the protein connexin-43. As a choice donor cells in the heart cell therapy, it is imperative that the donor SkMs should achieve morpho-functional integration with the host cardiomyocytes. Such integration of SkMs will ensure un-fluttered electrical conduction in the heart without arrhythmogenicity subsequent to SkMs engraftment. Indeed, N-cadherin and connexin-43 are expressed by SkMs in culture in their undifferentiated state but this expression is down-regulated following as soon as SkMs start to differentiate [102]. Using a novel micropatterned cell pair assay, Pedrotty and colleagues have shown that connexin43 and N-cadherin are expressed in different cell pairs [103]. Nevertheless, the frequency and spatial distribution of connexin-43 and N-cadherin significantly depend on multiple factors such as the coupling protein being studied, the length of the formed cell contact, and the cell types involved in coupling. Similarly, the microenvironmental factors in the infarcted heart also contribute to the downregulation of connexin-43 expression in SkMs post engraftment.

Engraftment of SkMs in normal and injured heart was initially motivated by the optimism that transplanted cells would undergo myogenic differentiation and integrate with the host tissue to actively participate in left ventricle contractile function. In order to achieve this end-point, the engrafted cells are required to adopt the right orientation to follow host myocardial architecture such that they synchronously contract with the host myocardium and increase its pump activity. Finally, the grafted cells should also express the appropriate electromechanical properties to couple with the host cardiomyocytes. On the contrary, analysis of the SkMs graft-host myocardium junction failed to demonstrate any evidence for coordinated mechanical or electrical coupling between neofibers of skeletal origin and host cardiomyocytes thus contributing passively in the contractile activity of the heart [104,105]. Consequently, side-effects have been reported in some patients after SkM transplantation in terms of transient period of electrical instability which leads to ventricular arrhythmias [57,106]. On the other hand, SkMs transplantation has also been reported as event free procedure without any complications [87,107]. More so, even within the same study group of patients receiving SkMs treatment, only a few develop arrhythmia whereas the others have event free SkMs engraftment (Table **3**). The controversy regarding arrhythmogenic nature of SkMs continues unabated and carefully designed animal studies have been conducted to address this issue. In a canine model of postinfarction congestive heart failure, transplantation of autologous SkMs did not effect the rhythmic stability of the heart as was indicated by insignificant change in ventricular arrhythmias as compared to the controls animals [108]. The mechanism of arrythmogenicity after SkMs transplantation is generally related to the different electrophysiological characteristics of cardiomyocytes and SkMs. The newly formed electrically uncoupled skeletal myofibers in the heart offer a barrier to the electrical impulse propagation. Once SkMs have developed into skeletal myofibers with slow twitch characteristics which are well-suited for cardiac workload, myocardial electrical stability is restored. A recent study by Fouts et al has highlighted the fact that SkM injection into areas of normal myocardium results in slowing of conduction velocity, which may be pro-arrhythmic [109]. Hence, the results should motivate a careful assessment of injection sites in clinical trials of SkMs transplantation. One noteworthy contributory factor for arrhythmogenicity is related with patients' history. Patients resuscitated from a sustained ventricular arrhythmia have a high risk of recurrence. In order to decrease the incidence of ventricular arrhythmias, it has been advocated that the patients should be temporarily maintained on prophylactic anti-arrhythmic medication after SkMs transplantation. Oral amiodarone treatment for 3 months has been reported to decrease the incidence of cardiac arrhythmias [86]. Some other considerations include optimal cell number, route of administration and more importantly, selection of the patient population who are suitable candidates SkMs therapy.

In an interesting new development to exploit their myogenic potential, SkMs were transduced to over-express connexin-43 to facilitate improved electrical coupling of the donor SkMs with host cardiomyocytes. The results showed that the genetically modified SkMs for connexin-43 successfully formed intercalated discs with host CM [110]. Since significant improvement of damaged heart function has been well-documented even without the formation of gap junctions, the question remains that is it really necessary to over-express connexin-43 in SkMs [111].

SUMMARY AND FUTURE DIRECTIONS

SkMs engraftment into the infarcted myocardium is a potential therapeutic approach for mitigating pathological remodeling after myocardial infarction. Their inability to adopt cardiac phenotype may not be helpful in myocardial regeneration albeit their myogenic differentiation provide the much needed support as a scaffold to the infarcted left ventricle wall and prevents its dilatation. These beneficial effects have already been reported in pre-clinical and clinical studies. The urgency of its adoption for routine clinical practice will be determined by the outcome of the ongoing double blinded multi-center clinical trials with appropriate endpoints. Despite these inspiring results, impending skepticism on some of the fundamental but important issues has hampered its progress to the routine clinical application. The underlying mechanism of ventricular arrhythmias subsequent to SkMs engraftment and its relation especially with SkMs transplantation remains undefined. Whether occurrence of ventricular arrhythmia is cell-type dependent or it is a consequence of cell engraftment in general remains to be elucidated. Perfection in transplantation techniques and the development of novel strategies aimed at improved retention and survival of donor cells at the site of the graft would significantly contribute to the effect-tiveness of this approach. The optimal time for SkMs engraftment following myocardial infarction, the most efficient route of administration, number of cells to be injected, autologous *vs.* allogenic SkMs are some of the other issues which need to be defined. Combining SkMs engraftment with other modalities of intervention such as gene therapy for cardioprotection and angiogenesis may lead to significantly improved overall outcome in patients with heart failure [71,112,113].

ACKNOWLEDGEMENTS

This work was supported by National Institutes of Health grants # R37-HL074272; HL-23597; HL70062 and HL-080686 (to M.A).

REFERENCES

[1] Arjomand H, Cohen M, Ezekowitz MD. Combination antithrombotic therapy with antiplatelet agents and anticoagulants for patients with atherosclerotic heart disease. J Invasive Cardiol 2004; 16: 271-278.

[2] Sadoshima J, Izumo S. The cellular and molecular response of cardiac myocytes to mechanical stress. Annu Rev Physiol 1997; 59: 551-571.

[3] Beltrami AP, Urbanek K, Kajstura J, *et al.* Evidence that human cardiac myocytes divide after myocardial infarction. N Engl J Med 2001; 344: 1750-1757.

[4] Kajstura J, Leri A, Finato N, Di Loreto C, Beltrami CA, Anversa P. Myocyte proliferation in end-stage cardiac failure in humans. Proc Natl Acad Sci USA 1998; 95: 8801-8805.

[5] Leri A, Kajstura J, Anversa P. Cardiac stem cells and mechanisms of myocardial regeneration. Physiol Rev 2005; 85: 1373-1416.

[6] Dawn B, Guo Y, Rezazadeh A, *et al.* Postinfarct cytokine therapy regenerates cardiac tissue and improves left ventricular function. Circ Res 2006; 98: 1098-1105.

[7] Weisel RD, Li RK, Mickle DA, Yau TM. Cell transplantation comes of age. J Thorac Cardiovasc Surg 2001; 121: 835-836.

[8] Mickle, D.; Li, R.; Weisel, R.D.: US20070031389A1 (**2007**).

[9] Chaudhry, H.W.; Wolgemuth, D.: US20070178075A1 (**2007**).

[10] Soonpaa MH, Koh GY, Pajak L, *et al.* Cyclin D1 overexpression promotes cardiomyocyte DNA synthesis and multinucleation in transgenic mice. J Clin Invest 1997; 99: 2644-2654.

[11] Engelmann GL, Birchenall-Roberts MC, Ruscetti FW, Samarel AM. Formation of fetal rat cardiac cell clones by retroviral transformation: retention of select myocyte characteristics. J Mol Cell Cardiol 1993; 25: 197-213.

[12] Rosenthal N, Tsao L. Helping the heart to heal with stem cells. Nat Med 2001; 7: 412-413.

[13] Chande M. Stem cells get to the heart of the matter. Lancet 2001; 357: 1099.

[14] Anversa, P.: US20060239983A1 (**2006**).

[15] Lattanzi L, Salvatori G, Coletta M, *et al.* High efficiency myogenic conversion of human fibroblasts by adenoviral vector-mediated MyoD gene transfer. An alternative strategy for *ex vivo* gene therapy of primary myopathies. J Clin Invest 1998; 101: 2119-2128.

[16] Murry CE, Kay MA, Bartosek T, Hauschka SD, Schwartz SM. Muscle differentiation during repair of myocardial necrosis in rats via gene transfer with MyoD. J Clin Invest 1996; 98: 2209-2217.

[17] Kocher AA, Schuster MD, Szabolcs MJ, *et al.* Neovascularization of ischemic myocardium by human bone-marrow-derived angioblasts prevents cardiomyocyte apoptosis, reduces remodeling and improves cardiac function. Nat Med. 2001; 7: 430-436.

[18] Condorelli G, Borello U, De Angelis L, *et al.* Cardiomyocytes induce endothelial cells to trans-differentiate into cardiac muscle: implications for myocardium regeneration. Proc Natl Acad Sci USA 2001; 98: 10733-10738.

[19] Watanabe E, Smith DM Jr, Delcarpio JB, *et al.* Cardiomyocyte transplantation in a porcine myocardial infarction model. Cell Transplant 1998; 7: 239-246.

[20] Koh GY, Soonpaa MH, Klug MG, Field LJ. Long-term survival of AT-1 cardiomyocyte grafts in syngeneic myocardium. Am J Physiol 1993; 264: H1727-733.

[21] Muller-Ehmsen J, Whittaker P, Kloner RA, *et al.* Survival and development of neonatal rat cardiomyocytes transplanted into adult myocardium. J Mol Cell Cardiol 2002; 34: 107-116.

[22] Freund C, Mummery CL. Prospects for pluripotent stem cell-derived cardiomyocytes in cardiac cell therapy and as disease models. J Cell Biochem 2009;107: 592-599.

[23] Zhang J, Wilson GF, Soerens AG, *et al.* Functional cardiomyocytes derived from human induced pluripotent stem cells. Circ Res 2009; 104: e30-41.

[24] Yoo KJ, Li RK, Weisel RD, Mickle DA, Li G, Yau TM. Autologous smooth muscle cell transplantation improved heart function in dilated cardiomyopathy. Ann Thorac Surg 2000; 70: 859-865.

[25] Li RK, Jia ZQ, Weisel RD, Merante F, Mickle DA. Smooth muscle cell transplantation into myocardial scar tissue improves heart function. J Mol Cell Cardiol 1999; 31: 513-522.

[26] Krause DS, Theise ND, Collector MI, *et al.* Multi-organ, multi-lineage engraftment by a single bone marrow-derived stem cell. Cell 2001; 105: 369-377.

[27] Makino S, Fukuda K, Miyoshi S, *et al.* Cardiomyocytes can be generated from marrow stromal cells *in vitro*. J Clin Invest 1999; 103: 697-705.

[28] Goodell MA, Jackson KA, Majka SM, *et al.* Stem cell plasticity in muscle and bone marrow. Ann N Y Acad Sci 2001; 938: 208-218.

[29] Kinnaird T, Stabile E, Burnett MS, *et al.* Local delivery of marrow-derived stromal cells augments collateral perfusion through paracrine mechanisms. Circulation 2004; 109: 1543-1549.

[30] Tse HF, Kwong YL, Chan JK, Lo G, Ho CL, Lau CP. Angiogenesis in ischaemic myocardium by intramyocardial autologous bone marrow mononuclear cell implantation. Lancet 2003; 361: 47-49.

[31] Stamm C, Kleine HD, Westphal B, *et al.* CABG and bone marrow stem cell transplantation after myocardial infarction. Thorac Cardiovasc Surg 2004; 52: 152-158.

[32] Leor J, Gerecht-Nir S, Cohen S, *et al.* Human embryonic stem cell transplantation to repair the infarcted myocardium. Heart 2007; 93(10):1278-1284.

[33] Rufaihah AJ, Haider HK, Heng BC, *et al.* Directing endothelial differentiation of human embryonic stem cells via transduction with an adenoviral vector expressing the VEGF(165) gene. J Gene Med 2007; 9: 452-461.

[34] Behfar A, Perez-Terzic C, Faustino RS, *et al.* Cardiopoietic programming of embryonic stem cells for tumor-free heart repair. J Exp Med 2007; 204: 405-420.

[35] Davidson BP GR, Zweigerdt R, Xuiqin X, Mummery, CL, Sun W.: WO07070964A1 (**2007**).

[36] Haider H, Tan AC, Aziz S, Chachques JC, Sim EK. Myoblast transplantation for cardiac repair: a clinical perspective. Mol Ther 2004; 9: 14-23.

[37] Marelli D, Ma F, Chiu RC. Satellite cell implantation for neomyocardial regeneration. Transplant Proc 1992; 24: 2995.

[38] Atkins BZ, Lewis CW, Kraus WE, Hutcheson KA, Glower DD, Taylor DA. Intracardiac transplantation of skeletal myoblasts yields two populations of striated cells in situ. Ann Thorac Surg 1999; 67: 124-129.

[39] Farahmand P, Lai TY, Weisel RD, *et al.* Skeletal myoblasts preserve remote matrix architecture and global function when implanted early or late after coronary ligation into infarcted or remote myocardium. Circulation 2008; 118: S130-137.

[40] Formigli L, Perna AM, Meacci E, *et al.* Paracrine effects of transplanted myoblasts and relaxin on post-infarction heart remodelling. J Cell Mol Med 2007; 11: 1087-1100.

[41] Khan M, Kutala VK, Vikram DS, *et al.* Skeletal myoblasts transplanted in the ischemic myocardium enhance *in situ* oxygenation and recovery of contractile function. Am J Physiol Heart Circ Physiol 2007; 293: H2129-2139.

[42] US20070041909A1 (**2007**).

[43] Taylor DA, Atkins BZ, Hungspreugs P, *et al.* Regenerating functional myocardium: improved performance after skeletal myoblast transplantation. Nat Med 1998; 4: 929-933.

[44] Jain M, DerSimonian H, Brenner DA, *et al.* Cell therapy attenuates deleterious ventricular remodeling and improves cardiac performance after myocardial infarction. Circulation 2001; 103: 1920-1927.

[45] Tambara K, Sakakibara Y, Sakaguchi G, *et al.* Transplanted skeletal myoblasts can fully replace the infarcted myocardium when they survive in the host in large numbers. Circulation 2003; 108 (Suppl 1): II259-11263.

[46] Soykan, O.; DonoVan, M.G.: US20070106201A1 (**2007**).

[47] Stegemann, J.P.; Evan, L.J.: US20070116680A1 (**2007**).

[48] Hoashi T, Matsumiya G, Miyagawa S, *et al.* Skeletal myoblast sheet transplantation improves the diastolic function of a pressure-overloaded right heart. J Thorac Cardiovasc Surg 2009; 138: 460-467.

[49] Ghostine S, Carrion C, Souza LC, *et al.* Long-term efficacy of myoblast transplantation on regional structure and function after myocardial infarction. Circulation 2002; 106: I131-I136.

[50] Murry CE, Wiseman RW, Schwartz SM, Hauschka SD. Skeletal myoblast transplantation for repair of myocardial necrosis. J Clin Invest 1996; 98: 2512-2523.

[51] Reinecke H, Poppa V, Murry CE. Skeletal muscle stem cells do not transdifferentiate into cardiomyocytes after cardiac grafting. J Mol Cell Cardiol 2002; 34: 241-249.

[52] Ohno N, Fedak PW, Weisel RD, Mickle DA, Fujii T, Li RK. Transplantation of cryopreserved muscle cells in dilated cardiomyopathy: effects on left ventricular geometry and function. J Thorac Cardiovasc Surg 2003; 126: 1537-1548.

[53] Ott HC, Kroess R, Bonaros N, *et al.* Intramyocardial microdepot injection increases the efficacy of skeletal myoblast transplantation. Eur J Cardiothorac Surg 2005; 27: 1017-1021.

[54] Scorsin M, Hagege A, Vilquin JT, *et al.* Comparison of the effects of fetal cardiomyocyte and skeletal myoblast transplantation on postinfarction left ventricular function. J Thorac Cardiovasc Surg 2000; 119: 1169-1175.

[55] Agbulut O, Vandervelde S, Al Attar N, *et al.* Comparison of human skeletal myoblasts and bone marrow-derived CD133+ progenitors for the repair of infarcted myocardium. J Am Coll Cardiol 2004; 44: 458-463.

[56] Menasche P, Hagege AA, Scorsin M, *et al.* Myoblast transplantation for heart failure. Lancet 2001; 357: 279-280.

[57] Menasche P, Hagege AA, Vilquin JT, *et al.* Autologous skeletal myoblast transplantation for severe postinfarction left ventricular dysfunction. J Am Coll Cardiol 2003; 41: 1078-1083.

[58] Hagege AA, Carrion C, Menasche P, *et al.* Viability and differentiation of autologous skeletal myoblast grafts in ischaemic cardiomyopathy. Lancet 2003; 361: 491-492.

[59] Pagani FD, DerSimonian H, Zawadzka A, *et al.* Autologous skeletal myoblasts transplanted to ischemia-damaged myocardium in humans. Histological analysis of cell survival and differentiation. J Am Coll Cardiol 2003; 41: 879-888.

[60] Smits PC, van Geuns RJ, Poldermans D, *et al.* Catheter-based intramyocardial injection of autologous skeletal myoblasts as a primary treatment of ischemic heart failure: clinical experience with six-month follow-up. J Am Coll Cardiol 2003; 42: 2063-2069.

[61] Haider H, Jiang SJ, Lei Y, Law PK, Sim EKW. Effectiveness of transient immunosuppression using cyclosporine for xenomyoblast transplantation for cardiac repair. Transplant Proc 2004; 36: 232-235.

[62] Haider H, Ye L, Jiang S, *et al.* Angiomyogenesis for cardiac repair using human myoblasts as carriers of human vascular endothelial growth factor. J Mol Med 2004; 82: 539-549.

[63] Law PK, Fang G, Chua F, Kakuchaya T, Bockeria LA. First-in-Man myoblast allografts for heart degeneration. Int J Med Implants Dev 2003; 1: 100-155.

[64] Sim EK, Haider HK, Aziz S, Ooi OC, Law PK. Myoblast transplantation on the beating heart. Int Surg 2005; 90: 148-150.

[65] Hagege AA, Marolleau JP, Vilquin JT, *et al.* Skeletal myoblast transplantation in ischemic heart failure: long-term follow-up of the first phase I cohort of patients. Circulation 2006; 114: I108-I113.

[66] Murry CE, Soonpaa MH, Reinecke H, *et al.* Haematopoietic stem cells do not transdifferentiate into cardiac myocytes in myocardial infarcts. Nature 2004; 428: 664-668.

[67] Law, P.: EP1497410A2 (**2005**).

[68] Iijima Y, Nagai T, Mizukami M, *et al.* Beating is necessary for transdifferentiation of skeletal muscle-derived cells into cardiomyocytes. FASEB J 2003; 17: 1361-1363.

[69] Reinecke H, Minami E, Poppa V, Murry CE. Evidence for fusion between cardiac and skeletal muscle cells. Circ Res 2004; 94: e56-60.

[70] Rubart M, Soonpaa MH, Nakajima H, Field LJ. Spontaneous and evoked intracellular calcium transients in donor-derived myocytes following intracardiac myoblast transplantation. J Clin Invest 2004; 114: 775-783.

[71] Chancellor, M., Huard, J.: EP1113807A2 (**2001**).

[72] Ye L, Haider H, Jiang S, *et al.* Angiopoietin-1 for myocardial angiogenesis: a comparison between delivery strategies. Eur J Heart Fail 2007; 9: 458-465.
[73] Koh GY, Kim SJ, Klug MG, Park K, Soonpaa MH, Field LJ. Targeted expression of transforming growth factor-beta 1 in intracardiac grafts promotes vascular endothelial cell DNA synthesis. J Clin Invest 1995; 95: 114-121.
[74] Ye L, Haider H, Jiang S, *et al.* Reversal of myocardial injury using genetically modulated human skeletal myoblasts in a rodent cryoinjured heart model. Eur J Heart Fail 2005; 7: 945-952.
[75] Yau TM, Kim C, Li G, *et al.* Enhanced angiogenesis with multimodal cell-based gene therapy. Ann Thorac Surg 2007; 83: 1110-1119.
[76] Ye L, Haider H, Jiang S, *et al.* Improved angiogenic response in pig heart following ischaemic injury using human skeletal myoblast simultaneously expressing VEGF165 and angiopoietin-1. Eur J Heart Fail 2007; 9: 15-22.
[77] Ye L, Haider H, Tan R, *et al.* Transplantation of nanoparticle transfected skeletal myoblasts overexpressing vascular endothelial growth factor-165 for cardiac repair. Circulation 2007; 116: I113-I120.
[78] Ye L, Haider H, Esa WB, *et al.* Nonviral vector-based gene transfection of primary human skeletal myoblasts. Exp Biol Med (Maywood) 2007; 232: 1477-1487.
[79] Lungwitz U, Breunig M, Blunk T, Gopferich A. Polyethylenimine-based non-viral gene delivery systems. Eur J Pharm Biopharm 2005; 60: 247-266.
[80] Fischer D, Bieber T, Li Y, Elsasser HP, Kissel T. A novel non-viral vector for DNA delivery based on low molecular weight, branched polyethylenimine: effect of molecular weight on transfection efficiency and cytotoxicity. Pharm Res 1999; 16: 1273-1279.
[81] Elmadbouh I, Haider H, Jiang S, Idris NM, Lu G, Ashraf M. *Ex vivo* delivered stromal cell-derived factor-1alpha promotes stem cell homing and induces angiomyogenesis in the infarcted myocardium. J Mol Cell Cardiol 2007; 42: 792-803.
[82] Schwarz ER, Speakman MT, Patterson M, *et al.* Evaluation of the effects of intramyocardial injection of DNA expressing vascular endothelial growth factor (VEGF) in a myocardial infarction model in the rat--angiogenesis and angioma formation. J Am Coll Cardiol 2000; 35: 1323-1330.
[83] Lee RJ, Springer ML, Blanco-Bose WE, Shaw R, Ursell PC, Blau HM. VEGF gene delivery to myocardium: deleterious effects of unregulated expression. Circulation 2000; 102: 898-901.
[84] Su H, Arakawa-Hoyt J, Kan YW. Adeno-associated viral vector-mediated hypoxia response element-regulated gene expression in mouse ischemic heart model. Proc Natl Acad Sci USA 2002; 99: 9480-9485.
[85] Pouzet B, Vilquin JT, Hagege AA, *et al.* Intramyocardial transplantation of autologous myoblasts: can tissue processing be optimized? Circulation 2000; 102: III210-215.
[86] Herreros J, Prosper F, Perez A, *et al.* Autologous intramyocardial injection of cultured skeletal muscle-derived stem cells in patients with non-acute myocardial infarction. Eur Heart J 2003; 24: 2012-2020.
[87] Chachques JC, Herreros J, Trainini J, *et al.* Autologous human serum for cell culture avoids the implantation of cardioverter-defibrillators in cellular cardiomyoplasty. Int J Cardiol 2004; 95 (Suppl 1): S29-33.
[88] Yaeger, P.; Stewart, J.D.; Wentworth, B.M.: US20070086987A1 (**2007**).
[89] Pouzet B, Vilquin JT, Hagege AA, *et al.* Factors affecting functional outcome after autologous skeletal myoblast transplantation. Ann Thorac Surg 2001; 71: 844-850.
[90] Qu Z, Balkir L, van Deutekom JC, Robbins PD, Pruchnic R, Huard J. Development of approaches to improve cell survival in myoblast transfer therapy. J Cell Biol 1998; 142: 1257-1267.
[91] Merly F, Huard C, Asselin I, Robbins PD, Tremblay JP. Anti-inflammatory effect of transforming growth factor-beta1 in myoblast transplantation. Transplantation 1998; 65: 793-799.
[92] Guerette B, Asselin I, Vilquin JT, Roy R, Tremblay JP. Lymphocyte infiltration following allo- and xenomyoblast transplantation in mdx mice. Muscle Nerve 1995; 18: 39-51.
[93] Skuk D, Caron N, Goulet M, Roy B, Espinosa F, Tremblay JP. Dynamics of the early immune cellular reactions after myogenic cell transplantation. Cell Transplant 2002; 11: 671-681.
[94] Su CY, Chong KY, Chen J, Ryter S, Khardori R, Lai CC. A physiologically relevant hyperthermia selectively activates constitutive hsp70 in H9c2 cardiac myoblasts and confers oxidative protection. J Mol Cell Cardiol 1999; 31: 845-855.
[95] Suzuki K, Smolenski RT, Jayakumar J, Murtuza B, Brand NJ, Yacoub MH. Heat shock treatment enhances graft cell survival in skeletal myoblast transplantation to the heart. Circulation 2000; 102: III216-221.
[96] Hodgetts SI, Grounds MD. Complement and myoblast transfer therapy: donor myoblast survival is enhanced following depletion of host complement C3 using cobra venom factor, but not in the absence of C5. Immunol Cell Biol 2001; 79: 231-239.
[97] Pavlath GK, Rando TA, Blau HM. Transient immunosuppressive treatment leads to long-term retention of allogeneic myoblasts in hybrid myofibers. J Cell Biol 1994; 127: 1923-1932.

[98] Irintchev A, Zweyer M, Wernig A. Cellular and molecular reactions in mouse muscles after myoblast implantation. J Neurocytol 1995; 24: 319-331.
[99] Murry, C.; Laflamme, M.A.: US20070166288A1 (**2007**).
[100] Gurke L, Mattei A, Chaloupka K, *et al.* Mechanisms of ischemic preconditioning in skeletal muscle. J Surg Res 2000; 94: 18-27.
[101] Niagara MI, Haider H, Jiang S, Ashraf M. Pharmacologically preconditioned skeletal myoblasts are resistant to oxidative stress and promote angiomyogenesis via release of paracrine factors in the infarcted heart. Circ Res 2007; 100: 545-555.
[102] Balogh S, Naus CC, Merrifield PA. Expression of gap junctions in cultured rat L6 cells during myogenesis. Dev Biol 1993; 155: 351-360.
[103] Pedrotty DM, Klinger RY, Badie N, Hinds S, Kardashian A, Bursac N. Structural coupling of cardiomyocytes and noncardiomyocytes: quantitative comparisons using a novel micropatterned cell pair assay. Am J Physiol Heart Circ Physiol 2008; 295: H390-400.
[104] Leobon B, Garcin I, Menasche P, Vilquin JT, Audinat E, Charpak S. Myoblasts transplanted into rat infarcted myocardium are functionally isolated from their host. Proc Natl Acad Sci USA 2003; 100: 7808-7811.
[105] Reinecke H, MacDonald GH, Hauschka SD, Murry CE. Electromechanical coupling between skeletal and cardiac muscle. Implications for infarct repair. J Cell Biol 2000; 149: 731-740.
[106] Dib N, Michler RE, Pagani FD, *et al.* Safety and feasibility of autologous myoblast transplantation in patients with ischemic cardiomyopathy: four-year follow-up. Circulation 2005; 112: 1748-1755.
[107] Siminiak T, Grygielska B, Jerzykowska O, *et al.* Autologous bone marrow stem cell transplantation in acute myocardial infarction-report of two cases. Kardiol Pol 2003; 59: 502-510.
[108] Sherman W, He KL, Yi GH, *et al.* Myoblast transfer in ischemic heart failure: effects on rhythm stability. Cell Transplant 2009; 18: 333-341.
[109] Fouts K, Fernandes B, Mal N, Liu J, Laurita KR. Electrophysiological consequence of skeletal myoblast transplantation in normal and infarcted canine myocardium. Heart Rhythm 2006; 3: 452-461.
[110] Suzuki K, Brand NJ, Allen S, *et al.* Overexpression of connexin 43 in skeletal myoblasts: Relevance to cell transplantation to the heart. J Thorac Cardiovasc Surg 2001; 122: 759-766.
[111] Gutstein DE, Morley GE, Fishman GI. Conditional gene targeting of connexin43: exploring the consequences of gap junction remodeling in the heart. Cell Commun Adhes 2001; 8: 345-348.
[112] Toh R, Kawashima S, Kawai M, *et al.* Transplantation of cardiotrophin-1-expressing myoblasts to the left ventricular wall alleviates the transition from compensatory hypertrophy to congestive heart failure in Dahl salt-sensitive hypertensive rats. J Am Coll Cardiol 2004; 43: 2337-2347.
[113] Sugimoto T, Inui K, Shimazaki Y. Gene therapy for myocardial angiogenesis: with direct intramuscular gene transfer of naked deoxyribonucleic acid encoding vascular endothelial growth factor and cell transplantation of vascular endothelial growth factor transfected H9c2 myoblast. Jpn J Thorac Cardiovasc Surg 2003; 51: 192-197.
[114] Kim EJ, Li RK, Weisel RD, *et al.* Angiogenesis by endothelial cell transplantation. J Thorac Cardiovasc Surg 2001; 122: 963-971.
[115] Ruhparwar A, Tebbenjohanns J, Niehaus M, *et al.* Transplanted fetal cardiomyocytes as cardiac pacemaker. Eur J Cardiothorac Surg 2002; 21: 853-857.
[116] Huwer H, Winning J, Vollmar B, *et al.* Long-term cell survival and hemodynamic improvements after neonatal cardiomyocyte and satellite cell transplantation into healed myocardial cryoinfarcted lesions in rats. Cell Transplant 2003; 12: 757-767.
[117] Skobel E, Schuh A, Schwarz ER, *et al.* Transplantation of fetal cardiomyocytes into infarcted rat hearts results in long-term functional improvement. Tissue Eng 2004; 10: 849-864.
[118] Orlic D, Kajstura J, Chimenti S, Bodine DM, Leri A, Anversa P. Transplanted adult bone marrow cells repair myocardial infarcts in mice. Ann N Y Acad Sci 2001; 938: 221-229.
[119] Jiang S, Haider H, Idris NM, Salim A, Ashraf M. Supportive interaction between cell survival signaling and angiocompetent factors enhances donor cell survival and promotes angiomyogenesis for cardiac repair. Circ Res 2006; 99: 776-784.
[120] Kudo M, Wang Y, Wani MA, Xu M, Ayub A, Ashraf M. Implantation of bone marrow stem cells reduces the infarction and fibrosis in ischemic mouse heart. J Mol Cell Cardiol 2003; 35: 1113-1119.
[121] Robinson SW, Cho PW, Levitsky HI, *et al.* Arterial delivery of genetically labelled skeletal myoblasts to the murine heart: long-term survival and phenotypic modification of implanted myoblasts. Cell Transplant 1996; 5: 77-91.
[122] Chazaud B, Hittinger L, Sonnet C, *et al.* Endoventricular porcine autologous myoblast transplantation can be successfully achieved with minor mechanical cell damage. Cardiovasc Res 2003; 58: 444-450.
[123] Suzuki K, Murtuza B, Suzuki N, Smolenski RT, Yacoub MH. Intracoronary infusion of skeletal myoblasts improves cardiac function in doxorubicin-induced heart failure. Circulation 2001; 104: I213-1217.

[124] Rajnoch C, Chachques JC, Berrebi A, Bruneval P, Benoit MO, Carpentier A. Cellular therapy reverses myocardial dysfunction. J Thorac Cardiovasc Surg 2001; 121: 871-878.

[125] Zhang F, Chen Y, Yang Z, *et al.* Cellular cardiomyoplasty for a patient with heart failure. Cardiovasc Radiat Med 2003; 4: 43-46.

[126] Chachques JC, Acar C, Herreros J, *et al.* Cellular cardiomyoplasty: clinical application. Ann Thorac Surg 2004; 77: 1121-1130.

[127] Siminiak T, Kalawski R, Fiszer D, *et al.* Autologous skeletal myoblast transplantation for the treatment of postinfarction myocardial injury: phase I clinical study with 12 months of follow-up. Am Heart J 2004; 148: 531-537.

A Practical Approach to Diagnosis and Treatment of Symptomatic Thromboembolic Events in Children with Acute Lymphoblastic Leukemia: Recommendations of the "Coagulation Defects" AIEOP Working Group

Paola Giordano[†], Giovanni Carlo Del Vecchio[†], Paola Saracco°, Marco Zecca^, Angelo Claudio Molinari[#] and Domenico De Mattia[*,†]

[†]Department of Biomedicine of Evolutive Age, University of Bari, °Hematology Unit, Department of Pediatrics, University of Torino, ^Department of Pediatric Sciences, University of Pavia, [#]Thrombosis and Haemostasis Unit, Department of Haematology and Oncology, Giannina Gaslini Children's Hospital, Genova; Italy

[§]Domenico Del Principe (Roma), Moncilo Jankovic (Monza), Bruno Nobili (Napoli), Margherita Nardi (Modena), Ugo Ramenghi (Torino), Giovanna Russo (Catania), Nicola Santoro (Bari)

Abstract: Intensified treatments with multi-drug regimens are responsible for the continuously increasing survival of children with acute lymphoblastic leukaemia. However, together with the widespread use of central venous lines, they are also considered the main risk factors for the growing number of thromboembolic complications in this population.

The rate of thrombosis that was observed in 17 prospective studies was 5.2%. Due to the high survival rate, it is relevant to apply strategies to the long term survivors who overcome the disease but who experience thromboembolic complications. Specific treatment includes anticoagulants, especially unfractionated heparin and low molecular weight heparins, and thrombolytic drugs in few cases.

Guidelines for the treatment of thrombosis in childhood only became available recently, but they do not include specific clinical subsets such as children with acute lymphoblastic leukaemia. The problems involved in scheduling thrombosis treatment in children with malignancy have recently been discussed, however the paper does not provide practical diagnostic schemes or treatment schedules. Some important questions regarding optimal prevention and treatment are still unanswered. Moreover, antithrombotic therapy in these patients is quite challenging owing to the higher risk of bleeding. We believe it would be possible to propose reasoned appropriate recommendations for treating thrombosis in children with acute lymphoblastic leukaemia, looking forward for the effects of recent patents. This paper is an attempt to provide a practical guide to the diagnosis and treatment of thrombotic events in children with acute lymphoblastic leukaemia, and it is aimed at physicians who have no specific knowledge of the diagnosis and management of thrombosis and haemostasis alterations in children.

Keywords: Thromboembolism, diagnosis, treatment, pediatric, acute lymphoblastic leukaemia.

* Corresponding author: Tel: +39-080-5592276; Fax: +39-080-5592290; E-mail: demattia@bioetaev.uniba.it

[†]"Cougulation Defects" AIEOP working group

Atta-ur-Rahman / M. Iqbal Choudhary (Eds.)

1. INTRODUCTION

Average survival rates for childhood acute lymphoblastic leukaemia (ALL) increased to over 50% during the 1980s in Europe, ranging from 56% to over 90% [1, 2], due to the introduction of effective risk-adopted combination chemo-therapies. In the near future the usage of new prognostic factors such as outcome predictor in acute leukaemia 1 (OPAL1) [3, 4] will allow a better treatment.

Intensified treatments with multi-drug regimens are responsible for these results [2], but together with the widespread use of central venous lines (CVL), they are also considered the main risk factors for the increasingly observed thromboembolic complications in children with ALL [5, 6].

The prevalence of venous thromboembolic events (VTE) in children with ALL ranges from 1% to 40%, depending on how the VTE is diagnosed [7]. If it is diagnosed on the basis of clinical symptoms, the prevalence is in the 1.1%-11% range [8, 9], while x-ray screening provides a 37.5% [10] and 40% [11] prevalence rate.

A retrospective Italian study showed an 0.95% prevalence of symptomatic VTE in children with ALL who were treated according to the Associazione Italiana di Ematologia e Oncologia Pediatrica (AIEOP) ALL 91 and 95 protocols [12]. Metanalysis by Caruso et al. on 1,752 children enrolled in 17 prospective studies showed that the rate of thrombosis was 5.2% (95% CI 4.2-6.4) [13]. Due to the high survival rate, it would be relevant to apply strategies to protect children who overcome the disease but experience thromboembolic complications from the long term complications of thrombosis [14, 15].

The most frequent clinical manifestations include: deep vein thrombosis (DVT), especially in the upper venous system, and cerebral sinus venous thrombosis (CSVT) [7, 16].

The treatment phase with the highest incidence of events is the induction phase (77% - 90%), whereas reinduction has a lower incidence [8, 12].

The exact etiology of thrombosis in association with ALL is not known. Thromboembolic events (TE) are thought to result from the interaction of various factors, including effects of cancer itself, central venous line, chemotherapy and associated complications (e.g. infections, dehydration), and acquired or inherited prothrombotic defects [17-19]. Tumour cells can synthesise molecules such as cancer procoagulant and fibrinolytic molecules. Furthermore, they can interact with monocytes or macrophages by releasing inflammatory cytokines and activating endothelial cells and platelets, thus resulting in the down-regulation of anticoagulant properties and the up-regulation of procoagulant properties [20, 21]. Some studies have shown increased thrombin activation at diagnosis in children with ALL [7, 22].

The presence of a CVL may increase the risk of a TE through various effects: the presence of intravascular foreign substances, changes in venous flow, endothelial damage, CVL-associated infections [5, 6, 23-25].

Associated infectious episodes, either local CVL-related or systemic, Gram positive or Gram negative mediated are likely to increase the chance of a TE by activating platelets, serine proteases, pro-inflammatory cytokines and by causing endothelial damage [26].

Chemotherapy can influence the haemostatic system either through the direct effect of the chemotherapeutic drug or through complications like infections [21, 27]. Corticosteroids activate platelet function, asparaginase reduces the synthesis of natural anticoagulants and in combination they increase the risk of TE in children with ALL [28, 29].

The role of congenital alterations, such as Factor V Leiden G1691A (FVL), Factor II G20210A, Protein C (PC) deficiency, Protein S (PS) deficiency, Antithrombin (AT) deficiency, disfibrinogenaemia, fibrinolytic system alterations, Heparin Cofactor II deficiency, and hyperhomocysteinaemia, is not well known in children with ALL. The differences that can be found in the prevalence of the gene mutations are difficult to explain. The variations may be due to the different study populations, the type of thrombophilia being studied and the chemotherapy protocol that is used [8, 9, 12, 13, 16, 27].

In short, the main risk factors for TE in children with ALL are the disease itself and the chemotherapy it requires, that hereditary or acquired factors may or may not act upon.

In this paper, we give recommendations that are suggestions regarding clinical behaviour, and are an attempt to help the paediatrician in the diagnostic process and to determine the most appropriate treatment for thromboembolic events occurring in children with ALL. They are not to be taken as a "must-follow" standard. Applying such recommen-dations does not ensure a successful outcome in every case. The definitive decision regarding the treatment of each patient will be made by the attending clinician after careful consideration of the patient's clinical data and of the available diagnostic and treatment options.

These recommendations are based on available literature and when not present on the opinions of authors. A search of the literature was carried out in the PubMed data directory to find using these keywords: thromboembolism, diagnosis, treatment, children, acute lymphoblastic leukaemia.

2. DIAGNOSIS

The clinical suspicion is the trigger of the diagnostic work-up, which is based on history, physical examination, and instrumental and laboratory testing.

2.1. History

Background information must include data on symptoms and other possible risk factors, both hereditary and acquired, and on the type of leukaemia and treatment phase as well.

As far as family anamnesis is concerned, special attention must be paid to any TE that may have occurred in a patient's relatives (especially parents) before the age of 45 years [30]. It must be pointed out that in childhood the difference between the thrombophilic factors associated with venous thrombosis and those associated with arterial thrombosis is not so evident [5].

In addition to the leukaemia and the given treatment (mainly steroids and asparaginase) some acquired conditions can increase the thrombotic risk: use of central venous line, especially when related to the upper venous system or right atrium thrombosis [23-25]; severe dehydration (venous sinus thrombosis); central or peripheral (femoral) arterial catheters (in the event of arterial TE) infection and surgery.

2.2. Clinical Features

Clinical signs of thromboembolic complications in children vary depending on the localisation of the thrombus, the patient's age, and the building speed of the thrombus.

2.2.1 Deep Venous Thrombosis (DVT)

Usually presents with pain, change in colour and swelling of the involved limb (40% of the time in the upper venous system due to the use of CVL).

Catheter Related Thrombosis

In *catheter related thrombosis,* other possible signs include acute symptoms related to catheter occlusion (cephalalgia and swelling of the face, persistent sepsis, and pulmonary embolism). Most CVL related thromboses are actually asymptomatic or show chronic, subtle symptoms: superficial cutaneous vein dilatation beyond the proximal tract of the affected limb and/or of the thorax /abdomen.

Right Atrium Thrombosis

Usually asymptomatic and discovered during echocardiography. Clinical signs may include: CVL malfunctioning, persistent sepsis, heart failure, and onset of a new cardiac murmur.

2.2.2 Pulmonary Embolism (PE)

Pulmonary embolism is characterised by chest pain, dyspnoea, cough gasping and hemoptysis. It may be overlooked at an early stage, or misinterpreted as a lower airway infection. PE should always be taken into consideration when respiratory symptoms occur in patients with CVL.

2.2.3. Cerebrovascular Thromboembolism

Cerebrovascular thromboembolism, or ictus, or "stroke" are vascular disorders whose neurological outcomes last longer than 24 hours [31].

Vascular thrombosis (TE originating in an intracranial or extracranial vessel, or from the heart) is responsible for ischaemic "stroke", which may then evolve into a haemorrhagic one.

A vascular focal neurological deficiency (thromboembolism or vasoconstriction lasting less than 24 hours) is called a transient ischaemic attack (TIA) [31].

Cerebrovascular TE also include cerebral sinus venous thrombosis. Clinical symptoms are often age-related. Young children show irritability, a decrease in consciousness, and seizures, while older children usually have increasing headache and signs of raised intracranial pressure, focal neurological failure (hemiparesis, worsening eyesight, cranial nerve palsy, language disorders, ataxia), and seizures [32, 33].

2.2.4. Arterial TE of the Limbs

Clinical manifestations include: low temperature and paleness of the limbs, with a 10 mmHg decrease in arterial pressure of the involved limb as compared to the controlateral limb.

2.3. Radiological Investigation

They include several types of imaging, ranging from ultrasound examination and veno or arteriography to computed tomography (CT) and magnetic resonance imaging (MRI). The main investigative support techniques used in paediatrics are shown in Table **1** [34].

Table 1. Instrumental Diagnosis of Thromboembolic Events in Childhood [34 Modified]

Site of Thrombosis	Gold Standard	Current Practice
DVT in Upper venous district	Venography	• Bilateral Venography • Ultrasound scan of internal jugular veins
Lower limb DVT	Venography	• Ultrasound scan (venography is needed if doppler ultrasonography is not diagnostic)
CVL Tip	Transthoracic echocardiography Transoesophageal echocardiography	• Echocardiography • Lineogram
Pulmonary Embolism	Ventilatory/perfusional scintigraphy	• Ventilatory/perfusional scintigraphy • Spiral CT is not validated in the paediatric age yet.
Cerebral TE	Angiography	• MRI • MR Angiography
Cerebral Sinus Venous Thrombosis		• MRI • MR Angiography
Arterial Thrombosis	Angiography	If clinical symptoms are evident, positive ultrasonographic evaluation suffices to start treatment

DVT= Deep Vein Thrombosis; TE= Thromboembolic Event; CVL = Central Venous Line; MRI = Magnetic Resonance Imaging.

2.3.1. Deep VenousThrombosis

Compressive and/or doppler ultrasound is often used as the initial test to study DVT in the lower limbs and in the distal upper venous system (neck, upper limbs). In the paediatric age several factors may interfere with these examinations: reduced blood vessel diameter, decreased pulsus, the possible presence of a CVL in the seat of the thrombus which hampers the compression of the involved vein. Therefore, *venography* should be performed when echography/ultrasound examination yields negative or dubious results despite a legitimate clinical suspicion. Venography (introduction of contrast medium into the vein) should not be mistaken for lineograms (introduction of contrast medium into the CVL). The latter may prove to be useful when attempting to localise either the tip of the CVL or a clot in the tip of the catheter, but it cannot show the presence of thrombi along its intravascular external surface. Venography is indeed considered the reference standard for the diagnosis of DVT in adult patients, while the need to find a venous access makes it unfeasible in paediatric patients. A prospective evaluation [35] was carried out on children with ALL by comparing venography to doppler ultrasound in the diagnosis of asymptomatic DVT in the upper venous system. It showed that there is no single "gold standard" for studying this topic. The sensitivity of each individual test was below 80%, and the combination of the two was required to obtain accurate screening and to study the upper venous system.

The diagnosis of intrathoracic vascular system thrombosis (proximal subclavian, anonymous, upper cava) requires the use of bilateral venography or, as an alternative, spiral CT or MR angiography, since echo-colour Doppler echography fails to detect thrombosis in this area with adequate sensitivity. Both spiral CT and MR angiography are worthwhile, less invasive alternatives, even though they require sedation in younger children.

Echocardiography is an excellent method for diagnosing thrombi in the right atrium. It should be outlined that transesophageal echocardiography (TEE) has higher sensitivity than conventional transthoracic echocardiography (TTE). Nevertheless, this technique requires far more resources and operator skill than does TTE, and is easiest to perform in the unconscious patient [36].

2.3.2. Pulmonary Embolism

There is no single "best" imaging technique for PE. A positive helical CT scan confirms the diagnosis of PE while a normal ventilation perfusion (VQ) scan rules it out. In the adult literature, CT is more often obtained in patients at high risk of PE while VQ is often performed on patients at_clinical low probability of PE and with negative D-dimers [37, 38].

Pulmonary angiography is reserved for interventional procedures and diagnostic dilemmas due to its invasiveness. TEE may be considered [36] but the above considerations make it rarely feasible.

2.3.3. Cerebral TE

Conventional CT has low sensitivity for acute cerebral ischaemia, nearly 75% in the first six hours, as compared to diffusion-MRI, and may fail to reveal a significant number of CSVT [33, 39]. On the other hand, CT can accurately reveal haemorrhages, thus making it a mandatory exam in order to choose which patients should be treated with fibrinolytic drugs. Performing CT long after the acute event allows us to visualise a distinct area that has been damaged by the stroke.

MRI provides the highest resolution for detecting ischaemic changes, both in TIA and in ischaemic stroke and, compared to CT, it shows greater sensitivity in revealing posterior fossa strokes. Its sensitivity for distinguishing intracranial haemorrhage is not yet known. Several new magnetic resonance techniques, such as diffusion/perfusion weighted-MR can be employed to evaluate ischaemic stroke in the early phase. It must be pointed out that due to the need for immobility, and on account of the duration of the MRI, sedation is often required.

Arteriography remains the standard method for defining the anatomy of intra and extracranial vessels. It is also useful for evaluating carotid stenosis and the subsequent risk of stroke, and for diagnosing aneurisms, arteriovenous malfor-mations, or vasospasm after subcranial haemorrhage. The use of this technique is, however, limited in the paediatric age [40].

In the future, *Positron Emission Tomography* (PET) will allow us to collect more data on cerebrovascular diseases.

2.4. Laboratory Investigation

Laboratory diagnostics include two essential aspects: on one hand, evaluation of the state of the on-going thrombosis, and on the other, evaluation of acquired and hereditary thrombophilia. The latter must be carried out on all children who have had venous or arterial thrombosis, regardless of the circumstances surrounding the thrombosis or of the severity of the clinical manifestations.

2.4.1 Laboratory Investigations to Prove the Existence of TE

Among the laboratory investigations that can prove the existence of TE, currently, the most commonly employed one is the measurement of D-Dimers (DD). DD are specific markers of fibrinolysis secondary to fibrin formation and do not appear in fibrinogenolysis (primary hyperfibrinolysis). The clinical use of DD is widespread owing to their high sensitivity, their relatively long half-life, and to the fact that they are easy to measure. They increase during deep vein thrombosis and in disseminated intravascular coagulation (DIC), as they do in ALL and hepatic diseases as well, even without the occurrence of thrombosis. Unfortunately, DD are not sensitive and specific enough in oncology since they may also show up as false negatives [41-44], and their usefulness for diagnosis of venous thromboembolism has not been validated in children [45].

Other markers of thrombin activation such as Thrombin-Antithrombin complexes (TAT), Prothrombin fragments 1+2 and Fibrinopeptide A are less useful in clinical practice since they require radioimmunologic assay or ELISA on plasma and furthermore, they are not readily available. Thus, they are more suitable for research purposes.

2.4.2. Evaluation of Hereditary and Acquired Thrombophilia

The need to carry out screening for hereditary thrombophilia after correctly diagnosing a TE in subjects with ALL in the paediatric age has long been under debate [8, 9, 11-13, 16, 27, 46]. Nevertheless, considering the effects of treatment (replacement therapy in the event of inhibitor deficiency), and the secondary prophylaxis, most clinicians would obtain a detailed family anamnesis and would carry out the laboratory exams shown in bold characters in Table **2**, since there are no global screening tests for hypercoagulability. Interpretation of the results should take into consideration age-related reference levels [47]. Possible drug induced alterations should also be taken into account (low AT levels during prolonged heparin therapy; low PC and PS levels during oral anticoagulant therapy; low AT, PC and PS levels during treatment with L-Asp), as should pathological conditions (reduced AT, PC and PS levels in case of hepatic damage). Diagnosis of hereditary AT, PC, or PS deficiency should be confirmed by an abnormal assay result 3-6 months after the acute event and at least one month after discontinuing anticoagulant or other (Asparaginase) therapy. Identifying another relative of the proband with low inhibitor levels would be helpful, since a large number of mutations have been reported for these defects, and consequently molecular studies are not feasible on a routine basis.

Table 2. Assays to Detect Congenital or Acquired Prothrombotic Conditions

Clotting Tests	Genetic Tests	Serological Tests
Antithrombin activity	FV G506Q	Anticardiolipin and antiphospholipid Antibodies
Protein C: activity	FII G20210A	Homocysteine
Protein S: free antigen		Lipoprotein(a)
Lupus anticoagulant		Cholesterol, LDL, HDL, Triglycerides,
Resistance to Activated Protein C		
FVIII activity		
Fibrinogen (Clauss)		
Plasminogen		

Tests printed in standard type should be performed on patients with normal or negative results to the tests printed in bold and who present more than one TE, or on patients with positive family history.

Thrombophilia test interpretation is quite difficult and often marred by diagnostic over- or under- estimation. Thus, it is highly recommended that an expert paediatric haematologist should evaluate the results.

3. TREATMENT

When deciding how to treat a TE in children with ALL the physician should respect the assigned chemotherapy protocol as closely as possible, and pay careful attention to any alterations in haemostatic parameters induced by the disease and the therapies. The treatment recommendations reported herein are based upon the few available data regarding the paediatric age [48-50] and are partially gleaned from adult protocols [51, 52], or are based on the experience of AIEOP centres [12, 16, 25, 53] and other paediatric centres [6, 54]. Beyond specific antithrombotic treatment, supportive therapy (both general and specific, such as antithrombin replacement when therapy induced deficiency occurs) and rehabilitation therapy should be undertaken in all cases of TEs in children with ALL.

3.1. Overall View

Specific treatment includes anticoagulants, especially unfractionated heparin (UH) and low molecular weight heparins (LMWHs), and sometimes, though rarely, thrombolytic drugs, mainly urokinase (UK) and recombinant tissue plasminogen activator (rt-PA).

To date, only one randomised controlled study (the REVIVE trial) has compared LMWHs to UH and to coumadin for the treatment of TE in children, and almost 30% of the enrolled patients had cancer [55]. The study was closed prematurely due to issues with enrolment, and however, did not show any differences among the treatment arms.

Information about such drugs will be provided further on, and can also be found in the references [48-50]. UH has long been used to treat TE, even in children [44] but LMWHs are probably the best choice for anticoagulation in children with cancer [6, 54] and similarly in children with ALL, both for attack and for maintenance therapy. Antagonists of Vitamin K oral anticoagulants (OA) are only rarely taken into consideration due to the possible interac-tions with drugs and the problems of nutrition which reflect problems in vitamin K stores [6]. Advantages and disadvantages of each anticoagulant are reported in Table **3**.

Table 3. Anticoagulants in Children with all

Drug	Advantages	Disadvantages
Unfractionated Heparin	• Short half-life • Complete reversibility by protamine sulphate • Low cost	• Frequent monitoring • Continuous venous infusion and possible interference with other solutions
Low Molecular Weight Heparins	• Minimal monitoring • No drug interference	• No complete reversibility by protamine sulphate • Discomfort by subcutaneous injection
Oral Anticoagulants	• Oral administration	• Potential interaction with chemiotherapy • Influence of vitamin K status and liver function • Frequent monitoring

3.2. Unfractionated Heparin

UH is given with a loading bolus injection and continuous infusion and require frequent monitoring, therefore it is not ideal for the treatment of TE in children with ALL. However, we should consider using UH when anticoagulation could potentially require prompt complete reversal due to its short half-life.

Considering monitoring, it is to be noted that aPTT aiming for a prolongation to 2 to 3 times the baseline value can be used only if the baseline aPTT is within the normal range, otherwise the anti Factor Xa (anti-FXa) activity level in a range of 0.35 to 0.70 IU/mL can be used.

Bolus doses of 75 to 100 IU/Kg result in therapeutic range in 90% of children; maintenance doses are 18-20 IU/Kg/h in children > year of age. Protocol for systemic UH administration and adjustment in children (< 1 yr and > 1 yr) have been published [49].

Discontinuing heparin administration usually suffices, due to its rapid clearance. If an immediate effect is required, intravenous protamine sulphate can rapidly neutralise heparin activity thanks to its positive charge. The dose of protamine sulphate ranges from 0.25 to 1 mg for 100 IU of UH, depending on the total amount of UH received in the preceding 2 h [49].

3.3. Low Molecular Weight Heparins

LMWHs are preferable for treating children with ALL because they are much handier due to a more predictable dose response, and therefore they require less monitoring. In addition, the risk of heparin induced thrombocytopenia and osteoporosis is significantly lower with LMWHs. Nevertheless, some issues about compliance should be taken into consideration. In particular, discomfort coming from subcutaneous injection can be overcame by subcutaneous device that lasts for about a week [48] or topic analgesic creams that may be applied about one hour prior to the injection [56].

The most relevant experience involving the use of LMWHs in the paediatric age involves enoxaparin and reviparin, while there is more limited experience with dalteparin, nadroparin and tinzaparin [49, 57-59], the latter of which is not available in Italy. Although dalteparin is more rarely used in childhood than enoxaparin, it seems to have longer bioavailability, thus requiring only one daily administration [49].

The doses are extrapolated from the adult's and are based on anti FXa activity levels that ought to be between 0.50 - 1.0 IU/mL in a sample taken 4-6 hours following a subcutaneous injection. Anti-F.Xa assay should be obtained from instruments which have been regulated for the administered drug.

The dose of enoxaparin for initial treatment in children $\geq$ 2 month of age is 1 mg/Kg q12h and initial prophylactic dose is 0.5 mg/Kg q12h [49].

Invasive procedures must be avoided during the attack therapy, whereas if an invasive procedure is planned during maintenance treatment, especially a lumbar puncture, it should be performed at least 24 hours after the last LMWH dose, and the following dose should be administered 12-24 hours after completing the procedure [54]. Frequent monitoring for signs and symptoms suggesting haemorrhage should be carried out after any invasive procedure. Following lumbar puncture, special attention should be paid to signs of neurological damage (sensory motor impairment, functional alterations of the bowel and bladder), which may suggest a spinal or epidural haematoma, possibly requiring spinal marrow decompression.

Protocols for treatment of LMWH-induced bleeding by using protamine sulphate have been reported [49], however a complete reversibility by using this drug cannot be obtained.

3.3.1. Interaction with Other Drugs

Unlike OAs, LMWHs do not interfere with diet and drugs. Nevertheless, any association which may increase the bleeding risk should be avoided. Salicylates and systemically administered NSAIDs, ticlopidin and other platelet anti-aggregating drugs should not be administered. Special care must be taken when administering systemic corticosteroids, since these drugs may increase the risk of haemorrhage (high doses and long term therapy >10 days, may damage the stomach mucosa). In these cases adequate gastroprotection is recommended and clinical surveillance must be increased. Caution is required when using dextran, since inhibiting platelet function may increase the risk of bleeding.

Thrombocytopenia may occur secondary to the disease or to the anticancer treatments. No data are available regarding the platelet count which may be considered safe for full anticoagulation. Some authors [6] proposed the following schedule:

For the first two weeks: treat children with TE in ALL with full dose LMWH, maintaining platelet count above 50 x 10^9/L.

After the first two weeks: if platelet count is between 20 and 50 x 10^9/L, halve the dose; if platelet count is below 20 x 10^9/L hold the anticoagulation until the platelet count recovers above 20 x 10^9/L.

3.4. Thrombolytic Therapy

Systemic thrombolytic therapy in children is still vexed, and there are no data that allow us to provide specific recommendations [49]. Therefore, in the presence of large thrombi that may induce life-threatening haemodynamic alterations, or that could cause organ failure, the treatment schedule should be personalised for each patient. Thrombolysis should only be undertaken if there are no contraindications, such as recent surgery or cerebral vascular accident in the previous 10 days, or invasive interventions (CVL placement, lumbar puncture, bone marrow biopsy) in the previous 72 hours. UK is the only thrombolytic drug licensed for the treatment of CVL-related thrombosis in Italy.

rt-PA has proven to be more efficient than UK in resolving CVL obstructions, it also proved to be effective when UK failed [60], and is faster at dissolving clots [61]. Therefore, it might shorten the period in which ALL patients are at increased risk for bleeding. The use of rt-PA in the paediatric age is not authorised in Italy.

Doses for fibrinolytic therapy have been reported: UK loading dose is 4,400 IU/Kg followed by a maintenance dose of 4,400 IU/Kg/h for 6-12 h; rt-PA is given without loading dose at 0.1-0.6 mg/Kg/h for 6 h [49].

Recently, the efficacy of administering a very low dose of rt-PA (0.01-0.06 mg/Kg/h) in continuous infusion for 12 to 96 hours was reported [62] in a small and varied series of children with thrombosis. This is an interesting schedule, which is probably worth using as a primary approach before switching to the standard doses in case of failure.

Appropriate replacement therapy can overcome the theoretical contraindications of platelet count below 50 x 10^9/L and fibrinogen levels lower than 100 mg/dl [48].

The management of bleeding during thrombolytic therapy is the following:

for minor bleedings, for which no transfusion is needed, press carefully and apply topic thrombin; in severe cases, for which transfusion is needed, discontinue thrombolytic therapy and infuse fresh frozen plasma (10 ml/Kg in 2h) or infuse lyophilised fibrinogen over 15 minutes (100mg/Kg) in order to increase fibrinogen activity by 70mg/dl. Administer antifibrinolytic therapy if possible.

Regardless of the dose that is administered, the size of the thrombus must be checked daily by objective imaging, and once clot dissolution is achieved thrombolytic drugs must be discontinued. Full dose therapy should be started with UH, though without bolus, or with LMWHs during or immediately after the end of thrombolysis, and should be continued for 3 months. Prolonged treatment is recommended in case of persisting risk factors (CVL, plasma or genetic thrombophilia, atrial fibrillation). See above in the LMWHs section.

Finally, some additional points are worth highlighting: PT, aPTT, fibrinogen and thrombin time should be checked 4 hours after beginning therapy and then every 12 hours afterwards; if there is no fibrinolytic response, plasminogen should be assayed and in case of low values, 15-20 ml/kg of frozen fresh plasma should be infused [48].

As far as symptomatic CVL related thrombosis is concerned, optimal management begins with CVL removal after a few days of anticoagulation. However, the child often needs the device for the management of the underlying disease. Thus if the CVL cannot be removed, initial treat-ment is suggested with thrombolytic therapy in case of symptomatic thrombosis, or with LMWH if clinical symptoms are absent [6, 25, 49].

3.5. Indications to Specific Treatment

The most common and relevant TEs requiring specific treatment (when they have recently occurred and are symptomatic) that may develop in children with ALL include: deep venous thrombosis and pulmonary embolism, thrombosis of the cerebral venous sinuses, CVL related right atrium thrombi, and arterial thrombosis. Treatment of venous thrombosis is recommended only when: 1) it is symptomatic 2) haemodynamic alterations are detectable 3) high risk for additional complications (sepsis and embolism) is confirmed.

Drugs of choice for commonest specific clinical manifestations are reported in Table **4**.

Table 4. Specific Treatment for DVT and CSVT

Clinical Manifestation	Thrombolysis	Anticoagulant Attack	Anticoagulant Maintenance
DVT	In selected cases. low dose rt-PA	LMWHs or UH	LMWHs
PE	In selected cases. UK or rt-PA	LMWHs or UH	LMWHs
CSVT	Not advisable	In absence of major cerebral haemorrhage LMWHs or UH	LMWHs

For details see text.

3.5.1. Deep Venous Thrombosis and Pulmonary Embolism

Anticoagulant Therapy

Initial treatment:	LMWHs or UH for at least ten days. [48, 49, 63]
Maintenance/secondary prophylaxis:	LMWHs for at least three months after diagnosis of the event. [48, 49, 63]

Treatment should be maintained if additional congenital or acquired risk factors are found following evaluation of each specific case. If thrombocytopenia is present, see above.

Thrombolysis should be taken into consideration in selected cases, especially in massive PE with severe haemodynamic involvement [63, 64]. Notably, a recently published paper reports the efficacy of thrombolysis with rt-PA at very low doses [62]. This report makes such a schedule feasible since it would allow patients with ALL who are at increased risk of bleeding to resume chemotherapy as soon as possible.

3.5.2 Cerebral Sinus Venous Thrombosis

Thrombolysis is not advisable for CSVT [49, 65], while anticoagulation is appropriate in the absence of major cerebral haemorrhage. According to published guidelines [49], small petechial or localised haemorrhages that are confined to an area of venous infarction are not necessarily a contraindication to anticoagulation.

Anticoagulant Therapy

Initial treatment:	LMWHs or UH for at least ten days [49, 66, 67]
Maintenance/secondary prophylaxis:	LMWHs for at least three months after diagnosis of the event [49, 66, 67]

Treatment should last longer if additional (congenital or acquired) risk factors are present, or if recanalisation is not completed after three months of therapy, following evaluation of each specific case. If thrombocytopenia is present, see above.

Instrumental monitoring (CT scan/MRI, overall view in the instrumental investigations section).

Periodic evaluation: first examination 10-15 days after diagnosis of the event. Afterwards: the patient should be evaluated again one and three months later, unless the situation requires otherwise. If no anticoagulants are administered (e.g., significant haemorrhage), then repeat MR angiography or CT at least 1 week after diagnosis in order to assess propagation of the initial thrombosis and reconsider anticoagulation.

Support therapy: support treatment should be evaluated by consulting the neurologist, and then specific rehabilitation for the neurological impairment should be taken into consideration.

3.5.3 Arterial Thrombosis

Drug of choice: UH; however, thrombolysis should be started in case of UH failure or if there is a life threatening situation or severe organ damage, but only in the absence of any contraindications [49, 50, 68].

4. PREVENTION

Few studies have addressed the possibility of preventing thrombosis in children with cancer in general, and in ALL in particular [11,55,69]. A recent study [70] comparing LMWHs and AT versus AT alone for the prevention of symptomatic venous TE in children with ALL showed that LMWHs were safe and effective in children with ALL. However based on the available information, routine prophylaxis in children with cancer is not advisable [6].

5. CURRENT AND FUTURE DEVELOPMENTS

Children are now surviving malignancies that previously resulted in mortality. Complications do however occur, including thrombosis, that result in mortality and morbidity. Many adults who have thrombosis have significant underlying illnesses (eg, cardiac disease, cancer) which decrease life expectancy. Conversely, despite underlying illnesses, children have an increasingly better chance of survival and are expected to live 6 to 8 decades following an episode of venous or arterial thrombosis. One of the most thoroughly invest-tigated areas of thrombosis in paediatric oncology is in patients with ALL, which has led to the availability of information on the additional risk factors for thrombosis in this subset. The most useful diagnostic procedures are more or less the same as in the general paediatric population. Treatment schedules however, are less well defined since antithrombotic therapy in these patients is challenging due to the higher risk of bleeding. urt ermore man important questions regarding optimal prevention and treatment are still unanswered The effect of recent and important patents on antithrombotic therapy in children are to be verified as a patent regarding an oral active factor Xa inhibitor [70] or dipyridamole [71] and other platelet antagonists [72, 73].

While properly designed studies are urgently needed to further define the epidemiology of thrombosis in different malignancies and to find the best way to diagnose and treat thrombosis in children, it is actually possible to propose suitable recommendations for treating TE in children with ALL.

6. APPENDIX: LEVELS OF EVIDENCE OF PRINCIPAL LITERATURE

The scientific soundness of sources was carefully evaluated using the grading of evidence, as previously described [74].

Principal References Dealing with Diagnosis

Level of Evidence	References
IV	[35]
V	[33, 39-41]

Principal References Dealing with Treatment

Level of Evidence	References
II	[51, 52, 55, 60, 61]
III	[59]
V	[48, 49, 52-54, 57, 61, 69]

REFERENCES

[1] Coebergh JW, Pastore G, Gatta G, Corazziari I, Kamps W. Variation in survival of European children with acute lymphoblastic leukaemia, diagnosed in 1978-1992: the EUROCARE study. Eur J Cancer 2001; 37: 687-694.

[2] Gatta G, Capocaccia R, Stiller C, Kaatsch P, Berrino F, Terenziani M. Childhood cancer survival trends in Europe: a EUROCARE Working Group study. J Clin Oncol 2005; 23: 3742-3751.

[3] Willman C.L., Helman P., Veroff R., Mosquera-Caro M., Davidson G.S., Martin S.B., Atlas S.R., Andries E., Kang H., Shuster J.J., Wang X., Harvey R.C., Haaland D.M., Potter J.W.: US20060063156A1 (**2006**)

[4] Willman, C.L., Helman, P., Veroff, R., Mosquera-Caro, M., Davidson, G.S., Martin, S.B., Atlas, S.R., Andries, E., Kang, H., Shuster, J.J., Haaland, D.M., Potter, J.W., Wang, X., Harvey, R.C.: WO2004053074A2 (**2004**).

[5] Journeycake JM, Manco-Johnson MJ. Thrombosis during infancy and childhood: what we know and what we do not know. Hematol Oncol Clin North Am 2004; 18: 1315-1413.

[6] Bajzar L, Chan AK, Massicotte MP, Mitchell LG. Thrombosis in children with malignancy. Curr Opin Pediatr 2006; 18: 1-9.

[7] Athale UH, Chan AK. Thrombosis in children with acute lymphoblastic leukemia: part I. Epidemiology of thrombosis in children with acute lymphoblastic leukemia. Thromb Res 2003; 111: 125-131.

[8] Nowak-Gottl U, Wermes C, Junker R, *et al.* Prospective evaluation of the thrombotic risk in children with acute lymphoblastic leukemia carrying the MTHFR TT 677 genotype, the prothrombin G20210A variant, and further prothrombotic risk factors. Blood 1999; 93: 1595-1599.

[9] Mauz-Korholz C, Junker R, Gobel U, Nowak-Gottl U. Prothrombotic risk factors in children with acute lymphoblastic leukemia treated with delayed E. coli asparaginase (COALL-92 and 97 protocols). Thromb Haemost 2000; 83: 840-843.

[10] Glaser DW, Medeiros D, Rollins N, Buchanan GR. Catheter-related thrombosis in children with cancer. J Pediatr 2001; 138: 255-259.

[11] Mitchell LG, Andrew M, Hanna K, *et al.* A prospective cohort study determining the prevalence of thrombotic events in children with acute lymphoblastic leukemia and a central venous line who are treated with L-asparaginase: Results of the prophylactic antithrombin replacement in kids with acute lymphoblastic leukemia treated with asparaginase (PARKAA) study. Cancer 2003; 97: 508-516.

[12] Giordano P, Santoro N, Del Vecchio GC, Rizzari C, Masera G, De Mattia D. T-immunophenotype is associated with an increased prevalence of thrombosis in children with acute lymphoblastic leukemia. A retrospective study. Haematologica 2003; 88: 1079-1080.

[13] Caruso V, Iacoviello L, Di Castelnuovo, *et al.* Thrombotic complications in childhood acute lymphoblastic leukemia. A meta-analysis of 17 prospective studies comprising 1,752 pediatric patients. Blood 2006; 108: 2216-2222.

[14] Manco-Johnson MJ. Postthrombotic syndrome in children. Acta Haematol 2006; 115: 207-213.

[15] Goldenberg NA, Manco-Johnson MJ. Pediatric hemostasis and use of plasma components. Best Pract Res Clin Haematol 2006; 19: 143-155.

[16] Santoro N, Giordano P, Del Vecchio GC, *et al.* Ischemic stroke in children treated for acute lymphoblastic leukemia: a retrospective study. J Pediatr Hematol Oncol 2005; 27:153-157.

[17] Athale UH, Chan AK. Thromboembolic complications in pediatric hematologic malignancies. Semin Thromb Hemost 2007; 33: 416-426.

[18] Horowitz N, Brenner B. Thrombophilia and cancer. Pathophisiol Haemost Thromb 2008; 36: 131-136.

[19] Appel IM, Hop WC, van Kessel-Bakvis C, Stigter R, Pieters R. L-Asparaginase and the effect of age on coagulation and fibrinolysis in childhood acute lymphoblastic leukemia. Thromb Haemost 2008; 100: 330-337.

[20] Rickles FR. Falanga A. Molecular basis for the relationship between thrombosis and cancer. Thromb Res 2001; 102: 215-224.

[21] Sutherland DE, Weitz IC, Liebman HA. Thromboembolic complications of cancer: epidemiology, pathogenesis, diagnosis, and treatment. Am J Hematol 2003; 72: 43-52.

[22] Giordano P, Del Vecchio GC, Saracco P, *et al.* Hemostatic alterations in pediatric leukemias. Pathophysiol Haemost Thromb 2003; 33: 97-98.

[23] Massicotte MP, Dix D, Monagle P, Adams M, Andrew M. Central venous catheter related thrombosis in children: Analysis of the canadian registry of venous thromboembolic complications. J Pediatr 1998; 133: 770-776.

[24] Male C, Chait P, Andrew M, Hanna K, Julian J, Mitchell L. Central venous line-related thrombosis in children: association with central venous line location and insertion technique. Blood 2003; 101: 4273-4278.

[25] Molinari AC, Castagnola E, Mazzola C, Piacentino M, Fratino G. Thromboembolic complications related to indwelling central venous catheters in children with oncological/haematological diseases: a retrospective study of 362 catheters. Support Care Cancer 2001; 9: 539-544.
[26] Bick RL. Cancer-associated thrombosis. N Engl J Med 2003; 349: 109-111.
[27] Athale UH, Chan AK. Thrombosis in children with acute lymphoblastic leukemia. Part II. Pathogenesis of thrombosis in children with acute lymphoblastic leukemia: effects of the disease and therapy. Thromb Res 2003; 111: 199-212.
[28] Nowak-Gottl U, Heinecke A, von Kries R, Nurnberger W, Munchow N, Junker R. Thrombotic events revisited in children with acute lymphoblastic leukemia: impact of concomitant *Escherichia coli* asparaginase/prednisone administration. Thromb Res 2001; 103: 165-172.
[29] Nowak-Gottl U, Ahlke E, Fleischhack G, *et al.* Thromboembolic events in children with acute lymphoblastic leukemia (BFM protocols): prednisone versus dexamethasone administration. Blood 2003; 101: 2529-2533.
[30] Manco-Johnson MJ, Nuss R. Thrombophilia in the infant and child. Adv Pediatr 2001; 48: 363-384.
[31] Kirkham FJ. Stroke in childhood. Arch Dis Child 1999; 81:85-89.
[32] deVeber G, Andrew M, Adams C, *et al.* Cerebral sinovenous thrombosis in children. N Engl J Med 2001; 345: 417-423.
[33] Lynch JK, Hirtz DG, deVeber G, Nelson KB. Report of the national institute of neurological disorders and stroke workshop on perinatal and childhood stroke. Pediatrics 2002; 109:116-123.
[34] Revel-Vilk S, Massicotte P. Thromboembolic diseases of childhood. Blood Rev 2003; 17:1-6.
[35] Male C, Chait P, Ginsberg JS, *et al.* Comparison of venography and ultrasound for the diagnosis of asymptomatic deep vein thrombosis in the upper body in children: results of the PARKAA study. Prophylactic antithrombin replacement in kids with all treated with asparaginase. Thromb Haemost 2002; 87: 593-598.
[36] Kearon C. Diagnosis of pulmonary embolism. CMAJ 2003; 168:183-194.
[37] Goldhaber SZ. Echocardiography in the management of pulmonary embolism. Ann Intern Med 2002; 136: 691-700.
[38] Fedullo PF, Tapson VF. Clinical practice. The evaluation of suspected pulmonary embolism. N Engl J Med 2003; 349: 1247-1256.
[39] Wintermark M, Bogousslavsky J. Imaging of acute ischemic brain injury: the return of computed tomography. Curr Opin Neurol 2003; 16: 59-63.
[40] Ganesan V, Savvy L, Chong WK, Kirkham FJ. Conventional cerebral angiography in children with ischemic stroke. Pediatr Neurol 1999; 20: 38-42.
[41] Gomes MP, Deitcher SR. Diagnosis of venous thromboembolic disease in cancer patients. Oncology 2003; 17: 126-135; 139.
[42] ten Wolde M, Kraaijenhagen RA, Prins MH, Buller HR. The clinical usefulness of D-dimer testing in cancer patients with suspected deep venous thrombosis. Arch Intern Med 2002; 162:1880-1884.
[43] Lee AY, Julian JA, Levine MN, *et al.* Clinical utility of a rapid whole-blood D-dimer assay in patients with cancer who present with suspected acute deep venous thrombosis. Ann Intern Med 1999; 131: 417-423.
[44] Schutgens RE, Esseboom EU, Haas FJ, Nieuwenhuis HK, Biesma DH. Usefulness of a semiquantitative D-dimer test for the exclusion of deep venous thrombosis in outpatients. Am J Med 2002; 112: 617-621.
[45] Young G. Diagnosis and treatment of thrombosis in children: general principles. Pediatr Blood Cancer 2006; 46: 540-546.
[46] De Stefano V, Rossi E, Paciaroni K, Leone G. Screening for inherited thrombophilia: indications and therapeutic implications. Haematologica 2002; 87:1095-1108.
[47] Andrew M, Monagle PT, Brooker LA. Thromboembolic complications during infancy and childhood. Hamilton, Ont; Lewiston, N.Y.: B.C. Decker 2000.
[48] Manco-Johnson MJ. How I treat venous thrombosis in children. Blood 2006; 107: 21-29.
[49] Monagle P, Chan A, Massicotte P, Chalmers E, Michelson AD. Antithrombotic therapy in children: The seventh ACCP conference on antithrombotic and thrombolytic therapy. Chest 2004; 126: 645S-687S.
[50] Hirsh J, Raschke R. Heparin and low-molecular-weight heparin: The seventh ACCP conference on antithrombotic and thrombolytic therapy. Chest 2004; 126: 188-203.
[51] Lee AY, Levine MN, Baker RI, *et al.* Low-molecular-weight heparin versus a coumarin for the prevention of recurrent venous thromboembolism in patients with cancer. N Engl J Med 2003; 349: 146-153.
[52] Lee AY. Treatment and secondary prophylaxis of VTE in the cancer patient: current status. Pathophysiol Haemost Thromb 2003; 1: 42-43.
[53] Molinari AC, Haupt R, Saracco P, Di Marco M, Castagnola E, Fratino G. Urokinase for restoring patency of malfunctioning or blocked central venous catheters in children with hemato-oncological diseases. Support Care Cancer 2004; 12: 840-843.

[54] Wiernikowski JT, Athale UH. Thromboembolic complications in children with cancer. Thromb Res 2006; 118: 137-152.

[55] Massicotte P, Julian JA, Gent M, *et al.* An open-label randomized controlled trial of low molecular weight heparin compared to heparin and coumadin for the treatment of venous thromboembolic events in children: the REVIVE trial. Thromb Res 2003; 109: 85-92.

[56] Castagnola E, Molinari AC, Fratino G, Viscoli C. Conditions associated with infections of indwelling central venous catheters in cancer patients: a summary. Br J Haematol 2003; 121: 233-239.

[57] Nohe N, Flemmer A, Rumler R, Praun M, Auberger K. The low molecular weight heparin dalteparin for prophylaxis and therapy of thrombosis in childhood: a report on 48 cases. Eur J Pediatr 1999; 158:134-139.

[58] White RH, Ginsberg JS. Low-molecular-weight heparins: are they all the same? Br J Haematol 2003; 121: 12-20.

[59] Massicotte MP. Low-molecular-weight heparin therapy in children. J Pediatr Hematol Oncol 2001; 23:189-194.

[60] Haire WD, Atkinson JB, Stephens LC, Kotulak GD. Urokinase versus recombinant tissue plasminogen activator in thrombosed central venous catheters: a double-blinded, randomized trial. Thromb Haemost 1994; 72: 543-547.

[61] Choi M, Massicotte MP, Marzinotto V, Chan AK, Holmes JL, Andrew M. The use of alteplase to restore patency of central venous lines in pediatric patients: a cohort study. J Pediatr 2001; 139:152-156.

[62] Wang M, Hays T, Balasa V, *et al.* Low-dose tissue plasminogen activator thrombolysis in children. J Pediatr Hematol Oncol 2003; 25: 379-386.

[63] Chan AK, deVeber G, Monagle P, Brooker LA, Massicotte PM. Venous thrombosis in children. J Thromb Haemost 2003; 1: 1443-1455.

[64] Manco-Johnson MJ, Nuss R, Hays T, Krupski W, Drose J, Manco-Johnson ML. Combined thrombolytic and anticoagulant therapy for venous thrombosis in children. J Pediatr 2000; 136: 446-453.

[65] Chalmers EA, Gibson BE. Thrombolytic therapy in the management of paediatric thromboembolic disease. Br J Haematol 1999; 104: 14-21.

[66] DeVeber G, Chan A, Monagle P, *et al.* Anticoagulation therapy in patients with sinovenous thrombosis. Arch Neurol 1998; 55: 1533-1537.

[67] Johnson MC, Parkerson N, Ward S, deAlarcon P. Pediatric sinovenous thrombosis. J Ped Hematol Oncol 2003; 25: 312-315.

[68] Streif W, Monagle P, South M, Leaker M, Andrew M. Spontaneous arterial thrombosis in children. J Pediatr 1999; 134:110-112.

[69] Elhasid R, Lanir N, Sharon R, *et al.* Prophylactic therapy with enoxaparin during L-asparaginase treatment in children with acute lymphoblastic leukemia. Blood Coagul Fibrinolysis 2001; 12: 367-370.

[70] Meister B, Kropshofer G, Klein-Franke A, Strasak AM, Hager J, Streif W. Comparison of low-molecular-weight heparin and antithrombin versus antithrombin alone for the prevention of symptomatic venous thromboembolism in children with acute lymphoblastic leukemia. Pediatr Blood Cancer 2008; 50: 298-303.

[71] Misselwitz, F., Kubitza, D., Park, S.-M., Wehling, K.: WO2006079474 (**2006**).

[72] Eisert, W., Serebruany, V.L.: WO2005113006 (**2005**).

[73] Boyer, J., Olins, G.M., Yerxa, B.R., Douglass, III, J.G.: US20067018985 (**2006**).

[74] De Mattia D, Del Principe D, Del Vecchio GC, *et al.* Acute childhood idiopathic thrombocytopenic purpura: AIEOP consensus guidelines for diagnosis and treatment. Haematologica 2000; 85: 420-424.

Recent Progress in Pharmacological Research of Antioxidants in Pathological Conditions: Cardiovascular Health

Milagros Rocha[1,2], Remedios García-Bou[2], Raul Herance[3], Antonio Hernandez-Mijares[2,4] and Victor M. Victor[*,1,2,5]

[1]*University Hospital Doctor Peset Foundation, Avda Gaspar Aguilar 90, 46017, Valencia, Spain*

[2]*University Hospital Doctor Peset, Endocrinology Service, Avda Gaspar Aguilar 90, 46017, Valencia, Spain*

[3]*High Technology Institute-PRBB, Barcelona, Spain*

[4]*Department of Medicine, University of Valencia, and Research group CIBER CB/06/02/0045 actions in Epidemiology and Public Health*

[5]*Department of Physiology and CIBER ehd, University of Valencia, Valencia, Spain*

Abstract: Antioxidants are essential, and are involved in several important biological processes such as immunity, protection against tissue damage, reproduction, growth and development. Antioxidants preserve adequate function of cells against homeostatic disturbances such as those caused by septic shock, aging and, in general, processes involving oxidative stress. Each year, many scientific articles are published describing the pharmacological and biological properties of antioxidants. This review article compiles recent findings on these properties, focusing mainly on the anti-inflammatory properties of antioxidants in different pathological areas, such as cardiovascular damage and sepsis. In relation to this process, this review focuses on the involvement of reactive oxygen and nitrogen species. Finally, the protective role of antioxidants against homeostatic disturbances such as those caused by endotoxin toxicity and cardiovascular damage, their potential clinical use, and the effects on the redox state of immune cells are discussed.

Keywords: Antioxidant, cardiovascular dysfunction, endotoxin, flavonoids, immune system, ischemia, mitochondria, *N*-acetylcysteine, NF-kB, nitric oxide, patent, peroxynitrite, reactive oxygen species, septic shock, vitamin.

INTRODUCTION

The presence of free radicals in biological materials was discovered about 50 years ago [1]. Today, there is a large body of evidence indicating that patients in hospital intensive

*Corresponding author: Tel: 0034961622497; Fax: 0034961622409; E-mail: victor.victor@uv.es

Atta-ur-Rahman / M. Iqbal Choudhary (Eds.)

care units (ICUs) are exposed to excessive free radicals from drugs and other substances that alter cellular reduction -oxidation (redox) balance, and disrupt normal biological functions [2, 3]. However, low levels of free radicals are also vital for many cell signaling events and are essential for proper cell function. Excess free radicals can result from a variety of conditions such as tissue damage and hypoxia (limiting oxygen levels), overexposure to environmental factors (tobacco smoke, ultraviolet radiation, and pollutants), a lack of antioxidants, or destruction of free radical scavengers. When the production of damaging free radicals exceeds the capacity of the body's antioxidant defenses to detoxify them, a condition known as oxidative stress occurs. The resultant cellular injury caused by oxidative stress has been linked to over 200 clinical disorders, many of which are seen in ICU patients units [4].

FREE RADICALS AND ANTIOXIDANTS: AN OVERVIEW

A free radical can be described as any atom or a group of atoms or molecules in which there is at least one unpaired electron in the outermost shell [5]. These free radicals are very reactive with adjacent molecules such as lipids, proteins, and carbohydrates and can cause cellular damage [6]. Paradoxically, free radicals can also be produced by many cells as a protective mechanism, for example neutrophils produce free radicals to attack and destroy pathogens, while the liver uses free radicals for detoxification [7]. However, the presence of free radicals within the body can also have a significant role in the development and progression of many disease processes for example heart disease, hypertension, cerebrovascular accidents, and diabetic complications. Any free radical involving O_2 is referred to as a reactive oxygen species (ROS) [8]. Normal cellular metabolism involves the production of ROS, and in humans, superoxide (O_2^-) is the most commonly produced free radical. Phagocytic cells such as macrophages and neutrophils are prominent sources of O_2^-. During an inflammatory response, these cells generate free radicals that attack invading pathogens such as bacteria and, because of this, the production of O_2^- by activated phagocytic cells in response to inflammation is one of the most studied free radical producing systems [5]. O_2^- produced from a one-electron reduction of O_2 can undergo either spontaneous or enzyme-catalyzed dismutation to hydrogen peroxide (H_2O_2). H_2O_2, although not technically considered an oxygen free radical, is a member of the ROS family and may selectively participate in free radical generation. The majority of the H_2O_2 is broken down to O_2 and water by the antioxidant enzyme catalase. In addition to catalase, glutathione peroxidase can also break down H_2O_2 and also any peroxides that form on lipids within the body [5]. When O_2^- reacts with nitric oxide (NO), the toxic product peroxynitrite ($ONOO^-$) is formed. Although it is true that most ROS originate from O_2^- generated as a by-product of oxidative phosphorylation (mitochondrial respiration), they differ in their mechanism of production, necessary cofactors, diffusion range, hydrophobicity, biological targets, detoxification pathways and breakdown products. O_2^- is membrane impermeant and its damaging reactions largely involve disassembly of iron-sulphur clusters in proteins. In fact, studies in rat liver lysates have shown that H_2O_2 or O_2^- alone lacked reactivity toward iron regulatory protein-1 (IRP-1), but a combined action of the two species induced reversible inactivation of IRP-1. Such an effect was attributed to direct interactions of O_2^- and H_2O_2 with a preformed pool of IRP-1, resulting in reversible modifications of -SH residues; in fact, its action would be limited to removing only iron atoms, an effect sufficient to abolish enzyme activity. The hydroxyl radical ($^{\cdot}OH$) is the most reactive of the free radical molecules [1]. $^{\cdot}OH$ damages cell membranes and lipoproteins by a process termed lipid peroxidation. In fact, lipid peroxidation can be defined as the process whereby free radicals "steal" electrons from the lipids in our cell membranes, resulting in cell damage and increased production of ROS. This process takes place in 3 stages: 1. Initiation: In a peroxide-free lipid system, the initiation of a peroxidation sequence refers to the attack of ROS (with sufficient reactivity) able to abstract a hydrogen (H) atom from a methylene group (- CH_2-), as these hydrogens have very high mobility. This attack easily generates free radicals from polyunsaturated fatty acids. ˙OH is the most efficient ROS for this attack, whereas O_2^- is insufficiently reactive.2. Propagation: A peroxyl radical is able to abstract H from another lipid molecule (adjacent fatty acid), especially in the presence of metals such as copper or iron, thus causing an autocatalytic chain reaction. The peroxyl radical combines with H to give a lipid hydroperoxide (or peroxide). This reaction characterizes the propagation stage. 3. Termination: formation of a hydroperoxide. Lipid peroxidative damage to lipids in low-density lipoprotein (LDL) plays an important role in atherosclerosis [9]. To protect against oxidative damage, organisms have developed a variety of antioxidant defenses that include proteins, compounds such as vitamins, and specialized antioxidant enzymes. Antioxidants can be described as substances capable of counteracting the damaging effects of oxidation in body tissues. Antioxidants are divided in general into two classes based on mechanisms of action: 1. chain-breaking antioxidants, such as Vitamin E and betacarotene, "break the chain" of free radical formation by donating an electron to stabilize an existing free radical. In general, they act by reacting with peroxyl radicals. 2. preventive antioxidants are enzymes that scavenge initiating radicals before they start an oxidation chain. Chain-breaking antioxidants are found in the blood and the fluids of the extracellular space, where preventive antioxidant enzymes are absent or present in very small quantities [8]. These small-molecule antioxidants include both water and lipid-soluble varieties. The lipid-soluble antioxidants are located in the cellular membranes and lipoproteins, whereas the water-soluble antioxidants are present in the aqueous environments, such as fluids inside cells and in the blood. Preventative antioxidant enzymes inside the cell are an important defense against free radicals. The main enzymatic "scavengers" responsible for the prevention of ROS formation and oxidation are superoxide dismutase (SOD), catalase, and glutathione peroxidase. SOD is found in virtually every oxygen-based organism, and its major function is to catalyze the dismutation of O_2^- to H_2O_2. This reaction is generally considered to be the body's primary antioxidant defense because it prevents further generation of free radicals. In humans, the highest levels of SOD are found in the liver, adrenal gland, kidney, and spleen [10]. Catalase and glutathione peroxidase both work to detoxify O_2^- reactive radicals by catalyzing the formation of H_2O_2 derived from O_2^-. The liver, kidney, and red blood cells possess high levels of catalase, which helps to detoxify chemicals in the body. The water-soluble tripeptide-thiol glutathione also plays an important role in a variety of detoxification processes. Glutathione is found in millimolar concentrations in the cell cytosol and other aqueous phases, and readily interacts with free radicals, especially the hydroxyl radical, by donating a hydrogen atom. This reaction provides protection by neutralizing reactive hydroxyl radicals that are thought to be a major source of free radical pathology, including cancer [11]. Glutathione is also an essential co-factor for antioxidant enzymes. Below, the data is summarized regarding some of the most frequently antioxidants in pathologies which implicate free radicals production such as sepsis and cardiovascular dysfunction. These pathogenesis generally involve impairment in endothelial function.

SEPSIS AND SIGNALING PATHWAYS

Serious infections trigger systemic inflammatory response and can result in sepsis. It is believed that sepsis and therefore septic shock are due to the inappropiate increase in the innate immune response *via* circulating and tissue inflammatory cells, such as monocytes/ macrophages and neutrophils. These cells normally exist in a nonactivated state but are rapidly activated in response to bacteria, their products or inflammatory mediators, to become highly active phagocytes. In doing so, they can contribute to the development of injuries by producing mediators such as cytokines and ROS. In fact, sepsis induces a dysfunction in immune cells [12-14]. As most infections occur primarily in the tissue and not in the blood stream, extravasation of leukocytes is essential to bring inflammatory cells and foreign pathogens into contact. This requires both a chemotactic gradient and coordinated up-regulation of endothelial and inflammatory cell adhesion molecule expression (ICAM). Leukocytes have only a finite life-span at the inflammation site. Neutrophils rapidly undergo apoptosis to be cleared by inflammatory macrophages, which themselves emigrate from the inflamed site during the resolution phase. Thus, a successful inflammatory event requires not only appropriate activation of cells and mediators with subsequent phagocytosis and removal of the exciting stimulus, but also a consequent elimination of the inflammatory cells and debris to allow the tissues to reform a normal architecture and function.

LIPOPOLYSACCHARIDE (LPS) SIGNALING

The molecular mechanisms by which LPS induces gene activation, and hence inflammatory mediator expression, have been reviewed recently [15]. LPS of Gram-negative organisms induces macrophages to secrete cytokines, which in turn activate T, and B cells to upregulate the adaptive immune responses. Toll-like receptor 4 (TLR4) is the LPS receptor and its stimulation induces nuclear factor kB (NF-κB) activation. The activation of NF-κB involves phosphorylation and degradation of IkB, an inhibitor of NF-κB, which allows the translocation of NF-κB heterodimers to the nucleous to bring about its action. The NF-κB/IkB system exerts transcriptional regulation on proinflammatory genes encoded for various adhesion molecules and cytokines. Most of these genes have functional NF-κB binding elements in their promoter regions. Activation of NF-κB leads to the induction of NF-κB binding elements in their promoter regions. Activation of NF-κB leads to the induction of NF-κB dependent effector genes such as TNFα, IL-1, chemokines, adhesion molecules and also ROS production. All these biologically active molecules/factors produce modifications in blood flow, and aggregation of neutrophils, and platelets. This results in damaged endothelium and also coagulation abnormalities often seen in patients with sepsis and septic shock. Therefore, NF-κB is reported to be an O_2 sensor in LPS-induced endotoxemia. A schematic representation of the LPS/NF-κB pathway is illustrated in (Fig. **1**).

Accordingly, there is a need to improve our understanding of IkB degradation and for the identification of modulators of this degradation process for use in treating diseases associated with activation of NF-κB. Some patent compounds satisfy these needs and further provide other related advantages by using modulating agents that comprise a recognition domain for E3 ubiquitin ligase, a necessary factor for ubiquitin-controlled IκB degradation [16, 17]. In addition, some patents have been developed in order to counteract the effect of other important mediator in sepsis, TNFα. For example, [18] shows that anti-TNF antibodies, fragments and regions thereof, which are specific for human TNFα, are useful for *in vivo* diagnosis and therapy of a number of TNFα-mediated pathologies and conditions. Further, polynucleotides coding for murine and chimeric antibodies, methods of producing the antibody, methods of use of the anti-TNF antibody, or fragment, region or derivative thereof, in immunoassays and immunotherapeutic approaches are described.

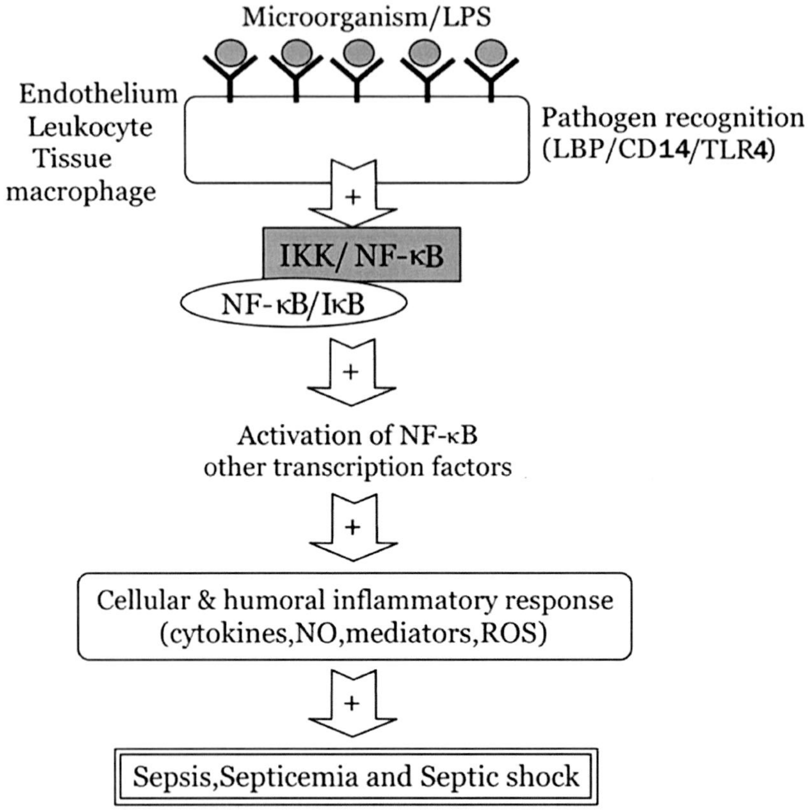

Fig. (1). Schematic diagram of LPS-induced signalling pathway of the host inflammatory response in monocytes, macrophages and neutrophils. For a detailed explanation of this figure see text. NF-κB, nuclear factor κB; LPS, lipopolysaccharide; LBP, LPS-binding protein; CD14, CD14 surface receptor; TLR4, Toll like receptor 4; IKK-NF-κB, IκB kinase-NFκB pathway; NF-κB-IkB, NF-κB inhibitory protein IκB; complex MAPK, mitogen-activated protein kinase pathway.

FREE RADICALS AND ANTIOXIDANTS IN SEPSIS

The pathogenetic sequence of reactions mediated by endotoxin (LPS) leading to the development of sepsis involves ROS [12-13, 19]. Among ROS, ˙OH either singly or in combination with $ONOO^-$, leads to tissue damage often observed during septic injury. Inactivation of these damaging radicals by antioxidants or NO inhibitor(s) may be helpful application of these agents as drugs in humans has not been fully successful.

The sources of ROS during sepsis are: (1) the mitochondrial respiratory chain. (2) the metabolic cascade of arachidonic acid. (3) the protease-mediated enzyme xanthine oxidase. (4) granulocytes and other phagocytes activated byco complement, bacteria, endotoxin, lysosomal enzymes, etc. (5) Other oxidases mainly NADPH oxidase. Under normal physiological conditions, the majority of ROS are formed during cellular respiration and by activated phagocytic cells, including neutrophils, involved in the inflammatory response. ROS have physiologically essential roles in mitochondrial respiration, prostaglandin production pathways and host defense [20]. The electron reduction of O_2 occurs in the mitochondrial electron transport system of all aerobically respiring cells. The enzyme catalyzing this reaction (cytochrome c oxidase or Complex IV) contains the transition metals iron and copper in its active site. These ions can be paramagnetic and contain stable unpaired electrons. By using the unpaired electrons in these transition metals to control the O_2 reactions, mitochondria prevent the unwanted release of ROS. In sepsis, there are several potential sources of ROS, including the mitochondrial respiratory electron transport chain, xanthine oxidase activation as a result of ischemia and reperfusion, the respiratory burst associated with immune cell activation, arachidonic acid metabolism and NADPH oxidase. In fact, activated immune cells produce O_2^- as a cytotoxic agent as part of the respiratory burst *via* the action of membrane-bound NADPH oxidase on O_2. The increase of ROS after LPS challenge has been demonstrated in different models of septic shock in peritoneal macrophages and lymphocytes [12-13,19]. This disturbance in the balance between pro-oxidants (ROS) and antioxidants in favor of the former is characteristic of oxidative stress in immune cells in response to endotoxin. In this context, a typical behavior of these cells under an oxidative stress situation implies changes in different immune functions such as an increase in adherence and phagocytosis and a decrease in chemotaxis [12-15,19]. Neutrophils play a crucial role in the primary immune defense against infectious agents. They have several well established functions, which include phagocytosis and the production of ROS. However, in addition to the microbicidal activity, neutrophils can also damage the host by disrupting tissue integrity and function. In fact, neutrophils are activated and increased in number during sepsis as a means to control infection, but may, also be destructive to the tissue. Because of this dual role, targeting therapies for sepsis may involve inhibiting or enhancing neutrophil function. Neutrophils and macrophages also produce NO, which can react with O_2^- to produce peroxynitrite ($ONOO^-$), itself a powerful oxidant, which may decompose to form $HO^{\cdot}$. Under ischemic conditions followed by subsequent reperfusion, the enzyme xanthine oxidase catalyzes the formation of uric acid with the co-production of O_2^-, whose release results in the recruitment and activation of neutrophils and their adherence to endothelial cells. During oxidative stress, damage mediated by ROS can occur. Oxidation of DNA and proteins takes place, along with membrane damage due to lipid peroxidation, leading to alterations in membrane permeability, modification of protein structure and functional changes [21].

ANTIOXIDANT DEFENSES

Antioxidants are central to the redox balance in the human body. They do not act in isolation, but synergistically with other classes of molecules. Primary antioxidants prevent oxygen radical formation, by either removing free radical precursors or by inhibiting catalysis, e.g. the enzymes glutathione peroxidase and catalase. Secondary antioxidants react with ROS which have already been formed, either to remove or inhibit them, e.g. vitamins C and E. Endogenous antioxidant defenses exist in a number of locations, namely intracellularly, on the cell membrane and extracellularly [5]. The immune system is highly reliant on accurate cell-cell communication for optimal function, and any damage to the signaling systems involved will result in an impaired immune responsiveness. Oxidant-mediated tissue injury is a particular hazard to the immune system, since phagocyte cells produce ROS as part of the defense against infection. Therefore, adequate amounts of neutralizing antioxidants are required to prevent damage to the immune cells themselves. For example, vitamin A deficiency can affect the function of different cells in the immune system. Different studies have reported defects in phagocytic activity (defect in chemotaxis, adhesion and the ability to generate ROS in neutrophils) and impairment of T and B cell function. In general, improvement of immune function and increased resistance to infection is observed in vitamin A-deficient hosts after supplementation [22]. Several patents have described antioxidant treatment in order to improve immune function by diet before or during oxidative stress situations such as: U.S. Pat. No. 4,981,844 [23] discloses a method of improving the immune response in patients comprising the ingestion of a diet that provides 20-60 kilo calories per kg of patient body weight and wherein 20-80% of the calories are derived from linoleic acid. The Alexander *et al.* patent also teaches the consumption of from 100-1000 IU per day of vitamin E. U.S. Pat. No. 5,556,644 [24] discloses a multi-nutrient nutritional supplement designed to be effective in increasing immunity and decreasing the instances and severity of infection among the elderly. This patent specifically teaches the consumption of a nutritional supplement having recited levels of various vitamins and minerals. The patent more specifically teaches the consumption of the nutritional supplement by the elderly to improve their immunological status.

U.S. Pat. No. 5,444,054 [25] discloses a nutritional product for patients suffering from ulcerative colitis or inflammation of the colon. The nutritional product utilizes an oil blend containing specified fatty acids and a source of indigestible carbohydrate. The indigestible carbohydrate is disclosed as being metabolized to short-chain fatty acids by microorganisms present in the human colon. U.S. Pat. No. 5,223,285 [26] discloses a liquid nutritional product that contains a specific lipid blend for pulmonary patients. This patent discloses that the lipid should have a particular ratio of n-6 to n-3 fatty acids. Further, this reference describes a nutritional product containing quantities of nutrients having antioxidative properties *in vivo*. Examples of such antioxidative nutrients include b- carotene, vitamin E, vitamin C, selenium and taurine.

U.S. Pat. No. 4,871,768 [27] describes a dietary supplement that contains a structured glyceride comprising n-3 fatty acids and medium chain fatty acids. This patent describes synthetic triglycerides or structured lipids that provide a high energy fat source and fatty acids that assist in fighting infection. This patent also describes a method of minimizing the effects of infection and minimizing the effects of subsequent infection by administering a diet containing 10-80% by weight of an oil-based fraction comprising glycerol, fatty acids and combinations thereof, wherein 50-90% of the fatty acids are caprylic acid, capric acid or mixtures thereof and 10-50% by weight of n-3 fatty acids. This reference teaches that the dietary supplement will not prevent the onset of infections, however, it will promote survival of infected patients. This patent fails to suggest that stress-induced down regulation of the immune system can be lessened by a nutritional composition that comprises (1) a structured glyceride; and (2) an antioxidant system comprising of at least vitamin E, vitamin C, selenium and β-carotene. Other patents have included similar compounds in order to treat diabetes or other pathologies [28]. U.S. Pat. No. 4,607,052 [29] describes triglycerides wherein specific polyunsaturated acyl fragments are present at the sn-2 position of the glycerol molecule. The structured lipids of Mendy *et al.* are described as being useful for the treatment of lipid digestion problems, metabolic diseases, nutritional deficiencies, hypertension and in conditions where immune modulation is desired. There is neither teaching nor suggestion in the Mendy *et al.* patent that a structured glyceride, when combined with a specific antioxidant system, would be effective in reducing the immunosuppression typically seen in animal models subjected to stress. De Michele *et al.* [30] describes a patent directed to the discovery of immunonutritional products that are useful in reducing the immunological system suppression that results from stress. The stress may be in the form of physical exertion, mental exhaustion, disease states and the like. In one embodiment, the invention relates to a nutritional composition comprising a structured glyceride component and an antioxidant system. This nutritional composition has been shown to be highly effective in reducing immune system downregulation or dysregulation as a result of stress. As previously described, the SOD enzymes are a family of metalloenzymes which rapidly promote the conversion of O_2^- to H_2O_2. Three forms of SOD are recognized to be important: copper-zinc SOD (cytoplasmic-located), manganese SOD (mitochondrial-located) and extracellular SOD (extracellular matrix-located). Catalase and glutathione peroxidase, a selenium containig enzyme which requires the presence of reduced GSH for its action, both catalyze the conversion of H_2O_2 to H_2O. GSH also has direct antioxidant activity, through donation of hydrogen ions, to repair damaged DNA. Oxidative stress and modulation on GSH/GSSG (GSSG=oxidized GSH) levels also up-regulate gene expression of several other antioxidant proteins, such as manganese SOD, glutathione peroxidase, thioredoxin (Trx) and metallothionein. The hydrophobic lipid interior of membranes require a different spectrum of antioxidants. Fat-soluble vitamin E (α-tocopherol) is the most important antioxidant in this environment. β-carotene, lycopene and co-enzyme Q have also been implicated as membrane antioxidants. Lipid soluble antioxidants are important in preventing membrane polyunsaturated fatty acids from undergoing lipid peroxidation, which leads to loss of membrane integrity. ROS may also be present in the extracellular compartment, especially as a result of neutrophil activation. The plasma and red cell components of blood both act as antioxidants; red cells have a copper-zinc SOD-dependent pathway for the inactivation of O_2^-, and catalase and glutathione peroxidase for dealing with H_2O_2. A number of metal-binding plasma proteins function as valuable antioxidants in addition to their transport roles, including apotransferrin, lactoferrin and caeruloplasmin. Albumin is also effective *via* its oxidizable thiol group, which permits radical scavenging, and the binding of reactive transition metal ions. A number of important smaller molecules are present in the plasma, which act as secondary antioxidants. These include vitamin E, vitamin C, uric acid and bilirubin. Vitamin C interacts with O_2^- to form dehydroascorbic acid. Vitamin C may also reduce Fe^{3+} to Fe^{2+}, which can then be involved in iron-catalyzed hydroxyl generation, thereby implicating vitamin C as both pro-oxidant and an antioxidant. Vitamin C exerts anti-inflammatory effects in human and animal studies. Vitamin E is an important nutrient for maintaining the immune system, and plays a role in the differentiation of immature T cells in the thymus. Many groups have investigated the possibilities of quenching ROS production in different pathologies which involve oxidative stress. In this regard, there are several approximations to modulate arachidonic acid metabolism. For example, the compounds heterocyclo-alkylsulfonyl pyrazoles and sulfonyl heteroaryl triazoles have demonstrated anti-inflammatory/analgesic properties [31]. Both compounds are reported to control cycloxygenase (COX) in different pathogenic situations. Other approximations to control free radical production, include compounds such as hydroxyguanidines which control the enzyme xanthine oxidase in different pathogenic situations that include sepsis as well as ischemic diseases, hypoxia or arrhytmias [32]. In reference to another important source of free radicals, NADPH oxidase, there are several patents which have demonstrated excellent results to modulate this enzyme such as o-methoxycatechol (apocynin) [33], as well as in another method [34], another patent has demonstrated that compositions derived from low molecular weight GTPbinding proteins (LMWG), mastaparan, GAP proteins, and related peptides can regulate the oxidative burst [35]. This method contemplates compositions useful in inhibiting activation of NADPH oxidase or in promoting GDP/GTP exchange and therefore inhibits O_2^- production in phagocytic cells, reducing the severity of inflammation and inflammatory disorders.

EFFECTS OF NITRIC OXIDE

NO is synthesized from L-arginine by different isoenzymes of (NOS) [36], and is implicated in a wide range of disease processes, exerting both detrimental and beneficial effects at the cellular and vascular levels. To date, three main isoforms of NOS are known: neuronal NOS (NOS-1 or nNOS), inducible NOS (NOS-2 or iNOS), and endothelial NOS (NOS-3 or eNOS). NO has been shown to play a key role in the pathogenesis of septic shock [37]. Hyperproduction of NO induces excessive vasodilation, changes in vascular permeability, and inhibition of noradrenergic nerve transmission, all characteristics of human septic shock. The recogniton of NO production by activated macrophages as part of the inflammatory process was an important milestone for assesing both the biological production of NO and the phenomenon of induction of NOS activity [38]. The observation has been extended to neutrophils [39], lymphocytes [40], and other cell types. The role of NO in the pathophysiology of endotoxic shock was advanced by Thiemermann and Vane [41], who observed that administration of the specific NOS inhibitor *N*-methyl-L-arginine (L-NMMA) decreased the severe hypotension produced by administration of LPS. Other groups simultaneously reported similar results indicating that endotoxin increases NO production [42,43] and prompted the idea that pharmacological inhibition of NOS may be useful in the treatment of inflammation and septic shock [44]. However, clinical trials using L-NMMA failed to show a beneficial effect in septic shock patients [45]. The major limitation for the use of NOS inhibitors in clinical studies is the development of pulmonary hypertension as a side effect of NOS blockade, which can be alleviated by the use of inhaled NO. However, several compounds which modulate NO synthesis have been patented in recent years, such as various inflammatory mediators that have been implicated in the induction and activation of iNOS, particularly IFNγ, TNFα, IL-1β, and platelet-activating factor (PAF) alone or synergistically [46,47]. In addition to the activation of iNOS, cytokines and endotoxin may increase NO release by increasing arginine availability through the opening of the specific y+ channels and the expression of the cationic aminoacid transporter (CAT), or by increasing tetrahydrobiopterin levels, a key cofactor in NO synthesis. Several experimental studies have demonstrated a decrease in NOS activity resulting in an impairment in endothelial-dependent relaxation during endotoxemia and experimental sepsis [48], possibly as the result of a cytokine-or hypoxia-induced shortened half-life of NOS mRNA [49], or of altered calcium mobilization [50]. Other investigators have shown increased endothelial NO release immediately after endotoxin administration either directly [51] or indirectly as suggested by the lack of effect of a specific iNOS inhibitor on the initial hypotension after endotoxin administration. NO exerts *in vitro* toxic effects including nuclear damage, protein and membrane phospholipid alterations, and the inhibition of mitochondrial respiration in several cell types. Mitochondrial impairment could also be considered as an adaptive phenomenon, decreasing cellular metabolism when the energy supply is limited. The relevance of mitochondrial impairment is, however, questionable, as administration of the NO donor SIN-1 in a canine model of endotoxic shock increased O_2 extraction capabilities [52]. The toxicity of NO itself may be enhanced by the formation of $ONOO^-$ from the reaction of NO with O_2^- [53]. Therefore, the multiple organ failure syndrome (MOFS) that often accompanies severe sepsis may be related to the cellular effects of excess NO or $ONOO^-$. In contrast, NO may protect cells from oxidative damage by scavenging ROS [54]. NO has effects in vascular tone. During sepsis and endotoxemia, convincing data suggest a pivotal role for NO in the endotoxin-induced [51] vasodilation and vascular hyporeactivity to vasoconstrictors. Both pharmacological inhibition and iNOS gene deficiency are associated with a loss of endotoxin-induced vasodilation [55]. The increased NO release has also been implicated in the diminished response to vasoconstrictors [56]. Some patents have been designed in order to modulate the levels of NO and pro-inflammatory cytokines, such as described by Singh *et al.* [57]. This invention first provides a method for suppressing the induction of iNOS and/or proinflammatory cytokines in a cell comprising contacting said cell with an effective amount of at least one induction suppressor and/or inhibitor of iNOS. Preferred cells throughout the various embodiments of the invention are lymphocytes, macrophages, endothelial cells, astrocytes, masengial cells, myocytes, Kuffer cells, epithelial cells, microglia, oligodendrocytes and neurons. Proinflammatory cytokines that are preferred include TNF-α, IL-1β, IL-2, IL-6, IL-8 and IFNγ. Inhibition of NO cytotoxicity includes inhibition of iNOS activity, production of iNOS protein, production or translation of iNOS mRNA, and inhibition of LPS- or cytokine-induced NF-κB activation in a cell. In preferred aspects of the invention, the induction suppressor and/or inhibitor of iNOS and/or proinflammatory cytokines may be selected from the group including, but not limited to, lovastatin, mevastatin, FPT inhibitor II, forskolin, rolipram, phenylacetate (NaPA), N-acetyl cysteine (NAC), pyrolidine dithiocarbamate (PDTC), 4-phenylbutyrate (4PBA), 5-aminoimidazole-4-carboxamide ribonucleoside (AICAR), theophylline, papaverine, cAMP, 8-bromo-cAMP, (S)-cAMP, and salts, analogs, or derivatives thereof. Other patents have described amidino compounds useful as NOS inhibitors in inflammation disorders [47]. Apart from this, the following individual publications disclose compounds that inhibit NO synthesis and preferentially inhibit the iNOS [58-64].

INVOLVEMENT OF NITROGEN SPECIES

ROS and reactive nitrogen species (RNS) play an important role in inflammatory processes as mediators of injury. RNS is a collective name that includes NO, $ONOO^-$, nitrogen dioxide radical (NO_2.), other oxides of nitrogen and products arising when NO reacts with O_2^-, RO. and RO2. NO reacts rapidly with ferrous iron, and at physiological concentrations, NO also binds to soluble guanylate cyclase and to another hemoprotein, cytochrome c oxidase (Complex IV), the terminal enzyme of the mitochondrial respiratory chain. NO can therefore control cellular functions *via* the reversible inhibition of respiration [65]. There are a number of reactive NO species, such as N_2O_3 and $ONOO^-$ that can also alter critical cellular components. During the first hours after injury, iNOS-mediated NO production is upregulated, producing a burst of NO that far exceeds basal levels. This overabundance of NO produces significant cellular injury *via* several mechanisms. First NO may directly promote overwhelming peripheral vasodilation, resulting in vascular decomposition; second, NO may upregulate the transcription NF-κB initiating an inflamma tory signaling pathway that, in turn, triggers numerous inflammatory cytokines [66]. NO also interacts with the O_2^- to yield $ONOO^-$, a highly reactive compound that exacerbates the injury produced by either O_2^- alone or NO alone [67]. These investigators have proposed that the $ONOO^-$ generation which occurs during fluid resuscitation in the injured subject produces cellular death by enhancing DNA single strand breakage, activating the nuclear enzyme polyADP ribose synthetase (PARS), which in turn leads to cellular energy depletion and cellular necrosis [68]. The detrimental effects of $ONOO^-$ in shock and resuscitation have been attributed to oxidation of sulfhydryl groups, the nitration of tyrosine, tryptophane, and guanine, as well as inhibition of the membrane sodium-potassium adenosine triphosphatase. In addition, PARS activation depletes NAD and thus alters electron transport, ATP synthesis, and glycolysis; more recently, studies have shown that PARS activates the caspase cascade, which results in DNA fragmentation and cellular apoptosis [66,69]. The activation of monocytes, macrophages and endothelial cells by LPS results in the expression of iNOS, and consequently increases the transformation of L-arginine to NO, which can combine with O_2^- to form $ONOO^-$, causing tissue injury during shock, inflammation and ischemia reperfusion [70]. NO also stimulates H_2O_2 and O_2^- production by mitochondria [71], possibly by inhibiting COX, thus increasing leakage of electrons from the respiratory chain. H_2O_2, in turn, participates in the upregulation of iNOS expression *via* NFkB activation [72]. Cultured astrocytes and macrophages expressing iNOS produce up to 1 mM NO, and so it is possible that catalase in these cells could be inhibited. Indeed, iNOS expression in activated astrocytes leads to increased H_2O_2 levels [73], as well as inhibition of cellular respiration at the level of COX [74]. $ONOO^-$ has also been shown to stimulate H_2O_2 production by isolated mitochondria [75]. Paradoxically, NO can also decrease ROS-produced damage that occurs at physiological levels of NO [76]. The high reactivity of NO with radicals might be beneficial *in vivo*, for example, by scavenging peroxyl radicals and inhibiting peroxidation. Additionally, it has been suggested that $ONOO^-$ may also be a signal transmitter and can mediate vasorelaxation, similarly to NO [77]. Apart from $ONOO^-$, other RNS such as nitrogen oxides and nitryl chloride are believed to cause several different pathophysiological events, including inflammation [78]. Inflammatory reactions play an important role in endotoxin-induced tissue injury. The latter is mediated by adhesion and migration of leukocytes through the endothelium, generation of ROS and RNS [79], and release of several proinflammatory cytokines by monocytes/macrophages. Local generation of RNS contributes to tissue injury. Recent studies have demonstrated that activation of the nuclear enzyme poly(ADP-ribose) polymerase-1 by RNS-mediated DNA damage is an important pathway of tissue injury in conditions associated with oxidative stress [80]. Increased formation of RNS in response to endotoxin challenge is organ specific [81]. Some authors have described different methods to avoid the harmful effects of $ONOO^-$. For example Szabo *et al.* [82] have shown that mercaptoethylguanidine and guanidine inhibitors of NOS react with ONOO and protect against $ONOO^-$ induced oxidative damage.

CARDIOVASCULAR DYSFUNCTION

There is mounting evidence for involvement of oxidative stress in the mechanism of cardiovascular disease (stroke, congestive heart failure, hypertension and coronary artery disease). Among the most numerous causes of mortality is cardiac arrest. In relation to the heart, a principal deleterious influence is arrhythmia, resulting from toxic action on membranes that are concerned with cardiac conduction. Impaired myocardial contractile function is a well documented feature in both experimental and human septic shock [83] that greatly contributes to the mortality associated with this pathological condition [84]. Several hypotheses have been proposed to explain endotoxin-induced cardiovascular failure, including microvascular dysfunction, the presence of activated leukocytes, and the effects of various circulating and/or locally produced proinflammatory cytokines, such as TNFα and IL-1β [85]. Most of the deleterious effects of proinflammatory cytokine release have been attributed to the production of large amounts of NO, which may exert detrimental effects on the myocardium in animal models, isolated hearts, and isolated cardiac myocytes [86]. Deleterious effects of NO have been mainly reported in biological conditions in which ROS generation is also enhanced [87]. The relevance of these biological events in mediating myocardial dysfunction is further illustrated by the finding that antioxidant therapy [79] and inhibition of NO synthase activity can improve endotoxin and cytokine induced contractile dysfunction [79,88]. In the cardiovascular system, endothelium, which separates the vascular wall from the circulation and the blood components, plays a key role, because it regulates vascular homeostasis by elaborating a variety of factors that act locally in the blood vessel wall and lumen, such as NO, prostacyclin and endothelin. Endothelium, in fact plays important roles in maintaining a normal vascular tone and blood fluidity, reduced platelet activity and leukocyte adhesion, and limiting vascular inflammatory reactions. In sepsis, NO may exert direct and indirect effects on cardiac function. Sustained generation of NO occurs in systemic inflammatory reactions, such as septic shock with involvement in circulatory failure. In fact, myocardial iNOS activity has been reported in response to endotoxin and cytokines and inversely correlated with myocardial performance [89]. Recently, several studies have added to the confusion surrounding the role of NO by demonstrating no effect of NO or NOS inhibition on the myocardium or on β-adrenergic responsiveness [90]. Nevertheless, in most studies, low-to-moderate doses of iNOS inhibitors restore myocardial contractility in hearts exposed to proinflammatory cytokines, whereas at higher doses, the effects are reversed. This finding may indicate that small amounts of NO produced by iNOS may be necessary to maintain contractility [90] and can be cardio-protective in experimental sepsis [91]. Systemic sepsis is associated with cardiovascular dysfunction through its effects on the myocardium, endothelium and vascular smooth muscle [92]. Moreover, during septic shock, ventricular function is altered despite normal or increased cardiac output. The number of endogenously produced inflammatory mediators which can potentially contribute to septic myocardial depression is extensive. The list includes arachidonic acid metabolites, PAF, histamine, and endorphins. Some evidence also suggests that ROS may increase the left ventricular diameter and decrease left ventricular contractility [93]. The most proposed mechanism implicated in the pathogenesis of endothelial dysfunctions is related to an increased production of ROS. This would deplete the bioavailability of NO and exacerbate local oxidative stress by directly reacting with NO to form $ONOO^-$, which in turn, would further sustain an oxidative injury to the endothelium. In human neutrophils, $ONOO^-$ triggers the downregulation of L-selectin expression, and upregulation of CD11/CD18 expression [94]. These effects are likely to be mediated by the ability of $ONOO^-$ to trigger nuclear factor NF-κB activation [95]. The development of $ONOO^-$ neutralizers has provided a more direct approach to assess the role of $ONOO^-$ in organ injury in a variety of inflammation states [82]. For example, mercaptoethylguanidine (MEG), a $ONOO^-$ scavenger and iNOS inhibitor [82] and 5,10,15,20-tetrakis(4-sulfonatophenyl)-porphyrinato iron (III) (FeTPPS), which catalyzes the isomerization of ONOO to nitrate anion [96], may decrease the generation of highly reactive intermediates such as nitrogen dioxide and OH radicals. Besides, $ONOO^-$ neutralizers may attenuate inflammatory processes associated with ischemia reperfusion [97], and infection [98]. Future investigations are necessary to see the effects in endotoxin-induced cardiovascular inflammation.

ROLE OF OXIDATIVE STRESS IN HEART FAILURE

The pathological mechanism of heart failure is complex and involves the activation of numerous secondary pathways (cytokines, oxidative stress and nitrosative stress) (Fig. **2**), which leads to: (i) abnormalities in various signaling processes, cardiac receptors and Ca^{2+} homeostasis; (ii) contractile protein desensitization; and (iii) endothelial dysfunction. Experimental and clinical studies demostrate increased production of ROS in the pathogenesis of acute heart failure. In fact, malondyaldehyde (a marker of lipid peroxidation), is increased in patients with ischemic cardiomyopathy. The generation of ROS in the myocardium is triggered by ischemia and reperfusion and by exposure of the heart to inflammatory cytokines. Source of ROS in failing myocardium includes, among

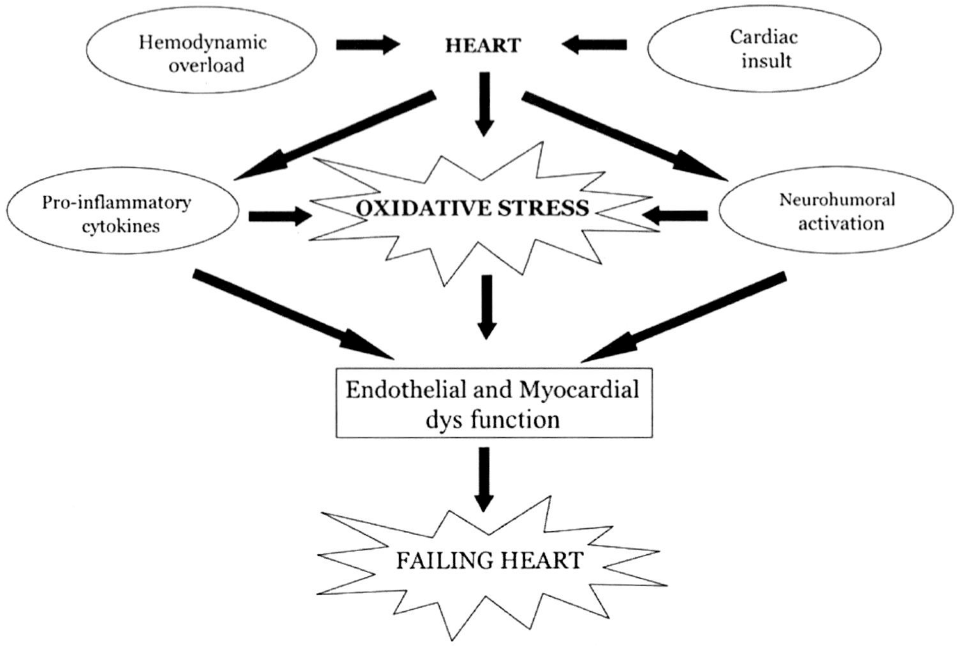

Fig. (2). Progression of heart failure and the role of oxidative and nitrosative stress.

others, xanthine and NADPH oxidoreductases, the mitochondrial electron transport chain and activated neutrophils [99]. The generation of $ONOO^-$ has been demonstrated in acute heart failure. In fact, the pathogenesis of endothelial dysfunction associated with acute heart failure involves enhanced oxidative stress from various local sources. A potential additional source of ROS is iNOS, which, paradoxically, can produce O_2. There are several mechanisms of $ONOO^-$-induced cardiac and vascular dysfunction (Fig. **3**). For example, $ONOO^-$ -induced tyrosine nitration can lead to dysfunctional nitrated proteins, whereas $ONOO^-$-induced oxidation of sulfydryl groups can inhibit important enzymes in the mitochondrial respiratory chain. Furthermore, ONOO-modified cellular proteins are subject to accelerated degradation via the proteasome and $ONOO^-$ inhibits a variety of ion pumps [100]. $ONOO^-$ also potently oxidizes various molecules including BH4, a crucial cofactor of NOS, to quinoid 5,6-dihydropterin. The generation of $ONOO^-$ also decreases the availability of NO for G-protein stimulation and vasodilation, thus further contributing to endothelial dysfunction. In addition, $ONOO^-$ can inhibit SOD, glutaredoxin and other antioxidant molecules and systems, which leads to positive feedback cycles of intracellular oxidant generation and oxidative injury [100]. $ONOO^-$ can also activate matrix metalloproteinases (MMPs) [101] and the nuclear enzyme poly(ADP-ribose) polymerase (PARP) [102]. $ONOO^-$ also triggers the expression of P-selectin, ICAM-1 and Mac-1, and mediates the cytokine-induced expression of IL-8 in human leukocytes via enhancement of NF-kB activation [100], thereby promoting proinflammatory responses. Some patents have been designed in order to modulate cardiovascular damage, by supplementing with antioxidants. For example, Zeng *et al.* (2004) [103], describe an invention with antioxidant composition comprising the constituents of a-thioctacid and vitamin E, which prevents cardiovascular and cerebrovascular diseasess. Other patents describe inventions which include an antioxidant cocktail designated to treat and prevent heart disease and stroke [104-106].

Besides heart failure, ROS and vascular oxidative stress have been involved in hypertension and atherogenesis. Compelling experimental evidence indicates that ROS play an important pathophysiological role in the development in atherogenesis and therefore in hypertension. This is due, in large, to oxidative stress and decreased NO bioavailability in the vasculature and to ROS-mediated cardiovascular remodeling. Atherosclerosis, a chronic inflammatory disease of the arterial wall, is a major cause of morbidity and mortality from cardiovascular disease in much of the world's population. For this reason, we would like to mention some important patents in the treatment of these pathologies. For example, Morawalla *et al.* [107] describes the medicinal properties of *Terminalia arjuna* in alleviation of various health related disorders, showing cardio-protective principles. In other patent, De Simone [108] describes an antioxidant combination composition to protect from oxidative stress in cardiovascular damage. The composition includes: L-carnitine inner salt, acetyl L-carnitine inner salt, α-lipoic acid, coenzyme Q10, vitamin E and selenomethionine.

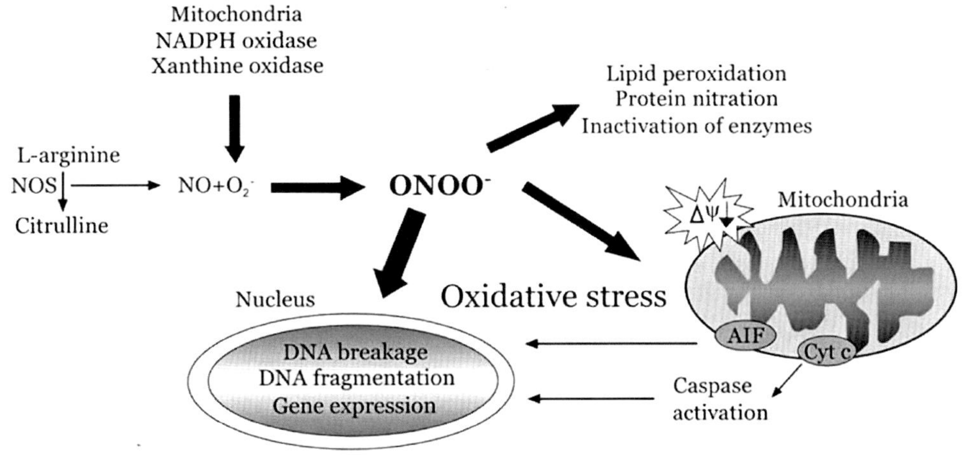

Fig (3). Role of oxidative stress in oxidant-induced cellular dysfunction and necrosis. Nitric oxide (NO) and superoxide (O_2^-), induce cell damage *via* lipid peroxidation, inactivation of enzymes by oxidation and nitration. Peroxynitrite (ONOO-) also acts on mitochondria decreasing the membrane potential (Δψ), triggering the release of pro-apoptotic factors such as cytochrome c (Cyt c) and apoptosis-inducing factor (AIF). These factors mediate caspase-dependent and caspase-independent apoptotic death pathways, respectively. Moreover, peroxynitrite, causes strand breaks in DNA.

ANTIOXIDANT PROTECTION IN SEPSIS

It has been reported that sepsis increases markers of oxidative stress in different animal models and in humans. This effect is correlated with an imbalance of antioxidant amount [109]. The clear evidence for oxidative stress in sepsis and the link with inflammatory gene expression has provided a foundation for intervention to either reduce oxidative stress or inhibit transcriptional activation. For this reason, the protective role of antioxidants against endotoxin toxicity and their potential clinical use is discussed. Endogenous and synthetic antioxidants, such as ironchelating agents, *N*-acetyl-L-cysteine (NAC), apocynin, probucol, and edaravone, are useful in preventing cardiovascular injury and diseases. Endogenous antioxidants in the myocardium include vitamins C and E, cysteine and the enzymes, SOD, catalase and glutathione peroxidase. In cases where events such as ischemia and hypoxia have compromised the cardiac cell's natural defense mechanisms, synthetic antioxidants such as NAC, a thiol containing compound, have proved successful in protection against oxidative stress on reperfusion. Secondary plant metabolites containing flavonoids and coumaric acid derivatives from spinach are effective against oxidative stress in the rat heart [79]. Targets for antioxidant therapy include NADPH oxidase, a source of O_2^- and peroxides. GSH comprises more than 90% of the nonprotein low molecular weight reduced thiols in cells and is one of the most important intracellular mechanisms protecting normal cells from oxidative injury. GSH linked redox homeostasis controls the levels of ROS that are constantly formed during cellular metabolism. It is recognized that the antioxidant GSH plays a very important role in several biological processes, and is implicated in the modulation of immune function and inflammatory response [110]. One of the treatments to enhance the GSH pool is NAC supplementation, which, of course, also has direct antioxidant activity [111]. NAC has been used safely to treat acetaminophen overdose for two decades [112]. NAC shows an *in vitro* and *in vivo* stimulatory effect on the phagocytic process of macrophages, and controls the functions of lymphocytes [113-116]. The regulation of redox state by NAC in immune cells and in animals with endotoxic shock [117], can lead to decreased NFκB activation [118], TNF-α release and increased survival [119]. In the clinical setting, NAC alone or in combination with other antioxidants has been shown to have variable results. An early acute study, in which NAC was administered in conjunction with vitamin C and α-tocopherol in patients with septic shock, did not measure NFκB activation, and neither total antioxidant capacity nor lipid peroxidation was changed [120].

Victor *et al.* [117] demonstrated that NAC treatment in animals with endotoxic shock decreased ROS, TNF, MDA levels, the GSSG/GSH ratio and iNOS levels, and increased the antioxidant defenses in peritoneal macrophages and lymphocytes. Moreover, NAC treatment prevented the activation of NF-κB, improved the redox state of these immune cells and increased survival. Byrne *et al.* [121] have demonstrated the therapeutic antioxidant effects of glutamine and NAC composition. Compositions comprising glutamine in combination with other ingredients such as NAC are disclosed. Such compositions can be administered to treat patients with certain disease states. In fact, glutamine and other amino acids have been given to patients with immune-compromised states, both alone and in combination with an immunopotentiator such as levitinan, OK-432, or sizofiran [122]. Vitamin C is a powerful electron donor, reacting with both O_2^- and OH. Vitamin C plays an important role in the defence against oxidative damage especially in leukocytes. The main role of vitamin C in the organism is linked to its function as a reductor, but it also participates in the modulation of complex biochemical pathways which are an essential part of the normal metabolism of immune cells. This antioxidant also inhibits the activation of the nuclear transcription factor NF-κB produced by endotoxin [123], which could result in a decrease of TNFα. These results suggest that early administration of vitamin C may be a valuable adjunct treatment in sepsis. Although several investigations revealed no association between vitamin C intake and lower risk of coronary disease, high doses of this supplement are reported to improve vascular function in some cases. Cardiovascular disease is the leading cause of death in the United States and many other countries. Nutritional factors are widely recognized as playing a role in preventing, delaying the onset of and/or slowing the progression of atherosclerosis and coronary heart disease. Attempts have been made in the prior art to design multivitamin supplements specifically for heart health. For example, U.S. Pat. No. 5,770,215 [124] discloses, a multivitamin composition containing various vitamins, minerals, and acetylsalicylic acid. Boulos *et al.* [125] have recently patented a multivitamin/multimineral optimized for cardiovascular health containing increased levels of Vitamin E and Folic Acid, low levels of iron, as well as containing mixed carotenoids. There have been several studies which have reported low circulating vitamin E (α-tocopherol) levels in sepsis. Vitamin E has been shown to have several additional biologically important effects apart from its role as an antioxidant. These include the inhibition of arachidonic acid oxidative metabolism and the inhibition of protein kinase C (PKC) activity. A steady decrease in circulating α-tocopherol levels in plasma was reported in a pig septic shock model in both survivor and non-survivor animals. This was accompanied by a simultaneous increase of markers of oxidative injury in the animals which subsequently died [126]. Vitamin E has been shown to be protective in reducing the effects of oxidative stress in sepsis in a number of animal studies [127]. Taken together, these studies reveal vitamin E to be a potent immunomodulator [128] agent that can interrupt the activation of inflammatory cells at the level of signal transduction. One strategy for preventing oxyradical-induced damage is to inhibit the formation of oxyradicals such as O_2^-. Iron chelators, such as desferrioxamine (also called deferoxamine or Desferol) and others, inhibit iron ion-dependent OH generation and thus act as inhibitors of free radical formation [129]. Amino-steroid-based antioxidants such as the 21-aminosteroids termed "lazaroids" (e.g., U74006F) have also been proposed as inhibitors of ROS formation. Desferrioxamine, allopurinol, and other pyrazolopyrimidines such as oxypurinol, have also been tested for preventing oxyradical formation in a myocardial stunning model system and following hemorrhagic and endotoxic shock [130]. However, each of these compounds has notable drawbacks for therapeutic usage. For example, deferoxamine is not an ideal iron chelator and its cellular penetration is quite limited. Another strategy for preventing oxyradical-induced damage is to catalytically remove oxyradicals such as superoxide once they have been formed. SOD and catalase have been extensively explored, with some success, as protective agents when added to reperfusates in many types of experiments or when added pre-ischemia [131]. The availability of recombinant SOD has allowed more extensive evaluation of the effect of administering SOD in the treatment or prevention of various medical conditions including reperfusion injury of the brain and spinal cord [132], endotoxemia [133], and myocardial infarction [134], and for osteoarthritis and intestinal ischemia [135]. SOD also has been reported to have positive effects in treating systemic lupus erythematosus, Crohn's disease, gastric ulcers, oxygen toxicity, burns patients, renal failure attendant to transplantation, and herpes simplex infection. An alternative strategy for preventing oxyradical-induced damage is to scavenge oxyradicals such as O_2^- once these have been formed, typically by employing small molecule scavengers which act stoichiometrically rather than catalytically. Congeners of GSH have been used in various animal models to attenuate oxyradical injury. For example, *N*-2-mercaptopropionylglycine has been found to confer protective effects in a canine model of myocardial ischemia and reperfusion [136] and NAC ("Mucomyst") has been used to treat endotoxin toxicity in sheep [137]. Dimethyl thiourea (DMTU) and butyl-phenylnitrone (BPN) are believed to scavenge OH, and have been shown to reduce ischemiareperfusion injury in rat myocardium and in rabbits [138]. Mannitol has also been used as a free radical scavenger to reduce organ injury during reoxygenation [139]. Thus, application of inhibitors of oxyradical formation and/or enzymes that remove O_2^- and H_2O_2 and/or small molecule oxyradical scavengers have all shown promise for preventing reoxygenation damage present in a variety of ischemic pathological states and for treating or preventing various disease states associated with free radicals. However, each of these categories contains several drawbacks. For example, inhibitors of oxyradical formation typically chelate transition metals which are used in essential enzymatic processes in normal physiology and respiration; moreover, even at very high doses, these inhibitors do not completely prevent oxyradical formation. SOD and catalase are large polypeptides which are expensive to manufacture, do not penetrate cells or the blood-brain barrier, and generally require parenteral routes of administration. Free radical scavengers act stoichiometrically and are thus easily depleted and must be administered in high dosages to be effective. The complex formed between the chelator desferroxamine and manganese has SOD activity and has shown some activity in biological models, but the instability of the metal ligand complex apparently precludes its pharmaceutical use. Porphyrin-manganese complexes have been shown to protect bacteria from paraquat toxicity and to promote the aerobic survival of SOD-deficient *E. coli* mutants. Based on the foregoing studies, it is clear that a need exists for antioxidant agents which are efficient at removing dangerous oxyradicals, particularly O_2^- and H_2O_2, and which are inexpensive to manufacture, stable, and possess advantageous pharmacokinetic properties, such as the ability to cross the blood-brain barrier and penetrate tissues. Such versatile antioxidants would find use as pharmaceuticals, chemoprotectants, and possibly as dietary supplements. In fact, for example Malfroy-Camine *et al.* [140] describes synthetic catalytic free radical scavengers useful as antioxidants for prevention and therapy of disease. In this patent, they provide antioxidant salen metal complexes, compositions of such antioxidant salen-metal complexes having O_2^- activity, catalase activity, and/or peroxidase activity, compositions of salen-metal complexes in a form suitable for pharmaceutical administration to treat or prevent a disease associated with cell or tissue damage produced by free radicals such as O_2^-, and cosmetic and free radical quenching formulations of salen metal compounds. Therefore, many groups of researchers have focused their attention on the biological activity of antioxidants and its active principles. Many scientific articles are published every year in different international journals related to the pharmacological properties of new antioxidants in order to counteract the effect of ROS in different pathologies. For example, Rao *et al.* have synthesized and used antioxidants such as (-)-mesquitol from natural sources (*Dichrostachys cinerea*), as well as (-)-Olivil from the plant *Stereospermum personatum*. Both compounds have demonstrated antioxidant, activity [141, 142]. Other studies have implicated mitochondria-targeted antioxidants which have also been shown to modulate the role of mitochondrial ROS production in redox signaling pathways [143].

CURRENT AND FUTURE DEVELOPMENTS

In an approach to design more optimally effective antioxidant regimes by targeting cells rather normal systemic route, Michael Murphy *et al.* have recently embarked on a program of work to deliver antioxidant moieties (for example vitamin E and ubiquinone) specifically to the mitochondrion, the major site of oxidative stress [144]. By using a lipophilic cationic group as a carrier, to facilitate targeting to the highly charged mitochondrion, Murphy *et al.* have shown that in principle, this method is very effective at combating oxidative stress in a variety of *in vitro* scenarios such as NFkB activation [145], Friedreich Ataxia complications [146], and stress-related teleomere shortening [147]. The first *in vivo* demonstration (proof-of-principle) of mitochondrially-targeted antioxidants in the area of cardiac ischemia reperfusion was recently reported [148]. These successes now open the doorway for novel treatments for clinical conditions in which oxidative stress plays a major role [149]. In this regard, the patent WO9926582A2 [150] relates to antioxidants having a lipophilic cationic group and to uses of these antioxidants, for example, as pharmaceuticals. This can be to prevent the elevated mitochondrial oxidative stress associated with particular diseases, or diseases associated with mitochondrial DNA mutations. Accordingly, they have the potential to be used as an adjunct to cell transplant therapies for e.g. neurodegenerative diseases, as a means to increase survival rates of the implanted cells. In addition, these compounds could be used as prophylactics to protect organs during transplantation, or ameliorate the ischemia reperfusion injury that occurs during surgery. The compounds of the invention could also be used to reduce cell damage following stroke and heart attack. As these therapies use the selectivity of mitochondria, one can for see that a major advantage over current antioxidant therapies is that the antioxidant is taken to the cellular compartment under the greatest oxidative stress. It is thought that this should increase the efficacy of the therapy. In conclusion, antioxidants are involved in several important biological processes such as immunity, protection against tissue damage, reproduction, growth and development. Antioxidants preserve adequate function of cells against homeostatic disturbances such as processes involving oxidative stress such as septic shock and cardiovascular dysfunction. Many groups of researchers have focused their attention on the biological activity of antioxidants and its active principles. The protective role of antioxidants against homeostatic disturbances such as those caused by endotoxin toxicity and cardiovascular damage have been patented, their potential clinical use and the effects on the redox state of have been discussed. Although there are a large number of patents which describe beneficial effects of antioxidant treatment in several oxidative stress disorders, in general, the results obtained so far are slightly disappointing. From our point of view, the use of novel targeted antioxidants, such as those described by Murphy *et al.* appears to be an exciting new leap into the use of antioxidant therapy.

ACKNOWLEDGEMENTS

We thank B Normanly for his editorial assistance.

FUNDING

This study was financed by grant PI070091 and CIBERehd. VMV and MR are the recipients of FIS contracts (CP07/00171 and CA07/00366 respectively).

REFERENCES

[1] Drogue W. Free radicals in the physiological control of cell function. Physiol Rev 2002; 82: 47-95.
[2] Kehrer JP. Free radicals as mediators of tissue injury and disease. Crit Rev Toxicol 1993; 23: 21-48.
[3] Dalton TP, Shertzer HG, Puga A. Regulation of gene expression by reactive oxygen. Annu Rev Pharmacol Toxicol 1999; 39: 67-101.
[4] Kohen R, Nyska A. Oxidation of biological systems: oxidative stress phenomena, antioxidants, redox reactions, and methods for their quantification. Toxicol Pathol 2002; 30: 620-650.
[5] Victor VM, Apostolova N, Herance R, Hernandez-Mijares A, Rocha M. Oxidative stress and mitochondrial dysfunction in atherosclerosis: mitochondria-targeted antioxidants as potential therapy. Curr Med Chem 2009; 16(35): 4654-67.
[6] Kuhn MA. Oxygen free radicals and antioxidants. Am J Nurs 2003; 103: 58-62.
[7] Lunec J, Holloway KA, Cooke MS, Faux S, Griffiths HR, Evans MD. Urinary 8-oxo-2′-deoxyguanosine: redox regulation of DNA repair *in vivo*?. Free Radic Biol Med 2002; 33: 875-885.
[8] McDermott JH. Antioxidant nutrients: current dietary recommendations and research update. J Am Pharm Assoc 2000; 40: 785-799.
[9] Halliwell B. Oxidation of low-density lipoproteins: questions of initiation, propagation, and the effects of antioxidants. Am J Clin Nutr 1995; 61: 670-677.
[10] Halliwell B. Oxidative stress, nutrition and health. Experimental strategies for optimization of nutritinal antioxidant intake in humans. Free Radic Res 1996; 25: 57-74.
[11] Cadenas E, Davies KJ. Mitochondrial free radical generation, oxidative stress, and ageing. Free Radic Biol Med 2000; 29: 222-230.
[12] Victor VM, Miñano M, Guayerbas N, Del Rio M, Medina S, De la Fuente M. Effects of endotoxic shock in several functions of murine peritoneal macrophages. Mol Cell Biochem 1998; 189: 25-31.

[13] Victor VM, De la Fuente M. Comparative study of peritoneal macrophages functions in mice receiving lethal and non-lethal doses of LPS. J Endotox Res 2000; 6: 235-241.

[14] Victor VM, De la Fuente M. Changes in the superoxide production and other macrophage functions could be related with the mortality of mice with endotoxin-induced oxidative stress. Physiol Res 2003; 52: 101-110.

[15] Victor VM, Rocha M, De la Fuente M. Immune cells: free radicals and antioxidants in sepsis. Int Immunopharmacol 2004; 4: 327-347.

[16] Ben-Neriah, Y., Alkalay-Snir, I., Hatzubai, A. Ada, H., Shushan, E.B., Davis, M., Yaron, A. Ada, H., Shushan, E.B., Davis, M., Yaron, A.: US6905836 (**2005**).

[17] Alkalay-Snir, I., Ben-Neriah, Y., Ciechanover, A., Manning, A., Mercurio, F., Yaron, A.: US5932425 (**1999**).

[18] Le, J., Vilcek, J., Dadbona, P., Ghrayeb, J., Knight, D., Siegel, S.: US6835823 (**2004**).

[19] Victor VM, De la Fuente M. Immune cells redox state from mice with endotoxin-induced oxidative stress. Involvement of NF-kB. Free Radic Res 2003; 37: 19-27.

[20] Webster NR, Nunn JF. Molecular structure of free radicals and their importance in biological reactions. Br J Anaesth 1988; 60: 98-108.

[21] Zimmerman JJ. Defining the role of oxyradicals in the pathogenesis of sepsis. Crit Care Med 1995; 23: 616-617.

[22] Meydani SN, Erickson KL. Nutrients as regulators of immune function: Introduction. FASEB J 2001; 15: 2555.

[23] Alexander, J.W., Peck, M.D.: US4981844 (**1991**).

[24] Chandra, R.K.: US5556644 (**1996**).

[25] Garleb, K.A., Demichele, S.J.: US5444054 (**1995**).

[26] DeMichele, S.J.: Gregory, T.J.: US5223285 (**1993**).

[27] Bistrian, B.R., Babayan, V.K., Blackburn, G.L., Mascioli, E.A.: US4871768 (**1989**).

[28] Katz, D.P., Komorowski, J.R.: US6809115 (**2004**).

[29] Mendy, F., Barthelemy, P.: US4607052 (**1986**).

[30] De Michele, S.J., McEwen, J.W., Wood, S.M.: US6444700 (**2002**).

[31] Sakya, S.M., Rast, B.: US6900230 (**2005**).

[32] Wikberg, J., Prusis, P., Dambrova, M., Uhlen, S.: US6599943 (**2004**).

[33] Gehlsen, K.R.: US6350785 (**2002**).

[34] Hellstrand, K., Hermodsson, S., Gehlsen, K.R.: US6730692 (**2004**).

[35] Bokoch, G.M., Curnutte, J.T.: US6184203 (**2001**).

[36] Knowles RG, Moncada S. Nitric oxide synthases in mammals. Biochem J 1994; 298: 249-258.

[37] Vincent JL, Zhang H, Szabo C, Preiser JC. Effects of nitric oxide in septic shock. Am J Respir Crit Care Med 2000; 161: 1781-1785.

[38] Forman HJ, Torres M. Redox signaling in macrophages. Mol Aspects Med 2001; 22: 189-216.

[39] Carreras MC, Pargament GA, Catz S, Poderoso JJ, Boveris A. Kinetics of nitric oxide and hydrogen peroxide production and formation of peroxynitrite during the respiratory burst of human neutrophils. FEBS Lett 1994; 341: 65-68.

[40] Valdez LB, Boveris A. Nitric oxide and superoxide radical production in human mononuclear leukocytes. Antioxid Redox Signal 2001; 3: 505-513.

[41] Thiemermann C, Vane JR. Inhibition of nitric oxide synthesis reduces the hypotension induced by bacterial lipopolysacharide in the rat *in vivo*. Eur J Pharmacol 1990; 182: 591-595.

[42] Kilbourn RG, Jubran A, Gross SS, *et al.* Reversal of endotoxinmediated shock by NG-methyl-L-arginine, an inhibitor of nitric oxide synthesis. Biochem Biophys Res Commun 1990; 172: 1132-1138.

[43] Gray GA, Julou-Schaeffer G, Oury K, Fleming I, Parrat JR, Stoclet JC. An L-arginine-derived factor mediates endothelininduced vascular hyposensitivity to calcium. Eur J Pharmacol 1990; 191: 89-92.

[44] Hobbs AJ, Higgs A, Moncada S. Inhibition of nitric oxide synthase as a potential therapeutic target. Annu Rev Pharmacol Toxicol 1999; 39: 191-220.

[45] Ruetten H, Thiemermann C. Nitric oxide and septic shock. In: Ignarro L, Ed. Nitric oxide: biology and pathobiology. San Diego: Academic Press 2000; 747-758.

[46] Arnaiz, D.O., Baldwin, J.J., Davey, D.D., Vevlin, J.J., Dolle, R.E., Erickson, S.D., McMillan, K., Morrisey, M.M., Ohlmeyer, M.H., Pan, G., Paradkar, M., Parkinson, J., Phillips, G.B., Ye, B., Zhao, Z.: US6887865 (**2005**).

[47] Webber, R.K., Durley, R.C., Awasthi, A.K., Bergmanis, A.A., Fok, K.F., Ganser, S.S., Hagen, T.J.; Hallinan, E.A., Hansen, D.W., Hickory, B.S., Manning, P.T., Mao, M., Moormann, A.E., Pitzele, B.S., Promo, M.A., Schartman, R.R., Sholten, J.A., Snyder, J.S., Toth, M.V., Trivedi, M., Tsymbalov, S., Tjoeng, F.S.: US6914158 (**2005**).

[48] Umans JG, Wylam ME, Samsel RW, Edwards J, Schumacker PT. Effects of endotoxin *in vivo* on endothelial and smoothmuscle function in rabbit and rat aorta. Am Rev Respir Dis 1993;148: 1638-1645.

[49] Liao JK, Zulueta JJ, Yu FS, Peng HB, Cote CG, Hassoun PM. Regulation of bovine endothelial constitutive nitric oxide synthase by oxygen. J Clin Invest 1995; 96: 2661-2666.

[50] Graier WF, Myers PR, Rubin LJ, Adams HR, Parker JL. *Escherichia coli* endotoxin inhibits agonist-mediated cytosolic Ca2+ mobilization and nitric oxide biosynthesis in cultured endothelial cells. Circ Res 1994; 75: 659-668.

[51] Salvemini DR, Korbut R, Anggard E, Vane J. Immediate release of a nitric oxide-like factor from bovine aortic endothelial cells by *Escherichia coli* lipopolysaccharide. Proc Natl Acad Sci USA 1990; 87: 2593-2597.

[52] Zhang H, Rogiers P, Smail N., *et al.* Effects of nitric oxide on blood flow distribution and oxygen extraction capabilities during endotoxic shock. J Appl Physiol 1997; 83: 1164-1173.

[53] Szabo C, Cuzzocrea S, Zingarelli B, O'Connor M, Salzman AL. Endothelial dysfunction in a rat model of endotoxic shock Importance of the activation of poly (ADP-ribose) synthetase by peroxynitrite. J Clin Invest 1997; 100: 723-735.

[54] Wink DA, Hanbauer I, Krishna MC, DeGraff W, Gamson J, Mitchell JB. Nitric oxide protects against cellular damage and cytotoxicity from reactive oxygen species. Proc Natl Acad Sci USA 1993; 90: 9813-9817.

[55] Gunnett CA, Chu Y, Heistad DD, Loihl A, Faraci FM. Vascular effects of LPS in mice deficient in expression of the gene for inducible nitric oxide synthase. Am J Physiol 1998; 275: H416-421.

[56] Hollenberg SM, Cunnion RE, Zimmerberg J. Nitric oxide synthase inhibition reverses arteriolar hyporesponsiveness to catecholamines in septic rats. Am J Physiol 1993; 264: H660-663.

[57] Singh, I.: US6511800 (**2003**).

[58] Griffth, O.W.: US5132453 (**1991**).

[59] Hallinan, E.A., Hansen, D.W., Tsymbalov, S.: US5684008 (**1994**).

[60] Moore, W.M., Hallinan, E.A.: US5830917 (**1998**).

[61] Hallinan, A.E., Hansen, D.W., Donald, W., Tsymbalov, S.: US5854251 (**1998**).

[62] Beams, R.M., Hodson, H.F., Palmer, R.M.J.: US5863931 (**1999**).

[63] Webber, R.K., Tjoeng, F.S., Manning, R.E.: US5945408 (**1999**).

[64] Gapud, R.E., Hagen, T.J., Hallinan, A.E., Manning, R.E., Metz, S., Pitzele, B.S., Tjoeng, F.S., Toth, M.V., Keith, W.R.: US5981511 (**1999**).

[65] Clementi E, Brown GC, Foxwell N, Moncada S. On the mechanism by which vascular endothelial cells regulate their oxygen consumption. Proc Natl Acad Sci USA 1999; 96: 1559-1562.

[66] Szabo C. Role of nitric oxide in endotoxic shock. An overview of recent advances. Ann NY Acad Sci 1998; 851: 422-425.s

[67] Szabo C, Billiar T. Novel roles of nitric oxide in hemorrhagic shock. Shock 1999; 12: 1-9.

[68] Szabo C, Oshima H. DNA damage induced by peroxynitrite: subsequent Biological effects. Nitric Oxide 1997; 1: 373-385.

[69] Virag L, Scott G, Cuzzocrea S, Marmer D, Salzman AL, Szabo C. Peroxynitrite-induced thymocyte apoptosis: the role of caspases and poly (ADP-ribose) synthetase (PARS) activation. Immunology 1998; 94: 345-355.

[70] Brown GC. Regulation of mitochondrial respiration by nitric oxide inhibition of cytocrome c oxidase. Biochim Biophys Acta 2001; 1504: 46-57.

[71] Poderoso JJ, Carreras MC, Lisdero C, Riobo N, Schopfer F, Boveris A. Nitric oxide inhibits electron transfer and increases superoxide radical production in rat heart mitochondria and submitochondrial particles. Arch Biochem Biophys 1996; 328: 85-92.

[72] Han YJ, Kwon YG, Chung HT, *et al.* Antioxidant enzymes suppress nitric oxide production through the inhibition of Nfkappa B activation: role of H2O2 and nitric oxide in inducible nitric oxide synthase expression in macrophages. Nitric Oxide 2001; 5: 504-513.

[73] Bolanos JP, Peuchen S, Heales SJ, Land JM, Clark JB. Nitric oxide-mediated inhibition of the mitochondrial respiratory chain in cultures astrocytes. J Neurochem 1994; 63: 910-916.

[74] Brown GC. Reversible binding and inhibition of catalase by nitric oxide. Eur J Biochem 1995; 232: 188-191.

[75] Radi R, Rodriguez M, Castro L, Telleri R. Inhibition of mitochondrial electron transport by peroxynitrite. Arch Biophys Biochem 1994; 308: 89-95.

[76] Wink DA, Miranda KM, Espey MG, *et al.* Mechanisms of the antioxidant effects of nitric oxide. Antiox Redox Signal 2001; 3: 203-213.

[77] Graves JE, Lewis SJ, Kooy NW. Peroxynitrite-mediated vasorelaxation: evidence against the formation of circulating Snitrothiols. Am J Physiol 1998; 274: H1001-1008.

[78] Masuda M, Nishino H, Ohshima H. Formation of 8-nitrosoguanosine in cellular RNA as a biomarker of exposure to reactive nitrogen species. Chem Biol Interact 2002; 139: 187-197.

[79] Ben-Shaul V, Lomnitski L, Nyska A, Zurovsky Y, Bergman M, Grossman S. The effect of natural antioxidants, NAO and apocynin, on oxidative stress in the rat heart following LPS challenge. Toxicol Lett 2001; 123: 1-10.

[80] Liaudet L, Pacher P, Mabley JG, *et al.* Activation of poly(ADPribose) polymerase-1 is a central mechanism of lipopolysaccharide-induced acute lung inflammation. Am J Respir Crit Care Med 2002; 165: 373-377.

[81] Kozlov AV, Szalay L, Umar F, *et al.* EPR analysis reveals three tissues responding to endotoxin by increased formation of reactive oxygen and nitrogen species. Free Radic Biol Med 2003; 34: 1555-1562.

[82] Szabo C, Ferrer-Sueta G, Zingarelli B, Southan GJ, Salzman AL, Radi R. Mercaptoethylguanidine and guanidine inhibitors of nitric-oxide synthase react with peroxynitrite and protect against peroxynitrite-induced oxidative damage. J Biol Chem 1997; 272: 9030-9036.

[83] Natanson C, Eichenholz PW, Danner RL, *et al.* Endotoxin and tumor necrosis factor challenges in dogs simulate the cardiovascular profile of human septic shock. J Exp Med 1989; 169: 823-832.

[84] Kumar A, Haery C, Parrillo JE. Myocardial dysfunction in septic shock. Crit Care Clin 2000; 16: 251-287.

[85] Grocott-Mason RM, Shah AM. Cardiac dysfunction in sepsis: new theories and clinical implications. Intensive Care Med 1998; 24: 286-295.

[86] Finkel MS, Oddis CV, Jacob TD, Watkins SC, Hattler BG, Simmons RL. Negative inotropic effects of cytokines on the heart mediated by nitric oxide. Science 1992; 257: 387-389.

[87] Joe EK, Schussheim AE, Longrois D, *et al.* Regulation of cardiac myocyte contractile function by inducible nitric oxide synthase (iNOS): mechanisms of contractile depression by nitric oxide. J Mol Cell Cardiol 1998; 30: 303-315.

[88] Lancel S, Tissier S, Mordon S, *et al.* Peroxynitrite decomposition catalysts prevent myocardial dysfunction and inflammation in endotoxemic rats. J Mol Cell Cardiol 2004; 43: 2348-2358.

[89] Flesch M, Kilter H, Cremers B, *et al.* Effects of endotoxin on human myocardial contractility involvement of nitric oxide and peroxynitrite. J Am Coll Cardiol 1999; 33: 1062-1070.

[90] Panas D, Khadour FH, Szabo C, Schulz R. Proinflammatory cytokines depress cardiac efficiency by a nitric oxide-dependent mechanism. Am J Physiol 1998; 275:H1016-1023.

[91] Price S, Mitchell JA, Anning PB, Evans TW. Type II nitric oxide synthase is cardio-protective in experimental sepsis. Eur J Pharmacol 2003; 472: 111-118.

[92] Parrillo JE. Pathogenetic mechanisms of septic shock. N Engl J Med 1993; 328: 1471-1477.

[93] Goode HF, Cowley HC, Walker BE, Howdle PD, Webster NR. Decreased antioxidant status and increased lipid peroxidation in patients with septic shock and secondary organ dysfunction. Crit Care Med 1995; 23: 646-651.

[94] Zouki C, Zhang SL, Chan JS, Filep JG. Peroxynitrite induces integrin-dependent adhesion of human neutrophils to endothelial cells via activation of the Raf-1/MEK/Erk pathway. FASEB J 2001; 15: 25-27.

[95] Lush CW, Cepinskas G, Kvietys PR. Regulation of intestinal nuclear factor-kappa B activity and E-selectin expression during sepsis: a role for peroxynitrite. Gastroenterology 2003; 124: 118-128.

[96] Salvemini D, Wang ZQ, Stern MK, Currie MG, Misko TP. Peroxynitrite decomposition catalysts: therapeutics for peroxynitrite-mediated pathology. Proc Natl Acad Sci USA 1998; 95: 2659-2663.

[97] Cuzzocrea S, Misko TP, Costantino G, *et al.* Beneficial effects of peroxynitrite decomposition catalysts in a rat model of splachnic artery occlusion and reperfusion. FASEB J 2000; 14: 1061-1072.

[98] Zingarelli B, Cuzzocrea S, Szabo C, Salzman AL. Mercaptoethylguanidine, a combined inhibitor of nitric oxide synthase and peroxynitrite scavenger, reduces trinitrobenzene sulfonic acid-induced colonic damage in rats. J Pharmacol Exp Ther 1998; 287: 1048-1055.

[99] Pacher P, Schulz R, Liaudet L, Szabo C. Nitrosative stress and pharmacological modulation of heart failure. Trends Pharmacol Sci 2005; 26: 302-310.

[100] Szabo C. Multiple pathways of peroxynitrite cytotoxicity. Toxicol Lett 2003; 140-141: 105-112.

[101] Okamoto T, Akaike T, Sawa T, Miyamoto Y, van der Vliet A, Maeda H. Activation of matrix metalloproteinases by peroxynitrite-induced protein S-glutathiolation via disulfide Soxide formation. J Biol Chem 2001; 276: 29596-29602.

[102] Virag L, Szabo C. The therapeutic potential of poly(ADP-ribose) polymerase inhibitors. Pharmacol Rev 2002; 54: 375-429.

[103] Zeng, F., Wang, Y., Wang, L.: CN1524447A (**2004**).

[104] Gorsek, W.F.: US6551629 (**2003**).

[105] Hsia, H.S., Fan, D.: US6620440 (**2003**).

[106] Wechter, W.J.: US6908943 (**2005**).

[107] Patell-Villo, M., Vyas, D.: WO05016361A1 (**2005**).

[108] De Simone, C.: US6923960 (**2005**).

[109] Poon BY, Raharjo E, Patel KD, Tavener S, Kubes P. Complexity of inducible nitric oxide synthase: cellular source determines benefit versus toxicity. Circulation 2003; 108: 1107-1112.

[110] De Flora S. Mechanisms of inhibitors of mutagenesis and carcinogenesis. Mutat Res 1998; 402: 151-158.

[111] Aruoma OI, Halliwell B, Hoey BM, Butler J. The antioxidant action of *N*-acetylcysteine: its reaction with hydrogen peroxide, hydroxyl radical, superoxide, and hypochlorous acid. Free Radic Biol Med 1989; 6: 593-597.

[112] Vale JA, Proudfoot AT. Paracetamol (acetaminophen) poisoning. Lancet 1995; 346: 547-552.

[113] Victor VM, Guayerbas N Garrote D, Del Rio M, De la Fuente M. Modulation of murine macrophage function by N-acetylcysteine in a model of endotoxic shock. BioFactors 1999; 10: 347-357.

[114] De la Fuente M, Victor VM. Anti-oxidants as modulators of immune function. Immunol Cell Biol 2000; 78: 49-54.

[115] Victor VM, De la Fuente M. *N*-acetylcysteine improves *in vitro* the function of macrophages from mice with endotoxin-induced oxidative stress. Free Radic Res 2002; 36: 33-45.

[116] De la Fuente M, Victor VM. Ascorbic acid and *N*-acetylcysteine improve *in vitro* the function of lymphocytes from mice with endotoxin-induced oxidative stress. Free Radic Res 2001; 35: 73-84.

[117] Victor VM, Rocha M, De la Fuente M. *N*-acetylcysteine protects mice from letal endotoxemia by regulating the redox state of immune cells. Free Radic Res 2003; 37: 919-929.

[118] Blackwell TS, Blackwell TR, Holden EP, Christman BW, Christman JW. *In vivo* antioxidant treatment suppresses nuclear factor-kB activation and neutrophilic lung inflammation. J Immunol 1996; 157: 1630-1637.

[119] Zhang H, Spapen H, Nguyen DN, Benlabed M, Buurman WA, Vincent JL. Protective effects of *N*-acetyl-L-cysteine in endotoxemia. Am J Physiol 1994; 266: H1746-1754.

[120] Galley HF, Howdle PD, Walker BE, Webster NR. The effects of intravenous antioxidats in patients with septic shock. Free Radic Biol Med 1997; 23: 768-774.

[121] Byrne, T.A., Somerville, J.A.: US6797729 (**2004**).

[122] Aoki, T., Miyakoshi, H.: US5491150 (**1996**).

[123] Staal FJ, Roederer M, Raju PA, Anderson MT, Ela SW, Herzenberg LA. Antioxidants inhibit stimulation of HIV transcription. AIDS Res Hum Retroviruses 1993; 9: 299-306.

[124] Moshyedi, E.P.: US5770215 (**1998**).

[125] Boulos, A., Desai, J., Martin, N., Stillman, R., Udwin, M.: US6914073 (**2005**).

[126] Basu S, Eriksson M. Vitamin E in relation to lipid peroxidation in experimental septic shock. Postaglandins Leuk Essent Fatty Acids 2000; 62: 195-199.

[127] Goode HF, Webster NR. Free radicals and antioxidants in sepsis. Crit Care Med 1993; 21: 1770-1776.

[128] Bulger EM, Maier RV. An argument for vitamin E supplementation in the management of systemic inflammatory response syndrome. Shock 2003; 19: 99-103.

[129] Van der Kraaij AM, van Eijk HG, Koster JF. Prevention of postischemic cardiac injury by the orally active iron chelator 1,2-dimethyl-3-hydroxy-4-pyridone (L1) and the antioxidant (+)-cyanidanol-3. Circulation 1989; 80: 158-164.

[130] Bolli R, Jeroudi MO, Patel BS, *et al* . Marked reduction of free radical generation and contractile dysfunction by antioxidant therapy begun at the time of reperfusion. Evidence that myocardial "stunning" is a manifestation of reperfusion injury. Circ Res 1989; 65: 607-622.

[131] Gutteridge JM, Mitchell J. Redox imbalance in the critically ILL. Br Med Bull 1999; 55: 49-75.

[132] Uyama O, Shiratsuki N, Matsuyama T, *et al.* Protective effects of superoxide dismutase on acute reperfusion injury of gerbil brain. Free Radic Biol Med 1990; 8: 265-268.

[133] Schneider J, Friderichs E, Heintze K, Flohe L. Effects of recombinant human superoxide dismutase on increased lung vascular permeability and respiratory disorder in endotoxemic rats. Circ Shock 1990; 30: 97-106.

[134] Patel BS, Jeroudi MO, O'Neill PG, Roberts R, Bolli R. Effect of human recombinant superoxide dismutase on canine myocardial infarction. Am J Physiol 1990; 258: H369-380.

[135] Vohra K, Rosenfeld W, Singh I, Anderson V. Ischemic injury to newborn rabbit ileum: protective role of human superoxide dismutase. J Pediatr Surg 1989; 24: 893-898.

[136] Mitsos SE, Askew TE, Fantone JC, *et al.* Protective effects of N-2-mercaptopropionyl glycine against myocardial reperfusion injury after neutrophil depletion in the dog: evidence for the role of intracellular-derived free radicals. Circulation 1986; 73: 1077-1086.

[137] Bernard GR, Lucht WD, Niedermeyer ME, Snapper JR, Ogletree ML, Brigham KL. Effect of *N*-acetylcysteine on the pulmonary response to endotoxin in the awake sheep and upon *in vitro* granulocyte function. J Clin Invest 1984; 73: 1772-1784.

[138] Heide VRS, Sobotka PA, Ganote CE. Effects in the free radical scavenger DMTU and mannitol on the oxygen paradox in perfused rat hearts. J Mol Cell Cardiol 1987; 19: 615-625.

[139] Fox RB. Prevention of granulocyte-mediated oxidant lung injury in rats by a hydroxyl radical scavenger, dimethylthiourea. J Clin Invest 1984; 74: 1456-1464.

[140] Malfroy-Camine, B., Doctrow, S.R.: US6900198 (**2005**).

[141] Rao, J.M., Tiwari A.K., Kumar, U.S., Yadav, J.S., Raghavan, K.V.: US6592911 (**2003**).

[142] Rao, J.M., Rao, R.J., Tiwari A.K., Yadav, J.S., Raghavan, K.V.: US6781002 (**2004**).

[143] San Juan-Pla A, Cervera AM, Apostolova N, *et al.* A targeted antioxidant reveals the importance of mitochondrial reactive oxygen species in the hypoxic signaling of HIF-alpha. FEBS Lett 2005; 579: 2669-2674.

[144] Kelso GF, Porteous CM, Coulter CV, *et al.* Selective targeting of a redox-active ubiquinone to mitochondria within cells: antioxidant and antiapoptotic properties. J Biol Chem 2001; 276: 4588-4596.

[145] Hughes G, Murphy MP, Ledgerwood EC. Mitochondrial reactive oxygen species regulate the temporal activation of nuclear factor kappaB to modulate tumour necrosis factor-induced apoptosis: evidence from mitochondria-targeted antioxidants. Biochem J 2005; 389: 83-89.

[146] Jauslin ML, Meier T, Smith RA, Murphy MP. Mitochondria targeted antioxidants protect Friedreich Ataxia fibroblasts from endogenous oxidative stress more effectively than untargeted antioxidants. FASEB J 2003; 17: 1972-1974.

[147] Saretzki G, Murphy MP, von Zglinicki T, Mito Q. Counteracts telomere shortening and elongates lifespan of fibroblasts under mild oxidative stress. Aging Cell 2003; 2: 141-143.

[148] Adlam VJ, Harrison JC, Porteous CM, *et al.* Targeting an antioxidant to mitochondria decreases cardiac ischemiareperfusioin injury. FASEB J 2005; 19: 1088-1095.

[149] Victor VM, Rocha M, Esplugues JV, De la Fuente M. Role of free radicals in sepsis: antioxidants therapy. Curr Pharm Des 2005; 11: 3141-3158.

[150] Murphy, M.P., Smith R.: WO9926582A2 (**1999**).

Author Index to Volume 1

†"Cougulation Defects" AIEOP working group